PEDIATRIC
DERMATOLOGY

PEDIATRIC DERMATOLOGY

FIFTH EDITION

Bernard A. Cohen, MD

Professor of Pediatrics and Dermatology
Johns Hopkins Children's Center
Johns Hopkins University School of Medicine
Baltimore, Maryland

ELSEVIER

For additional online content visit expertconsult.com

Elsevier
1600 John F. Kennedy Blvd.
Ste 1800
Philadelphia, PA 19103-2899

Content Strategist: Charlotta Kryhl
Content Development Specialist: Laura Klein
Publishing Services Manager: Shereen Jameel
Project Manager: Aparna Venkatachalam
Design Direction: Brian Salisbury

Printed in India

Last digit is the print number: 9 8 7 6 5 4 3 2 1

Since I began taking clinical photographs during my residency training over 30 years ago, I have been impressed by the virtually unlimited variation in the expression of skin disease. However, with careful observation, clinical patterns that permit the development of a reasonable differential diagnosis emerge. In collaboration with my colleagues in the fifth edition, we have been able to use over 600 images, a third of which are new, to demonstrate the diverse variations and common patterns that are fundamental to an understanding of skin eruptions in children. The algorithm at the end of each chapter is designed as a practical approach to evaluating pediatric patients.

Pediatric Dermatology is designed for the pediatric and primary care provider with an interest in dermatology and the dermatology practitioner who cares for children. The text is organized around practical clinical problems. This book should not be considered an encyclopedic text of pediatric dermatology; it should be used in conjunction with the further reading list suggested at the end of Chapter 1. Classic papers and more recent literature are included in the further reading lists at the end of each chapter.

I have been fortunate to work with oral pathologists on the dermatology faculty in the roles of teacher and consultant. With their help, the importance of recognizing oral lesions in the care of children is reflected in Chapter 9, which is devoted to oral pathology.

Although the focus of this chapter is on primary lesions of the oral mucosa, a discussion of clues of systemic disease is included. I am also excited to introduce the new Chapter 10 that focuses on urologic, gynecologic, and anogenital findings in children. Chapter 2, which is devoted to dermatologic disorders of newborns and infants, remains the longest chapter in the book as a result of the continued blossoming of neonatology as a respected pediatric discipline. I never cease to be amazed by how human beings manipulate their skin accidentally, deliberately, secretly, and/or therapeutically. With this in mind, Chapter 11, Psychodermatology, focuses on psychodermatoses and concludes with disorders that are triggered, exacerbated, or caused primarily by external factors.

Finally, the format of the text should be user friendly. The pages and legends have been numbered in a standard textbook fashion, and the index was again revised to include all of the disorders listed in the text and legends. The text and images incorporate advances made in diagnosis, evaluation, and treatment during the last eight years, since the publication of the fourth edition. I only hope that students of pediatric dermatology will enjoy reading the book as much as I enjoyed working with my colleagues in pediatric dermatology completing this new edition.

Bernard A. Cohen
2021

ACKNOWLEDGMENTS

This book would not have been possible without the help of the children and parents who allowed me to photograph their skin eruptions and the practitioners who referred them to me. I am particularly indebted to the faculty, especially my colleague Annie Grossberg; residents, nurse practitioners; nurses; physicians assistants; and students at the Johns Hopkins Children's Center and the Departments of Pediatrics and Dermatology at the Johns Hopkins University School of Medicine for their inspiration and support. I would again like to thank my friends at the Children's Hospital of Pittsburgh where this book was first conceived.

Although we have been involved with online dermatology for over a decade, the craziness associated with the COVID pandemic has allowed for a dramatic expansion of virtual visits and high-quality clinical imaging. Many primary care providers, patients, and parents have learned how to organize online consultation, which will undoubtedly revolutionize the acquisition of data for clinical evaluation and teaching. This is all reflected in the fifth edition.

I am also indebted to the oral pathology faculty who call dermatology their home. They have taught me to seek clues for dermatologic and systemic disease from evaluation of the mucous membranes, and to respect oral pathology in its own right. Without them, the conception of Chapter 9 and the most recent updates would not have been possible.

I am also excited to thank Drs. Tina Ho and Kalyani S. Marathe who encouraged us to include a new chapter focused on urologic and anogenital lesions, which are often misdiagnosed in this age group.

I continue to be grateful for the persistent prodding and sensitive guidance of the editors at Elsevier who are responsible for completion of this book in a timely fashion. I would also like to thank Tracy Shuford for keeping the lines of communication open between the publisher and my office, despite the 6-hour time difference.

I will be forever indebted to the coauthors of the chapters in the fifth edition including Katherine Brown Püttgen for Chapter 2 Neonatal Dermatology, Jessica L. Feig for Chapter 3 Papulosquamous Eruptions, A. Yasmine Kirkorian and Nidhi Shah for Chapter 4 Vesiculopustular Eruptions, Kaiane Anoush Habeshian for Chapter 5 Nodules and Tumors, Daren J. Simkin for Chapter 6 Pigmentary Disorders, George O. Denny for Chapter 7 Reactive Erythema, Saleh Rachidi for Chapter 8 Disorders of the Hair and Nails, Nikhil Shyam for Chapter 9 Oral Cavity, and Sherry Guralnick Cohen for Chapter 11 Psychodermatology.

I would like to thank the residents in dermatology and pediatrics, who by their questions and consultations, have helped me prioritize topics for inclusion in this book.

Finally, I would like to again acknowledge Dr. Nancy Esterly who contributed the foreword to the second edition (reprinted in the subsequent editions). I think of her often and would like to honor her by using her foreword in this edition as well. Dr. Esterly taught me that pediatric dermatology could be exciting and academically challenging. As a role model and one of the mothers of pediatric dermatology, her memory continues to guide all of us in pediatric dermatology. I would also like to acknowledge Dr. Frank Oski who brought me home to Baltimore, where he incorporated pediatric dermatology into the pediatric training program. Hopefully, we can continue to live up to the high standards that he demanded.

FIGURE CREDITS

The following figures have been reprinted from Zitelli BJ, Davis HW (eds). Atlas of pediatric physical diagnosis, 3rd edn. Mosby, St Louis, 1997:

4.10, 7.8, 7.9, 8.1, 8.15, 8.49, 11.7, 11.9, 11.10, 11.13, 11.15.

I am grateful for the use of images contributed by Dr. Russ Corio and Dr. Gary Warnock for contributing additional images to the chapter on the Oral Cavity (Chapter 9).

To Sherry for her continued patience, love, understanding, and contributions to this edition, which took longer than I thought!

To Michael, Jared, and Jennie for keeping me young and laughing. It has been exciting to see them mature into young adults who now contribute to the care of children and adults in their own ways.

To Zeke and Thea who keep me honest!

To all of the children who made this project possible.

FOREWORD

NOTE FROM DR. COHEN

I have asked the managing editor to reprint the Foreword from the second edition (also reprinted in subsequent editions) written by Dr. Nancy Esterly to honor her for her contributions to pediatric dermatology, the training of many practitioners of the specialty, and my own career. In the spring of 1983 when I was desperately searching for a mentor in pediatric dermatology, Nan adopted me during my elective month at Children's Memorial Hospital in Chicago.

Dr. Esterly has been the quintessential practitioner of pediatric dermatology since her pediatric and dermatology training in Baltimore over 40 years ago. She was one of the founders of the Society for Pediatric Dermatology and embodies the tripartite mission of pediatric dermatology of patient care, resident teaching, and clinical research.

FOREWORD TO THE SECOND EDITION

It is not often that one encounters a single-author textbook that is outstanding in both text and illustrations. But, once again, Bernard Cohen has crafted an exceptional basic pediatric dermatology text liberally illustrated with photographs depicting a wide range of skin problems in infants and children.

In this fourth edition of *Pediatric Dermatology*, the text has been expanded to include a 20-page chapter devoted entirely to mucosal lesions and accompanied by more than 50 new photographs of patients with problems ranging from the common herpes simplex infection to the uncommon ectodermal dysplasias. In keeping with the very successful style of previous editions, the requisite algorithm, diagrams of the oral cavity and up-to-date references are included in this chapter. In addition, new photographs have been added and some old ones replaced throughout the book.

For beginners in this discipline, Dr. Cohen's text is an excellent place to start. For those of us who practice pediatric dermatology, there is still much to be learned from a well-put-together text such as this one.

Nancy B. Esterly, MD
Professor Emeritus
Medical College of Wisconsin
Milwaukee, Wisconsin

Anna M. Bender, MD
Assistant Professor of Dermatology
Department of Dermatology
Weill Cornell Medical College
New York, New York

Bernard A. Cohen, MD
Professor of Pediatrics and Dermatology
Johns Hopkins Children's Center
Johns Hopkins University School of Medicine
Baltimore, Maryland

Sherry Guralnick Cohen, MS, CRNP
Nurse Practitioner
Dermatology
Skin Care Specialty Physicians
Lutherville, Maryland

George O. Denny, MD, MS
Physician—Fellow
Dermatology
Johns Hopkins University School of Medicine
Baltimore, Maryland

Jessica L. Feig, MD, PhD
Attending Physician
Dermatology
Dermatology Laser and Surgery
New York, New York

Kaiane Anoush Habeshian, MD
Assistant Professor of Dermatology and Pediatrics
Children's National Hospital
George Washington University School of Medicine and Health Sciences
Washington, District of Columbia

Tina Ho, MD, PhD
Resident Physician
Department of Dermatology
University of Cincinnati
Cincinnati, Ohio

A. Yasmine Kirkorian, MD
Associate Professor of Dermatology and Pediatrics
Children's National Hospital
George Washington University School of Medicine and Health Sciences
Washington, District of Columbia

Kalyani S. Marathe, MD
Division Director
Division of Dermatology
Associate Professor
Department of Pediatrics
University of Cincinnati
Cincinnati, Ohio

John C. Mavropoulos, MD MPH PhD
Resident in Dermatology
Department of Dermatology
Johns Hopkins University School of Medicine
Baltimore, Maryland

Katherine Brown Püttgen, MD
Director, Pediatric Dermatology
Dermatology
Intermountain Healthcare
Salt Lake City, Utah
Adjunct Associate Professor
Dermatology
Johns Hopkins University School of Medicine
Baltimore, Maryland

Saleh Rachidi, MD, PhD
Resident Physician
Dermatology
Johns Hopkins University School of Medicine
Baltimore, Maryland

Nidhi Shah, BS
Medical Student
Department of Dermatology
George Washington University School of Medicine and Health Sciences
Washington, District of Columbia

Dr. Nikhil Shyam, MD, FAAD
Board-certified Dermatologist
Private Practice
Wayne, PA

Daren J. Simkin, MD
Assistant Professor
Department of Dermatology
Johns Hopkins University School of Medicine
Baltimore, Maryland

CONTENTS

Introduction to Pediatric Dermatology

Bernard A. Cohen

ANATOMY AND FUNCTION OF THE SKIN

Most of us think of skin as a simple, durable covering for the skeleton and internal organs. Yet skin is actually a very complex and dynamic organ consisting of many parts and appendages (Fig. 1.1). The outermost layer of the epidermis, the stratum corneum, is an effective barrier to the penetration of irritants, toxins, and organisms, as well as a membrane that holds in body fluids. The remainder of the epidermis, the stratum granulosum, stratum spinosum, and stratum basale, manufactures this protective layer. Melanocytes within the epidermis are important for protection against the harmful effects of ultraviolet light, and the Langerhans cells and other dendritic cells are one of the body's first lines of immunologic defense and play a key role in systemic and cutaneous diseases such as drug reactions and infections.

The dermis, consisting largely of fibroblasts and collagen, is a tough, leathery, mechanical barrier against cuts, bites, and bruises. Its collagenous matrix also provides structural support for a number of cutaneous appendages. Hair, which grows from follicles deep within the dermis, is important for cosmesis, as well as protection from sunlight and particulate matter. Sebaceous glands arise as an outgrowth of the hair follicles. Oil produced by these glands helps to lubricate the skin and contributes to the protective function of the epidermal barrier. The nails are specialized organs of manipulation that also protect sensitive digits. Thermoregulation of the skin is accomplished by eccrine sweat glands and changes in the cutaneous blood flow regulated by glomus cells. The skin also contains specialized receptors for heat, pain, touch, and pressure. Sensory input from these structures helps to protect the skin surface against environmental trauma. Beneath the dermis, in the subcutaneous tissue, fat is stored as a source of energy and also acts as a soft protective cushion.

EXAMINATION AND ASSESSMENT OF THE SKIN

The skin is the largest and most accessible and easily examined organ of the body, and it is often the organ of most frequent concern and quality of life for the patient. Therefore all practitioners should be able to recognize basic skin diseases and dermatologic clues to systemic disease.

Optimal examination of the skin is best achieved in a well-lit room. The clinician should inspect the entire skin surface, including the hair, nails, scalp, and mucous membranes. This may present particular problems in infants and teenagers, because it may be necessary to examine the skin in small segments to prevent cooling or embarrassment, respectively. Although no special equipment is required, a hand lens and side lighting are useful aids in the assessment of skin texture and small, discrete lesions. In many offices, the otoscope can be adapted for this purpose by removing the plastic speculum.

There are also a number of relatively inexpensive portable dermatoscopic devices, which can also be used to enhance the examination (also known as epiluminescence microscopy). These instruments have traditionally provided a magnified (×10) view of the skin with a nonpolarized light source, a transparent plate, and a liquid medium between the dermatoscope and the skin. This allows for a view of the superficial structures in the skin without interference from surface reflections. Dermatoscopic heads can be purchased for otoscope/ophthalmoscope handpieces, and mineral oil or alcohol gel can be applied directly to the skin lesion. Newer devices allow for toggling between nonpolarized and polarized light, which provides visualization of deeper structures in the dermis. (Fig. 1.2).

Despite the myriad of conditions affecting skin, a systematic approach to the evaluation of a rash facilitates and simplifies the process of developing a manageable differential diagnosis. After assessing the general health of a child, the practitioner should obtain a detailed history of the cutaneous symptoms, including the date of onset, inciting factors, evolution of lesions, and presence or absence of pruritus. Recent immunizations, infections, drugs, and allergies may be directly related to new rashes. The family history may suggest a hereditary or contagious process, and the clinician may need to examine other members of the family. A review of nursery records and images provided by parents and in the electronic record will help document the presence and evolution of congenital and acquired lesions.

Attention should then turn to the distribution and pattern of the rash. The distribution refers to the location of the skin findings, while the pattern defines a specific anatomic or physiologic arrangement. For example, the distribution of a rash may include the extremities, face, or trunk, while the pattern could be flexural or intertriginous areas (Fig. 1.3a). Other common patterns include sun-exposed sites, acrodermatitis (predilection for the distal extremities), pityriasis rosea (truncal, following the skin cleavage lines), clothing-protected sites, acneiform rashes, lines of Blaschko, and segmental lesions (Fig. 1.3b–h).

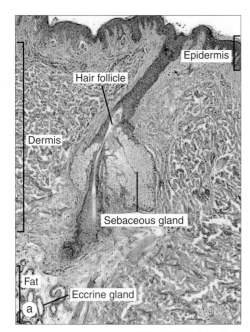

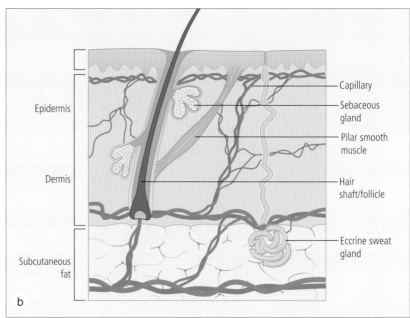

Fig. 1.1 (a) Skin photomicrograph and (b) schematic diagram of normal skin anatomy.

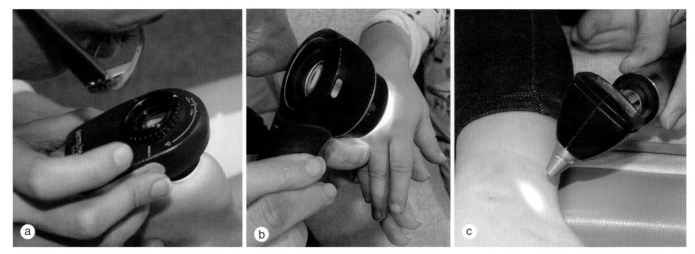

Fig. 1.2 Examination of pigmented nevi with (a) handheld DermLite dermatoscope by 3Gen, (b) DermLite DL4W dermatoscope by 3Gen, and (c) Welch Allyn otoscope.

Next, the clinician should consider the local organization and configuration of the lesions, defining the relationship of primary and secondary lesions to one another in a given location (Table 1.1) and the shape of the lesions. Are the lesions diffusely scattered or clustered (herpetiform)? Are they dermatomal, linear, serpiginous, circular, annular, or reticulated?

The depth of the lesions in the skin, as noted by both observation and palpation, may also give further clues (Table 1.2). Disruption of the normal skin markings by scale, papules, vesicles, or pustules points to the involvement of the epidermis. Alterations in skin color alone can occur in epidermal and dermal processes. In disorders of pigmentation, the color of the pigment may suggest the anatomic depth of the lesion. Shades of brown are present in flat junctional nevi, lentigines,

and café-au-lait spots, where the increased pigment resides in the epidermis or superficial dermis. In Mongolian spots and nevus of Ota, the Tyndall effect results in bluish-green to gray macules from melanin uniformly distributed in the mid-dermis. If the epidermal markings are normal but the lesion is elevated, the disorder usually involves the dermis. Dermal lesions have well-demarcated firm borders. Nodules and tumors deep in the dermis or subcutaneous tissue can distort the surface markings, which are otherwise intact. Some deep-seated lesions can only be appreciated by careful palpation.

Lesion color can provide important clues for diagnosis and the pathophysiology of the underlying process (Table 1.3). Brown, blue, gray, bronze, and black lesions are associated with disorders that alter normal pigmentation, while white lesions

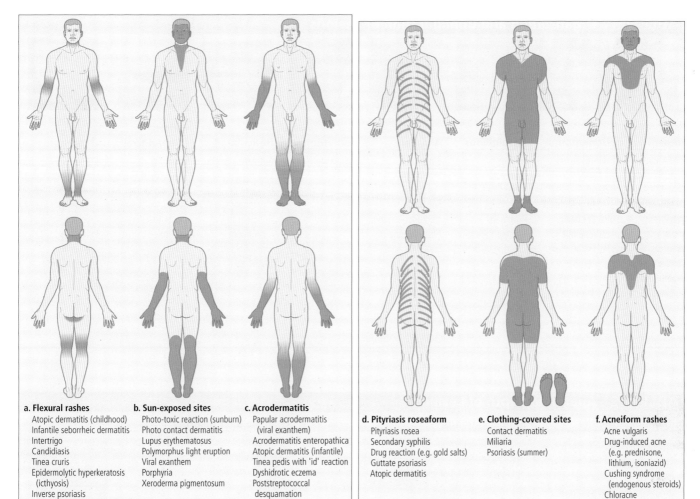

a. Flexural rashes
Atopic dermatitis (childhood)
Infantile seborrheic dermatitis
Intertrigo
Candidiasis
Tinea cruris
Epidermolytic hyperkeratosis
  (icthyosis)
Inverse psoriasis

b. Sun-exposed sites
Photo-toxic reaction (sunburn)
Photo contact dermatitis
Lupus erythematosus
Polymorphus light eruption
Viral exanthem
Porphyria
Xeroderma pigmentosum

c. Acrodermatitis
Papular acrodermatitis
  (viral exanthem)
Acrodermatitis enteropathica
Atopic dermatitis (infantile)
Tinea pedis with 'id' reaction
Dyshidrotic eczema
Poststreptococcal
  desquamation

d. Pityriasis roseaform
Pityriasis rosea
Secondary syphilis
Drug reaction (e.g. gold salts)
Guttate psoriasis
Atopic dermatitis

e. Clothing-covered sites
Contact dermatitis
Miliaria
Psoriasis (summer)

f. Acneiform rashes
Acne vulgaris
Drug-induced acne
  (e.g. prednisone,
  lithium, isoniazid)
Cushing syndrome
  (endogenous steroids)
Chloracne

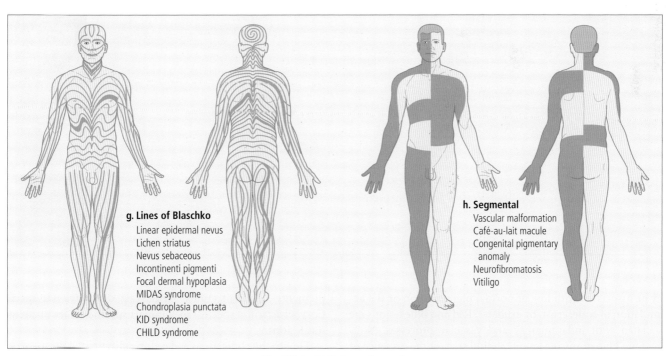

g. Lines of Blaschko
Linear epidermal nevus
Lichen striatus
Nevus sebaceous
Incontinenti pigmenti
Focal dermal hypoplasia
MIDAS syndrome
Chondroplasia punctata
KID syndrome
CHILD syndrome

h. Segmental
Vascular malformation
Café-au-lait macule
Congenital pigmentary
  anomaly
Neurofibromatosis
Vitiligo

Fig. 1.3 (a–h) Pattern diagnosis.

TABLE 1.1   Organization and Configuration of Lesions

Linear	Dermatomal	Serpiginous	Annular	Herpetiform	Reticulated	Filiform (Thread-like)	Geographic
Epidermal nevi	Herpes zoster	Psoriasis	Ringworm	Herpes simplex infection	Cutis marmorata	Wart	Psoriasis
Lichen striatus	Vitiligo	Erythema marginatum	Granuloma annulare	Herpes zoster	Livedo reticularis	Dermatosis papulosa nigra	Geographic tongue
Contact dermatitis	Nevus depigmentosus	Cutaneous larvae migrans	Subacute cutaneous lupus	Dermatitis herpetiformis	Congenital phlebectasia	Syringocystadenoma papilliferum	Nummular eczema
Warts	Becker nevus	Elastosis perforans serpiginosa	Atopic dermatitis		Reticulated and confluent papillomatosis	Skin tag	Erythema annulare centrifugum
Ichthyosis	Café-au-lait spot		Erythema annulare centrifugum		Erythema ab igne	Pigmented nevus	
Psoriasis	Port-wine stain		Erythema chronicum migrans				
Porokeratosis			Erythema marginatum				
Incontinentia pigmenti							

TABLE 1.2   Anatomic Depth of Lesions

Cutaneous Structure	Physical Findings	Specific Skin Disorder	
Epidermis	Altered surface markings Scale, vesicle, crust Color changes (black, brown, white)	Impetigo Café-au-lait spot Atopic dermatitis Vitiligo Freckle	
Epidermis + dermis	Altered surface markings Scale, vesicle, crust Distinct borders Color changes (black, brown, white, and/or red) Edema	Psoriasis Atopic dermatitis Cutaneous lupus erythematosus	
Dermis	Normal surface markings Color changes Altered dermal firmness	Urticaria Granuloma annulare Hemangioma Blue nevus	
Subcutaneous tissue	Normal surface markings Normal or red skin color Altered skin firmness	Hematoma Cold panniculitis Erythema nodosum	

may be associated with loss of normal pigmentation or the accumulation of scale, crust, or exudates. Red and blue lesions are associated with inflammatory and vascular processes. Non-blanching blue or purple lesions should suggest the presence of purpura. Yellow lesions occur when the skin is infiltrated with inflammatory or tumor cells containing lipid. Other pigments from topical agents (e.g. silver, gold), oral medications (e.g. minocycline, amiodarone), foreign bodies (e.g. asphalt, tattoo pigments), and infectious agents (e.g. *Pseudomonas* species, *Corynebacterium* species) may impart specific colors to cutaneous lesions.

Finally, the clinician may develop a differential diagnosis using the morphology of the cutaneous lesions. Primary lesions (macules, papules, plaques, vesicles, bullae, pustules, wheals, nodules, and tumors) arise *de novo* in the skin (Fig. 1.4). Secondary lesions (scale, crust, erosions, ulcers, scars with atrophy

TABLE 1.3   Lesion Color

Red	Purple	Brown	Gray	Blue	Bronze	Green	Yellow
Inflammatory disorders, such as eczema, psoriasis, urticaria, erythema chronicum migrans, and other figurate erythemas	Purpura, vascular malformations, hemangiomas, hematoma	Pigmented nevus, post-inflammatory hyperpigmentation, lentigo, ephiled (freckle), café-au-lait spot, epidermal nevus	Mongolian spot, graphite tattoo, nevus of Ota	Tattoo, vascular malformation, hemangiomas, blue nevus, Mongolian spot	Progressive-pigmented purpuric dermatosis, resolving hematoma, phyto-photodermatitis	Tattoo, pseudomonas infection, deposition of minocycline, Mongolian spot, resolving hematoma	Xantho-granuloma, xanthoma, sebaceous hyperplasia, epidermal inclusion cyst

and/or fibrosis, excoriations, and fissures) evolve from primary lesions or result from scratching of primary lesions by the patient (Fig. 1.5).

The practitioner who becomes comfortable with dermatology will integrate all of these approaches into their evaluation of a child with a skin problem. This will be reflected in the clinically focused format of this text.

Each chapter will finish with an algorithm that summarizes the material in a differential diagnostic flow pattern. The limited bibliography includes comprehensive, historically significant, and/or well-organized reviews of the subject. Readers may also find some of the texts and online further reading listed at the end of this chapter useful.

DIAGNOSTIC TECHNIQUES

Potassium Hydroxide Preparation

There are a number of rapid, bedside diagnostic procedures in dermatology. One of the most useful techniques is a wet mount of skin scrapings for microscopic examination (Fig. 1.6). Potassium hydroxide (KOH) 20% is used to change the optic properties of skin samples and make scales more transparent. The technique requires practice and patience.

The first step is to obtain the material by scraping loose scales at the margin of a lesion, nail parings, subungual debris, or the small, pearly globules from a molluscum body. Short residual hair stubs (black dots in tinea capitis) may also be painlessly shaved off the scalp with a #15 blade. Scale is placed on the slide and moved to the center with a cover slip. One or two drops of KOH are added and gently warmed with a match or the microscope light. Boiling the specimen will introduce artifacts and should be avoided, so sitting the specimen aside for 5 min is an alternative to gentle heating. Excess KOH can be removed with a paper towel applied to the edge of the cover slip. Thick specimens may be more easily viewed after gentle but firm pressure is applied to the cover slip with a pencil eraser. Thick scale will also dissolve after being set aside for 15–20 min.

View the preparation under a microscope, with the condenser and light at low levels to maximize contrast, and with the objective at ×10. Focus up and down as the entire slide is rapidly scanned. True hyphae are long branching green hyaline rods of uniform width that cross the borders of epidermal cells. They often contain septae. False positives may be vegetative fibers, cell borders, or other artifacts. Yeast infections show budding yeast and pseudohyphae. Molluscum bodies are oval discs that have homogeneous cytoplasm and are slightly larger than keratinocytes. In hair fragments, the fungi appear as small, round spores packed within or surrounding the hair shaft (see Fig. 8.19e in Chapter 8). Hyphae are only rarely seen on the hair.

Scabies Preparation

A skin scraping showing a mite, its egg, or feces is necessary to diagnose infestation with *Acarus scabiei* because many other skin rashes resemble scabies clinically (Fig. 1.7). The most important factor for obtaining a successful scraping is the choice of site. Burrows and papules, which are most likely to harbor the mite, are commonly located on the wrists, fingers, and elbows. In infants, primary lesions may also be found on the trunk, palms, and soles. A fresh burrow can be identified as a 5–10 mm elongated papule, with a vesicle or pustule at one end. A small, dark spot resembling a fleck of pepper may be seen in the vesicle. This spot is the mite, and it can be lifted out of its burrow with a needle or the point of a scalpel. Usually, it is best to hold the skin taut between the thumb and index finger while vigorously scraping the burrow. Although this may induce a small amount of bleeding, if performed with multiple, short, rapid strokes, it is usually painless. A drop of mineral oil should be applied to the skin before scraping to ensure adherence of the scrapings to the blade. The scrapings are then placed on the slide, another drop of mineral oil is added, and a cover slip is applied. Gentle pressure with a pencil eraser may be used to flatten thick specimens.

Mites are eight-legged arachnids easily identified with the scanning power of the microscope. Care must be taken to focus through thick areas of skin scrapings so as not to miss any camouflaged mites. The presence of eggs (smooth ovals, approximately one half the size of an adult mite) or feces (brown pellets, often seen in clusters) are also diagnostic. If eggs or feces

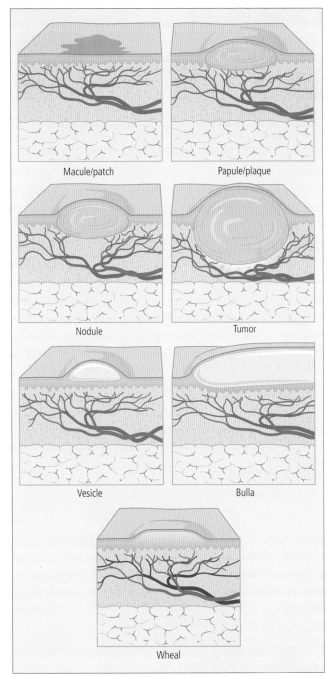

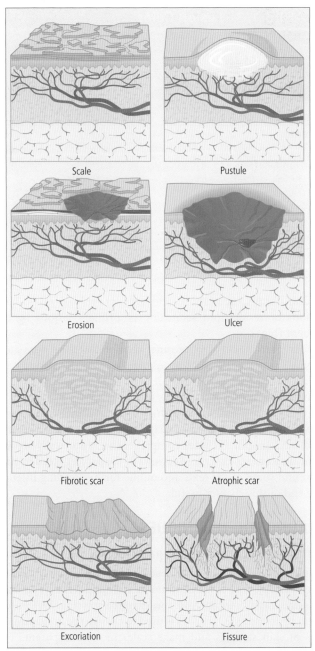

Fig. 1.4 Primary skin lesions. Macule: a small (usually 1 cm), flat lesion showing an alteration in color or tone. Large macule is a patch. Papule: a small (1 cm), sharply circumscribed, elevated lesion. An elevated lesion over 1 cm is referred to as a plaque. Nodule: a soft or solid mass in the dermis or subcutaneous fat. Tumor: a large nodule, localized and palpable, of varied size and consistency. Vesicle: a blister containing transparent fluid. Bulla: a large blister. Wheal: an evanescent, edematous, circumscribed, elevated lesion that appears and disappears quickly. (Adapted from CIBA.)

Fig. 1.5 Secondary skin lesions. Scale: dry and/or greasy fragments of adherent epidermis. Pustule: a sharply circumscribed lesion containing free pus. Crust: a dry mass of exudate from erosions or ruptured vesicles/pustules, consisting of serum, dried blood, scales, and pus. Erosion: well-defined partial-thickness loss of epidermis. Ulcer: a clearly defined, full-thickness loss of epidermis that may extend into the subcutis. Scar: a permanent skin change resulting from new formation of connective tissue after destruction of the epidermis and cutis. When the loss of dermis and/or fat is prominent, the lesion may be atrophic. Fibrosis may result in firm, thickened papules or plaques. Excoriation: any scratch mark on the surface of the skin. Fissure: any linear crack in the skin, usually accompanied by inflammation and pain. (Adapted from CIBA.)

are found first, perusal of the entire slide usually reveals the adult mite.

The dermatoscope can also be used to visualize the female mite whose mouth parts appear as an elongated triangle-shaped spot referred to as a delta sign.

Lice Preparation

Lice are six-legged insects visible to the unaided eye that are commonly found on the scalp (Fig. 1.8), eyelashes, and pubic areas. Pubic lice are short and broad, with claws spaced far apart for grasping the sparse hairs on the trunk, pubic area, and

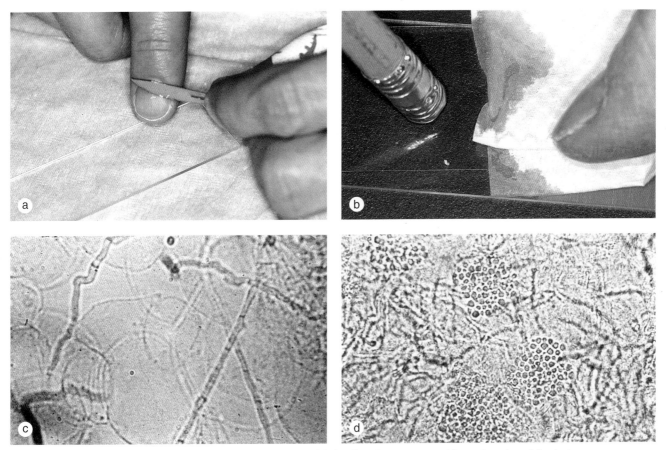

Fig. 1.6 Potassium hydroxide (KOH) preparation. **(a)** Small scales are scraped from the edge of the lesion onto a microscopic slide. **(b)** The scales are crushed to form a thin layer of cells in order to visualize the fungus easily. **(c)** In this positive KOH preparation of skin scrapings, fungal hyphae are seen as long septate, branching rods at the margins and center of the scales. **(d)** Pseudohyphae and spores typical of tinea versicolor give the appearance of spaghetti and meatballs.

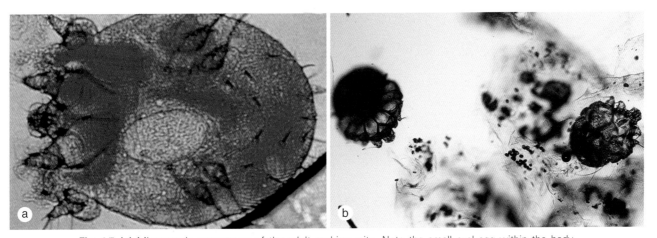

Fig. 1.7 (a) Microscopic appearance of the adult scabies mite. Note the small oval egg within the body. **(b)** Scraping from an adolescent with crusted scabies shows two mites and multiple fecal pellets.

eyelashes, whereas scalp lice are long and thin, with claws closer together to grasp the denser hairs found on the head. The lice are best identified close to the skin, where their eggs are more numerous and more obvious. Diagnosis can be made by identifying the louse, or by plucking hairs and confirming the presence of its eggs or "nits" by microscopic examination.

A dermatoscope or magnifying glass can also be used for confirmation of lice infestation.

Tzanck Smear

The Tzanck smear is an important diagnostic tool in the evaluation of blistering diseases. It is most commonly used to

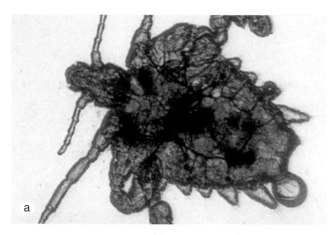

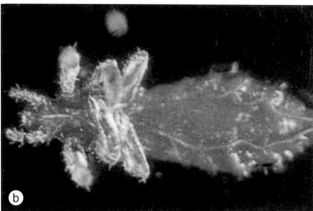

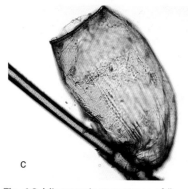

Fig. 1.8 Microscopic appearance of lice. **(a)** The crab louse has a short, broad body, with claws spaced far apart. **(b)** The head louse has a long, thin body, with claws closer together. **(c)** A hatched nit is tightly cemented to the hair shaft.

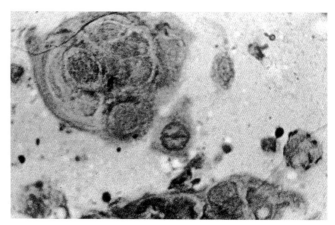

Fig. 1.9 Tzanck Smear. Note the multinucleated giant cells characteristic of viral infection with herpes simplex and varicella/zoster.

with multiple overlapping nuclei; it is much larger than other inflammatory cells. A giant cell may be mistaken for multiple epidermal cells piled on top of each other. If a microscope and stain are available, the Tzanck smear can be used for rapid confirmation of the clinical suspicion of infection, while more sensitive studies like polymerase chain reaction are pending.

Wood Light

Wood light is an ultraviolet source that emits at a wavelength of 365 nm. Formerly, its most common use was in screening patients with alopecia for tinea capitis, as the most common causative organisms, *Microsporum audouinii* and other *Microsporum* species, were easily identified by blue-green fluorescence under Wood light. However, today in North America, *Trichophyton* species are the most common fungi associated with tinea capitis, but it does not fluoresce. In the United States, fewer than 10% of cases are caused by *M. canis* and other *Microsporum* species. In Europe, Africa, and Asia, organisms that cause ectothrix scalp infection and which fluoresce include *M. ferrugineum*, *M. audouinii*, and *M. canis*.

Wood light is still of value in diagnosing a number of other diseases. Erythrasma is a superficial bacterial infection of moist skin in the groin, axilla, and toe webs. It appears as a brown or red flat plaque and is caused by a *Corynebacterium* that excretes a pigment that contains a porphyrin. This pigment fluoresces coral red or pink under Wood light. Tinea versicolor, a superficial fungal infection with hypopigmented macules and plaques on the trunk, also fluoresces under Wood light with a green-yellow color. *Pseudomonas* infection of the toe web space and colonization of the skin in burn patients will fluoresce yellow-green. Patients with porphyria cutanea tarda excrete uroporphyrins in their urine, and examination of a urine specimen will show an orange-yellow fluorescence. Adequate blood levels of tetracycline produce yellow fluorescence in the opening of hair follicles, while lack of fluorescence indicates poor intestinal absorption or poor patient compliance. Positive fluorescence in the skin is diagnostically useful, but many of the pigments that fluoresce are water soluble and readily removed by swimming or bathing.

distinguish viral diseases, such as herpes simplex, varicella, and herpes zoster, from nonviral disorders (Fig. 1.9). It is important to note that Tzanck smears from vesicles of vaccinia and small-pox do not demonstrate multinucleated giant cells. The smear is obtained by removing the "roof" of the blister with a curved scalpel blade or scissors, and scraping the base to obtain the moist, cloudy debris. The material is then spread onto a glass slide, air dried, and stained with Giemsa or Wright stain. The diagnostic finding of viral blisters is the multinucleated giant cell. The giant cell is a syncytium of epidermal cells,

Wood light also emits purple light in the visible spectrum. This wavelength can be used to accentuate subtle changes in pigmentation. The purple light is absorbed by melanin in the epidermis, and variably reflected by patches of hypopigmentation and depigmentation. It can be helpful to distinguish increased pigmentation in the epidermis that will be enhanced by the purple light from increased pigmentation in the dermis that does not enhance. Purple light may be particularly useful in evaluating light-pigmented individuals with vitiligo or ash leaf macules (congenital hypopigmented macules).

DERMATOLOGIC THERAPEUTICS

General Principles

Single component generic preparations are often effective and inexpensive. Fixed multiple component preparations are occasionally useful and may increase adherence to the treatment regimen, but the practitioner must be aware of all the constituent agents and the increased risk of adverse drug reactions. Specially formulated medications are often prohibitively expensive and seldom indicated in general practice. Fortunately, there are now some special formulating pharmacies that follow Food and Drug Administration guidelines, prepare safe and cost effective products, and obtain insurance preauthorization.

The practitioner must calculate the quantity of medication required for the patient to comply with instructions. In a child, 15–30 g of an ointment is needed to cover the entire skin surface once. This quantity will vary with the vehicle used and the experience of the individual applying the preparation.

Topical Vehicles

Two variables are particularly important in the selection of effective topical therapy: the active medication and the vehicle. No matter how effective the active medication, adherence to the recommended regimen will require that the clinician consider the selection of a vehicle carefully. In infants and young children, ointments tend to be better tolerated than other vehicles, while in older children, adolescents, and young adults, more elegant vehicles (e.g. creams, foams, sprays, solutions) that are free of lingering odors, color residues, or tackiness, will encourage adherence.

Ointments

In general, ointments are occlusive and allow for high transcutaneous penetration of the active drug. Ointments are stable for long periods and require few preservatives and bacteriostatic additives. As a consequence, they are least likely to cause contact allergy or irritation. These vehicles are well tolerated when the skin is cracked or fissured, particularly in young children with chronic skin disease (e.g. atopic dermatitis, psoriasis). Unfortunately, ointments tend to be messy and may stain clothing, so they are not often welcome by older children and adolescents.

Open Wet Dressings

Open wet dressings, using tap water or normal saline, provide symptomatic relief by cooling and drying acute inflammatory lesions. They cleanse the skin by loosening exudates and crusts that can be painlessly removed before the dressing dries. Various astringents and antiseptics, such as vinegar or 5% aluminum acetate solution (e.g. Burrow solution), may be added to compression solutions in a 1:20–40 dilution. Bleach baths and chlorine swimming pools can also be used as gentle antiseptics and anti-inflammatory agents in patients prone to chronic or recurrent infection such as atopic dermatitis and epidermolysis bullosa. The concentration of chlorine in bleach baths (1/4 cup of household bleach or 59 mL to a 40-gallon bathtub to give a concentration of sodium hypochlorite of 6–8.25%) is designed to reproduce the concentration of chlorine recommended for supervised swimming pools.

Powders and Lotions

Powders promote drying and are especially useful in the intertriginous areas. Lotions are powders suspended in water (e.g. calamine lotion). When these preparations dry, they cool the skin and provide a uniform covering of the suspended agent. The clinician should warn patients and parents against the use of combination products that might result in irritation or percutaneous absorption of the active ingredients (e.g. calamine and diphenhydramine).

Gels

Gels are aqueous preparations that liquefy on contact with the skin and leave a uniform film on drying. Gels are well tolerated in hair-bearing areas. Water-based gels are best tolerated by children, while alcohol-containing products are more likely to cause burning or irritation. Gels are well tolerated in hair-bearing areas.

Aerosols

Aerosols and sprays act in a manner similar to lotions and gels. Active ingredients are incorporated into an aqueous phase. A convenient delivery system usually allows for easy dispersion over the skin surface. Aerosols are also particularly useful on the scalp.

Creams

Traditional creams are suspensions of oil in water. As the proportion of oil increases, the preparation approaches the consistency of an ointment, which is the most lubricating vehicle. Creams are water washable and hygroscopic. They may be drying and occasionally sensitizing.

Pastes

Pastes, which are mixtures of powder in ointment, are messy and may be difficult to remove from the skin. They are used to protect areas prone to irritation, such as the diaper area. Pastes can be removed with mineral oil.

Foams

Foams represent a novel vehicle, which enhances percutaneous absorption of medication in a cosmetically acceptable elegant preparation. Foams remain stable until applied to the skin, where warming from natural body heat results in volatilization of inert contents with deposition of the active medication on the skin surface. Because foams contain minimal solid ingredients, there is little residue, making them particularly attractive vehicles for products designed for the scalp and intertriginous areas. A number of topical steroid foams have been approved for the treatment of atopic dermatitis and psoriasis, while other agents have been approved for seborrheic dermatitis and ichthyosis.

Shampoos and Washes

Short contact therapy with medicated shampoos and washes may also enhance adherence, particularly in adolescents with busy schedules and little time for topical therapy. These formulations contain insoluble particulate drugs such as benzoyl peroxide, salicylic acid, corticosteroids, and antifungal agents, some of which remain after showering or washing. Shampoos and washes may also be particularly useful when longer periods of contact are likely to result in burning or irritation.

Topical Corticosteroids

Topical steroids are available in every type of vehicle. A good approach is to become familiar with one or two products in each of the potency ranges (Table 1.4). A check of local pharmacies is useful in determining the availability and cost of medications.

Most childhood skin eruptions requiring topical steroids can be readily managed with twice-daily applications of low- or medium-potency preparations. Moreover, a number of studies have shown that twice-daily applications of mid-potency agents can be applied to most areas of the skin in children for long periods of time safely. With few exceptions, low-potency medications should be used on the face and intertriginous areas because more potent preparations may produce atrophy, telangiectasias, and hypopigmentation. Regardless of

TABLE 1.4 **Topical Corticosteroids**		
	Generic Name	**Trade Name**
Super high-potency topical steroids—class 1	Betamethasone dipropionate augmented 0.05%	Diprolene ointment 0.05%
	Clobetasol propionate 0.05%	Clobex lotion, spray, shampoo 0.05%
		Olux E foam 0.05%, Olux foam 0.05%
		Temovate cream, ointment, solution 0.05%
	Fluocinonide 0.1%	Vanos cream 0.01%
	Halobetasol propionate 0.05%	Ultravate cream, ointment 0.05%
High-potency topical steroids—class 2	Amcinonide 0.1%	
	Desoximetasone 0.25%, 0.05%	Topicort cream, ointment 0.25%, gel 0.05%
	Diflorasone diacetate 0.05%	ApexiCon E cream 0.05%
		Maxiflor ointment 0.05%
	Halcinonide 0.1%	Halog, Halog E ointment, cream 0.1%
	Fluocinonide 0.05%	Lidex cream, gel, ointment 0.05%
	Mometasone furoate 0.1%	Elocon ointment 0.1%
Topical steroids—class 3	Amcinonide 0.1%	Cyclocort cream, lotion 0.01%
	Betamethasone dipropionate 0.05%	Diprosone cream 0.05%
	Betamethasone valerate 0.1%	Valisone ointment 0.1%
		Betacap 0.1% (UK)
	Clobetasone butyrate 0.05%	Eumovate ointment, cream 0.05% (UK)
	Fluocinonide 0.05%	Lidex ointment, cream, gel 0.05%
	Fluticasone propionate 0.05%	Cutivate 0.05%, cream, lotion
Topical steroids—class 4	Betamethasone valerate 0.1%	Luxiq foam 0.1% ointment, cream, lotion
	Clocortolone pivalate 0.1%	Cloderm cream 0.1%
	Desoximetasone 0.05%	Topicort LP cream 0.05%
	Fluocinolone acetonide 0.025	Synalar ointment 0.025%
	Flurandrenolide 0.05%	Cordran ointment, lotion 0.05%
	Hydrocortisone probutate 0.1%	Pandel cream 0.1%
	Hydrocortisone valerate 0.2%	Westcort ointment 0.2%
	Prednicarbate 0.1%	Dermatop ointment 0.1%
	Triamcinolone acetonide 0.1%, 0.025%	Kenalog ointment 0.1%, 0.025%

TABLE 1.4 Topical Corticosteroids—cont'd

	Generic Name	Trade Name
Topical steroids—class 5	Betamethasone dipropionate 0.05%	Diprosone lotion 0.05%
	Betamethasone valerate 0.1%	Valisone cream, lotion 0.1%
	Fluocinolone acetonide 0.025%	Synalar 0.025%, cream 0.01%
	Fluticasone propionate 0.05%	Cutivate cream, lotion 0.05%
	Hydrocortisone butyrate 0.1%	Locoid Lipocream, ointment, lotion, solution 0.1%
	Hydrocortisone valerate 0.2%	Westcort cream 0.2%
	Prednicarbate 0.1%	Dermatop ointment, cream 0.1%
	Triamcinolone acetonide 0.1%	Kenalog cream, lotion 0.1%
Topical steroids—class 6	Alclometasone dipropionate 0.05%	Aclovate ointment, cream 0.05%
		Modrasone ointment, cream 0.05%
	Desonide 0.05%	DesOwen ointment, cream, lotion 0.05%
		Desonate Gel 0.05%
		Tridesilon cream 0.05%
	Fluocinolone acetonide 0.01%	Synalar cream, solution 0.1%
		Derma-Smoothe/FS oil
Topical steroids—class 7	Hydrocortisone 2.5%	Hytone cream, lotion 2.5%
		Cobadex 1%
		Dioderm 0.1%
		Mildison 1%
		Hydrocortisyl 1%
		Hytone ointment 1%
	Dexamethasone 0.04%	Hexadrol cream 0.04%
	Methylprednisolone acetate 0.25%	Medrol ointment 0.25%
	Prednisolone 0.5%	Meti-derm cream 0.5%
Topical steroids—class 8	Hydrocortisone 0.5%, 1%	Hytone, Cortaid, Synacort, Nutracort 0.5% ointment, cream, lotion

the potency of a medication, patients should be followed carefully for steroid-induced changes, even though they are only rarely produced by therapy restricted to 2–4 weeks. Patients receiving chronic therapy to sensitive areas should take frequent "time-outs" from their topical steroids (e.g. 1 week per month) and should taper them when possible. Tapering may be achieved by decreasing the frequency of application, as well as by mixing the active preparation with a bland emollient such as petrolatum.

Steroids may mask infections and suppress local and systemic immune responses. Consequently, they are contraindicated in most patients with viral, fungal, bacterial, or mycobacterial infections.

Topical Calcineurin Inhibitors

The topical nonsteroidal anti-inflammatory agents, pimecrolimus (Elidel) and tacrolimus (Protopic), provide an alternative for the treatment of atopic dermatitis. These calcineurin inhibitors selectively suppress the release of inflammatory mediators from lymphocytes without compromising the function of melanocytes, fibroblasts, or endothelial cells. As a consequence, they are not associated with the development of pigment alteration, atrophy, or telangiectasias. They can be applied at any site including the genital skin, breasts, and face. However, they are contraindicated in erythrodermic conditions, where significant percutaneous absorption may occur.

The nonsteroidal agents are approved for use in children over 2 years of age, but recent studies on a large number of patients from 3 months to 2 years old demonstrate safety and efficacy similar to older children.

A black box warning cautions prescribers and patients against using these agents in children under 2 years of age and long term in any patient. However, when used judiciously, they offer a safe alternative to topical steroids particularly in sensitive areas of the skin. Before using these agents, it is imperative that the practitioner discuss the black box warning and the rationale for prescribing them.

Emollients (Lubricants)

Another topical non-steroidal agent crisaborole ointment 2%, which is anti-inflammatory phosphodiesterase-4 inhibitor, is safe and approved for children with eczema down to 3 months of age. Any preparation that reduces friction and leaves a smooth, occlusive film that prevents drying is classified as a lubricant (Table 1.5). In patients with chronic dermatitis, ointments (or water-in-oil–based products) provide the best lubrication, especially during the dry winter months. Less oily preparations (oil-in-water creams, lotions, foams, aerosols) are

TABLE 1.5 Emollients

Types of Skin	Moisturizing Base Type	Product Name
1. Extremely dry skin	Ointment or oil-based	Bag Balm
		Blue Star ointment
		Elta Swiss skin cream
		Johnson's Baby Oil
		Palmer's Cocoa Butter
		Theraplex Emollient
		Vaseline Petroleum Jelly
		Mineral Oil
		A+D ointment
		Alpha Keri Moisture Rich Baby Oil
		Aquaphor Healing ointment
2. Dry	Water-in-oil emulsion	A+D ointment with zinc oxide
		Acid Mantle cream
		Elta Light moisturizing cream
		Eucerin Original moisturizing cream/lotion
		Jergens All-Purpose Face Cream
		Olay Body lotion
		Restoraderm lotion
		St. Ives Swiss Formula products
		Sween Cream
		Theraplex Clear lotion
		Vanicream
		Vaseline Intensive Care lotion
3. Normal to dry	Oil-in-water	Alpha hydroxy cream/lotion
		Aqua Care cream
		Biore Balancing Moisturizer Normal to Dry
		Caress Body Silkening lotion
		Carmol 40 cream
		Complex 15 lotion
		Curél Moisturizing lotion
		Cutemol cream
		Gold Bond Moisturizing Body Lotion
		Jergens Original Scent lotion
		Keri lotion
		LactiCare lotion
		Lubriderm Skin Therapy
		Moisturel cream/lotion
		Neutrogena lotion
		Nivea Body Creamy Conditioning Oil
		Nutraderm lotion
		Olay Active Hydrating Original Cream
		Pacquin Plus skin cream
		Pond's Age Defying lotion/cream
		Purpose Alpha Hydroxy Moisture cream/lotion
		Sarna lotion
4. Normal to oily	Oil-free	Carmol 10 Deep Moisturizing lotion
		CeraVe lotion or cream
		Cetaphil lotion or cream
		Corn Huskers lotion
		Epilyt lotion
		Gerber Baby Lotion
		Johnson's Baby Lotion
		Lubriderm Skin Therapy
		Neutrogena Combination Skin Moisture
		Olay Regenerist Facial Moisturizer
		Walgreens Glycerin and Rosewater

often preferred by patients during the spring and summer. More elegant products should be considered in older children and young adults, especially for use on the scalp or intertriginous areas. Cultural preferences should also be taken into account when selecting a lubricant. Preparations containing topical sensitizers such as fragrance, neomycin, and benzocaine should be avoided, particularly in patients with inflamed skin.

Sun Protective Agents

These agents (Table 1.6) include sunscreens (light-absorbing compounds) and sunblocks (inert compounds that reflect light). Although the long-awaited guidelines from the Food and Drug Administration have not yet been finalized, in 2019 the Food and Drug Administration recently described two sun-blocking ingredients, titanium dioxide and zinc oxide, as generally recognized as safe and effective (GRASE). The Food and Drug Administration also listed two other ingredients para-aminobenzoic acid (PABA) and trolamine salicylate as not GRASE and 12 other ingredients as potentially safe ingredients pending the presentation of more data on safety and efficacy (see Table 1.6 for listing of GRASE and potentially GRASE ingredients). Most experts recommend the use of broad-spectrum sun protective agents (protective against both ultraviolet A and B light) with an SPF of at least 30. Parents should also be counseled to purchase products that are water resistant. See Chapter 7 Photodermatoses for further discussion of these agents.

TABLE 1.6 Sun Protection

Sunlight Type	Ultraviolet Spectrum (nm)	Sun Protection Agent
Visible light	>400	Titanium dioxide
UVA	320–400	Zinc oxide
		Dioxybenzone
		Titanium dioxide
		Zinc oxide
		Avobenzone
		Octocrylene
		Avobenzone
		Meradimate
		Cinoxate
UVB	290–320	Titanium dioxide
		Zinc oxide
		Oxybenzone
		Sulisobenzone
		Octocrylene
		Cinoxate
		Padimate
		Homosalate
		Octisalate
		Ensulizole
UVC	<290	Filtered out by ozone, does not reach the Earth's surface

UVA, Ultraviolet light A; *UVB,* ultraviolet light B; *UVC,* ultraviolet light C.

FURTHER READING

Bologna JL, Schaeffer JV, Cerroni L. Dermatology, 4th edn. Elsevier, China, 2018.

Baran R, de Berker D, Holzberg M, et al. Diseases of the nails and their management, 5th edn, Wiley & Sons, Ltd, India, 2019.

Cragi FE, Smith E, Williams H. Bleach baths to reduce severity of atopic dermatitis colonized by staphylococcus. Arch Dermatol 2010:146:541-543.

Eichenfield LF, Frieden IJ. Neonatal and infant dermatology, 3rd edn. Elsevier, Saunders, China, 2015.

Elder DE, Elenitsas R, Rosenbach M, et al. Lever's Histopathology of the skin, 11th edn. Lippincott, Wolters Kluwer, China, 2015.

Habif TP. Clinical dermatology: a color guide to diagnosis and therapy, 6th edn. Saunders, St Louis, 2016.

Harper JH, Oranje A, Prose N. Harper's textbook of pediatric dermatology, 3rd edn. Wiley-Blackwell Science, London, 2011.

Hordinsky MK, Sawaya ME, Scher RK. Atlas of hair and nails. Churchill Livingstone, Philadelphia, 2000.

Kang S, Amagai M, Bruckner AL, et al. Fitzpatrick's dermatology, 9th edn. McGraw Hill, New York, 2019.

Kristal L, Prose N. Color atlas of pediatric dermatology, 5th edn. McGraw Hill, China, 2017.

Neville BW, Damm DD, Allen CM, Chi AC. Oral and maxillofacial pathology, 4th edn. Elsevier, Canada, 2016.

Paller AS, Mancini AJ. Hurwitz clinical pediatric dermatology, 5th edn. Elsevier, Canada, 2016.

Patterson JW. Weedon's skin pathology, 4th edn. Churchill Livingstone, Elsevier, China, 2016.

Schachner LA, Hansen RC. Pediatric dermatology, 4th edn. CV Mosby, New York, 2011.

USEFUL WEBSITES

A good resource for skin diseases, conditions, and treatments: https://www.dermnetnz.org

General medical reference with data from a number of medical texts: https://www.emedicine.com

National Library of Medicine: https://www.nlm.nih.gov

PubMed: National Library of Medicine reference journal database: https://www.ncbi.nlm.nih.gov/pubmed

Online Mendelian Inheritance in Man: https://www.ncbi.nlm.nih.gov/omim

A good resource for pediatricians and families: https://www.aad.org › public › kids

See section for patients and families: https://pedsderm.net

2

Neonatal Dermatology

Katherine Brown Püttgen and Bernard A. Cohen

INTRODUCTION

Newborn skin differs from adult skin in several important ways (Table 2.1). It has less hair and fewer sweat and sebaceous gland secretions, is thinner, has fewer intercellular attachments, and has fewer melanosomes. These differences are magnified in the preterm neonate. As a consequence, newborns are not as well equipped to handle thermal stress and sunlight, have increased transepidermal water loss (TEWL) and penetration of toxic substances and medications, and are more likely to develop blisters or erosions in response to heat, chemical irritants, mechanical trauma, and inflammatory skin conditions. An algorithmic approach to diagnosis for neonatal dermatology is summarized at the end of the chapter (see Fig. 2.95).

BARRIER PROPERTIES AND USE OF TOPICAL AGENTS

The barrier properties of the skin reside primarily in the stratum corneum, the compact layer of flattened keratinocytes that cover the surface. Although keratinization begins at 24 weeks, it is not complete until close to term. TEWL and drug absorption through the epidermis at term are similar to those in older children and adults. Skin barrier properties in babies of gestational age 36 weeks approximate those of term infants within several days but may be delayed by 14–21 days in children of gestational age less than 32–34 weeks. Barrier maturation may be further delayed when epidermal injury, inflammation, or hyperemia are present. Sepsis, ischemia, and acidosis in the severely ill newborn may also compromise barrier function. Moreover, even in healthy term infants, the increased surface-to-volume ratio compared with older children and adults may result in relatively high transcutaneous penetration of topical agents.

Percutaneous absorption of toxic substances in newborns, particularly preterm infants and term infants with disruption of barrier function, has been well documented. Aniline dyes used to mark diapers have caused methemoglobinemia and death. Topical corticosteroids may produce adrenal suppression and systemic effects. Vacuolar encephalopathy has been demonstrated in infants bathed with hexachlorophene, particularly premature infants exposed repeatedly.

Pentachlorophenol poisoning occurred in 20 infants who were accidentally exposed to this chemical in nursery linens. Topical application of povidone-iodine to the perineum before delivery and the umbilical cord after delivery has resulted in elevated plasma iodine levels and thyroid dysfunction in the neonate. Other substances, which include isopropyl alcohol, ethyl and methyl alcohol, and chlorhexidine, are readily absorbed and may produce toxic reactions.

In general, topical agents should be used in newborns and infants only if systemic administration of the agent is not associated with toxicity. Antiseptic agents must be used only with great caution and to limited areas of the skin, particularly in premature infants under 30 weeks' gestational age during the first several weeks of life. Injuries to the skin induced by tape, monitors, adhesives, and cleansing agents must be kept to a minimum, as these tend to compromise barrier function. When lubrication is necessary, small amounts of petrolatum or other fragrance-free, bland emollients are adequate. Some investigators advocate the routine use of barrier products (e.g. petrolatum, Aquaphor) in low birth weight, premature infants to reduce heat and insensible water loss. Bubble blankets and humidified air also help minimize energy requirements. There is evidence that the early institution of daily use of petrolatum-based emollients in infants at high risk for atopic dermatitis prevents atopic dermatitis development in these children.

At birth, the skin is covered with vernix caseosa, a greasy white material of pH 6.7–7.4 (Fig. 2.1). It contains lipids, protein, lanugo hairs, shed skin cells, and water. It also helps to minimize TEWL and has antibacterial and antioxidant properties. Beneath the vernix, the skin has a pH of 5.5–6.0. Overwashing of the baby, particularly with harsh soaps, may result in irritation, alkaline pH, and a decrease in normal barrier function of the stratum corneum. As a consequence, bathing is done gently a few times a week with tap water. Mild, soap-free syndet (synthetic detergent) cleansers with neutral to slightly acidic pH (5.5–7.0) are restricted to areas in which cutaneous bacteria are most numerous, such as the umbilicus, diaper area, neck, and axillae. In ill newborns, bathing may be limited to saline compresses of areas of irritated, macerated skin, which occur commonly in intertriginous areas.

Thermoregulation

Cold stress is the major risk to naked preterm infants nursed in a dry incubator. Decreased epidermal and dermal thicknesses result in increased heat loss from radiation and conduction. Minimal subcutaneous fat and an immature nervous system also decrease the premature infant's ability to respond to cooling. Although heat loss may be minimized by increasing ambient

TABLE 2.1	Structural and Functional Differences of Adult, Term, and Preterm Infant Skin			
	Adult	Term	Preterm (30 Weeks)	Significance
Epidermal thickness	50 μm	50 μm	27.4 μm	Permeability to topical agents ↑ Transepidermal water loss
Cell attachments (desmosome, hemidesmosome)	Normal	Normal	Fewer	↑ Tendency to blister
Dermis	Normal	↓ Collagen and elastic fibers	↓↓ Collagen and elastic fibers	↓ Elasticity ↑ Blistering
Melanosomes	Normal	Fewer Delayed activity for 1–7 days	One-third term infant	↑ Photosensitivity
Eccrine glands	Normal	↓ Neurologic control for 2–3 years	Total anhidrosis	↓ Response to thermal stress
Sebaceous glands	Normal	Normal	Normal	Barrier properties Lubricant Antibacterial
Hair	Normal	↓ Terminal hair	Persistent lanugo	Helpful in assessing gestational age

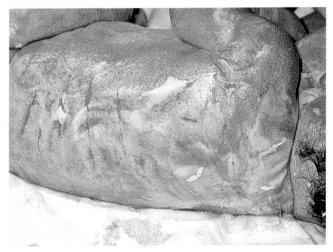

Fig. 2.1 Vernix caseosa covered the skin surface of this healthy newborn at delivery.

humidity and temperature in a humidified Isolette, increasing postnatal age and weight approaching 2000 g are associated with maintenance of normal body temperature.

In growing premature and full-term infants, hyperthermia may be a problem in warm climates, particularly when additional thermal stresses such as insulated clothing and phototherapy are present. Although sweat glands are anatomically complete at 28 weeks' gestation, they may not be fully functional until several weeks after delivery, even in the full-term neonate. At birth, sweating has been demonstrated in response to thermal stress in term babies. However, it may not be detectable in infants under 35 weeks' gestational age for several weeks. Consequently, sweating may not be an effective mechanism for thermoregulation in term or premature infants for at least several weeks, so thermal stress must be minimized.

Pigmentation and Photoprotection

Although melanocytes are actively synthesizing and transferring pigment to epidermal keratinocytes by 20–24 weeks of intrauterine life, the skin surface tends to be less pigmented during the first few postnatal months than in later childhood. As a consequence, infants have less natural protection from sunlight and are more likely to develop sunburn.

The use of sunscreen is not approved by the U.S. Food and Drug Administration (FDA) in infants under 6 months of age. However, as these infants are not ambulatory, sun avoidance and protective clothing are effective barriers to excessive sun exposure. If, however, sun exposure cannot be strictly avoided, it is likely best to use a sunscreen that is fragrance-free and which contains the physical sunscreen ingredients zinc oxide and/or titanium dioxide.

Certain children are particularly sensitive to sunlight, and for these children, prolonged sun avoidance beyond infancy and aggressive use of sunscreens may be mandatory (see Chapter 7). Hereditary porphyrias, xeroderma pigmentosum, Bloom syndrome, Cockayne syndrome, and a number of other photosensitivity disorders may present with exaggerated sunburn reactions in infancy. In some infants, tingling and burning of the skin may occur after sun exposure with no obvious physical findings. In neonatal lupus erythematosus, the skin rash is often triggered by sun exposure. Although some of these children benefit from broad-spectrum sunscreens or sunscreens with sun protective factors above 30, photoreactions may be caused by wavelengths of light that are not absorbed by currently available sunscreens. A number of products achieve broad-spectrum coverage and high sun protection factors by incorporating cosmetically elegant formulations of inert physical blocking agents, such as zinc oxide and titanium dioxide.

CUTANEOUS COMPLICATIONS OF THE INTENSIVE CARE NURSERY

Scars and burns are frequent complications of nursery care and monitoring. Careful management of the skin in the nursery and after discharge minimizes the risk of serious functional impairment and cosmetic disfigurement.

Surgical Scars

Wounds from subclavian and jugular venous lines generally heal with barely noticeable scars. Occasionally, scars are more obvious,

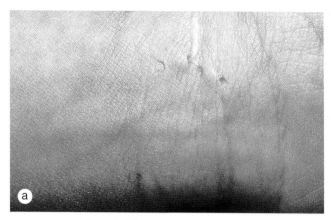
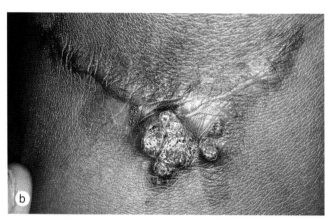

Fig. 2.2 Effect of surgical scars. **(a)** Scar from an arterial cut down site. Recurrent drainage ended after a small fistulous tract in the scar was excised from the wrist of this 2-year-old girl. **(b)** This 6-year-old girl has a hypertrophic scar in the right antecubital space. She developed prurigo nodules in the center of the scar from chronic scratching.

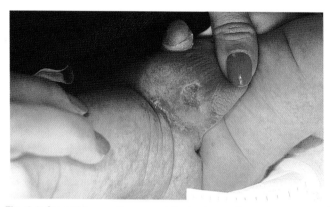

Fig. 2.3 Several hours after an umbilical artery catheter was removed from this infant, a purple area developed unilaterally on the scrotum, perineum, and perirectal skin. After 1 day, the area became ulcerated. Note the formation of granulation tissue and early scarring 1 week later.

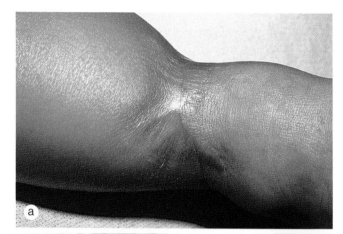
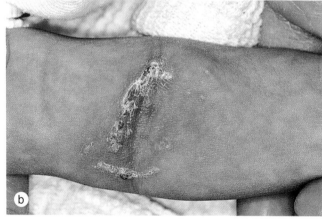

Fig. 2.4 (a) Infiltration of the antecubital skin with 20% glucose resulted in an ulcer that healed with severe scarring. The scar was surgically revised at 4 years of age. **(b)** Infiltration of calcium resulted in a painful red patch that healed with an annular red calcified plaque.

but usually they fade over the first 2 years of life, particularly if the wounds conform to the normal skin lines. However, dimpling may result from sutures used to keep the lines in place (Fig. 2.2). Scarring and dimpling may also be minimized by gentle massage of the area.

Frequently, chest tubes are placed in emergencies with little time taken to consider optimal site selection. Unnecessary scars or injury to sensitive breast tissue may require later surgical repair. Lateral placement beyond the breast tissue may eliminate the need for later surgery. Gentle massage after removal may prevent the formation of adhesions and dimpling. As with other surgical scars, these lesions tend to improve spontaneously over the first several years of life.

Arterial Catheters

In addition to local scarring, arterial catheters may be associated with serious systemic and cutaneous complications in the areas distal to their placement. Extensive ischemia and necrosis of the genital and buttock skin is an unusual complication of umbilical artery spasm and thromboembolism. Ensuing ulcerations may take months to heal and require surgical repair (Fig. 2.3). Radial artery catheters have rarely been associated with the necrosis of digits. However, more subtle findings, such as discrepancies in hand size, may not be evident for a year.

Chemical and Thermal Burns

Infiltration of the soft tissues by intravenous fluids often produces cutaneous inflammation and necrosis. Hypertonic fluids, such as glucose and calcium, may result in full-thickness sloughing of the skin and in contractures (Fig. 2.4). These lesions usually heal over weeks to months and may require splinting,

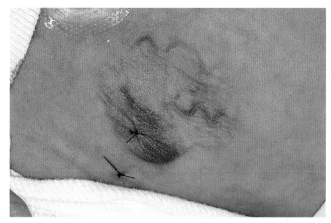

Fig. 2.5 Repeated trauma from removal of monitor leads produced a round, atrophic patch on the lower abdominal wall of this 29-week premature infant. Note the wrinkling of the skin, prominent vessels, and purpura (which was present before a biopsy was taken).

physical therapy, and surgical repair, particularly if they are located over joints.

Removal of adhesives used with dressings, of endotracheal and nasotracheal tubes, and of monitor leads results in extensive trauma to the skin (Fig. 2.5). Although full-thickness sloughs may rarely develop, postinflammatory hyperpigmentation and hypopigmentation are common. Pigmentary changes may persist for years, particularly in dark-pigmented individuals, but usually fade markedly within the first year of life. Other topical agents, such as iodophors, soaps, detergents, and solvents, may produce severe irritant reactions, particularly in premature infants or children with an antecedent cutaneous injury (Fig. 2.6).

Accidental thermal burns have been reported after exposure to heated water beds, radiant warmers, transcutaneous oxygen monitors, and heated, humidified air. Although cold stress must be minimized in the small premature infant, extensive burns that have cutaneous and airway involvement may be prevented by close monitoring of these devices.

Heel-Stick Nodules

Repeated blood sampling from the heel leads to the formation of papules and nodules in many graduates of the neonatal intensive care unit (Fig. 2.7a). Although the most prominent lesions occur in children who have had frequent heel sticks, these scars are also detected in infants who have had only a few. Lesions may be palpable at the time of discharge from the nursery. Over a period of several months, they generally become more superficial and resemble milia. Papules typically calcify over the ensuing months and resolve spontaneously in 18–30 months. During this time, most infants are asymptomatic, and walking is not delayed.

Similar lesions occur from injuries at other sites (Fig. 2.7b). Isolated calcified nodules (calcinosis cutis) may be present at birth and probably result from incidental intrauterine trauma to the skin. They are most common on the face and extremities.

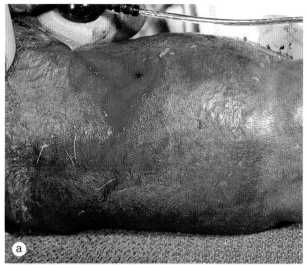

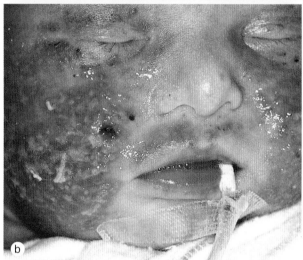

Fig. 2.6 Severe irritant reactions. **(a)** Application of a solution containing topical iodophor produced an erosive irritant dermatitis on the flank of a premature infant in the intensive care nursery. Fortunately, this area healed with only minimal scarring. **(b)** A chemical burn resulted from a solvent that was applied to this child's face to remove adhesive tape.

TRANSIENT ERUPTIONS OF THE NEWBORN

A number of innocent rashes occur in infants. Although they are usually transient, they may be very dramatic and a major source of parental anxiety. Early recognition is important to differentiate these lesions from more serious disorders and to provide appropriate counseling to parents.

Transient Vascular Phenomena

During the first 2–4 weeks of life, cold stress may be associated with acrocyanosis and cutis marmorata (Fig. 2.8). In acrocyanosis, the hands and feet become variably and symmetrically blue in color without edema or other cutaneous changes. Cutis marmorata is identified by the characteristic reticulated cyanosis or marbling of the skin, which symmetrically involves the trunk and extremities. Both patterns usually resolve with warming of the skin, and recurrence is unusual after 1 month of age.

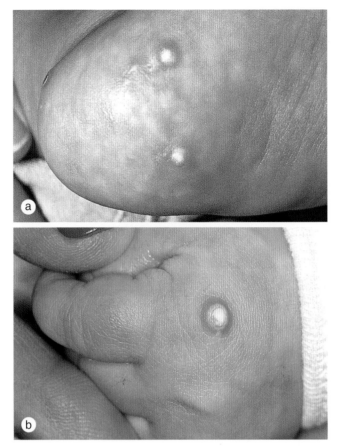

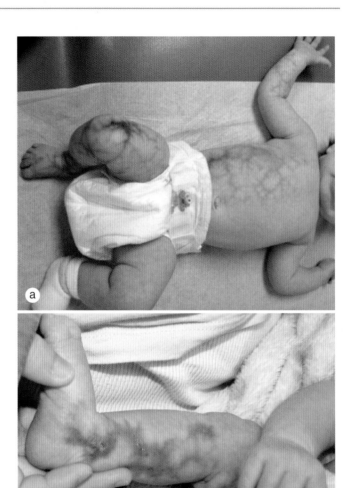

Fig. 2.7 Calcinosis cutis. **(a)** Heel-stick papules developed at 3 months of age on the feet of this graduate of the intensive care nursery. They cleared 9 months later without treatment. **(b)** This calcified nodule was present on the hand of a healthy newborn at birth.

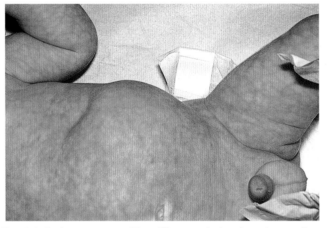

Fig. 2.8 Cutis marmorata. The diffuse, reticulated erythema disappeared with warming of this newborn.

Fig. 2.9 Cutis marmorata telangiectatica congenita (CMTC). **(a)** An otherwise healthy infant with extensive CMTC affecting the right arm, trunk, and leg with sharp midline cutoff. **(b)** The right leg of an affected infant demonstrating extensive marbling and some atrophy. (a, Courtesy Katherine B. Püttgen. b, Reprinted with permission from Bernard A. Cohen© DermAtlas, Johns Hopkins University; 2000–2012.)

Acrocyanosis is readily differentiated from persistent central cyanosis (cyanosis of the lips, face, and/or trunk), which occurs in association with pulmonary or cardiac disease. Cutis marmorata that persists beyond the neonatal period may be a marker for trisomy 18, Down syndrome, Cornelia de Lange syndrome, hypothyroidism, or other causes of central nervous system–induced neurovascular dysfunction.

Cutis marmorata telangiectatica congenita (CMTC) or congenital phlebectasia (Fig. 2.9) may mimic cutis marmorata. However, the lesions are persistent in a localized patch on the trunk or extremities. Location on the legs is most common, followed by truncal involvement. The eruption may extend in a Blaschkoid pattern, and occasionally widespread lesions and reticulated cutaneous atrophy are present. Although CMTC may be an isolated cutaneous finding, it may also occur in association with other mesodermal and neuroectodermal anomalies; reports of associated anomalies range from 20% to 70% of cases. Hypotrophy or hypertrophy of the affected site may occur.

The harlequin color change is noted when the infant lies horizontally, and the dependent half of the body turns bright red in contrast to the pale upper half (Fig. 2.10). The color shifts

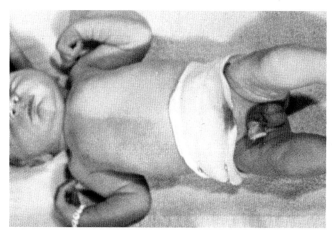

Fig. 2.10 The dependent side is bright red in this infant with the harlequin color change.

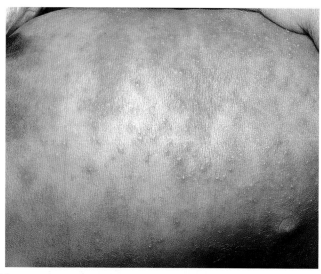

Fig. 2.11 Erythema toxicum neonatorum. Numerous yellow papules and pustules are surrounded by large, intensely erythematous rings on the trunk of this infant.

when the infant is rolled from side to side. This phenomenon lasts from seconds to 20 minutes, and recurrences are common until 3–4 weeks of life. The cause is unknown, and it is not associated with serious underlying disease.

Benign Pustular Dermatoses

Several innocent pustular eruptions must be differentiated from potentially serious infectious dermatoses.

Erythema Toxicum Neonatorum

Erythema toxicum neonatorum (ETN) is the most common pustular rash; it occurs in up to 70% of full-term infants (Fig. 2.11). Although lesions usually appear on the second or third day of life, onset has been reported up to 2–3 weeks of age. Typically, ETN begins with 2–3 mm diameter erythematous and blotchy macules and papules, which may evolve over several hours into pustules on a broad erythematous base to give affected infants a "flea-bitten" appearance. Lesions may be isolated or clustered on the face, trunk, and proximal extremities, and usually fade over 5–7 days. Recurrences, however, may occur for several weeks. A Wright stain of the pustule contents reveals sheets of eosinophils and occasional neutrophils, and 15–20% of patients have a circulating eosinophilia.

Transient Neonatal Pustular Melanosis

Transient neonatal pustular melanosis (TNPM) occurs in 4% of newborns, particularly in black male infants (Fig. 2.12). Unlike ETN, lesions are usually present at birth and probably evolve in many children prenatally. Characteristically, TNPM appears as 2–5 mm diameter pustules on a non-erythematous base on the chin, neck, upper chest, sacrum, abdomen, and thighs. Over several days, lesions develop a central crust, which desquamates to leave a hyperpigmented macule with a collarette of fine scale. Lesions at different stages of development may be present simultaneously. Often, the only manifestation of the eruption is the presence of brown macules with a rim of scale at birth. In newborns with lighter pigmentation, little or no hyperpigmentation remains. A Wright stain of the pustular smear shows numerous neutrophils and rare eosinophils.

Acropustulosis of Infancy

Acropustulosis of infancy is a chronic, recurrent pustular eruption that appears on the palms and soles but may also involve the scalp, trunk, buttocks, and extremities (Fig. 2.13). Onset may occur during the newborn period or in early infancy, and episodes typically last 1–3 weeks with intervening remissions of 1–3 weeks. Disease-free periods tend to lengthen until the rash resolves by 2–3 years of age. During flares, infants are usually fussy and pruritus is severe.

Although the cause is unknown, in some infants, scabies infestation may precede the onset of the eruption. Histopathology of the lesions reveals sterile, intraepidermal pustules. A Wright stain shows numerous neutrophils and occasional eosinophils. Although oral dapsone (1–3 mg/kg per day) suppresses lesions and symptoms in 24–48 hours, brief courses of moderate- to high-potency topical corticosteroids to the palms and soles typically provide safe temporary relief.

Eosinophilic Pustular Folliculitis

Eosinophilic pustular folliculitis (EPF), or Ofuji disease, is a rare, self-limiting vesiculopustular eruption of infancy characterized by recurrent episodes of 2–3 mm diameter follicular white vesicles and pustules on a red base on the scalp and forehead (Fig. 2.14). Occasionally, lesions spread to the trunk. It occurs almost exclusively in boys of age 5–10 months and can recur for months to years. Several neonatal cases have also been described. Although affected infants experience intense pruritus and irritability, EPF is not associated with systemic disease, and treatment is symptomatic. Wright stain preparations of material from pustules show large numbers of eosinophils but no evidence of bacterial, fungal, or viral organisms. The strong association of EPF with human immunodeficiency virus infection seen in adults has not been noted in infants. EPF may be an early presenting feature in cases of hyper immunoglobulin E (IgE) syndrome. The clinical findings and course may overlap

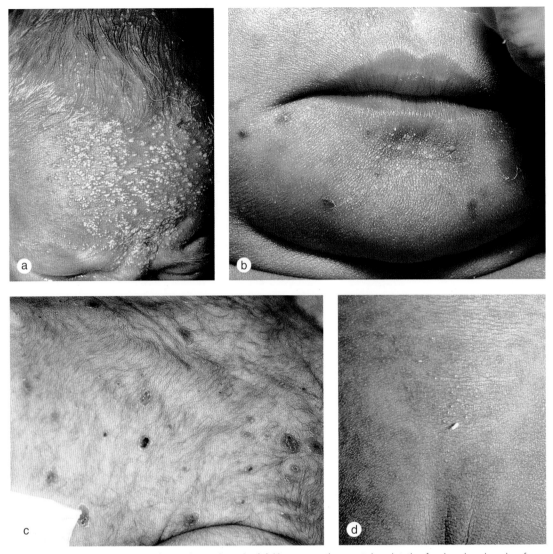

Fig. 2.12 Transient neonatal pustular melanosis. **(a)** Numerous tiny pustules dot the forehead and scalp of this light-pigmented neonate. **(b)** Healing pustules leave marked hyperpigmentation and scale on the chin of this dark-pigmented baby. **(c)** Dry, hyperpigmented crusts cover the back of this Asian newborn. **(d)** Healing pustules and brown macules dot the lower back and sacrum of this child at birth. Note the Mongolian spot on his gluteal cleft.

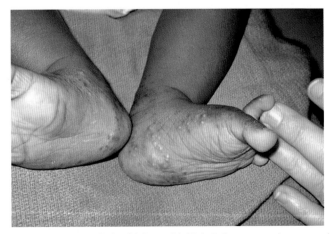

Fig. 2.13 Acropustulosis of infancy. Multiple 2–3 mm pustules covered the hands and feet of this otherwise healthy infant. Lesions recurred episodically until this child was 3 years old. (Courtesy Katherine B. Püttgen. Katherine B. Püttgen retains copyright of this figure.)

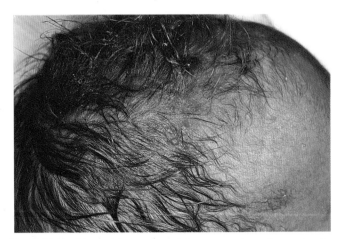

Fig. 2.14 Pruritic vesicles and pustules recurred on the scalp of a healthy 5-month-old boy for over a year. Histologic findings revealed eosinophilic folliculitis.

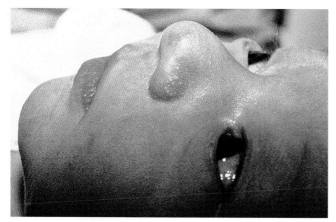

Fig. 2.15 Sebaceous gland hyperplasia. Note the yellow papules on the nose, forehead, and cheeks of this healthy newborn who also had a nodule that demonstrated the typical changes of Langerhans cell histiocytosis on histopathology. He had no evidence of systemic disease, and the nodule resolved without treatment over the first month of life.

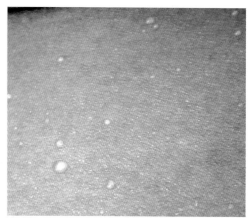

Fig. 2.16 Miliaria crystallina. Tiny, thin-walled vesicles quickly desquamated when this child was placed in a cooler environment. (Reprinted with permission from Bernard A. Cohen© DermAtlas, Johns Hopkins University; 2000–2012.)

with some cases of ETN and acropustulosis of infancy. Reported treatments include topical corticosteroids, oral erythromycin, dapsone, colchicine, indometacin, and cyclosporine.

Other Papulopustular Rashes

Benign pustular dermatoses can be differentiated from herpes simplex infection by the absence of multinucleated giant cells on Wright-stained smears of pustular contents. Negative Gram-stain and potassium hydroxide preparations exclude bacterial and candidal infection. However, in seriously ill infants, viral and bacterial cultures may be required to confirm the clinical impression. Serologic studies for syphilis and scrapings for ectoparasites exclude syphilis and scabies in children with acropustulosis.

The benign pustular dermatoses may also be confused with several other innocent papulopustular rashes, which include sebaceous gland hyperplasia, miliaria, milia, and acne.

Sebaceous gland hyperplasia. Sebaceous gland hyperplasia is a common finding over the nose and cheeks of term infants (Fig. 2.15). Lesions consist of multiple 1–2 mm diameter yellow papules that result from maternal or endogenous androgenic stimulation of sebaceous gland growth. The eruption resolves within 4–6 months.

Miliaria. Miliaria results from obstruction to the flow of sweat and rupture of the eccrine sweat duct. In miliaria crystallina, superficial, 1–2 mm diameter vesicles appear on noninflamed skin when the duct is blocked by keratinous debris just beneath the stratum corneum (Fig. 2.16). Small papules and pustules are typical of miliaria rubra (prickly heat), in which the obstruction occurs in the mid-epidermis (Fig. 2.17). Deep-seated papulopustular lesions of miliaria profunda occur only rarely in infancy, when the duct ruptures at the dermal–epidermal junction.

Miliaria occurs frequently in term and preterm infants after the first week of life in response to thermal stress. Lesions erupt in crops in the intertriginous areas, scalp, face, and trunk. In older infants, lesions appear most commonly in areas of skin occluded by tight-fitting clothing. Cooling the skin and loosening clothing results in prompt resolution of the rash.

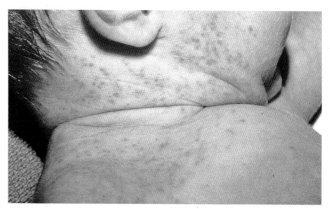

Fig. 2.17 Miliaria rubra. The red papules of prickly heat are readily visible on this infant.

Milia. Milia appear as pearly, yellow, 1–3 mm diameter papules on the face, chin, and forehead of 50% of newborns (Fig. 2.18a). Occasionally, they erupt on the trunk and extremities (Fig. 2.18b). Although milia usually resolve during the first month of life without treatment, they may persist for several months. Histology demonstrates miniature epidermal inclusion cysts that arise from the pilosebaceous apparatus of vellus hairs. Large numbers of lesions distributed over a wide area or persistence beyond several months of age suggest the possibility of the oral-facial-digital syndrome (Fig. 2.18c) or hereditary trichodysplasia (Marie Unna hypotrichosis). Increasing numbers of lesions, particularly in areas of normal trauma such as the hands, knees, and feet, may occur in patients with mild variants of scarring epidermolysis bullosa where blistering is subtle.

Neonatal acne. Mild acne develops in up to 20% of newborns, with an average onset at 3 weeks of age. Lesions may be present at birth or appear in early infancy. Inflammatory red papules and pustules predominate, and cysts may rarely occur. Absence of comedones distinguishes this condition from adolescent acne (Fig. 2.19). Although neonatal acne was once thought to be a result of androgen stimulation of sebaceous glands by maternal hormones, most now favor the term neonatal cephalic

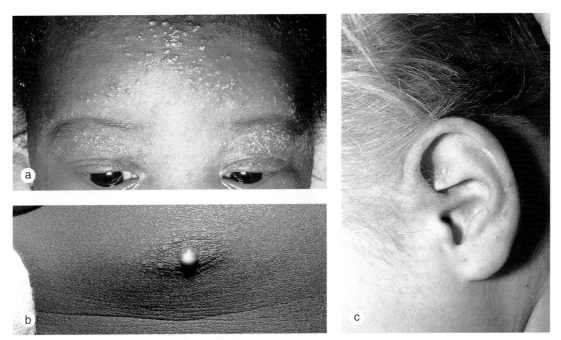

Fig. 2.18 Milia. **(a)** Widespread milia were noted on the forehead and eyelids of this vigorous newborn. The white papules resolved spontaneously before the 2-month pediatric check-up. **(b)** The milium on this infant's nipple also cleared without treatment. **(c)** Multiple congenital persistent milia on the sides of the cheeks and ears of this toddler were an early marker of oral-facial-digital syndrome.

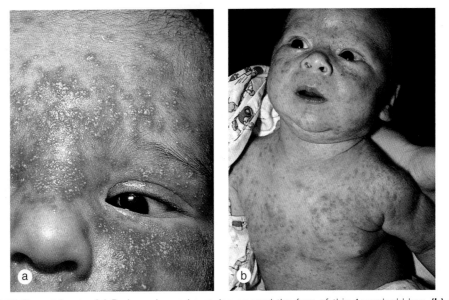

Fig. 2.19 Neonatal acne. **(a)** Red papules and pustules covered the face of this 4-week-old boy. **(b)** Acne spread to the trunk of this healthy infant. In both children, the eruption cleared by 4 months of age.

pustulosis to highlight that this condition in neonates is unlikely to be true acne. It has been suggested that colonization of the skin with *Malassezia* spp. causes an inflammatory reaction, though a direct correlation between burden and *Malassezia* and disease severity has been questioned.

Treatment is usually unnecessary, as lesions involute spontaneously within 1–3 months. However, topical acne preparations can be used with minimal risk in persistent or severe cases. Use of ketoconazole cream may also be of help. Risk of acne in adolescence does not seem to be increased.

Infantile acne. Occasionally, the onset of acne is delayed until 3–6 months of age, when it is referred to as infantile acne and is more common in boys. Lesions tend to be more pleomorphic, and inflammatory papules and pustules are common. Although infantile acne usually resolves by 3 years of age, lesions may rarely persist until puberty. Unlike neonatal acne, infantile acne is probably triggered by endogenous androgens, and open and closed comedones are seen. Children with early onset, persistent disease, and a positive family history of severe acne tend to have a more severe course with resurgence at puberty. Severe infantile acne should prompt a search for other signs of hyperandrogenism and an abnormal endogenous or exogenous source of androgens.

Subcutaneous Fat Necrosis of the Newborn

Fat necrosis is a rare, self-limited process that usually occurs in otherwise healthy full-term and post-mature infants (Fig. 2.20).

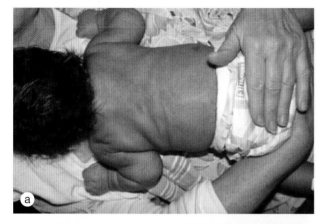

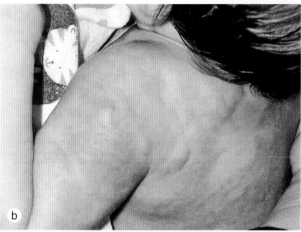

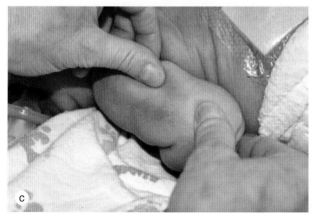

Fig. 2.20 Subcutaneous fat necrosis. **(a)** Red nodules are evident on the back of this neonate. **(b)** Multiple nodules covered the upper back of this newborn who developed hypercalcemia at 3 months of age as the lesions were resolving. **(c)** A deep reddish nodule on the left upper arm best appreciated on palpation. (a, Reprinted with permission from Bernard A. Cohen© DermAtlas, Johns Hopkins University; 2000–2012. c, Courtesy Katherine B. Püttgen. Katherine B. Püttgen retains copyright of this figure.)

It has been reported to occur after total body cooling for treatment of hypoxic ischemic encephalopathy. Discrete firm red or hemorrhagic nodules and plaques up to 3 cm in diameter appear most commonly over areas exposed to trauma, such as the cheeks, back, buttocks, arms, and thighs, during the first few weeks of life. Lesions are usually painless, but marked tenderness may be present. Although the cause is unknown, difficult deliveries, hypothermia, perinatal asphyxia, and maternal diabetes predispose to the development of fat necrosis, suggesting a role for mechanical, cold, and hypoxic injury to fat.

Nodules usually resolve without scarring in 1–2 months. However, lesions occasionally become fluctuant, drain, and heal with atrophy. Variable amounts of calcification develop and can be appreciated radiographically. Even in uncomplicated cases and occasionally after the lesions have resolved, hypercalcemia can develop 1–4 months after the initial detection of subcutaneous fat necrosis. Infants may present with nephrocalcinosis, poor weight gain, irritability, and seizures. Consequently, calcium should be monitored for the first 4–6 months of life in these infants at an interval of every 2–4 weeks. More rarely, thrombocytopenia, hyperlipidemia, and hyperglycemia may also occur.

Histopathology demonstrates necrosis of fat with a foreign body giant cell reaction. Remaining fat cells contain needle-shaped clefts, and calcium deposits are scattered throughout the subcutis. Occasionally, early lesions of sclerema neonatorum are confused with subcutaneous fat necrosis. However, in a severely ill newborn, sclerema is usually differentiated from fat necrosis by the presence of diffuse, wax-like hardening of the skin. Unlike subcutaneous fat necrosis, skin biopsy shows only minimal inflammation in the fat. Thickening of the skin occurs from the increased size of fat cells and interlacing bundles of collagen in the dermis and subcutis.

MINOR ANOMALIES

Minor anomalies occur in up to half of all newborns and are of no physiologic consequence. Their presence, particularly in association with other minor anomalies, prompts an evaluation for more serious multisystem disease.

Dimpling

Dimpling is a common finding over bony prominences, particularly the sacral area (Fig. 2.21a–c). Although skin dimples may be the first sign of several dysmorphic syndromes, these lesions are usually of only cosmetic consequence (Fig. 2.21d). Spinal anomalies should be excluded when deep dimples, sinus tracts, or other cutaneous lesions (e.g. lipomas, hemangiomas, nevi, and tufts of hair) involve the lumbosacral spine. This area is readily visualized by ultrasound during the first 8–12 weeks of life; after this time, ultrasound may suffice, but magnetic resonance imaging (MRI), which requires sedation, is typically necessary to obtain a clear view of the area of interest to exclude malformations.

Periauricular Sinuses, Pits, Tags, and Cysts

Periauricular sinuses, pits, tags, and cysts occur when brachial arches or clefts fail to fuse or close normally (Fig. 2.22). These

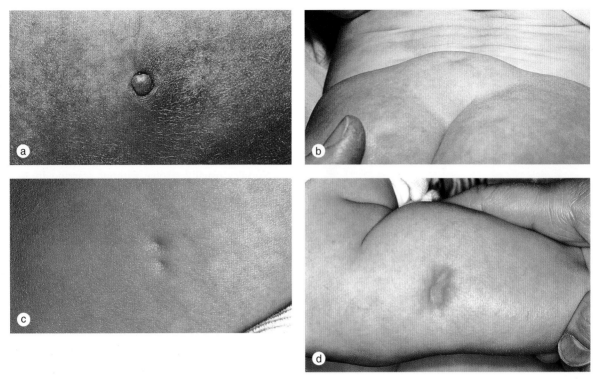

Fig. 2.21 Dimples. **(a)** A sacral dimple was noted in this healthy infant. Computed tomography scan of the lumbosacral spine was normal. **(b)** At birth, a spongy mass was palpable in the sacral area of this baby. A magnetic resonance image of this tumor revealed a lipoma and normal spine. **(c)** These dimples on the thigh of an otherwise healthy infant may have resulted from amniocentesis-induced trauma. **(d)** The cause of an isolated pit on the calf of this healthy infant was unknown. There was no history of amniocentesis.

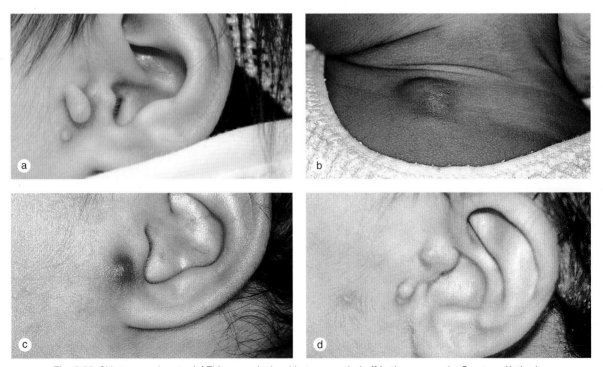

Fig. 2.22 Skin tags and cysts. **(a)** This preauricular skin tag was tied off in the nursery (a, Courtesy Katherine B. Püttgen. Katherine B. Püttgen retains copyright of this figure). **(b)** Congenital cyst on the supraclavicular area. **(c)** Congenital cyst on the preauricular area. The cysts on these children became apparent when they became infected. Both required surgical excision. **(d)** This healthy toddler exhibits two preauricular skin tags (accessory tragi). The lesions were broad-based and were eventually excised by a pediatric plastic surgeon.

lesions develop along a line from the preauricular area to the corner of the mouth. Defects may be unilateral or bilateral and are occasionally associated with other facial anomalies and rarely more complex malformation syndromes such as Goldenhar (oculoauriculovertebral) syndrome or branchio-oto-renal syndrome. Although occult lesions may be discovered when they present with secondary infection, many of these anomalies are noted at birth and readily excised during childhood.

Supernumerary Digits

Supernumerary digits appear most commonly as rudimentary structures at the base of the ulnar side of the fifth finger (Fig. 2.23). They are usually familial and asymptomatic. Histology demonstrates bundles of peripheral nerves extending in various directions and sharply demarcated from dermal connective tissue. A good cosmetic result is best achieved by local surgical excision.

Supernumerary Nipples

Supernumerary nipples may appear unilaterally or bilaterally anywhere along a line from the mid-axilla to the inguinal area (Fig. 2.24) and may develop without areolae, which results in their misdiagnosis as congenital nevi. Malignant degeneration rarely occurs, and many are excised for cosmetic purposes.

Some studies have demonstrated a relationship between accessory nipples and renal or urogenital anomalies, although other investigators have found no association. Ultrasound should be considered if clinical concern or physical findings warrant further evaluation.

Umbilical Granulomas

Umbilical granulomas occur commonly during the first few weeks of life. Normally, the cord dries and separates in 7–14 days. The open surface epithelializes and scars down in an additional 1–2 weeks. Excessive moisture and low-grade infection may result in the growth of exuberant granulation tissue to form an umbilical granuloma. Cauterization with silver nitrate or desiccation with repeated applications of isopropyl alcohol usually produces rapid healing of the granuloma. In some cases, a less friable, firmer nodule may be present (Fig. 2.25).

In some infants, secondary infection results in omphalitis (Fig. 2.26). Aggressive antibiotic therapy is necessary to prevent peritonitis and sepsis.

Umbilical granulomas must be differentiated from umbilical polyps, which result from persistence of the omphalomesenteric duct or urachus (Fig. 2.27). A mucoid discharge may occur

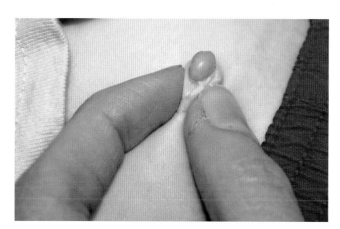

Fig. 2.25 An umbilical granuloma responded to shave removal with light cautery. (Courtesy Katherine B. Püttgen. Katherine B. Püttgen retains copyright of this figure.)

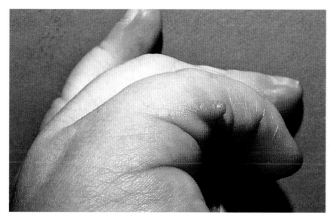

Fig. 2.23 This rudimentary, supernumerary digit was present at birth. It was surgically excised at 6 months of age.

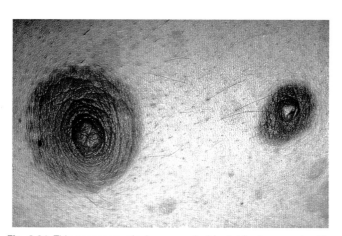

Fig. 2.24 This accessory nipple was an incidental finding on a healthy teenager with tinea versicolor.

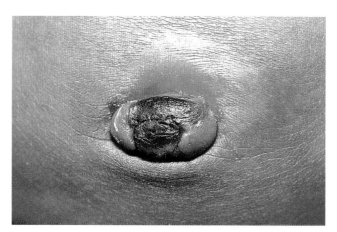

Fig. 2.26 Omphalitis developed in this 10-day-old infant shortly after the cord separated from the umbilicus. The infection cleared after a 10-day course of parenteral antibiotics.

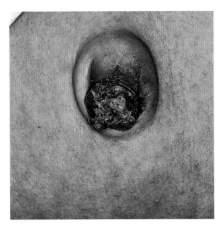

Fig. 2.27 This 2-week-old infant had a broad umbilical stump and chronic watery (urine) discharge. At surgery, the patent urachus was excised.

at the tip of the firm, red polyp, which histologically demonstrates gastrointestinal or urinary tract mucosa. Surgical excision is necessary.

THE SCALY NEWBORN

At delivery, the skin is smooth, moist, and velvety. Desquamation begins at 24–36 h of age and may not be complete for 3 weeks (Fig. 2.28). As peeling progresses, the underlying skin appears normal and cracking and fissuring are absent. Desquamation at birth or during the first day of life is abnormal and suggests postmaturity, intrauterine stress, or congenital ichthyosis.

Collodion Baby

Collodion infants are born encased in a thick, tight, cellophane-like membrane (Fig. 2.29). Although the collodion membrane may desquamate to leave normal skin, up to 70% of affected infants go on to develop autosomal recessive congenital ichthyosis (ARCI), most commonly lamellar ichthyosis. The congenital ichthyosiform erythroderma phenotype of ARCI may also occur. Less commonly, this membrane is a prelude to Netherton syndrome, Conradi–Hunermann syndrome, Sjögren–Larsson syndrome, or one of the ectodermal dysplasias, especially hypohidrotic ectodermal dysplasia. The association of collodion membrane with type II Gaucher disease and X-linked ichthyosis is less clear.

Although the horny layer is markedly thickened in collodion babies, barrier function is compromised by cracking and fissuring. Increased insensible water loss, heat loss, and risk of hypernatremic dehydration, cutaneous infection, and sepsis are minimized by placing affected newborns in a high-humidity (40–60% humidity), neutrally thermal environment. Debridement of the membrane is contraindicated, and topical applications should be restricted to bland emollients, such as petrolatum. Desquamation is usually complete by 2–3 weeks of life. A biopsy during the immediate newborn period before shedding of the membrane is not of value, and biopsy should be deferred until the membrane has fully desquamated.

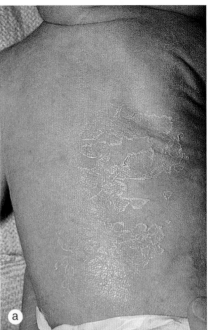

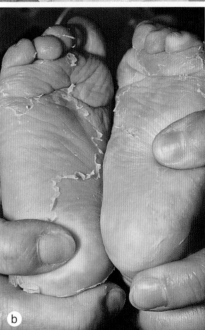

Fig. 2.28 Scaling in a 1-week-old healthy infant. **(a)** Scaling was present on the trunk. **(b)** Similar scaling was present on the hands and feet. A week later, the scaling had resolved completely.

A severe variant of ichthyosis, harlequin ichthyosis, occurs rarely (Fig. 2.30). Although these infants may appear normal at birth, within minutes they develop a thick, generalized membrane, deep cracks and fissures, and marked ectropion and eclabium. Most infants succumb to respiratory distress or infection, but children who survive the neonatal period may develop scale reminiscent of lamellar ichthyosis. Oral retinoids may be of benefit in the neonatal period.

Ichthyosis

The ichthyoses are a heterogeneous group of scaling disorders that may be differentiated by mode of inheritance, clinical features,

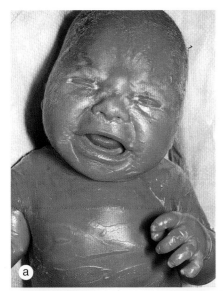

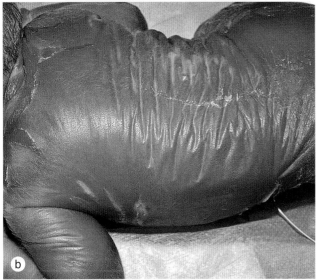

Fig. 2.29 Collodion baby. **(a)** A shiny, transparent membrane covered this baby at birth. **(b)** She later developed lamellar ichthyosis.

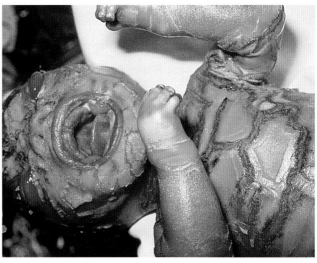

Fig. 2.30 Harlequin baby. This baby developed thick, plate-like scales immediately after drying in the delivery room. Respiratory failure resulted in death during the first week. Note the ectropion and eclabium.

histology, biochemical markers, and genetic mutational analysis (Table 2.2). Rarely, ichthyosis is a marker of multisystem disease in the newborn (Table 2.3).

Autosomal Recessive Congenital Ichthyosis

The phenotype of children with ARCI exists on a continuum from congenital ichthyosiform erythroderma (CIE) (Fig. 2.31), which presents with erythema and fine scale, to lamellar ichthyosis (LI) (Fig. 2.32), which presents with thick, brown scale involving the trunk, extremities, and flexural areas. Both CIE and LI present with a collodion membrane at birth. ARCI is rare and occurs in fewer than 1/100 000 deliveries. The erythroderma of congenital ichthyosiform erythroderma and the generalized, thick, brown scales of lamellar ichthyosis develop after the membrane desquamates at 2–4 weeks of age.

TABLE 2.2	Ichthyoses				
Variant	**Genetics**	**Incidence**	**Clinical Features**		**Onset**
Congenital ichthyosiform erythroderma MIM #242100	Autosomal recessive TGM-1, ABCA12, NIPAL4 (ICHTHYIN), ALOX12B, ALOXE3	1/50–1/100,000	Collodion baby Fine white scale on trunk, face, and scalp Large scale on legs Variable erythroderma		Birth
Lamellar ichthyosis MIM #242300	Autosomal recessive TGM-1, ABCA12, NIPAL4 (ICHTHYIN), CYP4F22, LIPN	1/100,000	Collodion baby Generalized large, dark plate-like scale Ectropion, eclabium Mild palmoplantar keratoderma		Birth
Epidermolytic hyperkeratosis MIM #113800	Autosomal dominant (most common) Autosomal recessive, sporadic KRT1, KRT10	Rare	Widespread blisters at birth Increase erythema, scale with age Marked scale in intertriginous areas, palms, soles Malodor from bacterial overgrowth		Birth
Ichthyosis vulgaris MIM #146700	Autosomal dominant FILAGGRIN	1/250 (may be higher)	Generalized mild scale sparing flexures Improves with age		After 3 months

Continued

TABLE 2.2   Ichthyoses—cont'd

Variant	Genetics	Incidence	Clinical Features	Onset
X-linked ichthyosis MIM #308100	X-linked recessive Steroid sulfatase gene	1/2000–1/6000 males	Large "dirty" scales on trunk, extremities sparing flexures Variable in female carriers Corneal opacities in Descemet's membrane Cryptorchidism Placental sulfatase deficiency with prolonged maternal labor	Within first 3 months
Harlequin ichthyosis MIM #242500	Autosomal recessive ABCA12	Very rare	Thick plates of "armor"-like scale in neonate Overall survival just over 50% Death in first 3 months of life most common	Birth

TABLE 2.3   Ichthyosis Syndromes

Syndrome/Disease	Genetics	Clinical Features
Netherton syndrome MIM #256500	Autosomal recessive SPINK5	Hair shaft anomaly (trichorrhexis invaginata most common), ichthyosis linearis circumflexa, severe atopic dermatitis, failure to thrive
Refsum disease, infantile MIM #266510	Autosomal recessive PEX1, PXMP3, PEX26	Retinitis pigmentosa, cerebellar ataxia, chronic polyneuritis with deafness, skin resembles ichthyosis vulgaris
Sjögren–Larsson syndrome MIM #270200	Autosomal recessive ALDH3A2 (fatty aldehyde dehydrogenase gene)	Spastic paralysis, mental retardation, seizures, glistening dots on retina, dental bone dysplasia, similar skin findings to congenital ichthyosiform erythroderma
Conradi–Hunermann syndrome (chondrodysplasia punctata type 2) MIM #302900	X-linked dominant EBP gene	Chondrodysplasia punctata, alopecia, skeletal anomalies, cataracts, dysmorphic facies, ichthyosiform erythroderma
KID (keratitis-ichthyosis-deafness) syndrome MIM #148210	Autosomal dominant (sporadic) GJB2 encoding connexin 26	Fixed keratotic plaques, keratoderma, atypical ichthyosis with prominent keratoses on extremities and head, neurosensory deafness, keratoconjunctivitis
CHILD syndrome MIM #308050	X-linked recessive NSDHL	Congenital hemidysplasia, unilateral ichthyosiform nevus (epidermal nevus), limb defects, cardiovascular and renal anomalies

Epidermolytic Ichthyosis

Infants with epidermolytic ichthyosis (formerly known as epidermolytic hyperkeratosis or bullous congenital ichthyosiform erythroderma; Fig. 2.33) demonstrate widespread blistering at birth and may be misdiagnosed as having a primary blistering dermatosis such as staphylococcal scalded-skin syndrome or epidermolysis bullosa. During the first few weeks and months of life, blisters give way to increasing hyperkeratoses, especially in intertriginous and flexural areas.

In these ichthyotic disorders, increased insensible water loss, temperature instability, and increased risk of infection may persist for weeks. Involvement of the face may result in ectropion formation, particularly in lamellar ichthyosis, and aggressive eye care is necessary to preserve visual acuity. Decreased sweating as a result of the obstruction of eccrine ducts in the epidermal scale often interferes with effective cooling of the skin. Aggressive management of fever, air conditioning, and cooling suits reduce the risk of hyperthermia associated with self-limited childhood illnesses and increased physical activity, especially during the summer.

Ichthyosis Vulgaris and X-linked Ichthyosis

Children with ichthyosis vulgaris (Fig. 2.34) and X-linked ichthyosis (Fig. 2.35) may not develop scaling until 3 months of age or later. The generally mild scales of ichthyosis vulgaris tend to spare the flexures and improve with age. The "dirty" brown scales of X-linked ichthyosis also spare the flexures, but typically involve much of the body surface. The skin lesions do not usually impair epidermal barrier function.

Mild scaling responds well to lubricants, urea-containing preparations (Carmol, Ureacin), and α-hydroxy acids in emollients (lactic acid [LactiCare, Lac-Hydrin], glycolic acid [Aqua Glycolic, Glycolix]). Irritation associated with these agents may be reduced by special formulation in bland vehicles such as petrolatum or hydrophilic ointment. Although topical salicylic acid is a potent keratolytic, its use is contraindicated in children less

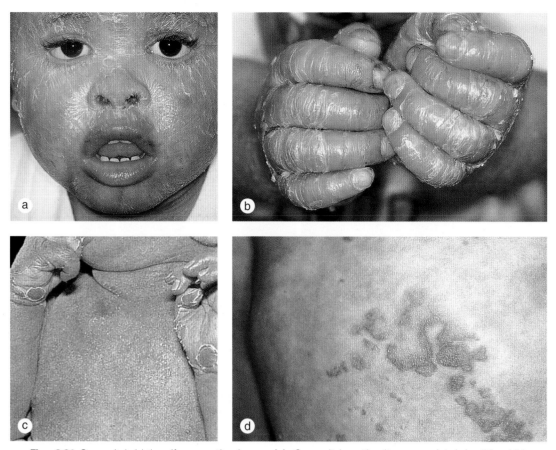

Fig. 2.31 Congenital ichthyosiform erythroderma. **(a)** Congenital erythroderma persisted in this child. **(b)** Note the marked scaling on her hands. **(c)** Generalized erythema with fine scaling was noted on the first day of life. **(d)** Shortly after his first birthday, he developed a new pattern of migrating, scaly, erythematous plaques typical of Netherton syndrome. Microscopic examination of his hair revealed trichorrhexis invaginata (bamboo hair).

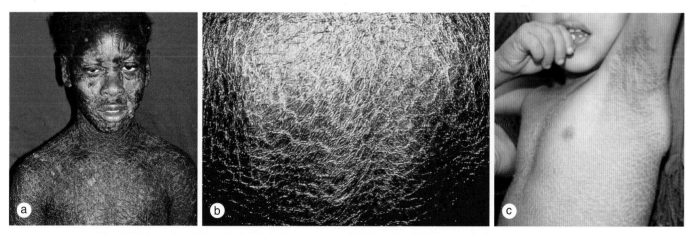

Fig. 2.32 Lamellar ichthyosis. **(a)** Typical appearance. **(b)** Note the thick, brown scales that cover the entire skin. This child was born with a collodion membrane. **(c)** Example of axillary and truncal scale in a patient with autosomal recessive congenital ichthyosis. (Courtesy Katherine B. Püttgen. Katherine B. Püttgen retains copyright of this figure.)

than 2 years of age because of the risk of transcutaneous absorption and systemic toxicity. Similarly, urea concentrations of 10% or greater should be avoided under a year of age except sparingly on palms and soles. Topical retinoids such as adapalene, tretinoin, and tazarotene can be useful on selected areas. Calcipotriol

has been shown to be useful in adults and N-acetylcysteine, a mucolytic compound, has shown benefit in small studies. The latter has a strong sulfur odor that can limit its use. Oral retinoids (isotretinoin, acitretin, etretinate) have demonstrated marked improvement of cutaneous lesions in severe ichthyosis.

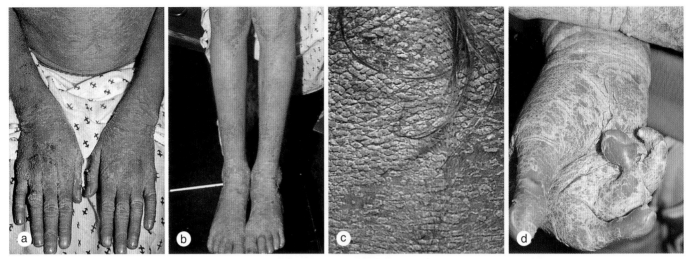

Fig. 2.33 Epidermolytic hyperkeratosis in a 6-year-old girl. **(a,b)** Generalized, thick, greasy scales accentuate the normal skin markings on the extremities. **(c)** Similar scales on the trunk and neck. Flexures were most severely involved. **(d)** This adult with epidermolytic hyperkeratosis from birth developed a severe keratoderma of the hands and feet, with constriction bands and autoamputation of several digits.

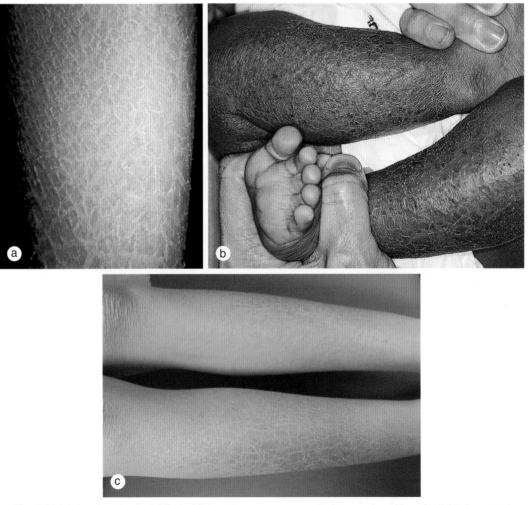

Fig. 2.34 Ichthyosis vulgaris. **(a)** Typical fish-scale appearance on the lower extremities of a light-pigmented child. **(b)** The appearance on a dark-pigmented child. Both children had at least one parent with similar findings. **(c)** Xerosis and ichthyotic scale on the bilateral lower legs. (Reprinted with permission from Bernard A. Cohen© DermAtlas, Johns Hopkins University; 2000–2012.)

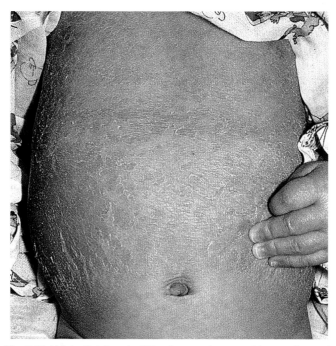

Fig. 2.35 X-linked ichthyosis: "Dirty" tan scales are evident on the trunk of this infant.

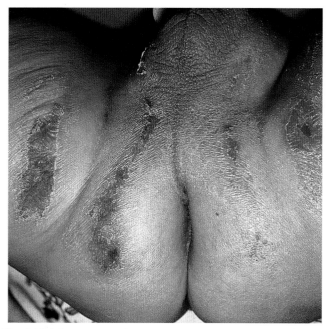

Fig. 2.36 Irritant contact dermatitis involves the convex surfaces and spares the creases in the diaper area.

However, clinical benefits must be weighed against the risk of systemic effects, particularly hepatic and skeletal toxicity, which can occur during prolonged use.

DIAPER DERMATITIS AND RELATED DISORDERS

The dermatitides are characterized by acute changes (erythema, edema, and vesiculation) and/or chronic changes (scale, lichenification, and increased or decreased pigmentation) in the skin. Microscopically, these disorders show infiltration of the dermis with inflammatory cells, variable thickening of the epidermis, and scale.

Irritant Contact Dermatitis

Diaper dermatitis is one of the most common skin disorders of infancy. In its most usual form, it is an irritant contact dermatitis (Fig. 2.36). The diaper area is a prime target for an irritant dermatitis because it is bathed in urine and feces and occluded by diapers. Although ammonia from urine was first thought to play a leading role in the pathogenesis of diaper dermatitis, current evidence points to feces as the principal culprit. Once the epidermal barrier is disrupted, the skin may become sensitive to other irritants such as soap, powder, and detergents. Watery stools, particularly after antibiotic exposure or viral infections, often trigger severe dermatitis that is recalcitrant to conservative measures.

Red, scaly, and occasionally erosive irritant reactions are usually confined to convex surfaces of the perineum, lower abdomen, buttocks, and proximal thighs. The intertriginous areas are invariably spared. Gentle, thorough cleansing of the area and the application of lubricants (e.g. petrolatum) and barrier pastes (e.g. zinc oxide) usually result in clearing of the dermatitis. A tapering course of low-potency topical corticosteroid ointment (e.g. hydrocortisone or desonide) in severe dermatitis may speed resolution of symptoms and clinical findings.

Allergic Contact Dermatitis

Although less common than irritant dermatitis, allergic contact dermatitis may account for occasional diaper rashes. Fragrances, preservatives, and emulsifiers such as methylisothiazolinone, mercaptobenzothiazole, fragrance mix, disperse dye, cyclohexylthiophthalimide, p-tert-butyl-phenol-formaldehyde resin, and sorbitan sesquioleate in topical baby products and diapers may be associated with allergic reactions in the diaper area, as well as on the face, trunk, and extremities. Avoidance of the offending agent, aggressive use of emollients, and judicious use of topical corticosteroids clear these reactions within several days.

Infected Contact Dermatitis

Contact diaper dermatitis is occasionally complicated by secondary staphylococcal infection, or pustules may appear as primary lesions, especially in the first few weeks of life (Fig. 2.37). The presence of thin-walled pustules on an erythematous base should alert the clinician to the diagnosis of staphylococcal pustulosis. Typically, the lesions rupture rapidly and dry to produce a collarette of scale around a denuded red base. Gram-stain of pustule contents demonstrates Gram-positive cocci in clusters and neutrophils. Bacterial cultures are confirmatory.

Seborrheic Dermatitis

Persistent diaper dermatitis may result from other disorders, such as seborrheic dermatitis, infantile psoriasis, and candidiasis. In particular, these should be considered when the intertriginous areas are involved.

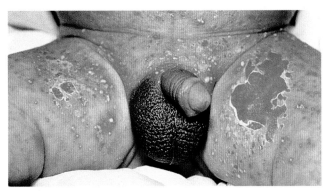

Fig. 2.37 Staphylococcal diaper dermatitis. Numerous, intact, thin-walled pustules surrounded by red halos are present, as well as multiple areas in which pustules have ruptured to leave a collarette of scaling around a denuded red base.

Seborrheic dermatitis is characterized by salmon-colored patches with greasy, yellow scale beginning in the intertriginous areas, especially the diaper area, axillae, and scalp (Fig. 2.38). Fissuring, maceration, and weeping develop occasionally. Thick, adherent scales on the occiput are referred to as "cradle cap." Although oval, red patches may spread to the trunk, proximal extremities, and postauricular areas, affected infants remain healthy and asymptomatic. In dark-pigmented children, postinflammatory hypopigmentation is marked but transient, resolving over a period of months.

In the diaper area, red, greasy, scaly patches extend from the skin creases to involve the genitals, perineum, suprapubic area, and thighs. Secondary candidiasis or impetigo may mask the underlying process.

The cause of seborrheic dermatitis is unknown. However, the yeast *Pityrosporum* has been implicated in adult seborrhea

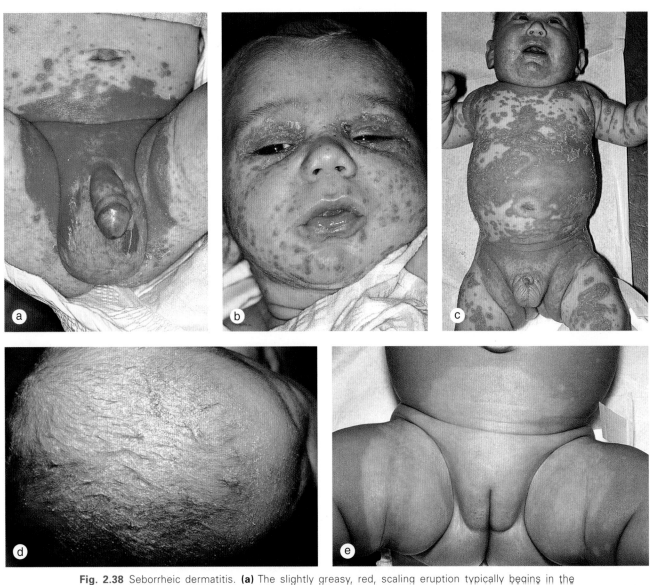

Fig. 2.38 Seborrheic dermatitis. **(a)** The slightly greasy, red, scaling eruption typically begins in the groin creases and spreads throughout the diaper area. **(b,c)** In florid cases, the dermatitis involves the trunk, face, and creases of the neck and extremities. **(d)** "Cradle cap" consists of thick, tenacious scaling of the scalp. **(e)** Postinflammatory hypopigmentation may be marked, particularly in darkly pigmented individuals.

and identified in the scalp of infants with cradle cap. This organism tends to proliferate in areas where sebaceous glands are most numerous and active, which probably explains the timing and distribution of the eruption. Seborrheic dermatitis may clear without treatment by 2–3 months of age but often persists until 8–12 months. Mild keratolytics found in antiseborrheic shampoos (zinc pyrithione, sulfur, and salicylic acid) are helpful in the management of cradle cap. Emollients and low-potency topical corticosteroids hasten the resolution of cutaneous lesions. Topical ketoconazole has been approved for treating adult seborrheic dermatitis and may be useful in infants, particularly in patients with associated candidiasis.

Psoriasis

Psoriasis occasionally begins as a persistent diaper dermatitis (Fig. 2.39), and there may be considerable clinical overlap with seborrheic dermatitis. Although lesions may disseminate to the trunk and extremities, the rash may continue in the diaper area alone for months. The eruption is typically bright red, scaly, and well-demarcated at the diaper line. Although topical corticosteroids result in temporary improvement, lesions tend to persist or recur for months, and occasionally short-term use of mid- to high-potency topical corticosteroids is necessary. The topical calcineurin inhibitors approved for atopic dermatitis, pimecrolimus (Elidel) and tacrolimus (Protopic), are helpful in treating psoriasis at sensitive sites such as the diaper area. Infants remain well, and the eruption may be asymptomatic. Skin biopsy is the only way to confirm the diagnosis, though clinical impression guides management of most cases.

Candidiasis

Candidiasis appears as a brilliant red eruption with sharp borders, satellite red papules, and pustules (Fig. 2.40). Lesions typically involve the skin creases. *Candida* is a common complication of systemic antibiotic therapy, seborrheic dermatitis, psoriasis, and chronic irritant dermatitis. Examination of material from a pustule by Gram-stain or potassium hydroxide preparation reveals pseudohyphae and/or budding yeast. Diaper candidiasis may be accompanied by oral thrush, candidal paronychia of the fingers or toes, and candidiasis of other intertriginous areas such as the neck and axillae. Diaper candidiasis responds rapidly to topical antifungals such as nystatin, ciclopirox olamine, and the imidazoles (miconazole, clotrimazole, econazole, sulconazole, ketoconazole). Although a brief course of topical corticosteroids (1–2 times a day for 3–4 days) may speed clinical improvement, high-potency agents can produce atrophy in a short period of time. Several products that incorporate a combination of moderate- to high-potency topical corticosteroids and antifungal agents are available and should be avoided.

Langerhans Cell Histiocytosis

Severe multisystem disease may begin with a progressive diaper dermatitis. A severe seborrheic dermatitis-like eruption is characteristic of Langerhans cell histiocytosis (LCH) (Fig. 2.41). The rash tends to become hemorrhagic and erosive, particularly in the diaper area. Scaly, crusted, purpuric plaques also develop on the scalp, trunk, and extremities. LCH is rare, with an incidence

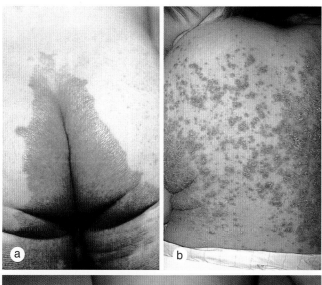

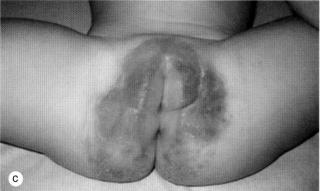

Fig. 2.39 Psoriasis. This diaper dermatitis failed to respond to routine topical therapy. **(a)** A skin biopsy demonstrated histologic changes of psoriasis. **(b)** In some infants with psoriasis, thick, disseminated plaques appear. **(c)** Confluent, beefy red and pink plaques in the diaper area consistent with psoriasis; the eruption required short courses of mid- to high-potency topical steroids to control it. (Courtesy Katherine B. Püttgen. Katherine B. Püttgen retains copyright of this figure.)

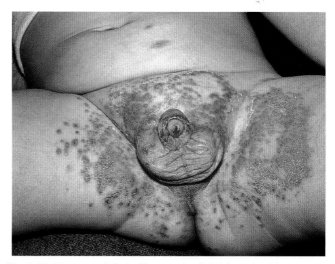

Fig. 2.40 Diaper candidiasis. The eruption is bright red, with numerous pinpoint satellite papules and pustules. The urethra and intertriginous areas are prominently involved.

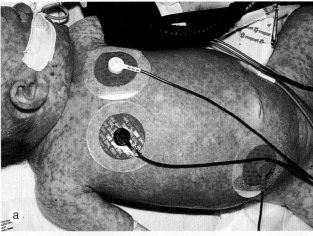

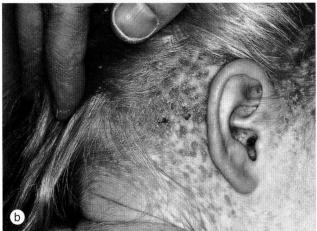

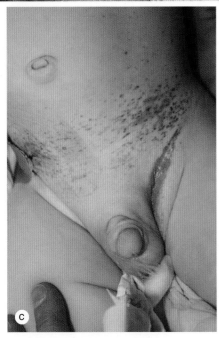

Fig. 2.41 Langerhans cell histiocytosis (LCH). **(a)** A hemorrhagic diaper dermatitis rapidly generalized to the entire skin surface in this 2-week-old infant with diarrhea, poor weight gain, lymphadenopathy, and hepatosplenomegaly. This child died of disseminated LCH at 6 weeks of age. **(b)** This toddler with chronic LCH had an episodic, erosive diaper dermatitis associated with papules and plaques in the scalp. **(c)** This young child had petechial papules and diaper dermatitis classic for LCH. (Courtesy Katherine B. Püttgen. Katherine B. Püttgen retains copyright of this figure.)

of 2–9 cases/million children under the age of 18, although the majority of affected children are 1–3 years of age at diagnosis. Diagnostic skin biopsies demonstrate infiltrates of atypical S100 protein OKT6-positive histiocytes containing Langerhans cell (Birbeck) granules. Similar infiltrates may involve the bone marrow, liver, lungs, kidneys, and nervous system, resulting in severe organ dysfunction and death. LCH is classified according to the extent of organ involvement (single organ vs. multiple organ) and by the presence of high-risk organ involvement (liver, spleen, bone marrow). Up to 50% of infants presenting with skin disease will go on to develop internal organ involvement. Infants suspected of having LCH require a thorough work-up including full physical examination, skin biopsy, laboratory work-up including complete blood count, complete metabolic panel including liver function tests, serum osmolality, urine osmolality, and initial imaging to include chest x-ray and skeletal survey. Early involvement of hematology/oncology and close follow-up is mandatory.

Benign Cephalic Histiocytosis

A non-LCH, benign cephalic histiocytosis is characterized by scattered yellow-brown papules and macules concentrated on face, scalp, neck, and upper trunk that appear in the first 2 years of life, though typically after birth. No systemic involvement occurs. It has been proposed that benign cephalic histiocytosis (BCH) may be a variant of micronodular juvenile xanthogranulomas with early onset. BCH lacks markers typical for LCH, such as S100 and Birbeck granules. No treatment is necessary as lesions regress over the first few years of life, though there can be scar tissue left behind in some cases (Fig. 2.42).

Acrodermatitis Enteropathica

Acrodermatitis enteropathica (AE) classically presents with an erosive diaper dermatitis, diarrhea, and hair loss during the first few months of life (Fig. 2.43). Weeping, crusted, erythematous patches also appear in a periorificial, acral, and intertriginous distribution. Affected infants are irritable, grow poorly, and are prone to infection and septicemia.

Because AE is an autosomal-recessive disorder of zinc metabolism, affected infants have either defective or low levels of a zinc-binding protein in the gastrointestinal tract and resultant zinc malabsorption. Breast milk contains a compensatory zinc-binding ligand that facilitates absorption. Consequently, breast-fed infants do not develop symptoms until nursing is discontinued. Zinc is stored in the fetal liver, particularly during the last month of gestation. As a result, affected premature infants who are not breastfed become zinc deficient quickly. Normal infants who require hyperalimentation, as well as those with zinc losses from other malabsorption states (e.g. cystic fibrosis, chronic infectious diarrhea, short bowel syndrome), also develop an AE-like rash if they do not receive zinc supplementation. Rare cases of zinc-deficient breast milk resulting in a zinc-deficiency eruption have been reported. Similar rashes have also been described with biotin deficiency, essential fatty acid deficiency, methylmalonic acidemia, propionic acidemia, type 1 glutaric aciduria, ornithine transcarbamylase deficiency, citrullinemia, maple syrup urine disease, and Hartnup disease.

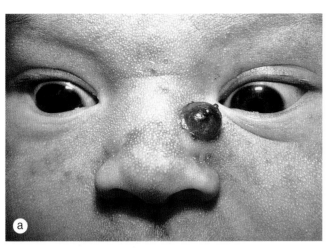
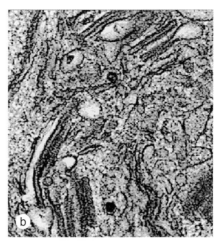

Fig. 2.42 Benign cephalic histiocytosis. **(a)** This healthy newborn with multiple congenital crusted papules was initially treated for herpes simplex infection. When the lesions did not respond to parenteral acyclovir, a skin biopsy that showed the typical changes of LCH on routine pathology and **(b)** electron microscopy was performed. Note the tennis racket–shaped Birbeck granules diagnostic of LCH. The lesions resolved without treatment within 2 weeks.

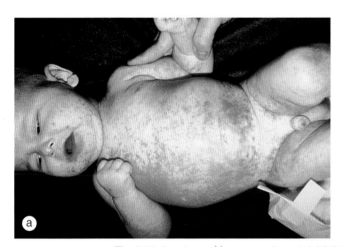
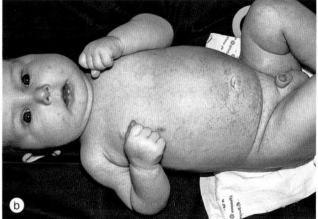

Fig. 2.43 Acrodermatitis enteropathica. **(a)** A bright red, scaling dermatitis spread to the intertriginous areas, face, and extremities of this 4-week-old infant. **(b)** After 4 days of zinc supplementation, many lesions were healing with desquamation.

AE responds dramatically to high doses of oral or intravenous zinc within several days. Although dietary zinc without supplementation may be adequate in older children with AE, these patients require close monitoring of growth and development. Some patients require lifelong zinc supplements.

CONGENITAL SYPHILIS

Although the incidence of neonatal syphilis decreased in the 1970s and 1980s, a resurgence has occurred, particularly in urban centers. Infants born to mothers who contract syphilis late in pregnancy are at high risk for contracting the disease. In the United States, rates of congenital syphilis decreased between 1991 and 2005, then showed slight increases from 2005 to 2008. Congenital syphilis rates decreased between 2008 and 2012 but then increased from 8.4 to 11.6 cases per 100 000 live births in 2014—the highest rate since 2001. Mothers with early syphilis have the highest risk of passing congenital infection to their offspring. Rates of transmission range from 40% to 70% across all trimesters of pregnancy, decreasing to about 10% in late-stage syphilis.

Although clinical manifestations of syphilis may be delayed until puberty (known as late congenital syphilis), common findings in early congenital syphilis, which encompasses disease diagnosed in children < 2 years of age, include mucocutaneous lesions, prematurity, anemia, poor growth, and hepatosplenomegaly. Occasionally, severe systemic disease presents with generalized lymphadenopathy, pneumonitis, nephritis, enteritis, pancreatitis, osteochondritis, hematologic abnormalities, and meningitis. The bones, teeth, and central nervous system are the most common sites of extracutaneous involvement.

Mucocutaneous lesions usually appear between 2 and 6 weeks of age. The most common finding in the skin is a papulosquamous eruption beginning on the palms and soles

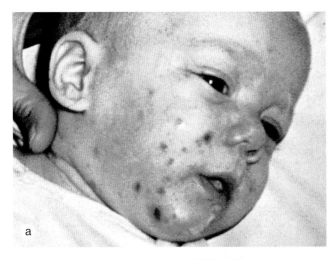

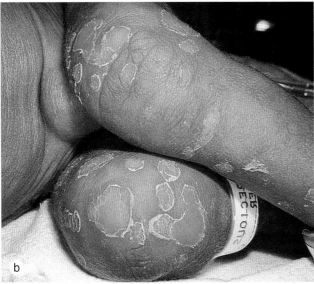

Fig. 2.44 Neonatal syphilis. **(a,b)** A scaly eruption reminiscent of the lesions of secondary syphilis appeared on the face, trunk, and extremities of these infants.

and spreading over the extremities, face, and trunk (Fig. 2.44). These lesions are comparable with the secondary syphilitic eruption of adults and may be associated with vesiculation, ulceration, and desquamation. Moist, warty excrescences may develop in the intertriginous and periorificial areas. Smooth, round, moist mucous patches are characteristic of early neonatal syphilis and commonly involve the mouth and perianal area. Such lesions are highly infectious. "Snuffles" or rhinitis with profuse and occasionally bloody rhinorrhea is invariably present in symptomatic babies.

Diagnosis may be confirmed by darkfield examination (though darkfield microscopy has limited availability now) of mucocutaneous lesions and serologic studies of the serum and cerebrospinal fluid. Screening of babies at risk for syphilis should include both specific *Treponema* (fluorescent treponemal antibody absorption tests) and nontreponemal (rapid plasma reagin or Venereal Disease Research Laboratory) studies. The most sensitive serologic method is detection of specific IgM, though a negative test does not exclude possible infection.

IgM can be detected in newborns using either 19S FTA-ABS tests, IgM immunoblots, or IgM enzyme-linked immunosorbent assays (ELISAs). Early diagnosis and treatment with high-dose penicillin prevents late complications of syphilis, including skeletal and dental anomalies, neurologic deterioration, eighth nerve deafness, and ophthalmologic disease.

VESICULOPUSTULAR DERMATOSES

Vesiculobullous and pustular eruptions may present a confusing clinical picture. Their diagnosis is critical, and early therapeutic intervention may be life-saving.

Infections and Infestations

Viral infections, including herpes simplex and varicella-zoster, produce characteristic vesiculopustular eruptions. Herpes simplex is a common cause of self-limited oral and cutaneous lesions in toddlers and older children. However, in neonates, there is a high risk of dissemination. Varicella is less common, but if lesions appear during the first week of life, the risk of mortality approaches 30%.

Neonatal Herpes Simplex Infection

The incidence of neonatal herpes simplex infection in a large Medicaid population is approximately 4.6 per 10 000 (or greater than 1 in 2200) deliveries. Inoculation occurs from ascending infection *in utero* (5% of cases) or from lesions on the cervix or vaginal area during delivery (85% of cases). However, the disease may be acquired postnatally from nursery personnel and family members (10% of cases). The incubation period varies from 2 to 21 days and peaks at 6 days. Consequently, infants may appear normal in the nursery and develop lesions after discharge home. Manifestations vary from subclinical disease to widely disseminated infection and death. Treatment delays of as short as 1 day are associated with a doubled risk of mortality. Of infected babies, 70% develop the skin rash, which can be quite subtle on presentation. The risk of transmission to an infant born during new maternal genital herpes simplex virus (HSV) infection is between 25% and 50%, compared with a rate of transmission of less than 1% if recurrent genital HSV is active during vaginal delivery. New maternal genital HSV infection accounts for 50–80% of neonatal HSV. The majority of mothers are asymptomatic at delivery. HSV has a higher incidence of transmission than syphilis, toxoplasmosis, and rubella.

Cutaneous lesions typically begin as 1–2 mm-diameter, clustered, red papules and vesicles, which may become pustular, denuded, crusted, and hemorrhagic over the following 2–3 days (Fig. 2.45). The first lesions commonly develop on the face and scalp in head deliveries and on the feet or buttocks after breech presentation.

Neonatal HSV can occur as skin, eyes, and mouth (SEM) disease, which accounts for 45% of neonatal HSV; central nervous system (CNS) disease, which accounts for 30% of neonatal HSV; or disseminated disease, which accounts for 25% of neonatal HSV. It is important to note that overlap does exist between these subtypes, and infants who present with skin disease only are at risk for dissemination to the CNS or other organs at any time during the acute infection. Infants with CNS and disseminated disease have a predictably worse outcome.

Blisters reveal multinucleated giant cells when their contents are prepared on a glass slide with Giemsa or Wright stain. Viral cultures from blister fluid or denuded areas of skin often demonstrate

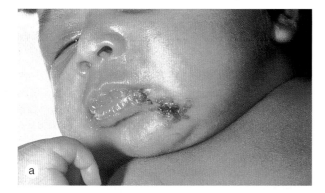

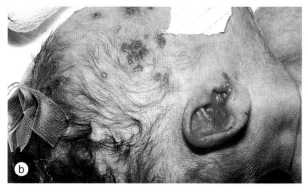

Fig. 2.45 Herpes simplex. **(a)** The eroded vesicles at the corner of the mouth were the first signs of herpes infection in this neonate. **(b)** An infant with respiratory distress and hepatitis developed herpetic vesicles on the face, scalp, and ear

a cytopathic effect within 12–24 hours. Diagnosis can be rapidly confirmed by double fluorescent antibody (DFA) or polymerase chain reaction (PCR) studies in some medical centers. Early intervention with parenteral acyclovir may decrease the risk of disseminated disease and of morbidity and mortality when dissemination has already occurred. Skin lesions are gently cleansed and excess blister fluid absorbed with a gauze pad to reduce cutaneous spread. Skin lesions may recur throughout childhood; recurrence prompts a trial of oral acyclovir, particularly when recurrences are frequent and skin lesions frighten caretakers at home or in a day care. Evidence suggests that a 6-month course of oral acyclovir after the acute infection may improve neurodevelopment scores in infants at 12 months of age.

Congenital Varicella Syndrome

Early exposure during the first 20 weeks' gestation—with highest risk (2%) between weeks 13 and 20—leads rarely to the development of the neonatal varicella syndrome, with linear scars, limb anomalies, ocular defects, and CNS involvement (Fig. 2.46).

Neonatal Varicella

When a mother has varicella within 3 weeks of delivery, her baby has a 25% risk of acquiring the disease during the neonatal period.

When neonates develop the rash before 5 days of life or mothers develop lesions at least 5 days before delivery, the disease in neonates tends to be mild because of the presence of protective transplacental antibody. Infection acquired by the mother <5 days before delivery to 2 days after delivery, or lesions that develop in the newborn between days 5 and 10 of life, tend to have more severe infection and are at risk for dissemination with resulting pneumonitis, encephalitis, purpura fulminans, widespread bleeding, hypotension, and death.

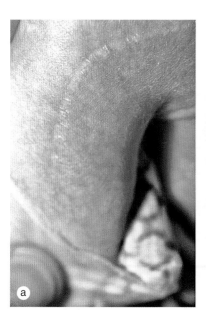

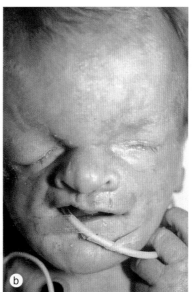

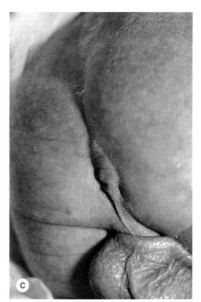

Fig. 2.46 Varicella. **(a)** A linear scar was evident on the arm of this newborn whose mother developed chickenpox during the first trimester. **(b,c)** This child also had multiple central nervous system, ocular, genitourinary, and gastrointestinal anomalies. Note the dysmorphic facies **(b)** and imperforate anus **(c)**.

Varicella-zoster immune globulin and parenteral acyclovir may improve the outcome and should be administered early in the course. As with herpes simplex, the Tzanck smear shows multinucleated giant cells. These two viral infections can only be definitively differentiated by culture of the blister contents or by molecular studies (DFA, PCR).

Impetigo and Staphylococcal Scalded-Skin Syndrome

Several common bacterial infections present with vesiculopustular eruptions in infancy. The rash tends to be localized in impetigo (see Fig. 4.12) and generalized in staphylococcal scalded-skin syndrome (SSSS) (Fig. 2.47; see also Fig. 4.13).

In classic streptococcal impetigo, honey-colored crusts overlie infected insect bites, abrasions, and other skin rashes, such as diaper dermatitis. Bullous impetigo, however, is characterized by slowly enlarging, blistering rings that surround central, umbilicated crusts. Lesions may appear anywhere on the skin surface. However, in young infants, areas prone to trauma, such as the diaper area, circumcision wound, and umbilical stump, are frequent sites of primary infection. Bullous lesions are caused by epidermal toxin-producing types of *Staphylococcus,* which produce exfoliative toxin A and exfoliative toxin B. Although lesions may remain localized, they are highly infectious and may be inoculated to multiple sites on the patient, as well as on other family members. In newborns and young infants, dissemination of the toxin may result in widespread erythema and blistering typical of SSSS (Fig. 2.47). Gentle pressure on the skin causes the upper epidermis to slide off, leaving a denuded base (Nikolsky sign).

In localized impetigo, bacteria are identified in Gram-stained material obtained directly from the rash. In SSSS, the practitioner may be unable to identify a primary cutaneous site of infection. In these children, noncutaneous sources, which include lungs, bone, meninges, conjunctivae, and ears, must be sought.

Small patches of impetigo respond well to topical antibiotic therapy (e.g. mupirocin, bacitracin, bacitracin-polymyxin B) and tepid tap water compresses. Healthy infants with recalcitrant or widespread impetigo require oral antibiotics with broad-spectrum Gram-positive coverage (dicloxacillin, cephalexin and other cephalosporins, cotrimoxazole, amoxicillin-clavulanate). Neonates and young infants may not localize infection to the epidermis and superficial dermis. Any signs of progressive cellulitis or visceral dissemination require immediate hospitalization, parenteral anti-staphylococcal antibiotics, and supportive care. When infants develop infection in the first 2–3 weeks of life, even after discharge from the hospital, a nursery source should be suspected. Breeches in nursery hygiene and skin colonization of personnel must be investigated.

Disseminated Candidiasis

Disseminated candidiasis in the newborn may be confused with bacterial infection. In congenital candidiasis, which develops during the first day of life, generalized erythematous papules, vesicles, and pustules may slough to leave large, denuded areas reminiscent of SSSS. The organism is acquired by ascending vaginal or cervical infection. The presence of oral thrush in some infants at birth and the identification of pseudohyphae and spores from pustules and scale are diagnostic. When infants acquire infection at delivery, the onset of lesions may be delayed by 7–10 days and erosive patches with satellite pustules are usually limited to intertriginous areas. Full-term infants often go on to heal with desquamation without treatment, although topical antifungals may help. Preterm infants are at high risk for dissemination, and early diagnosis and initiation of parenteral amphotericin may be life-saving. As increasing numbers of tiny premature infants survive the first few weeks of life and undergo long-term systemic antibiotic therapy, infection with other opportunistic fungal organisms should be considered (Fig. 2.48).

Scabies

Scabies is a common, well-characterized infectious dermatosis produced by the *Sarcoptes scabiei* mite. The impregnated female burrows through the outer epidermis, where she deposits her eggs. The resultant diagnostic rash consists of pruritic, linear burrows on the finger webs, wrists, elbows, belt-line, areola, scrotum, and penis. In infants, burrows are widespread with

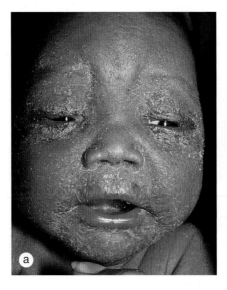
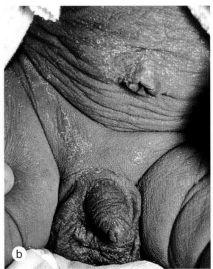

Fig. 2.47 Staphylococcal scalded-skin syndrome developed in this neonate who was being treated for mastitis. Erosive patches were most marked on the **(a)** face and **(b)** diaper areas.

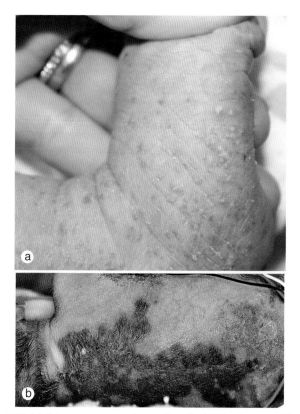

Fig. 2.48 (a) Primary cutaneous *Aspergillus* infection developed in this tiny premature infant who had extensive skin breakdown and was receiving parenteral antibiotics for pneumonia. The black eschars were loaded with hyphae. **(b)** This full-term neonate developed a diffuse, fine, red papular eruption evolving into pustules which showed budding yeast on KOH preparation and grew *Candida albicans* on culture.

involvement of the trunk, scalp, and extremities, including the palms and soles (Fig. 2.49). Although infants may be otherwise healthy and well grown, chronic infestation may result in poor feeding, fussiness, and failure to thrive. Chronic and recurrent infection, with pustules, crusting, and cellulitis, is a frequent complication.

The diagnosis is considered for any infant with a widespread dermatosis that involves the palms and soles, particularly if other family members are involved. The presence of burrows is pathognomonic, and an ectoparasite preparation is confirmatory. A drop of mineral oil is applied to a burrow, and the skin surface is stretched between the examiner's thumb and index finger. A #15 blade is used to scrape vigorously until the burrow is no longer palpable. This may leave a small bleeding point at the center of the burrow. The material is subsequently spread with the blade on a glass slide and pressed under a coverslip. The female mite, eggs, and fecal material are readily visualized under a scanning 10× lens (see Fig. 1.7).

Permethrin 5% cream is first-line therapy for scabies and may be used safely in children as young as 2 months. Alternative agents are either ineffective (crotamiton, benzyl benzoate), potentially toxic (lindane, sulfur ointment, benzyl benzoate), or cosmetically unacceptable (sulfur ointment).

At the start of therapy, parents are given careful instructions and limited quantities of the scabicide. The entire family and any others who have contact with the infant (e.g. babysitters) are treated simultaneously. Topical lubricants are necessary for several weeks after treatment to counteract drying and irritation produced by the scabicide and to resolve cutaneous lesions. Persistent pruritic nodules may arise from some burrows, par-

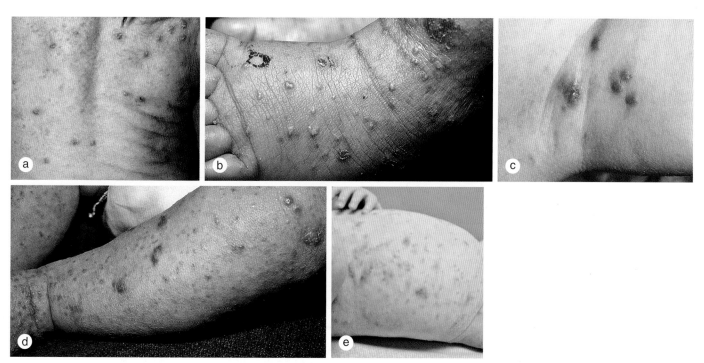

Fig. 2.49 Infants with widespread scabies. Burrows were present on **(a)** the trunk and **(b)** the feet. Nodules persisted on **(c)** the axillae and **(d)** the legs of these infants for 4 months. **(e)** This 10-week-old infant had been treated twice for scabies but continued to show evidence of burrows and papules until the entire family was treated. (Courtesy Katherine B. Püttgen. Katherine B. Püttgen retains copyright of this figure.)

ticularly in intertriginous areas. Nodular scabies requires symptomatic treatment only. The appearance of new inflammatory lesions suggests reinfestation or inadequate therapy. Secondary infection responds to tap water compresses and topical or oral antibiotics.

Some investigators advocated the use of oral ivermectin for the treatment of scabies at a dose of 200 μg/kg, but it is not recommended for children under 5 years of age or <15 kg because of lack of safety data. In older children, its efficacy is probably comparable with permethrin, and it may be particularly useful in patients with acquired immunodeficiency syndrome or crusted scabies.

Epidermolysis Bullosa

Epidermolysis bullosa (EB) comprises a heterogeneous group of blistering dermatoses characterized by the development of lesions after trauma to the skin. Variants of EB are differentiated by their inheritance pattern, specific genetic mutations, clinical presentation, histopathology, and biochemical markers (Table 2.4). Although blisters may appear at birth or in the neonatal period, in

TABLE 2.4 Selected Hereditary Mechanobullous Disorders

Type	Variant	Site of Blister	Inheritance	Molecular Defect	Onset	Clinical Features
Epidermolysis bullosa simplex (EBS)	EBS, localized	Basal layer for all EBS subtypes discussed here	Autosomal dominant	K5 (keratin 5), K14 (keratin 14)	Early childhood	Nonscarring blisters on hands and feet; hyperhidrosis
	EBS, Dowling–Meara		Autosomal dominant	K5 (keratin 5), K14 (keratin 14)	Birth	Grouped blisters, generalized denudation; nail dystrophy, milia, scarring may occur; keratoderma; improvement in adulthood
	EBS, other generalized		Autosomal dominant	K5 (keratin 5), K14 (keratin 14)	Birth	Nonscarring generalized blisters, worse on hands and feet
	EBS, muscular dystrophy		Autosomal recessive	PLEC1 (Plectin)	Birth (blisters); Muscular dystrophy (infant to adult)	Generalized blistering; muscular dystrophy; stenosis and granulation tissue in respiratory tract
	EBS, pyloric atresia		Possibly autosomal recessive	PLEC1 (Plectin), ITGA6, ITGB4 (α6β4-integrin)	Birth	Generalized blisters, aplasia cutis, pyloric atresia, deformities of pinnae and nasal alae, cryptorchidism
Junctional epidermolysis bullosa (JEB)	JEB–Herlitz	Lamina lucida for all JEB variants	Autosomal recessive for JEB all variants	LAMA3, LAMB3, LAMC2 (laminin-332)	Birth for all variants	Often lethal by 2 years; nonscarring widespread blisters; ≠ granulation tissue; nail dystrophy, loss; severe oral-dental involvement
	JEB–non-Herlitz			LAMA3, LAMB3, LAMC2 (laminin-332)		Localized blistering of hands, feet; nail dystrophy; enamel dysplasia
	JEB–pyloric atresia			ITGA6, ITGB4 (α6β4-integrin)		Generalized blisters, widespread aplasia cutis possible, genitourinary malformations, pyloric atresia
Dystrophic epidermolysis bullosa (DEB)	DDEB, generalized	Sublamina densa for all DEB variants	Autosomal dominant	COL7A1 (type VII collagen) for DEB all variants	Birth for all DEB variants	Albopapuloid skin lesions in some; mild esophageal, oral involvement; normal lifespan
	RDEB, severe generalized					Marked skin fragility; widespread blisters, atrophy, scarring; nail dystrophy, loss; risk of squamous cell carcinoma; severe oral, dental, esophageal, intestinal, genitourinary involvement
	RDEB, generalized other					Mild widespread lesions; mild oral involvement; normal life span

mild, localized forms, the onset of lesions is often delayed until later childhood or adult life.

Categorization of EB is into four major types: EB simplex, junctional EB, dystrophic EB, and Kindler syndrome. In EB simplex, blisters are intraepidermal, and the clinical course is usually mild (Fig. 2.50). In junctional EB, blisters form at the dermal–epidermal junction, usually through the lamina lucida in the basement membrane zone. Although patients may have mild disease comparable with EB simplex, in some children, progressive blistering with involvement of the mucous membranes and gastrointestinal tract leads to inanition, sepsis, and death in the first 2 years of life (Fig. 2.51). Dystrophic EB is characterized by scarring blisters that form in the dermis beneath the basement membrane zone. Blisters may be localized to the hands and feet or widespread, with involvement of the dentition, nails, airway, and esophagus (Fig. 2.52).

When infection has been excluded, EB should be considered in infants with recurrent blistering. Family history and examination of other family members aids in clinical diagnosis. A skin biopsy of an induced blister for immunofluorescent epitope mapping and/or electron microscopy provides precise identification of the cleavage plane in the skin (Fig. 2.53). Genetic counseling and prenatal diagnosis, particularly in severe variants, should be discussed with the family. Prenatal diagnosis is possible in some variants, using gene markers on amniocytes or electron microscopy on fetal skin biopsies.

In children with no family history of EB, it may be difficult to determine a prognosis in the newborn period. Infants with dystrophic EB may do very well, and children with junctional disease may develop a downhill course after a period of stabilization. In this setting, the practitioner should be reassuring and postpone discussion of prognosis until after a period of observation.

Treatment is dependent on the severity of EB. In mild variants, patients learn to avoid trauma that triggers bullae formation. Pain and progression of large blisters may be controlled by gently unroofing lesions or cutting a square skin window and covering with a topical antibiotic ointment and sterile gauze. Adhesives are applied from dressing to dressing and kept out of direct contact with the skin.

In severely affected children, the physician must orchestrate a multidisciplinary approach to management. The pediatrician, dermatologist, ophthalmologist, gastroenterologist, otolaryngologist, plastic surgeon, thoracic surgeon, dentist, and physical therapist may be involved in care. Preventive care includes avoidance of trauma to the skin and mucous membranes and early treatment of infection with topical and oral antibiotics. Iron may be required to replace chronic blood losses through the skin. Adaptic, Mepilex, Vaseline gauze, and Telfa dressings help retain moisture, reduce pain, and facilitate healing of erosions and ulcers. Topical dressings are gently held in place by clean wraps, such as gauze or Kling, and soaked off without tearing at fresh granulation tissue. Semipermeable dressings (N-Terface, Ensure, Vigilon, Mepilex, Mepitel) and occlusive dressings (DuoDERM, Comfeel) may be useful in the treatment of recalcitrant wounds. Good nutrition is mandatory for cutaneous healing and normal growth and development.

Aplasia Cutis Congenita

Aplasia cutis congenita is a heterogeneous group of disorders, the common feature of which is congenital absence of the skin.

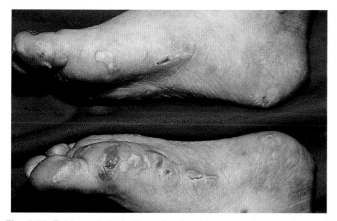

Fig. 2.50 Epidermolysis bullosa simplex. Numerous blisters form primarily in pressure areas on the hands and feet.

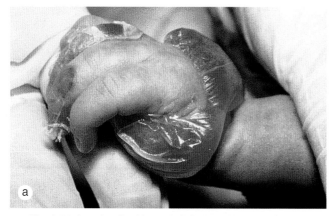
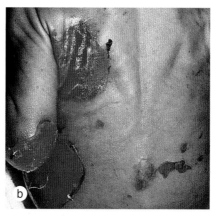

Fig. 2.51 Junctional epidermolysis bullosa. Widespread involvement was seen in this infant at birth. **(a)** Note the erosions and the large, intact blister over the thumb and dorsum of the hand. **(b)** Large, denuded areas occur over the back and buttocks.

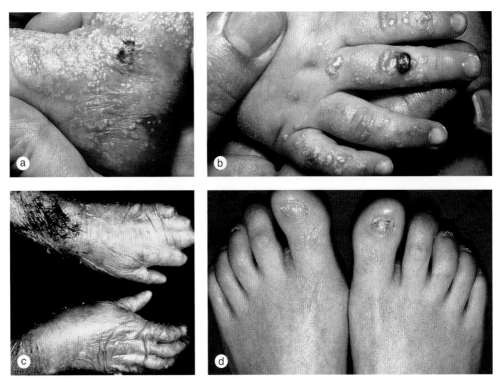

Fig. 2.52 Dystrophic epidermolysis bullosa. **(a)** Blisters, erosions, and hundreds of milia are seen on the foot and ankle and **(b)** hand of this newborn. **(c)** In this child, severe scarring encased the fingers, resulting in syndactyly. **(d)** Recurrent blistering resulted in scarring and permanent nail loss in this adolescent.

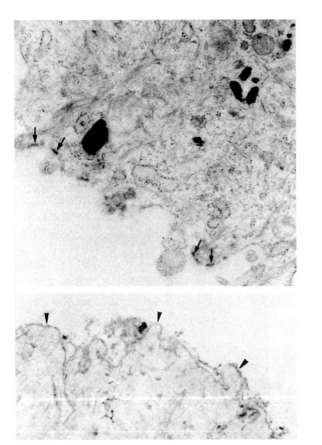

Fig. 2.53 Electron microscopic examination of a skin biopsy from a newborn with junctional epidermolysis bullosa revealed hypoplastic hemidesmosomes (*top, arrows*) in the basal keratinocyte and lamina densa (*bottom, arrowheads*) on the dermal side as a result of separation within the lamina lucida.

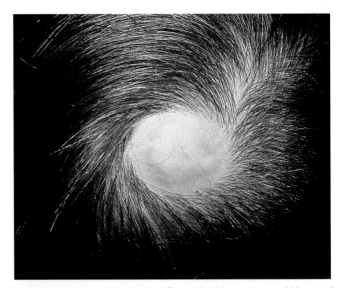

Fig. 2.54 Aplasia cutis congenita. This child, his mother, and his grandfather had similar hairless, atrophic plaques on the occiput. A thin, hemorrhagic membrane was noted at birth.

Although the cause is unknown, this entity has been recognized for over 250 years. In the classic form, one or several erosions or ulcerations covered with a crust or thin membrane involve the vertex of the scalp (Fig. 2.54). Healing with atrophic, hairless scars occurs over 2–6 months, depending on the size and depth of the ulceration (which may extend through the soft tissue into bone). This benign variant may be inherited as an autosomal-dominant trait or occur sporadically. Less commonly, the trunk

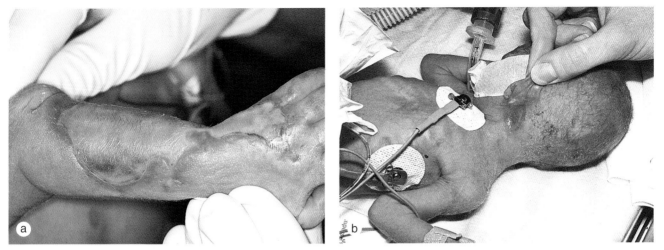

Fig. 2.55 Aplasia cutis congenita. **(a)** An isolated cutaneous defect was evident on the arm of this newborn. **(b)** This premature infant with a small defect on the back of the neck had hemiatrophy of the right side of the body (Adams–Oliver syndrome).

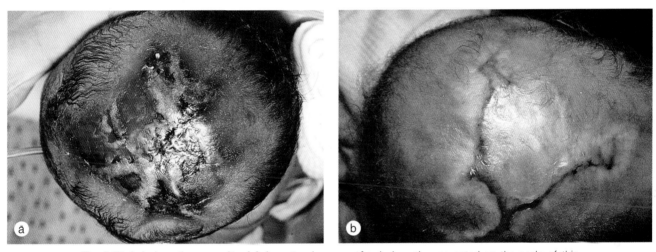

Fig. 2.56 Aplasia cutis congenita. **(a)** An extensive area of aplasia cutis was noted on the scalp of this newborn. **(b)** After 5 months, the scalp was almost completely healed. When the child was 5 years old, the residual scar was repaired after tissue expansion.

and extremities are involved, and lesions may be associated with limb defects, EB, and chromosomal aberrations (Fig. 2.55). Lesions occurring on the scalp with a ring of surrounding long, dark hairs, known as the hair collar sign, are a forme fruste of a neural tube defect (Fig. 2.59). MRI is warranted to evaluate for connection to the underlying brain and bone.

In uncomplicated aplasia cutis congenita, the defect is amenable to simple excision during later childhood or adult life. Large lesions may require staged excision and the use of tissue expanders (Fig. 2.56). In the newborn, care must be taken to evaluate the depth of the defect, prevent further tissue damage and infection, and search for associated anomalies. Gentle normal saline compresses, topical antibiotics, and sterile dressings are adequate for most patients. Large defects may respond to occlusive dressings. Occasionally, early surgical intervention is necessary.

Perinatal trauma to the scalp may result in similar defects noted at birth or within the first month of life. Scalp blood sampling, monitor electrodes, and forceps may produce small ulcers that heal with scarring (Fig. 2.57). Halo scalp ring is another form of localized scalp injury rarely associated with caput succedaneum and cephalohematoma, which occasionally resolves with a scarring alopecia (Fig. 2.58). Other nevoid malformations, which commonly present as hairless patches on the scalp, resemble aplasia cutis congenita. However, these birthmarks do not appear crusted or atrophic and usually develop distinctive clinical features (Fig. 2.59; see also Fig. 2.81 for epidermal nevi and Fig. 2.82 for sebaceous nevi). Some congenital melanocytic nevi on the scalp that are lightly pigmented can also mimic aplasia cutis congenita.

Congenital Erosive and Vesicular Dermatosis Healing With Supple Reticulated Scarring

Congenital erosive and vesicular dermatosis healing with supple reticulated scarring must be distinguished from EB and aplasia cutis congenita. Affected infants demonstrate widespread erythema, blistering, and erosions at birth involving >75% of body surface area, which heal within a few weeks to a

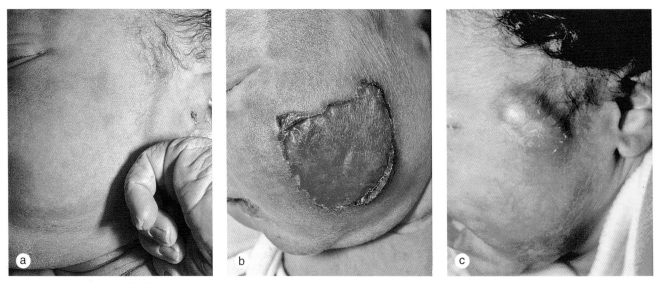

Fig. 2.57 Similar defects to aplasia cutis congenita. **(a)** Forceps injuries are most commonly associated with bruising. However, **(b)** superficial necrosis and **(c)** fat necrosis occur rarely.

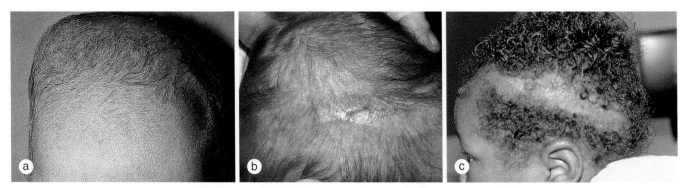

Fig. 2.58 Perinatal trauma. **(a)** Cephalohematoma, a subperiosteal bleed that usually resolves uneventfully. **(b,c)** Rarely, perinatal trauma to the scalp results in a "halo scalp ring," with scarring and permanent hair loss.

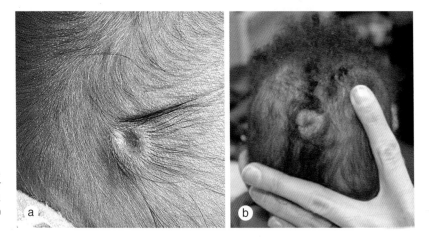

Fig. 2.59 (a) Hair collar sign on the scalp of a newborn. **(b)** This healthy 4-month-old infant presented with a hair collar sign. MRI showed no underlying abnormality. (b, Courtesy Katherine B. Püttgen. Katherine B. Püttgen retains copyright of this figure.)

few months, with widespread reticulated scars (Fig. 2.60). Nails, scalp, and the tongue and oral mucosa may be involved. The majority of children are born prematurely, and, in many cases, there is a history of maternal chorioamnionitis. Although most children grow and develop normally, abnormal neurodevelopment occurs in some cases.

Cases occur sporadically, and no inheritance pattern has been established. Extensive evaluations have excluded bacterial, fungal, and viral infections. Some infants have shown evidence of vascular insults in visceral sites and/or the placenta. However, the relationship between these findings and cutaneous lesions is unclear.

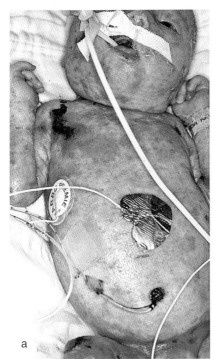

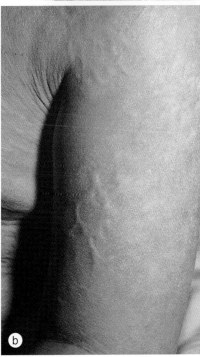

Fig. 2.60 Congenital erosive and vesicular dermatosis. **(a)** Extensive vesicles and erosions were noted on the skin of this child in the delivery room. **(b)** Erosions and crusts healed with widespread reticulated, supple scarring.

Unlike EB, new blisters do not occur except transiently in areas of old scarring. The pattern of blisters and erosions and subsequent scarring differs markedly from aplasia cutis congenita and incontinentia pigmenti.

Mastocytosis

Mastocytosis may first come to clinical attention when cutaneous lesions blister. The disorder typically presents at birth or in the first few months of life as a solitary mastocytoma or multiple lesions of urticaria pigmentosa, otherwise known as cutaneous mastocytosis (Fig. 2.61). Most patients present as sporadic cases, but rare families with multiple affected individuals have been reported. C-kit autoactivating mutations that allow for persistent mast cell development are thought to play a role in adult mastocytosis and some cases of childhood disease.

Although the trunk is most commonly involved, these benign macules, papules, and plaques that contain aggregates of mast cells may involve any cutaneous site, as well as the gastrointestinal tract, bone marrow, lungs, kidneys, and nervous system. Skin lesions range from less than 1 cm in diameter to large, infiltrated confluent plaques that cover the entire chest or back (Fig. 2.61d). Although the overlying epidermis may appear normal at birth, increasing age is associated with progressive localized hyperpigmentation and a leathery texture.

Nonspecific triggers of mast-cell degranulation, such as rubbing, hot water, vigorous physical activity, and certain medications (e.g. aspirin, anesthetic agents, radiography contrast material), may produce urtication of cutaneous lesions. Darier sign is a reliable physical finding in mastocytosis and refers to the hive that forms after stroking affected skin. If a Darier sign can be demonstrated, a skin biopsy to confirm the diagnosis is usually unnecessary. Infants are particularly prone to blister formation, and widespread blistering can be associated with fluid and electrolyte losses and increased risk of infection. Rarely, the release of histamine and other vasoactive mediators from mast cells triggers acute or chronic symptoms, including chronic diarrhea, gastric ulceration, uncontrolled pruritus, bleeding, and hypotension.

Pruritus and systemic symptoms are usually controlled with antihistamines. In infants with bullous mastocytosis and/or systemic disease, oral cromolyn sodium 20–30 mg/kg/day divided in 4 doses may be life-saving. In severe cases, topical corticosteroids under occlusion, systemic corticosteroids, or photochemotherapy (psoralen-ultraviolet A light [PUVA]) may be useful. In many children, the number of papules and plaques increases for 1–2 years. During childhood, mastocytomas usually become less reactive, and tan or brown overlying pigmentation fades slowly. Hyperpigmentation, urtication, and systemic symptoms may persist, however, in some individuals.

Incontinentia Pigmenti

Incontinentia pigmenti is a neurocutaneous syndrome named for the peculiar marble-cake swirls of brown pigment that appear on the trunk and occasionally the extremities in later infancy and early childhood. In the newborn, patches of erythema and blisters are scattered on the trunk, scalp, and extremities. Blisters are typically oriented in reticulated lines and swirls that follow the lines of Blaschko, special embryonic cleavage planes (Fig. 2.62a,b). Although inflammatory lesions may recur for months, they usually give way to hyperkeratotic, warty plaques by several weeks to several months of age (Fig. 2.62c). The hyperkeratotic stage is typically followed by increasing pigmentation at 2–6 months of age (Fig. 2.62d). During later childhood, brown streaks often fade to leave atrophic hypopigmented patches. Although these subtle scars may be the only manifestation of cutaneous disease in older

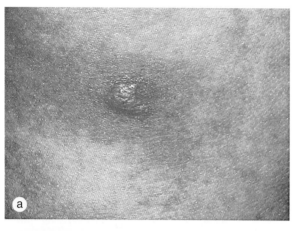

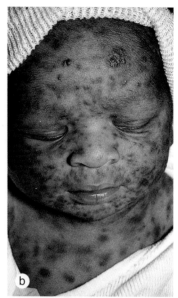

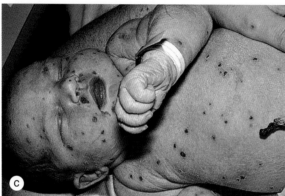

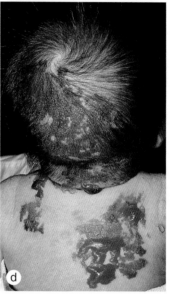

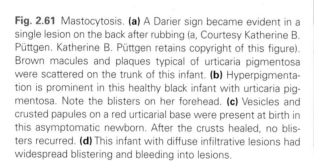

Fig. 2.61 Mastocytosis. **(a)** A Darier sign became evident in a single lesion on the back after rubbing (a, Courtesy Katherine B. Püttgen. Katherine B. Püttgen retains copyright of this figure). Brown macules and plaques typical of urticaria pigmentosa were scattered on the trunk of this infant. **(b)** Hyperpigmentation is prominent in this healthy black infant with urticaria pigmentosa. Note the blisters on her forehead. **(c)** Vesicles and crusted papules on a red urticarial base were present at birth in this asymptomatic newborn. After the crusts healed, no blisters recurred. **(d)** This infant with diffuse infiltrative lesions had widespread blistering and bleeding into lesions.

children and adults (Fig. 2.62e), missing teeth, dental malformations, and rarely nail dystrophy associated with recurrent or persistent subungual warty nodules may provide additional clues (Fig. 2.62f).

Histopathology of blisters in the newborn demonstrates characteristic intraepidermal edema and vesicles loaded with eosinophils. When incontinentia pigmenti is suspected, the child must be evaluated for associated defects, which may involve the CNS, heart, eye, skeletal system, and dentition. Incontinentia pigmenti is inherited as an X-linked dominant disorder that is lethal in males; 97% of affected infants are female. A careful examination of mothers often reveals subtle cutaneous findings. Mutations in the NEMO gene have been identified in 65% of patients tested.

NEVI/BIRTHMARKS

Nevus is a term used to describe a group of skin lesions that appear at birth or in the first months of life. Nevi are composed

of mature or nearly mature cutaneous elements organized in an abnormal fashion. These hamartomas may comprise virtually any epidermal or dermal structure.

Vascular Anomalies

For therapeutic and prognostic reasons, clinicians must distinguish between vascular malformations and infantile hemangiomas and other less common vascular tumors of infancy. This categorization of vascular birthmarks, which is now widely accepted, was first proposed by Mulliken in 1982 and modified by the International Society for the Study of Vascular Anomalies most recently in 2018. Accordingly, molecular and ultrastructural markers, histologic findings, and biological behavior help distinguish vascular malformations, which are composed of dysplastic vessels from proliferative, hyperplastic vascular tumors (Table 2.5).

Vascular malformations are further divided based on flow characteristics and the predominant type of vascular anomaly

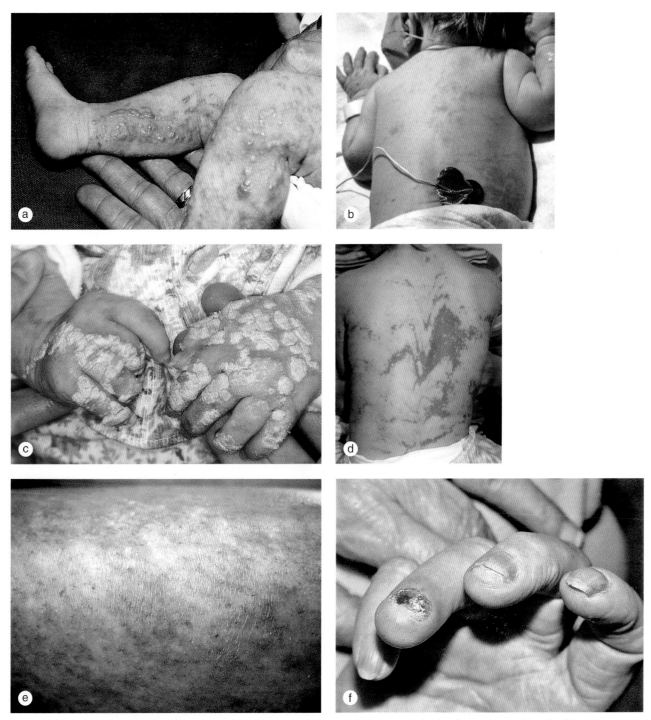

Fig. 2.62 Incontinentia pigmenti. Vesicles on an erythematous base extended in a linear pattern down the **(a)** legs and **(b)** trunk of an 8-day-old girl. **(c)** Warty papules developed on the fingers of this 4-month-old girl in the site of earlier vesicles. **(d)** Progressive "marble cake" hyperpigmentation was first noted on the trunk of this patient at 4 months of age. **(e)** Subtle scarring on the legs was the only sign of incontinentia pigmenti in the mother of the child. Note the absence of hair follicles in the linear scars. **(f)** This 60-year-old woman with incontinentia pigmenti has had recurrent warty subungual nodules and nail dystrophy since adolescence. A biopsy showed eosinophilic dermal inflammation and dyskeratosis.

into slow-flow capillary, venous, and lymphatic malformations and fast-flow arterial or arteriovenous malformations (Table 2.6). Complex malformations may include components of several different vascular structures. Although simple, uncomplicated lesions tend to be localized and well circumscribed, large segmental or widely disseminated lesions are often complex and associated with extracutaneous anomalies.

Infantile hemangiomas are the most common vascular neoplasm of infancy and occur in nearly 10% of Caucasian newborns by 12 months of age. They must be distinguished from

TABLE 2.5   Distinguishing Features of Hemangioma Versus Vascular Malformation

	Hemangioma	Vascular Malformation
Clinical features	Subtle at birth Early rapid growth Slow spontaneous regression	Usually visible at birth Proportionate growth
Sex ratio	3:1 female predominance	1:1
Pathology	Proliferative neoplasm Hyperplastic endothelial cells	Flat endothelial cells Mature vascular structures
Bone changes	Rarely mass effect	Variable distortion, thinning, invasion, rare destruction
Immunohistochemical markers	Markers of proliferative vascular tumors	Lack of expression of markers
Coagulopathy	None (usually associated with other vascular tumors, e.g. tufted angioma)	Slow-flow venous, lymphatic and combined lymphatic-venous malformations May develop coagulopathy

TABLE 2.6   Vascular Malformations

Vascular Anomaly	Flow Characteristics
Infantile hemangioma	Fast
Capillary malformation	Slow
Venous malformation	Slow
Lymphatic malformation	Slow
Arteriovenous malformation	Fast

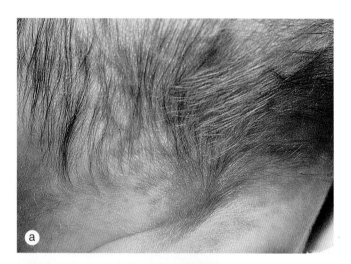

the rare kaposiform hemangioendothelioma and tufted angioma, which may be associated with the development of disseminated coagulopathy known as Kasabach–Merritt syndrome. A number of other tumors of infancy may present as bluish-purple lesions that may be confused with hemangiomas. Clinical features, course, and histopathologic findings help differentiate these lesions.

Vascular Malformations
Capillary Malformations

Salmon patches are common innocent capillary malformations which occur in 60–70% of newborns (Fig. 2.63). Lesions are usually located on the nape of the neck ("stork bite"), glabella, forehead ("angel kiss"), upper eyelids, and sacrum. Although salmon patches on the face usually fade during the first year of life and tend to be camouflaged by normal pigmentation, they may persist indefinitely when located on the neck and sacrum. The pink patches also darken with crying, breath holding, and physical exertion. These lesions are not associated with extracutaneous findings and do not usually require further evaluation.

At birth, 0.2–0.3% of newborns have port-wine stains (PWS). Unlike salmon patches, PWS represents a capillary malformation that tends to persist unchanged during childhood and to darken and thicken in adolescence and adulthood (Figs. 2.64–2.66). Progressive angiomatous papules and nodules and underlying soft tissue hypertrophy develop gradually over years (Fig. 2.66). Although unilateral lesions on the head and neck are most common, any part of the body surface and mucous membranes may be involved.

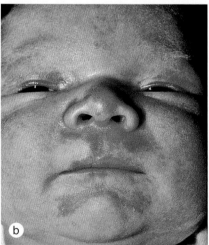

Fig. 2.63 Salmon patches. **(a)** Typical, light-red, splotchy patch at the nape of the neck in a healthy newborn. **(b)** Similar patches were present on this child's eyelids, nose, upper lip, and chin.

Occasionally, PWS provides a clue to extracutaneous defects. More than 35 named syndromes have been described in association with cutaneous vascular malformations.

Children with involvement of the forehead and upper eyelid may have a vascular malformation of the ipsilateral meninges,

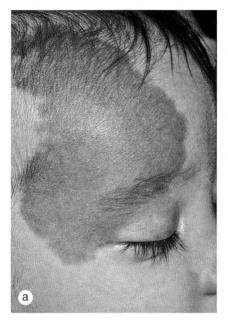
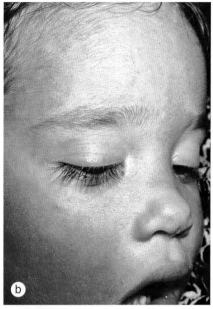

Fig. 2.64 Port-wine stains. **(a)** A port-wine stain involved the ophthalmic distribution of the trigeminal nerve on the face of this infant with Sturge–Weber syndrome. **(b)** After four treatments with the yellow pulsed-dye laser the lesion had almost completely resolved.

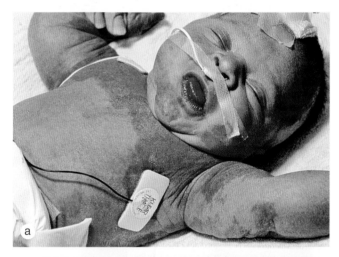

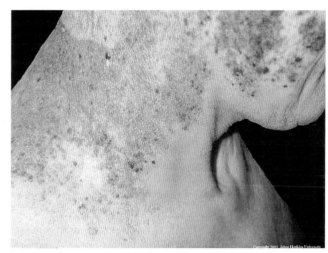

Fig. 2.66 Port-wine stain. Purple papules and nodules began to appear in this congenital port-wine stain on the neck of a 48-year-old man. The nodules disappeared with pulsed-dye laser therapy.

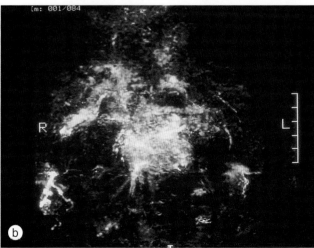

Fig. 2.65 Port-wine stains. **(a)** At birth, this newborn had a port-wine stain that involved his upper chest, neck, and portions of both arms and was associated with soft tissue hypertrophy (Klippel–Trénaunay–Weber syndrome) and high-output cardiac failure. **(b)** This composite magnetic resonance image of his body demonstrates increased blood flow to the right side of his neck and both upper extremities, with the greatest flow to the right shoulder and arm.

cerebral cortex, and eye (Sturge–Weber syndrome; Fig. 2.64). Seizures, mental retardation, hemiplegia, and glaucoma may develop during the first several years of life. Superficial vascular lesions associated with limb or segmental trunk hypertrophy are typical of Klippel–Trénaunay syndrome, which is the eponymous term for a capillary venous or capillary lymphatic venous malformation (Fig. 2.65). Up to 50% of these patients may have underlying malformations of the deep venous system as well.

Phakomatosis pigmentovascularis is a malformation syndrome in which a capillary malformation is associated with an epidermal nevus (type I), dermal melanocytosis (i.e., Mongolian spot) with or without nevus anemicus (type II), nevus spilus with or without nevus anemicus (type III), or dermal melanocytosis and nevus spilus with or without nevus anemicus (type IV). In Maffucci syndrome, superficial venous malformations are associated with deep complex venous and lymphatic malformations

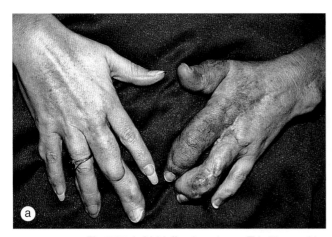
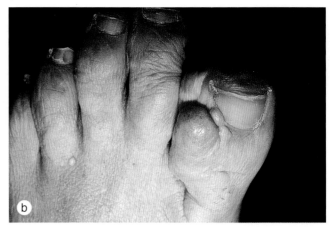

Fig. 2.67 **(a,b)** Maffucci syndrome. This 50-year-old woman had extensive port-wine stains and venous malformations on her trunk and extremities. She subsequently developed multiple firm nodules on her hands and feet.

and multiple enchondromas of bone, particularly the long bones (Fig. 2.67). There is a risk of malignant degeneration to chondrosarcomas, particularly affecting the skull.

CMTC presents with distinctive localized, segmental, or widespread reticulated blanching patches (Fig. 2.68). Although CMTC can involve any site, there is a preponderance of lesions on the extremities. Cases are usually sporadic, more common in girls, and more commonly reported in association with extracutaneous anomalies (musculoskeletal anomalies, coarctation of the aorta and other arterial and venous anomalies, cardiac defects, aplastic cutis congenita) than typical capillary malformations. However, this may represent a reporting bias; most lesions are probably restricted to the skin and contiguous soft tissue. Diffuse atrophy of the involved limb or reticulated atrophy after the course of vascular changes may develop, and erosions or ulcerations may follow with minor trauma.

Infants with PWS deserve a thorough physical examination for signs of systemic disease. Children with forehead and periorbital involvement require careful neurodevelopmental follow-up, regular eye examinations to exclude glaucoma, and further neurologic studies as indicated.

Rehabilitative cosmetics (e.g. Dermablend, Covermark) provide reasonable, safe, and temporary camouflage of PWS (Fig. 2.69). Definitive treatment eluded practitioners until approval of the pulsed-dye laser in the early 1980s (Fig. 2.64b); although refinements in laser technology continue to occur, the original physics of the pulsed-dye laser remain relatively unchanged from original models. Unlike previous modalities, including the argon and carbon dioxide lasers, the pulsed-dye laser has an extremely low risk of scarring. By selective photothermolysis, the yellow beam damages vascular structures while leaving the surrounding skin virtually unscathed. This device is safe, relatively painless, and effective in infants and children, as well as in adults. Maximal improvement of PWS requires multiple treatments separated by a 4–10-week healing period. Because the laser penetrates only 1.5–2 mm deep into the skin, it results in little improvement in those malformations with a deep component. Consequently, early treatment in childhood produces the best outcome with the fewest number of

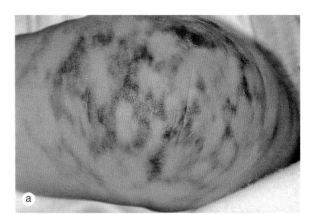

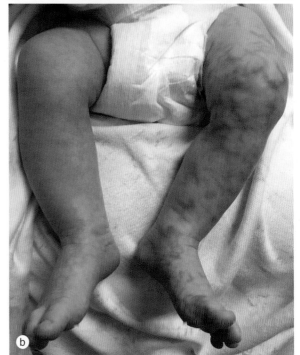

Fig. 2.68 Cutis marmorata telangiectatica congenital. Localized reticulated vascular malformations were present in these healthy infants with lesions on **(a)** the right knee and **(b)** the left leg. A complete medical evaluation failed to reveal other abnormalities.

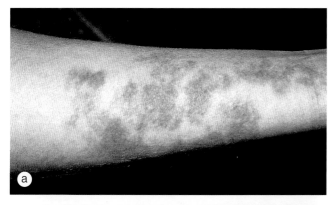

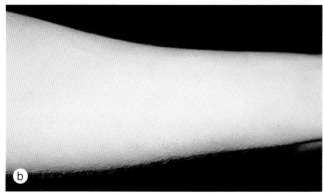

Fig. 2.69 Port-wine stains. **(a)** An extensive port-wine stain on the arm of this teenager. **(b)** It was readily camouflaged with a corrective cosmetic.

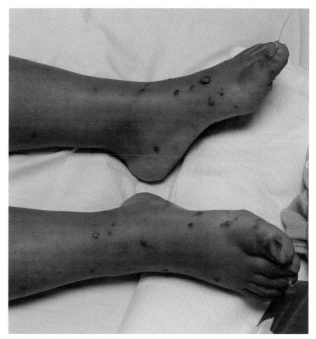

Fig. 2.70 Blue rubber bleb nevus syndrome. A 16-year-old girl was evaluated for multiple 3 mm–1 cm blue nodules on the skin. She had a history of similar lesions in the gastrointestinal tract, which were discovered during surgery for small bowel obstruction from intussusception.

treatments and the lowest cost. With increased use of lasers, recurrence of PWS has been documented, and patients should be counseled that further treatment may be required in the years after completion of laser therapy.

Venous Malformations

Venous malformations are slow-flow congenital anomalies composed of large dilated vascular channels lined by flat endothelium. The walls of these vessels are generally thin and fibrous. Although they may be found at any level in the skin or mucous membranes, they tend to occur in the mid to deep dermis and fat.

Superficial venous malformations present as scattered or grouped blue or purple papules and nodules (Fig. 2.70). Deeper lesions may demonstrate a subtle blue hue at the surface and are defined by the partially compressible ropy texture (Fig. 2.71). Small localized lesions usually occur as isolated malformations, but large or disseminated lesions should raise the possibility of a more complex malformation syndrome such as blue rubber bleb nevus syndrome or Maffucci syndrome.

Over time, venous malformations can produce distortion in underlying bone and significant disfigurement, whereas lesions located near joints may be associated with increasing swelling, pain, and functional impairment. Although many lesions can be managed with conservative measures such as compression garments, high-risk or symptomatic lesions may be ablated with a combination of percutaneous sclerotherapy and surgical excision.

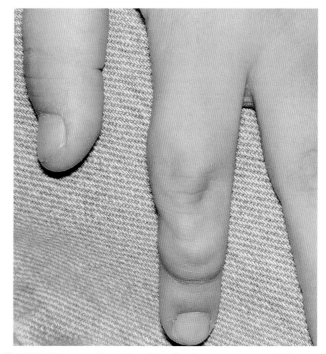

Fig. 2.71 Venous malformation. A small subcutaneous congenital venous malformation on the right second finger was associated with aching pain, particularly after intense physical activity in this 6-year-old boy.

Lymphatic Malformations

Microcystic lymphatic malformations, referred to in older literature as lymphangioma circumscriptum, are a group of localized congenital malformations of the lymphatic system, most of which become clinically evident at birth or during infancy. These

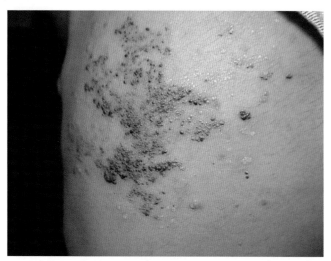

Fig. 2.72 Lymphangioma circumscriptum. A small cluster of grayish-purple vesicles on the knee of an adolescent demonstrates the typical "frog spawn" appearance.

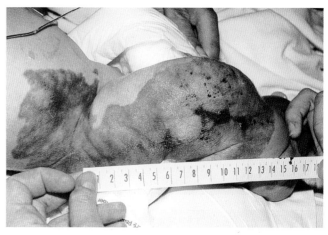

Fig. 2.73 Proteus syndrome. Massive hypertrophy of the leg was associated with an extensive cutaneous port-wine stain, soft tissue tumors, and a deep lymphangiohemangioma that involved the thigh, peritoneal cavity, and retroperitoneal space in this 1-month-old boy.

lesions may represent lymphatic structures that failed to link with the rest of the lymphatic or venous system. Clinically similar lesions may result from lymphedema secondary to tumor infiltration or surgical or accidental injury to normal lymphatics. Larger, deeper lesions characterized by larger lymph-filled cystic spaces are known as macrocystic lymphatic malformations; these have a predilection for the head and neck (see Fig. 9.13a) and may surround and compress vital structures in the anterior neck. Their presence may be marked by overlying superficial lymphatic malformations or capillary vascular malformations such as PWS. Combined microcystic and macrocystic lesions can occur. Some 90% of lymphatic malformations involve skin and soft tissue, and the remaining 10% involve viscera or bone.

Superficial lymphatic malformations consist of one or several patches of thick-walled skin-colored to gray vesicles that resemble fish eggs or frog spawn (Fig. 2.72). Thrombosis or bleeding into vesicles after trauma may result in purple or black discoloration. Lesions may be associated with an underlying soft-tissue fullness or extensive swelling of the involved area. Although there is a predilection for involvement of the proximal extremities and limb girdle regions, lesions may occur at any cutaneous or mucous membrane site.

Lymphatic malformations may be associated with complex congenital vascular malformations (Fig. 2.73). In Proteus syndrome, extensive dermal and subcutaneous lymphatic and venous malformations are associated with cutaneous PWS, soft-tissue tumors, and epidermal nevi. Vascular malformations may extend into the mediastinum, peritoneum, retroperitoneal space, and viscera. Organ dysfunction, recurrent soft-tissue infection, and musculoskeletal involvement may be debilitating and life-threatening.

Surgical management of lymphatic malformations is difficult because they often extend around vital structures, and recurrence rates are high. Superficial lesions may be ablated with the carbon dioxide laser, and deeper malformations may improve with sclerotherapy.

Arteriovenous Malformations

Arteriovenous malformations are uncommon fast-flow anomalies that arise most commonly on the head and neck; they represent the most dangerous of all vascular anomalies and are associated with significant potential morbidity. About half of the lesions are present at birth when they may be mistaken for capillary or venous malformations. In some patients, a tense vascular mass, palpable thrill, bruit, and infiltration of the overlying skin provide clues. Ultrasound and MRI studies will demonstrate the true character of these lesions. Arteriovenous malformations are potentially life-threatening anomalies that may suddenly expand after accidental trauma or partial surgical excision. Enlargement may also occur during puberty, during pregnancy, or after trauma.

Vascular Tumors
Hemangiomas

Although a recognizable lesion is only rarely present at birth, hemangiomas occur in up to 10% of Caucasian infants by 1 year of age (Fig. 2.74). Infantile hemangiomas (IH) are two to three times more common in girls. Prematurity has been shown to be the most significant risk factor for the development of IH. Lesions typically begin with a nascent phase as barely visible telangiectasias or red macules that rapidly grow into bright red, partially compressible tumors. The early telangiectasias with surrounding pallor are often present at birth or within the first few days of life and may be mistaken for capillary malformations or minor birth trauma. Many IH have a deep dermal or subcutaneous component (Fig. 2.75). Occasionally, lesions lack a superficial component altogether and can only be differentiated from vascular malformations by the growth pattern (Fig. 2.76). Histologically, early rapidly growing lesions are highly cellular and demonstrate small slit-like vascular lumina. As lesions mature, the vascular lumina become better defined, and the endothelium lining of vessels becomes flatter. Healing is mediated by apoptosis and a subsequent reduction in cell proliferation. Regression is associated with fibrosis and replacement of the vascular tissue with fat.

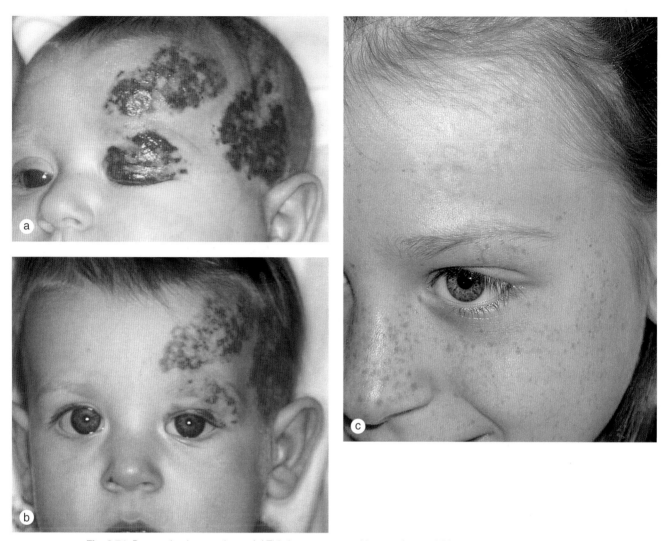

Fig. 2.74 Regressing hemangioma. **(a)** This large segmental hemangioma which appeared at 2 weeks of age was treated with high-dose oral steroids for 4 months because of obstruction of the left eye. **(b)** At 2 years later, the lesion had decreased dramatically, and **(c)** by age 7, there were only subtle residual changes.

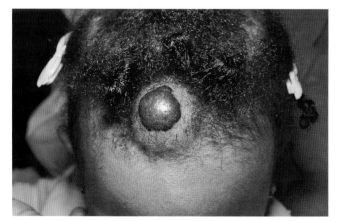

Fig. 2.75 The segmental infantile hemangioma on this child's forehead had both a superficial and a deep dermal component. The hemangioma involuted over 3 years without leaving a scar.

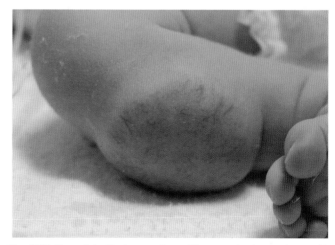

Fig. 2.76 Deep infantile hemangioma. The vessels that make up this large, partially compressible lesion are deep beneath the skin surface but still impart a bluish hue to the overlying skin. Note the indistinctness of the margins.

IH generally double in size in the first 2 months of life and reach 80% of their maximum size by 3–5 months of age (the early proliferative phase.) Proliferation may continue at a slower rate in some lesions until 6–12 months of age. Signs of early involution, such as graying of the surface and flattening of the deeper component, subsequently develop. Regression occurs in roughly 25% by age 2 years, 40–50% by age 4 years, 60–75% by age 6 years, and 95% by adolescence. Involution is independent of sex, location, and number of hemangiomas.

Unfortunately, scarring, loose skin, or telangiectasias remain in up to 50% of children. Both deep and segmental IH have a longer growth phase and subsequently take longer to regress. Another small group of hemangiomas is fully formed at birth and referred to as congenital hemangiomas, further subdivided into rapidly involuting congenital hemangiomas (RICH) and noninvoluting congenital hemangiomas (NICH). The majority of RICH begin to regress shortly after birth, and many disappear in 12–18 months, whereas NICH persist indefinitely. Some authors suggest a third categorization of partially involuting congenital hemangiomas (PICH).

Although IH are benign tumors and regression is the rule, these lesions may rarely compromise vital functions when they are located near the anus, urethra, airway, or eye. Hemangiomas around the eye or extending into the orbit may be associated with obstruction amblyopia or direct damage to orbital contents (Fig. 2.77). Multiple hemangiomas or single, large, rapidly growing lesions in young infants may be associated with high-output cardiac failure. In children with more than five cutaneous IH, lesions may involve internal organs, including the liver, gastrointestinal tract, lungs, kidneys, and CNS (Fig. 2.78).

In children in whom IH pose a threat to function of an organ or where they present with disfigurement severe enough to likely result in the need for future surgery, medical treatment is warranted. Propranolol, a nonselective beta blocker, is first-line

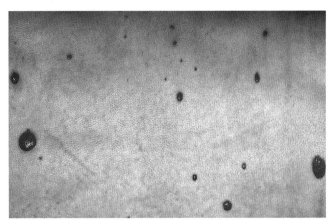

Fig. 2.78 Hemangiomatosis. Multiple hemangiomas dotted the back and extremities of this 3-month-old girl.

therapy and is FDA-approved for this indication. It is far more efficacious and safer that corticosteroids, the previous standard of care. Careful counseling is necessary to avoid hypoglycemia by coinciding doses with feedings. Risk of respiratory effects, such as wheezing and bronchospasm must also be discussed. Symptomatic hypotension and bradycardia are rare but may occur. Other beta blockers including atenolol and nadolol have been reported to have similar efficacy in smaller series. Thin, superficial IH may respond adequately to topical timolol maleate, which is available as an ophthalmic preparation; its use remains off-label at this time. Before the discovery of propranolol's utility, high-dose corticosteroids (prednisolone at 2–3 mg/kg per day and sometimes up to 5 mg/kg per day) were used for decades. Interferon-α and vincristine are now nearly never used for IH treatment. In selected lesions, there may be a role for intralesional steroids and/or early surgical excision during the proliferative phase of growth. However, in the majority of cases, surgery should be deferred until partial or complete involution has occurred.

Hemangiomas in the diaper area and other skin creases are prone to ulceration and infection (Fig. 2.79). Careful hygiene, topical and systemic antibiotics, occlusive dressings, barrier

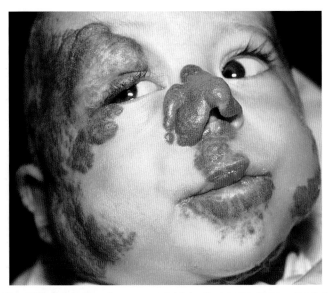

Fig. 2.77 This regressing segmental infantile hemangioma extended into the orbit and produced a large refractive difference between the two sides. The tumor also produced destruction of the nasal septum and obstructed the airway, which resulted in the need for tracheostomy.

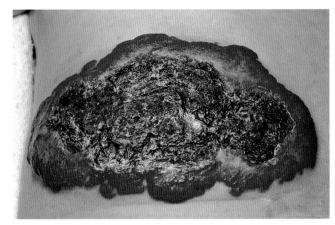

Fig. 2.79 A large hemangioma on the back of a 10-month-old girl developed an area of central necrosis that was associated with secondary bacterial infection and sepsis.

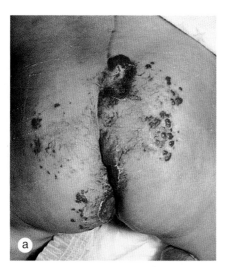
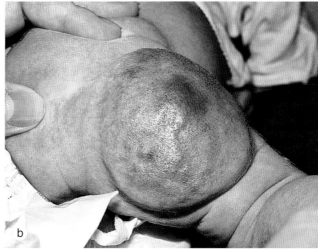

Fig. 2.80 Complicated hemangiomas. **(a)** This extensive sacral hemangioma was associated with a tethered cord. Note the scar from correction of the spinal defect. Ulceration of the hemangioma from irritation in the diaper area was a recurrent problem. **(b)** A violaceous patch on the back of the left thigh in a 3-week-old infant suddenly became firm and elevated. A complete blood count revealed a platelet count of 5000, and a biopsy showed a kaposiform hemangioendothelioma. The lesion did not improve with systemic steroids or interferon, but several months later it suddenly flattened and the platelet count jumped to over 1 000 000.

pastes, and pulsed dye laser may be required to prevent cellulitis and scarring. Failure of these conservative interventions should prompt discussion of systemic therapy in ulcerated IH associated with persistent pain, infection, and/or bleeding.

In general, IH are not associated with extracutaneous syndromes, but there are some notable exceptions. Midline hemangiomas, particularly in the lumbosacral area, with segmental morphology or large size may be associated with underlying vertebral and spinal cord anomalies (Fig. 2.80a). The association of lumbosacral IH and underlying genitourinary, spinal, and renal anomalies have been reported by various authors under the acronyms LUMBAR, SACRAL, and PELVIS syndromes. Ultrasound within the first 8–12 weeks may be used to exclude these anomalies; after this window of time, MRI is necessary. Some authors suggest that MRI should be used in all instances, given the risk of false-negative ultrasound studies. Large, segmental IH on the face and scalp have been associated with PHACE syndrome (**P**osterior fossa brain malformations, **H**emangiomas, **A**rterial anomalies, **C**ardiac defects, and **E**ye defects). MRI has proved particularly useful for delineating the extent of these defects and should include the face, orbits, brain, neck, and chest.

Although the pulsed-dye laser was originally approved for treating PWS, it appears to be useful in treating residual telangiectasias later in childhood and has occasional utility in early, thin hemangiomas. Pulsed-dye laser is also useful in treating some ulcerations that have failed to respond to topical measures. However, the pulsed-dye laser is not effective for preventing or eradicating the deeper component of hemangiomas.

Hemangiomas must be distinguished from other vascular tumors of infancy. Pyogenic granuloma is a common vascular tumor, composed of granulation-like tissue that usually arises after the newborn period, typically in older infants and toddlers. The lesion presents as a bloody, crusted nodule usually under 1 cm in diameter. Pyogenic granulomas are common on the face and are treated by destruction with electrocautery or laser. Tufted angiomas appear at birth or within the first few years of life as infiltrated red to purple plaques or large, firm exophytic nodules. Although many have a protracted course, some involute without treatment within the first 2 years of life or respond to oral steroids. A skin biopsy may be necessary to distinguish tufted angiomas from rare sarcomas of early infancy. Kasabach–Merritt syndrome is usually associated with kaposiform hemangioendothelioma (Fig. 2.80b).

Hamartomatous Nevi

Hamartomatous nevi include a number of birthmarks that contain various epidermal, dermal, and subcutaneous structures.

Epidermal Nevi

Epidermal nevi occur in 0.1–1% of children and consist of proliferating epidermal keratinocytes. Most epidermal nevi appear at birth or during early infancy as localized, linear, warty, subtly to markedly hyperpigmented plaques (Fig. 2.81). Lesions may involve any cutaneous site and extend onto mucous membranes. Epidermal nevi range in size from a few millimeters to extensive lesions that involve a large portion of the trunk and extremities. Infants with large lesions must be evaluated for associated defects, which include seizures, mental retardation, and skeletal and ocular defects (epidermal nevus syndrome). Occasionally, children with small epidermal nevi also demonstrate extracutaneous anomalies. Skin lesions may respond to the application of topical retinoids or keratolytics such as lactic acid, salicylic acid, and urea. Small lesions can be excised or ablated by carbon dioxide laser.

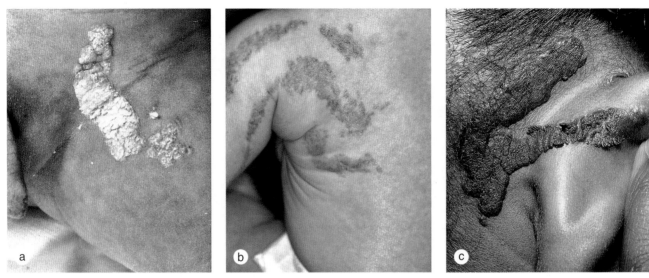

Fig. 2.81 Epidermal nevi. **(a)** An epidermal nevus on the upper thigh of a newborn still covered with vernix caseosa. **(b)** Three linear, warty plaques extend across the upper chest and down the arm of a healthy toddler. **(c)** A 10-year-old girl complained of itching from a congenital, V-shaped, warty plaque behind her ear.

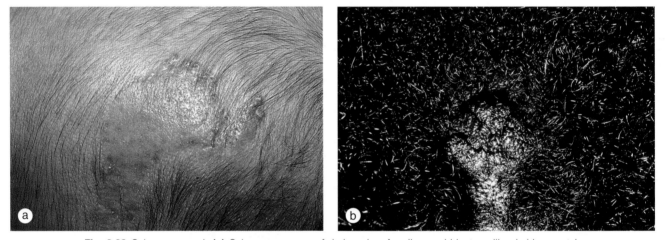

Fig. 2.82 Sebaceous nevi. **(a)** Sebaceous nevus of Jadassohn. A yellow, cobblestone-like, hairless patch present since birth. **(b)** Syringocystadenoma papilliferum arose in this sebaceous nevus on the scalp of a teenage boy. Local excision gave an excellent cosmetic result.

Sebaceous Nevi

Nevus sebaceous of Jadassohn is characterized by a linear, crescent-shaped, or round hairless, yellow, cobblestone-like plaque on the scalp (Fig. 2.82a). Although lesions usually involve the head and neck, nevi occasionally appear on the trunk and extremities. Rarely, lesions extend over a large portion of the body surface and are associated with multiple neuroectodermal and mesodermal defects (nevus sebaceous syndrome). Histology demonstrates multiple sebaceous glands, ectopic apocrine glands, and incompletely differentiated hair structures.

In the past, basal cell carcinomas were thought to be the most common neoplasm arising within sebaceous nevi, with an incidence in adults ranging from 10% to 20%. However, current evidence suggests that most basaloid neoplasms are actually benign trichoblastomas with basal cell carcinomas accounting for <1%. A number of other benign lesions have also

been reported primarily in adults (Fig. 2.82b). Benign hypertrophy of the sebaceous and apocrine components associated with the development of warty nodules and plaques can occur transiently at birth, but it is often progressive at puberty. Elective excision of problematic lesions can be delayed until puberty in most patients.

Smooth Muscle and Pilar Hamartomas

Smooth muscle and pilar hamartomas contain smooth muscle bundles and may be associated with prominent hair follicles (Fig. 2.83). Clinically, these innocent nevi are characterized by minimally hyperpigmented, supple 1.0–5.0 cm diameter plaques on the trunk. A pseudo-Darier sign or rippling of the skin occurs with rubbing. Hyperpigmentation and hair may become prominent. These lesions do not contain nevocellular nevus cells and pose no risk of malignancy. They may mimic

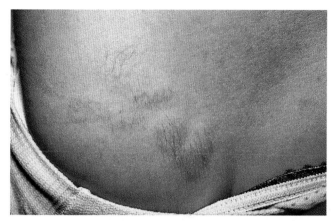

Fig. 2.83 Congenital smooth muscle hamartoma. This slightly hairy plaque on the left buttock of a 3-year-old girl demonstrates a pseudo-Darier's sign.

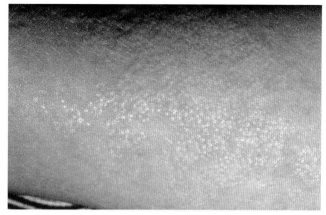

Fig. 2.84 Connective tissue nevus. This reticulated fibrotic plaque on the arm of a 10-year-old boy remained unchanged since birth. A medical evaluation for associated disorders was unrevealing.

the histologic and clinical features of Becker nevus, also known as hairy epidermal nevus.

Connective Tissue Nevus

Connective tissue nevus defines a group of hamartomas with increased quantities of dermal collagen and variable changes in elastic tissue (Fig. 2.84). Lesions appear in the newborn as 1.0–10 cm diameter plaques composed of fibrotic papules and nodules, which often give a *peau d'orange* texture to the skin. Although typically located on the trunk, lesions may be widely disseminated, and any cutaneous site may be involved.

Connective tissue nevi may occur as isolated skin findings or in association with asymptomatic osteopoikilosis or radiographic densities in the long bones and the bones of the hands and feet (Buschke–Ollendorff syndrome). The shagreen patch of tuberous sclerosis cannot be differentiated clinically and histologically from an innocent connective tissue nevus. Consequently, a careful search for other stigmata of tuberous sclerosis must be performed in all children with these hamartomas.

Congenital Melanocytic Nevi

Congenital melanocytic nevi are pigmented macules or plaques, often with dense hair growth noted at birth or during the first few months of life (Fig. 2.85). Melanocytic nevi contain nevomelanocytic nevus cells, cells derived from neural crest, and that share with normal skin melanocytes the ability to produce melanin. At birth, the lesions may be light tan with lightly pigmented vellus hairs. During infancy the nevus darkens and hair may become prominent. Occasionally, darkly pigmented lesions lighten during the first 1–2 years of life. Small, dark macules or nodules may also appear within the borders of the nevus (Fig. 2.85b).

Giant, congenital pigmented nevi may reach over 20 cm in diameter and are associated with a 2–6% lifetime risk of melanoma (Fig. 2.85c,d). The highest risk of malignant change occurs in the first 10 years of life, before puberty. Other tumors of neural-crest origin rarely arise within large lesions (Fig. 2.85c). Multistage procedures with tissue expansion may be feasible in selected patients. Unfortunately, large areas of the nevus may

not be amenable to surgical management, and close observation with photographs is required. Dermabrasion and laser surgery should be avoided. Regular examinations include careful palpation of the entire lesion because melanomas may arise deep within the nevus. Some practitioners recommend periodic MRI or computed tomography (CT) scans to follow large nevi. Radioimaging studies can also be used to document leptomeningeal involvement, which is commonly associated with giant melanocytic nevi that cover the scalp, neck, and/or back. The presence of inaccessible CNS lesions is important when assessing the risk of malignancy and planning surgical intervention.

Medium-sized (1.5–19.9 cm diameter) and small (under 1.5 cm diameter) congenital pigmented nevi may also be associated with a higher risk of malignant change than acquired moles. However, the incidence is unknown, and there are no uniformly accepted guidelines for their management. Small size and high parental anxiety may dictate early surgical excision, but removal of these nevi is usually safely left until later childhood when local anesthetic and outpatient surgery is possible. The vast majority of small congenital nevi follow a benign course, and observation throughout life is reasonable.

TUMORS

In addition to nevi, a number of other disorders present as lumps and bumps in the newborn. Many of these lesions are self-limited (fat necrosis, juvenile xanthogranuloma, hematoma) or innocent (dermoid cyst, lipoma), but some tumors herald the onset of serious systemic disease (leukemia, neuroblastoma, rhabdomyosarcoma).

Juvenile Xanthogranulomas

Juvenile xanthogranulomas (JXGs) commonly present at birth or within the first year of life (Fig. 2.86). Enlarging, 0.5–4.0 cm diameter, pink to yellow papules, plaques, and nodules with overlying telangiectasias involve the head, the neck, the trunk, and occasionally the extremities. Nearly half of the lesions are solitary, but multiple nodules may be scattered over the skin surface.

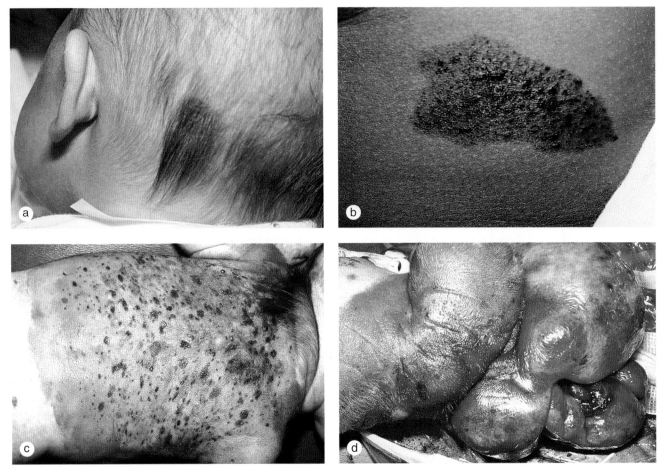

Fig. 2.85 Congenital pigmented nevi. **(a)** This small congenital pigmented nevus was associated with a tuft of dark hair on the scalp of an infant. **(b)** An innocent medium-sized 5 cm by 3 cm nevus uniformly studded with dark brown papules on the back of a 3-year-old boy was unchanged since birth. **(c)** A giant pigmented nevus contained numerous darkly pigmented nodules. This child had leptomeningeal involvement and developed a malignant melanoma in the central nervous system. **(d)** A large tumor developed within a giant pigmented nevus which involved the diaper area of this newborn. The tumor contained structures that arose from various neuroectodermal elements. The tumor was excised in several stages.

A confirmatory skin biopsy demonstrates characteristic lipid-laden histiocytes. Generally, JXGs are asymptomatic, and laboratory studies, which include a serum lipid profile, are normal. However, many clinicians recommend referral to a pediatric ophthalmologist in the presence of multiple cutaneous lesions, especially in a child presented at <2 years of age. JXGs are the most common cause of spontaneous anterior chamber hemorrhage (hyphema) in children. Further extracutaneous work-up should be based on symptoms.

In most children, no therapy is required. Surgical excision can lead to unnecessary scarring and, in early infancy, to recurrent lesions at the operative site; also, new lesions may continue to erupt for several months. After a period of growth in infancy, JXGs slowly flatten, and involution is often complete by mid-childhood (Fig. 2.86b).

Dermoid Cysts

Dermoid cysts appear as 1.0–4.0 cm diameter compressible or rubbery subcutaneous nodules at the site of closure of embryonic clefts. Although the lesions are usually noted in the newborn, subtle cysts may escape detection until they become inflamed in later infancy or early childhood. The forehead and periorbital area (Fig. 2.87a) are the most common sites of involvement, but dermoids occasionally present on the mid-chest, sacrum, perineum, and scrotum (Fig. 2.87b).

Dermoid cysts are lined by an epidermis that contains mature adnexal structures, which include sebaceous glands, eccrine glands, and apocrine glands. Although there is no risk of malignancy, lesions on the head may extend to the periosteum and cause erosion of the underlying bone. Cysts may be surgically excised during infancy or childhood.

Lesions on the head must be differentiated from hematomas, encephaloceles, and malignant tumors. Midline lesions require imaging before surgical excision. A CT scan and MRI of the head demonstrate the cystic nature of the dermoid cyst and exclude the possibility of communication with the CNS or infiltrative tumor. Dermoids that overlie the sacrum may be associated with occult defects of the vertebral column and spinal cord. The tumor and associated anomalies can be visualized with ultrasound and MRI.

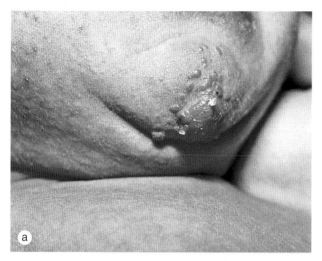

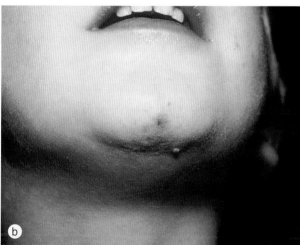

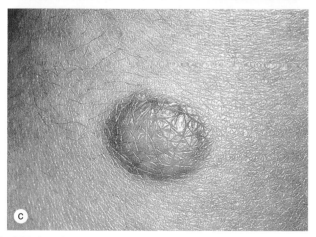

Fig. 2.86 Juvenile xanthogranuloma. **(a)** This tumor developed abruptly on the chin of a 3-month-old boy. Numerous tiny papules developed around the primary lesion. **(b)** After 1 year, the tumor and satellites had almost completely resolved without treatment. **(c)** A solitary xanthogranuloma on the leg of an infant shows the typical yellow plaque with surrounding telangiectasias.

Recurrent Infantile Digital Fibroma

In recurrent infantile digital fibroma, single or multiple fibrous nodules appear on the fingers and toes (Fig. 2.88). Although these tumors may occur in older children, 85% are diagnosed before 1 year of age, and many are noted at birth or in the first

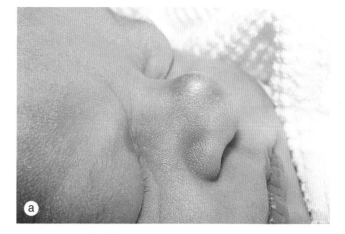

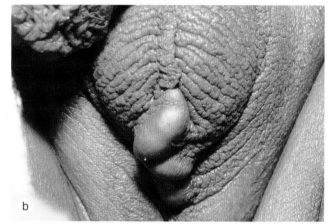

Fig. 2.87 Dermoid cyst. **(a)** This partially compressible mass was present on the nose at birth. A computed tomography scan of the head (to exclude a communication with the underlying central nervous system) was normal. **(b)** This cyst on the median raphe of the scrotum of a 4-month-old remained unchanged from birth.

month of life. Lesions rarely exceed 2.0 cm in diameter. Skin biopsy demonstrates numerous fibroblasts and interlacing collagen bundles. The presence of perinuclear intracytoplasmic inclusion bodies was considered to suggest a viral etiology, but this has been refuted by electron microscopy studies. Although excision is followed by recurrence in 75% of cases, most digital fibromas involute spontaneously within several years.

Infantile Myofibromatosis

Infantile myofibromatosis, also referred to as congenital fibromatosis, usually presents as a solitary, firm, red or blue, mobile, subcutaneous tumor (Fig. 2.89). However, multiple tumors may involve muscle and bone, and visceral lesions may produce organ dysfunction, particularly in the lungs. Histologically, these well-circumscribed tumors contain fibroblasts and smooth muscle cells with no cytologic atypia. Solitary lesions are usually excised without recurrence, but new tumors may erupt for the first several months of life. In the majority of infants who do not have severe visceral disease, spontaneous involution occurs in the first year of life.

Malignant Tumors

Malignant tumors rarely present at birth or in the newborn period. Of patients with neuroblastoma, 50% are diagnosed in

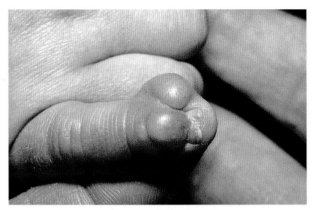

Fig. 2.88 Recurrent infantile digital fibroma. This tumor on the finger of a 7-month-old boy recurred after local excision. However, after an initial growth phase, it began to involute without further therapy.

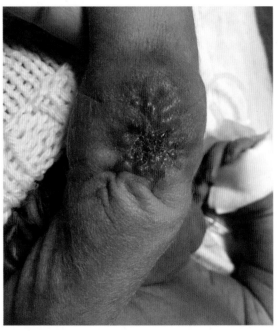

Fig. 2.89 Myofibromatosis. An infiltrating subcutaneous tumor on the thigh of a 1-month-old infant demonstrated histologic features of myofibromatosis. Other benign and malignant tumors, which include neuroblastoma, leukemia, and lymphoma, should be considered in the differential diagnosis.

Cutaneous plaques and tumors may also be the earliest finding in newborns with leukemia (Fig. 2.91), rhabdomyosarcoma (Fig. 2.92), lymphoma, and a number of other carcinomas and sarcomas. Skin biopsy of rapidly growing or infiltrative lesions is required to confirm diagnosis and dictate therapy.

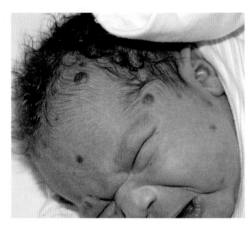

Fig. 2.90 Blueberry muffin rash. This infant with congenital rubella demonstrated the typical cutaneous lesions of extramedullary hematopoiesis. (Reprinted with permission from Bernard A. Cohen© DermAtlas, Johns Hopkins University; 2000–2012)

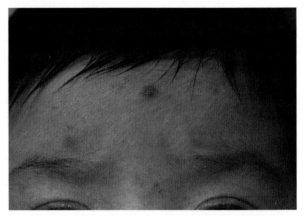

Fig. 2.91 Congenital leukemia cutis. This newborn presented with a hemoglobin of 5.0 g/dL (3.1 mmol/L) and infiltrative, pale pink, annular plaques on the extremities.

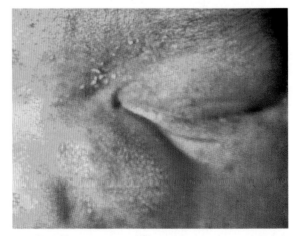

Fig. 2.92 Rhabdomyosarcoma. This rapidly growing congenital mass was part of an infiltrating rhabdomyosarcoma that involved the cheek, orbit, nose, and sinuses of this infant. This child was treated with surgical debulking of the mass and chemotherapy.

the first 2 years of life, and many develop clinical disease before 6 months of age. Although cutaneous metastases are seen in only about 3% of all patients with neuroblastoma, nearly one-third of affected newborns present with skin lesions as their initial manifestation. Metastases usually appear as 0.5–2.0 cm diameter, firm, bluish-red papules and nodules on the trunk and extremities. Stroking results in blanching and a red halo, probably because of the release of catecholamines from tumor cells. These "blueberry muffin" lesions must be differentiated from areas of extramedullary hematopoiesis seen in infants with congenital infections, such as rubella, cytomegalovirus, and toxoplasmosis (Fig. 2.90). Affected infants may also present with periorbital ecchymoses "raccoon eyes." In neonatal cases of neuroblastoma, cutaneous metastases portend a better prognosis than in older patients.

REACTIVE ERYTHEMAS

Reactive erythema refers to a group of disorders characterized by erythematous macules, plaques, and nodules, which vary in size, shape, and distribution. Unlike specific dermatoses, they represent reaction patterns in the skin triggered by a number of different endogenous and environmental factors. In infants, erythema multiforme, erythema nodosum, urticaria, and vasculitis occur after exposure to various infections and drugs. Just as in older children and adults, management of affected infants involves identification and elimination of the offending agent and supportive care. Several reactive erythemas, however, are peculiar to infancy.

Neonatal Lupus Erythematosus

Neonatal lupus erythematosus is the most common cause of congenital heart block. Although cutaneous lesions may not appear until a few months of age, they are frequently present at birth. Affected infants demonstrate annular erythematous plaques with a central scale, telangiectasias, atrophy, and pigmentary changes (Fig. 2.93). Lesions are typically in the range 0.5–3.0 cm in diameter and may spread from the scalp and face to the neck, upper trunk, and upper extremities. Although development of the cutaneous rash does not require sunlight, it may be triggered or exacerbated by sun exposure.

The cause of neonatal lupus is unknown. However, the presence of transplacentally acquired anti-ssA (Ro) and anti-ssB (La) antibodies is thought to play a primary role in the pathogenesis of the disorder. In adults, anti-ssA and anti-ssB antibodies are associated with Sjögren syndrome and the photosensitive lupus variant subacute cutaneous lupus erythematosus.

In addition to conduction defects and structural cardiac anomalies, affected infants may develop hepatosplenomegaly, anemia, leukopenia, thrombocytopenia, and lymphadenopathy. With the exception of cardiac involvement, neonatal lupus usually resolves spontaneously in 6–12 months, as transplacentally derived antibody wanes. The use of low- and medium-potency topical corticosteroids on intensely inflammatory cutaneous lesions for several weeks may reduce the risk of scarring. Subtle atrophy, telangiectasias, and pigmentary changes may persist indefinitely. Rarely, infants require systemic corticosteroids and supportive care. Parents are instructed to protect children with sunscreens and to ensure that the infant avoids direct sun exposure for at least 4–6 months. Mothers who have no clinical signs of lupus also require careful follow-up because they are at increased risk of developing overt disease.

Annular Erythema of Infancy

Annular erythema of infancy is an innocent gyrate erythema that presents during the first 6 months of life with red papules and plaques that enlarge in a centrifugal pattern (Fig. 2.94).

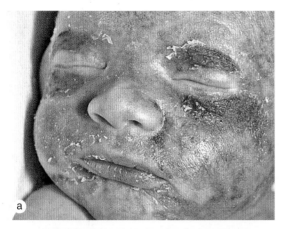

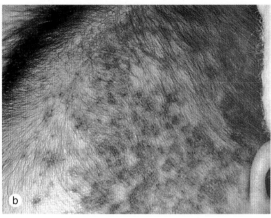

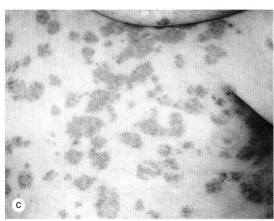

Fig. 2.93 Neonatal lupus erythematosus. **(a)** This newborn presented with extensive cutaneous atrophy and telangiectasias of the face, hepatosplenomegaly, and thrombocytopenia. **(b,c)** At 1 month of age, this infant developed an extensive eruption of annular red plaques with central atrophy. **(b)** Lesions first appeared on the scalp and face and **(c)** subsequently spread to the neck and trunk.

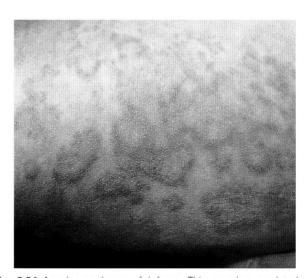

Fig. 2.94 Annular erythema of infancy. This eruption persisted for months on the trunk and extremities of an otherwise healthy infant.

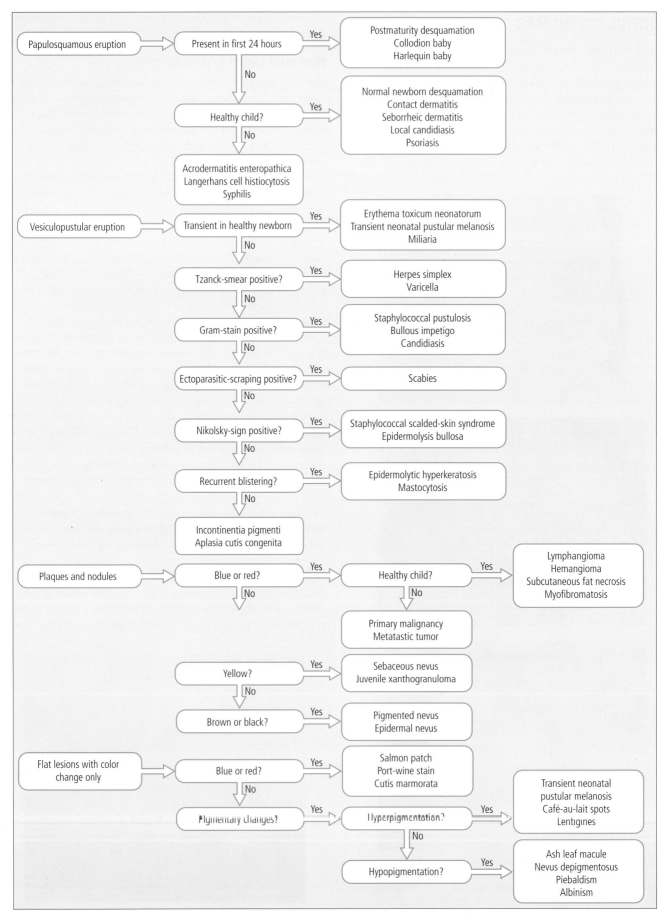

Fig. 2.95 Algorithm for evaluation of neonatal rashes.

Lesions may develop a dusky center and exceed 10 cm in diameter over 1–3 weeks. Plaques periodically fade, only to recur for months to years. Although this reaction may be triggered by infections, drugs, and malignancy, evaluation for an underlying disease is usually unrevealing. Fortunately, infants generally continue to thrive, and most lesions eventually resolve without treatment. However, in a subset of infants with familial annular erythema, lesions may persist indefinitely.

FURTHER READING

Barrier Properties and Topical Agents

Dollison EJ, Beckstrand J. Adhesive tape vs pectin-based barrier use in preterm infant. Neonatal Netw 1995; 14:35–39.

Maibach HI, Boisits EK. Neonatal skin structure and function. Marcel Dekker, New York, 1982.

Malloy-McDonald MB. Skin care for high risk neonates. J Wound Ostomy Continence Nurs 1995; 22:177–182.

Mancini AJ, Sookedo-Dorst S, Madison KC, et al. Semipermeable dressings: improved epidermal barrier function in preterm infants. Pediatr Res 1994; 36:306–314.

Marchini F, Lindow S, Brismar H, et al. The newborn infant is protected by an innate antimicrobial barrier: peptide antibiotics are present in the skin and vernix caseosa. Br J Dermatol 2002; 147:1127–1134.

Nachman RL, Esterly NB. Increased skin permeability in preterm infants. J Pediatr 1971; 79:628–632.

Paller AS, Hawk JL, Honig P, et al. New insights about infant and toddler skin: implications for sun protection. Pediatrics 2011; 128(1):92–102.

Blume-Peytavi U, Lavender T, Jenerowicz D, et al. Recommendations from a European Roundtable Meeting on Best Practice Healthy Infant Skin Care. Pediatr Dermatol 2016; 33:311–321.

Cutaneous Complications of the Intensive Care Nursery

Ballard RA. Pediatric care of the ICN graduate. Saunders, Philadelphia, 1988.

Cohen BA, Jones MD, Gleason CA, et al. Dermatology in hospital care of the recovering NICU infant. Williams and Wilkins, Baltimore, 1991.

Cutis Marmorata

Fitzsimmons JS, Starks M. Cutis marmorata telangiectatica congenita or congenital generalized phlebectasia. Arch Dis Child 1970; 45:724–726.

Kienast AK, Hoeger PH. Cutis marmorata telangiectatica congenita: a prospective study of 27 cases and review of the literature with proposal of diagnostic criteria. Clin Exp Dermatol 2009; 34(3):319–323.

O'Toole EA, Deasy P, Watson R. Cutis marmorata telangiectatica congenita associated with a double aortic arch. Pediatr Dermatol 1995; 12:348–350.

Pehr K, Moro ZB. Cutis marmorata telangiectatica congenita: long-term follow-up, review of the literature and report of a case with congenital hypothyroidism. Pediatr Dermatol 1993; 10:6–11.

Erythema Toxicum Neonatorum

Chang MW, Jiang SB, Orlow SJ. Atypical erythema toxicum neonatorum of delayed onset in a term infant. Pediatr Dermatol 1999; 16:137–141.

Kanada KN, Merin MR, Munden A, et al. A prospective study of cutaneous findings in newborns in the United States: correlation with race, ethnicity, and gestational status using updated classification and nomenclature. J Pediatr 2012; 161(2):240–245.

Maffei FA, Michaels MG, Wald ER. An unusual presentation of erythema toxicum scrotal pustules present at birth. Arch Pediatr Adolesc Med 1996; 150:649–650.

Monteagudo B, Labandeira J, Cabanillas M, et al. Prospective study of erythema toxicum neonatorum: epidemiology and predisposing factors. Pediatr Dermatol 2012; 29(2):166–168.

Treadwell PA. Dermatoses in newborns. Am Fam Physician 1997; 56:443–450.

Wagner A. Distinguishing vesicular and pustular disorders in the neonate. Curr Opin Pediatr 1997; 9:396–405.

Transient Neonatal Pustular Melanosis

Barr RJ, Globerman LM, Werber FA. Transient neonatal pustular melanosis. Int J Dermatol 1979; 18:636–638.

Laude TA. Approach to dermatologic disorders in black children. Semin Dermatol 1995; 14:15–20.

Ramamurthy RS, Reveri M, Esterly MB, et al. Transient neonatal pustular melanosis. J Pediatr 1976; 88:831–835.

Van Praag ML, Van Rooij RW, Folkers E, et al. Diagnosis and treatment of pustular diseases in the neonate. Pediatr Dermatol 1997; 14:131–143.

Acropustulosis of Infancy

Dorton DW, Kaufmann M. Palmoplantar pustules in an infant. Acropustulosis of infancy. Arch Dermatol 1996; 132:1365–1366.

Jarratt M, Ramsdell W. Infantile acropustulosis. Arch Dermatol 1979; 115:834–836.

Kahn G, Rywlin AM. Acropustulosis of infancy. Arch Dermatol 1979; 115:831–834.

Eosinophilic Folliculitis

Buckley DA, Munn SE, Higgins EM. Neonatal eosinophilic pustular folliculitis. Clin Exp Dermatol 2001; 26:251–255.

Garcia-Patos V, Pujol RM, DeMoragas JM. Infantile eosinophilic pustular folliculitis. Dermatology 1994; 189:33–38.

Finelt N, Kristal L. Patient characteristics of neonatal eosinophilic pustulosis. Pediatr Dermatol 2013; 30(6):e204–207.

Hernández-Martín Á, Nuño-González A, Colmenero I, et al. Eosinophilic pustular folliculitis of infancy: a series of 15 cases and review of the literature. J Am Acad Dermatol. 2013; 68(1):150–155.

Miliaria

Feng E, Janniger CK. Miliaria. Cutis 1995; 55:213–216.

Haas N, Henz BM, Weigel H. Congenital miliaria crystallina. J Am Acad Dermatol 2002; 45(5 Suppl):S270.

Holzle E, Kligman AM. The pathogenesis of miliaria rubra: role of the resident microflora. Br J Dermatol 1978; 99:117–137.

Milia

Epstein W, Kligman AM. The pathogenesis of milia and benign tumors of the skin. J Invest Dermatol 1956; 26:1–11.

Neonatal and Infantile Acne

Bergman JN, Eichenfield LF. Neonatal acne and cephalic pustulosis: is Malassezia the whole story? Arch Dermatol 2002; 138:255–257.

Bernier V, Weill FX, Hirigoyen V, et al. Skin colonization with Malassezia in neonates: a prospective study and relationship with neonatal cephalic pustulosis. Arch Dermatol 2002; 138:215–218.

Forest MG, Cathaird AM, Bertrand JA. Evidence of testicular activity in early infancy. J Clin Endocrinol Metab 1973; 37:148–151.

Friedlander SF, Baldwin HE, Mancini AJ, et al. The acne continuum: an age-based approach to therapy. Semin Cutan Med Surg 2011; 30(3 Suppl):S6–11.

Hernane MI, Ando I. Acne in infancy and acne genetics. Dermatology 2003; 206:24–28.

Janniger CK. Neonatal and infantile acne vulgaris. Cutis 1993; 52:16.

Jansen T, Burgdorf WHC, Plewig G. Pathogenesis and treatment of acne in childhood. Pediatr Dermatol 1997; 14:17–22.

Katsambas AD, Katoulis AL, Stavropoulos P. Acne neonatorum: a study of 22 cases. Int J Dermatol 1999; 38:128–130.

Lucky AW. A review of infantile acne and pediatric acne. Dermatology 1998; 196:95–97.

Subcutaneous Fat Necrosis of the Newborn

Akcay A, Akar M, Oncel MY, et al. Hypercalcemia due to subcutaneous fat necrosis in a newborn after total body cooling. Pediatr Dermatol 2013; 30:120–123.

Beneggi A, Adamoli P, Conforto F, et al. Fat necrosis of the newborn. Pediatr Med Chir 1995; 17:281–282.

Chuang SB, Chin HC, Chuang CC. Subcutaneous fat necrosis of the newborn complicating hypothermic cardiac surgery. Br J Dermatol 1995; 132:805–810.

Dudink J, Walther FJ, Beekman RP. Subcutaneous fat necrosis of the newborn: hypercalcemia with hepatic and atrial myocardial calcification. Arch Dis Child Fetal Neonatal Ed 2003; 88:343–345.

Norwood-Galloway A, Lebwohl M, Phelps RG, et al. Subcutaneous fat necrosis of the newborn with hypercalcemia. J Am Acad Dermatol 1987; 16:435–439.

Tran JT, Sheth AP. Subcutaneous fat necrosis of the newborn: a case report and review of the literature. Pediatr Dermatol 2003; 20:257–261.

Minor Anomalies

Steele MW, Golden WL. Syndromes of congenital anomalies. In: Kelley VC (ed.), Practice of pediatrics. Lippincott, Philadelphia, 1984.

Wang RY, Earl DL, Ruder RO, et al. Syndromic ear anomalies and renal ultrasounds. Pediatrics 2001; 108(2):E32.

Collodion Baby

deDobbeleer G, Heenen M, Song M, et al. Collodion baby skin. Ultrastructural and autoradiographic study. J Cutan Pathol 1982; 9:196–202.

Lareque M, Gharbi R, Daniel J, et al. Le bebe collodion evolution a propos de 29 cas. Ann Dermatol Venereol 1976; 103:31–56.

Sybert, V. Genetic skin disorders, 2nd ed. Oxford University Press, New York, 2010.

Taieb A, Labreze C. Collodion baby: what's new. J Eur Acad Dermatol Venereol 2002; 16:436–437.

Van Gysel D, Lijnen RL, Meokti SS, et al. Collodion baby: a followup study of 17 cases. J Eur Acad Dermatol Venereol 2002; 16:472–475.

Prado R, Ellis LZ, Gamble R, et al. Collodion baby: an update with a focus on practical management. J Am Acad Dermatol 2012; 67(6):1362–1374.

Ichthyosis

DiGiovanna JJ, Robinson-Bostom L. Ichthyosis: etiology, diagnosis, management. Am J Clin Dermatol 2003; 17:81–95.

Niemi KM, Kanerva L, Kuokkanen K, et al. Clinical, light and electron microscopic features of recessive congenital ichthyosis type I. Br J Dermatol 1994; 130:626–633.

Parmentier L, Blanchet-Bardon C, Nguyen S, et al. Autosomal recessive lamellar ichthyosis: identification of a new mutation transglutaminase and evidence for genetic heterogeneity. Hum Mol Genet 1995; 4:1391–1395.

Rand RE, Baden HP. The ichthyoses—a review. J Am Acad Dermatol 1983; 8:285–305.

Smith DL, Smith JG, Wong SW, et al. Netherton syndrome: a syndrome of elevated IgE and characteristic skin and hair findings. J Allergy Immunol 1995; 95:116–123.

Mazereeuw-Hautier J, Vahlquist A, Traupe H, et al. Management of congenital ichthyoses: European guidelines of care, part one. Br J Dermatol 2019; 180(2):272–281.

Diaper Dermatitis

Benoit S, Hamm H. Childhood psoriasis. Clin Dermatol 2007; 25(6):555–562.

Ferrazzini G, Kaiser RR, Hirsig Cheng SK, et al. Microbiologic aspects of diaper dermatitis. Dermatology 2003; 206:136–141.

Giusti F, Massone MD, Bertoni L, et al. Contact sensitization to disperse dyes in children. Pediatr Dermatol 2003; 20:393–397.

Prasad HR, Srivastava P, Verma KK. Diaper dermatitis: ammonia. Indian J Pediatr 2003; 70:635–637.

Smith WJ, Jacob SE. The role of allergic contact dermatitis in diaper dermatitis. Pediatr Dermatol 2009; 26:369–370.

Stein H. Incidence of diaper rash when using cloth and disposable diapers. J Pediatr 1982; 101:721–723.

Fölster-Holst R. Differential diagnoses of diaper dermatitis. Pediatr Dermatol 2018; 35 (1 Suppl):s10–s18.

Seborrheic Dermatitis

Cohen S. Should we treat infantile seborrheic dermatitis with topical antifungals or topical steroids? Arch Dis Child 2004; 89:288–289.

Skinner RB Jr, Noah PW, Taylor RM, et al. Double blind treatment of seborrheic dermatitis with 2% ketoconazole cream. J Am Acad Dermatol 1985; 12:852–856.

Yates VM, Kerr EI, Mackie RM. Early diagnosis of infantile seborrheic dermatitis and atopic dermatitis—clinical features. Br J Dermatol 1983; 108:633–645.

Langerhans Cell Histiocytosis

Chu T. Langerhans cell histiocytosis. Australas J Dermatol 2001; 42:237–242.

Esterly NB, Maurer HS, Gonzales-Crussi F. Histiocytosis X: a seven year experience at a children's hospital. J Am Acad Dermatol 1985; 13:481–496.

Roper SS, Spraker MK. Cutaneous histiocytosis syndromes. Pediatr Dermatol 1985; 3:19–30.

Wright TS. Cutaneous manifestations of malignancy. Curr Opin Pediatr 2011; 23(4):407–411.

Krooks J, Minkov M, Weatherall AG. Langerhans cell histiocytosis in children: history, classification, pathobiology, clinical manifestations, and prognosis. J Am Acad Dermatol 2018; 78(6):1035–1044.

Acrodermatitis Enteropathica

Campo AG Jr, McDonald CJ. Treatment of acrodermatitis enteropathica with zinc sulfate. Arch Dermatol 1976; 112:687–689.

Danbolt N, Closs K. Acrodermatitis enteropathica. Acta Dermatol Venereol (Stockh) 1942; 23:127–169.

Ghali FE, Steinberg JB, Tunnessen WW Jr. Picture of the month: acrodermatitis enteropathica-like rash in cystic fibrosis. Arch Pediatr Adolesc Med 1996; 150:99–100.

Gonzalez JR, Botet MV, Sanchez JL. The histopathology of acrodermatitis enteropathica. Am J Dermatopathol 1982; 4:303–311.

Perafan-Riveros C, Franca LF, Alves AC, et al. Acrodermatitis enteropathica: a case report and review of the literature. Pediatr Dermatol 2002; 19:426–431.

Sehgal VN, Jan S. Acrodermatitis enteropathica. Clin Dermatol 2000; 18:745–748.

Congenital Syphilis

Bowen V, Su J, Torrone E, et al. Increase in incidence of congenital syphilis — United States, 2012-2014. MMWR Morb Mortal Wkly Rep 2015; 64(44):1241–1245.

Carey JC. Congenital syphilis in the 21st century. Curr Womens Health Rep 2003; 3:299–302.

Cooper JM, Sánchez PJ. Congenital syphilis. Semin Perinatol 2018; 42(3):176–184.

Dorfman DH, Glaser JH. Congenital syphilis presenting in infants after the newborn period. N Engl J Med 1990; 323:1299–1301.

Herremans T, Kortbeek L, Notermans DW. A review of diagnostic tests for congenital syphilis in newborns. Eur J Clin Microbiol Infect Dis 2010; 29(5):495–501.

Mascola L, Pelosi R, Blount JH, et al. Congenital syphilis revisited. Am J Dis Child 1985; 139:575–580.

McIntosh K. Editorial: Congenital syphilis—breaking through the safety net. N Engl J Med 1990; 323:1339–1340.

Stafford IA, Sánchez PJ, Stoll BJ. Ending congenital syphilis. JAMA 2019 Dec 3;322(21):2073-2074. doi: 10.1001/jama.2019.17031.

Herpes Simplex

Corey L, Wald A. Maternal and neonatal herpes simplex virus infections. N Engl J Med 2009; 361(14):1376–1385.

Enright AM, Prober CG. Neonatal herpes infection: diagnosis, treatment, and prevention. Semin Neonatol 2002; 7:283–291.

Gaensbauer J, Grubenhoff JA. Neonatal herpes simplex virus infections: new data, old conundrum. Pediatrics 2019; 143(4):e20190159.

Jones CA, Walker KS, Badawi N. Antiviral agents for treatment of herpes simplex virus infection in neonates. Cochrane Database Syst Rev 2009; 2009(3):CD004206.

Kimberlin DW. Neonatal herpes simplex infection. Clin Microbiol Rev 2004; 17:1–13.

Kimberlin DW, Lin CY, Jacobs RF, et al. National Institute of Allergy and Infectious Diseases Collaborative Antiviral Study Group. Natural history of neonatal herpes simplex virus infections in the acyclovir era. Pediatrics 2001; 108(2):223–229.

Kimberlin DW, Whitley RJ, Wan W, et al. National Institute of Allergy and Infectious Diseases Collaborative Antiviral Study Group. Oral acyclovir suppression and neurodevelopment after neonatal herpes. N Engl J Med 2011; 365(14):1284–1292.

Mahant S, Hall M, Schondelmeyer AC, et al. Neonatal herpes simplex virus infection among Medicaid-enrolled children: 2009-2015. Pediatrics 2019; 143(4):e20183233.

Sauerbrei A, Wutzler P. Herpes simplex and varicella-zoster virus infections during pregnancy: current concepts of prevention, diagnosis and therapy. Part 1: herpes simplex virus infections. Med Microbiol Immunol 2007; 196(2):89–94.

Varicella

Isaacs D. Neonatal chickenpox. J Paediatr Child Health 2000; 36:76–77.

La Foret E, Lynch CL. Multiple congenital defects following maternal varicella. N Engl J Med 1947; 236:534–537.

Sauerbrei A, Wutzler P. Neonatal varicella. J Perinatol 2001; 21: 545–549.

Smith CK, Arvin AM. Varicella in the fetus and newborn. Semin Fetal Neonatal Med 2009; 14(4):209–217.

Staphylococcal Scalded-Skin Syndrome

Elias PM, Fritsch P, Epstein EH Jr. Staphylococcal scalded skin syndrome (review). Arch Dermatol 1977; 113:207–219.

Gemmell CG. Staphylococcal scalded skin syndrome. J Med Microbiol 1995; 43:318–327.

Ginsburg CM. Staphylococcal toxin syndromes. Pediatr Infect Dis 1983; 2(Suppl):23.

Lina G, Gillet Y, Vandenesch F, et al. Toxin involvement in staphylococcal scalded skin syndrome. Clin Infect Dis 1997; 25:1369–1373.

Lyell A. Toxic epidermal necrolysis (the scalded skin syndrome): a reappraisal. Br J Dermatol 1979; 100:69–86.

Stanley JR, Amagai M. Pemphigus, bullous impetigo, and the staphylococcal scalded-skin syndrome. N Engl J Med 2006; 355(17):1800–1810.

Candidiasis

Chapel TA, Gagliardi C, Nichols W. Congenital cutaneous candidiasis. J Am Acad Dermatol 1998; 6:926–928.

Gibrey MD, Siegfried EC. Cutaneous congenital candidiasis: a case report (see comments). Pediatr Dermatol 1995; 12:359–363.

Johnson DE, Thompson TR, Ferrieri P. Congenital candidiasis. Am J Dis Child 1981; 135:273–275.

Scabies

Currie BJ, McCarthy JS. Permethrin and ivermectin for scabies. N Engl J Med 2010; 362(8):717–725.

Meinking TL, Taplin D, Hermida JL, et al. The treatment of scabies with ivermectin. N Engl J Med 1995; 333:26–30.

Orkin M, Maibach HI. Scabies treatment: current considerations. Curr Prob Dermatol 1996; 24:151–156.

Taplin D, Meinking TL, Chen JA, et al. Comparison of crotamiton 10% cream (Eurax) and permethrin 5% cream (Elimite) for the treatment of scabies in children. Pediatr Dermatol 1990; 7:67–73.

Epidermolysis Bullosa

Bello YM, Falabella AF, Schachner LA. Management of epidermolysis bullosa in infants and children. Clin Dermatol 2003; 21:278–282.

Fine JD, Eady RA, Bauer EA, et al. The classification of inherited epidermolysis bullosa (EB): Report of the Third International Consensus Meeting on Diagnosis and Classification of EB. J Am Acad Dermatol 2008; 58(6):931–950.

Fine JD. Inherited epidermolysis bullosa: recent basic and clinical advances. Curr Opin Pediatr 2010; 22(4):453–458.

Hintner H, Stingl G, Schuler G, et al. Immunofluorescence mapping of antigen determinants within the dermal-epidermal junction in mechanobullous diseases. J Invest Dermatol 1981; 76:113–118.

Intong LR, Murrell DF. Inherited epidermolysis bullosa: new diagnostic criteria and classification. Clin Dermatol 2012; 30(1):70–77.

Lin AN. Management of patients with epidermolysis bullosa. Dermatol Clin 1996; 14:381–387.

Mitsuhashi Y, Hashimoto I. Genetic abnormalities and clinical classification of epidermolysis bullosa. Arch Dermatol Res 2003; 295(Suppl 1):529–533.

Trent JI, Kirsner RS. Epidermolysis bullosa: identification and treatment. Adv Skin Wound Care 2003; 16:284–290.

Aplasia Cutis Congenita

Cohen BA, Esterly NB, Nelson PF. Congenital erosive and vesicular dermatosis healing with reticulated supple scarring. Arch Dermatol 1985; 121(3):361–367.

Drolet B, Prendiville J, Golden J, et al. 'Membranous aplasia cutis' with hair collars. Congenital absence of skin or neuroectodermal defect? Arch Dermatol 1995; 131(12):1427–1431.

Evers ME, Steijlen PM, Hamel BC. Aplasia cutis congenita and associated disorders: an update. Clin Genet 1995; 47:295–301.

Frieden IJ. Aplasia cutis congenita: a clinical review and proposal for classification. J Am Acad Dermatol 1986; 14:646–660.

Harrington BC. The hair collar sign as a marker for neural tube defects. Pediatr Dermatol 2007; 24(2):138–140.

Mashiah J, Wallach D, Leclerc-Mercier S, et al. Congenital erosive and vesicular dermatosis: a new case and review of the literature. Pediatr Dermatol 2012; 29:756–758.

Stevens CA, Galen W. The hair collar sign. Am J Med Genet A 2008; 146A(4):484–487.

Mastocytosis

Caplan RM. The natural course of urticaria pigmentosa. Arch Dermatol 1983; 87:146–157.

Guzzo C, Lavker R, Roberts LJ, et al. Urticaria pigmentosa: systemic evaluation and successful treatment with topical steroids. Arch Dermatol 1991; 127:191–196.

Hartmann K, Henz BM. Mastocytosis: recent advances in defining the disease. Br J Dermatol 2001; 144:208–209.

Heide R, Tank B, Oranje AP. Mastocytosis in childhood. Pediatr Dermatol 2002; 19:375–381.

Simon RA. Treatment of mastocytosis. N Engl J Med 1980; 302: 231–232.

Smith ML, Orton PW, Chu H, et al. Photochemotherapy of dominant, diffuse, cutaneous mastocytosis. Pediatr Dermatol 1990; 7:251–255.

Soter NA, Austen KF, Wasserman SL. Oral sodium cromoglycate in the treatment of systemic mastocytosis. N Engl J Med 1979; 401:465–469.

Incontinentia Pigmenti

Berlin AL, Paller AS, Chan LS. Incontinentia pigmenti: a review and update on the molecular basis of pathophysiology. J Am Acad Dermatol 2002; 47:169–187.

Carney RG. Incontinentia pigmenti, a world statistical analysis. Arch Dermatol 1976; 112:535–542.

Cohen BA. Incontinentia pigmenti. Neurol Clin North Am 1987; 5:361–377.

Francis JS, Sybert VP. Incontinentia pigmenti. Semin Cutan Med Surg 1997; 16:54–60.

Smahi A, Courtois G, Rabia SH, et al. The NF-kappaB signalling pathway in human diseases: from incontinentia pigmenti to ectodermal dysplasias and immune-deficiency syndromes. Hum Mol Genet 2002; 11(20):2371–2375.

Vascular Malformation

Enjolras O, Mulliken J. Vascular tumors and vascular malformations, new issues. Adv Dermatol 1997; 13:375–423.

Huikeshoven M, Koster PH, de Borgie CA, et al. Redarkening of port-wine stains 10 years after pulsed-dye-laser treatment. N Engl J Med 2007; 356(12):1235–1240.

Maclean K, Hanke CW. The medical necessity for treatment of port-wine stains. Dermatol Surg 1997; 23:663–667.

Mulliken JB, Flowacki J. Hemangiomas and vascular malformations in infants and children: a classification based on endothelial characteristics. Plast Reconstr Surg 1982; 69:412–420.

Requena L, Sangueza OP. Cutaneous vascular proliferations. II. Hyperplasias and benign neoplasms. J Am Acad Dermatol 1997; 37:887–920.

Reyes BA, Geronemus R. Treatment of port-wine stains during childhood with the flashlamp-pumped pulsed dye laser. J Am Acad Dermatol 1990; 23:1142–1148.

Tallman B, Tan O, Morelli JG, et al. Location of port-wine stains and the likelihood of ophthalmic and/or central nervous system complications. Pediatrics 1991; 87:323–327.

Lymphatic Malformations

Hilliard RI, McKendry JBJ, Phillips MJ. Experience and reason—briefly recorded: congenital abnormalities of the lymphatic system: a new clinical classification. Pediatrics 1990; 86:988–994.

Padwa BL, Hayward PG, Ferrero NF, et al. Cervicofacial lymphatic malformation: clinical course, surgical intervention, and pathogenesis of skeletal hypertrophy. Plast Reconstr Surg 1995; 95:951–960.

Hemangiomas

Bruckner AL, Frieden IJ. Hemangiomas of infancy. J Am Acad Dermatol 2003; 48:477–493.

Chang LC, Haggstrom AN, Drolet BA, et al. Hemangioma Investigator Group. Growth characteristics of infantile hemangiomas: implications for management. Pediatrics 2008; 122(2):360–367.

Drolet BA, Chamlin SL, Garzon MC, et al. Prospective study of spinal anomalies in children with infantile hemangiomas of the lumbosacral skin. J Pediatr 2010; 157(5):789–794.

Drolet BA, Swanson EA, Frieden IJ. Hemangioma Investigator Group. Infantile hemangiomas: an emerging health issue linked to an increased rate of low birth weight infants. J Pediatr 2008; 153(5): 712–715, 715.e1.

Enjolas O, Riche MC, Merland JJ, et al. Management of alarming hemangiomas in infancy: a review of 25 cases. Pediatrics 1990; 85:491–498.

Ezekowitz RAB, Mulliken JB, Folkman J. Interferon α-2a therapy for life-threatening hemangiomas of infancy. N Engl J Med 1992; 326:1456–1463.

Frieden IJ, Reese V, Cohen D. PHACE syndrome. The association of posterior fossa brain malformations, hemangiomas, arterial anomalies, coarctation of the aorta and cardiac defects, and eye abnormalities. Arch Dermatol 1996; 132(3):307–311.

Girard C, Bigorre M, Guillot B, et al. PELVIS Syndrome. Arch Dermatol 2006; 142(7):884–888.

Haggstrom AN, Drolet BA, Baselga E, et al. Prospective study of infantile hemangiomas: clinical characteristics predicting complications and treatment. Pediatrics 2006; 118(3):882–887.

Hemangioma Investigator Group, Haggstrom AN, Drolet BA, et al. Prospective study of infantile hemangiomas: demographic, prenatal, and perinatal characteristics. J Pediatr 2007; 150(3):291–294.

Metry D, Heyer G, Hess C, et al. PHACE Syndrome Research Conference. Consensus statement on diagnostic criteria for PHACE syndrome. Pediatrics 2009; 124(5):1447–1456.

Sadan N, Wolach B. Treatment of hemangiomas of infants with high dose prednisone. J Pediatr 1996; 128:141–146.

Stockman A, Boralevi F, Taïeb A, et al. SACRAL syndrome: spinal dysraphism, anogenital, cutaneous, renal and urologic anomalies, associated with an angioma of lumbosacral localization. Dermatology 2007; 214(1):40–45.

Epidermal Nevus

Happle R. Epidermal nevus syndromes. Semin Dermatol 1995; 14:111–121.

Losee JE, Serletti JM, Pennino RP. Epidermal nevus syndrome: a review and a case report. Ann Plast Surg 1999; 43:211–214.

Rogers M. Epidermal nevus and the epidermal nevus syndromes: a review of 233 cases. Pediatr Dermatol 1992; 9:342–344.

Sebaceous Nevus

Cribier B, Scrivener Y, Grosshans E. Tumors arising in nevus sebaceous: a study of 596 cases. J Am Acad Dermatol 2000; 42(2 Pt 1):263–268.

Domingo J, Helwig EB. Malignant neoplasms associated with nevus sebaceus of Jadassohn. J Am Acad Dermatol 1979; 1:545.

Morioka S. The natural history of nevus sebaceus. J Cutan Pathol 1985; 12:200–213.

Santibanez-Gallerani A, Marshall D, Duarte AM, et al. Should nevus sebaceus of Jadassohn in children be excised? A study of 757 cases and literature review. J Craniofac Surg 2003; 14:658–680.

Smooth Muscle Nevus

Bronson DM, Fretzin DF, Farrell LN. Congenital pilar and smooth muscle nevus. J Am Acad Dermatol 1983; 8:111–114.

Connective Tissue Nevus

Gantan RK, Kar HK, Jain RK, et al. Isolated collagenoma: a case report with a review of connective tissue nevi of the collagen type. J Dermatol 1996; 23:476–478.

Schorr WF, Opitz JM, Reyes CN. The connective tissue nevus-osteopoikilosis syndrome. Arch Dermatol 1972; 106:208–214.

Verbov J, Graham R. Buschke-Ollendorff syndrome—disseminated dermatofibrosis with osteopoikilosis. Clin Exp Dermatol 1986; 11:17–26.

Pigmented Nevi

Everett MA. Histopathology of congenital pigmented nevi. Am J Dermatopathol 1989; 11:11–12.

Leeich SN, Bell H, Linand N, et al. Neonatal giant congenital nevi with proliferative nodules: a clinicopathologic study and literature review of neonatal melanoma. Arch Dermatol 2004; 140:83–88.

Makkas HS, Frieden IJ. Congenital melanocytic nevi: an update for the pediatrician. Curr Opin Pediatr 2002; 14:397–403.

Marghoob AA, Borrego JP, Halpern AC. Congenital melanocytic nevi: treatment modalities and management. Semin Cut Med Surg 2003; 22:21–32.

Marghoob AA, Schoenbach P, Kopf AV, et al. Large congenital melanocytic nevi and the risk for the development of malignant melanoma: a prospective study. Arch Dermatol 1996; 132:170–175.

Shah KN. The risk of melanoma and neurocutaneous melanosis associated with congenital melanocytic nevi. Semin Cutan Med Surg 2010; 29(3):159–164.

Slutsky JB, Barr JM, Femia AN, et al. Large congenital melanocytic nevi: associated risks and management considerations. Semin Cutan Med Surg 2010; 29(2):79–84.

Swerdlow AJ, English JS, Qiao Z. The risk of melanoma in patients with congenital nevi: a cohort study. J Am Acad Dermatol 1995; 32:595–599.

Juvenile Xanthogranuloma

Cohen BA, Hood A. Xanthogranuloma: report on clinical and histologic findings in 64 patients. J Pediatr Dermatol 1989; 6:262–266.

Dehner LP. Juvenile xanthogranuloma in the first 2 decades of life: a clinicopathologic study of 174 cases with cutaneous and extracutaneous manifestations. Am J Surg Pathol 2003; 27:579–593.

Sangueza OP, Salmon JK, White CR Jr, et al. Juvenile xanthogranuloma: a clinical, histologic and immunohistochemical study. J Cutan Pathol 1995; 122:327–335.

Dermoid Cyst

Kennard CD, Rasmussen JE. Congenital midline nasal masses: diagnosis and management. J Dermatol Surg Oncol 1990; 16:1025–1036.

Smirniotopoulos JG, Chiechi MV. Teratomas, dermoids and epidermoids of the head and neck. Radiographics 1995; 15:1437–1455.

Recurrent Infantile Digital Fibroma

Burgert S, Jones DH. Recurring digital fibroma of childhood. J Hand Surg Br 1996; 21:400–402.

Falco NA, Upton J. Infantile digital fibroma. J Hand Surg Am 1995; 20:1014–1020.

Infantile Myofibromatosis

Spraker MK, Stack C, Esterly NB. Congenital generalised fibromatosis. J Am Acad Dermatol 1984; 10:365–371.

Variend S, Bax NM, van Gorp J. Are infantile myofibromatosis, congenital fibrosarcoma and congenital haemangiopericytoma histogenetically related? Histopathology 1995; 26:57–62.

Venecie PV, Bigel P, Desgruelles C, et al. Infantile myofibromatosis. Br J Dermatol 1987; 117:255–259.

Malignant Tumors

Abdesalam AR, Heyn R, Tefft M, et al. Infants younger than 1 year of age with rhabdomyosarcoma. Cancer 1986; 58:2606–2610.

Bhatt S, Schreck R, Graham JM, et al. Transient leukemia with trisomy 21: description of a case and review of the literature. Am J Genet 1995; 58:310–314.

Boyd TK, Schonfield DE. Monozygotic twins concordant for congenital neuroblastoma: case report and review of the literature. Pediatr Path Lab Med 1995; 15:931–940.

Francis JS, Sybert VP, Benjamin DR. Congenital monocytic leukemia: report of a case with cutaneous involvement, and review of the literature. J Pediatr Dermatol 1989; 6:306–311.

Resnik KS, Brod BB. Leukemia cutis in congenital leukemia. Arch Dermatol 1993; 129:1301–1306.

Schneider KM, Becker GM, Krasna IH. Neonatal neuroblastoma. Pediatrics 1965; 36:359–366.

Xue H, Horwitz JR, Smith MB, et al. Malignant solid tumors in neonates: a 40 year review. J Pediatr Surg 1995; 30:543–545.

Neonatal Lupus Erythematosus

Burch JM, Lee LA, Weston WL. Neonatal lupus erythematosus. Dermatol Nurs 2002; 14:157–160.

Buyon JP, Clang RM. Neonatal lupus: a review of proposed pathogenesis and clinical data from the US-based research registry for neonatal lupus. Autoimmunity 2003; 36:33–40.

Izmirly PM, Llanos C, Lee LA, et al. Cutaneous manifestations of neonatal lupus and risk of subsequent congenital heart block. Arthritis Rheum 2010; 62(4):1153–1157.

Martin V, Lee LA, Askanase AD, et al. Long-term followup of children with neonatal lupus and their unaffected siblings. Arthritis Rheum 2002; 46:2377–2383.

Watson RM, Lane AT, Barnett NK, et al. Neonatal lupus erythematosus. A clinical, serological and immunogenetic study with review of the literature. Medicine (Baltimore) 1984; 63:362–378.

Annular Erythema of Infancy

Helm TN, Bass J, Chang LW, et al. Persistent annular erythema of infancy. Pediatr Dermatol 1993; 10:46–48.

Peterson AQ Jr, Jarratt M. Annular erythema of infancy. Arch Dermatol 1981; 117:145–148.

Stachowitz S, Abeck D, Schmidt T, et al. Persistent annular erythema of infancy associated with intestinal Candida colonization. Clin Exp Dermatol 2000; 25:404–405.

Wang LC, Kakakios A, Rogers M. Congenital annular erythema persisting in a 15-year-old girl. Australas J Dermatol 2002; 43:55–61.

3

Papulosquamous Eruptions

Jessica L. Feig and Bernard A. Cohen

INTRODUCTION

Papulosquamous eruptions comprise a group of disorders characterized by the presence of superficial papules and scale. These conditions account for a large number of patients in both pediatric dermatology and pediatric primary-care practice. In disorders of keratinization (psoriasis, pityriasis rubra pilaris, keratosis follicularis, ichthyosis, hyperkeratosis of the palms and soles, and porokeratosis), cutaneous lesions develop as a result of either genetically programmed retention or increased production of scale in the epidermis. In the inflammatory dermatoses (dermatitides, pityriasis rosea, pityriasis lichenoides, lichenoid dermatoses, and fungal infections), clinical findings result from epidermal response to dermal inflammation. An algorithmic approach to diagnosis for the papulosquamous disorders is summarized at the end of the chapter (see Fig. 3.55).

DISORDERS OF KERATINIZATION

Psoriasis

Psoriasis is a common disorder characterized by red, well-demarcated plaques with a dry, thick, silvery scale (Fig. 3.1). The condition affects 1–3% of Americans, of whom an estimated 40% develop the eruption before the age of 20 years. Psychosocial impairment in addition to physical symptoms make early diagnosis and intervention critical in children and adolescents.

Psoriasis is a multifactorial disorder with both hereditary and environmental components. In more than one-third of patients, other family members are affected. A number of human leukocyte antigen (HLA) (e.g. HLA Cw6) types have been associated with psoriasis in different populations. Several genetic loci have been under investigation, and studies suggest a major susceptibility region for early-onset psoriasis on chromosome 6p21.3. Although the factors that initiate the rapid turnover in epidermal cells, which contributes to psoriatic plaques, are unknown, upper respiratory tract viral and streptococcal infections, urinary tract infections, and other infections are known to precipitate outbreaks in genetically predisposed individuals. Triggers of psoriasis also include drugs (interferon, lithium, carbamazepine, indomethacin, beta-blockers, terfenadine, terbinafine, isotretinoin, antimalarials), climate, cigarette smoking, alcohol, psychologic stress, and malignancy. Once the process is initiated, keratinocytes within the epidermis, under the influence of Th1 cytokines and cells of the immune system, amplify the psoriatic cascade, resulting in angiogenesis, hyperproliferation, and altered cell differentiation.

Cutaneous lesions tend to locate on the scalp, the sacrum, and the extensor surfaces of the extremities. About 50% of children present with large plaques over the knees and elbows. Thickening and fissuring of the skin of the palms and soles (keratoderma) may also be present (Fig. 3.1c,d). In one-third of children, many drop-like lesions (guttate psoriasis) are scattered over the body, including the face, trunk, and extremities (Fig. 3.1e). In infancy, psoriasis may present as a persistent diaper dermatitis. In older children, the eyelids, genitals, and periumbilical areas are commonly involved (Fig. 3.2). Scalp disease may develop as an isolated finding but is often seen with other variants (Fig. 3.1b). Itchy, red plaques with thick, tenacious scale are often evident at the frontal hairline and around the ears. Nail changes, which may also occur as the first manifestation of psoriasis, include onycholysis (separation of the nail plate from the nail bed to produce "oil drop changes"), nail pitting, yellowing, increased friability, and subungual hyperkeratosis (see Fig. 8.58a,b).

Of psoriasis patients, close to 10% suffer from psoriatic arthritis, one of the seronegative spondyloarthropathies. In half of these individuals, arthritis develops before the skin rash. Examination of the joints characteristically demonstrates heat, pain, and swelling of multiple joints of the hands and feet, particularly the distal interphalangeal joints. The arthritis tends to be progressive with the development of flexure deformities and contractures. In addition to the typical lesions of plaque psoriasis, patients often demonstrate severe psoriatic involvement of the hands, nails, and feet (Fig. 3.3). The HLA B-27 antigen is usually positive.

Rarely, children develop erythrodermic psoriasis with acute widespread erythema and scaling or pustular psoriasis with generalized erythema and pustule formation (Fig. 3.4). These variants are associated with high fevers, chills, arthralgias, myalgias, and severe, cutaneous tenderness. Fluid and electrolyte losses and leukocytosis may be marked. Secondary bacterial infection and sepsis can occur.

Psoriatic lesions are often induced in areas of local injury, such as scratches, surgical scars, or sunburn, a response termed the Koebner or isomorphic phenomenon (Fig. 3.5). In areas of thick scale, tortuous capillary loops proliferate close to the surface. Gentle removal of the scale results in multiple, small bleeding points, referred to as the Auspitz sign (Fig. 3.6).

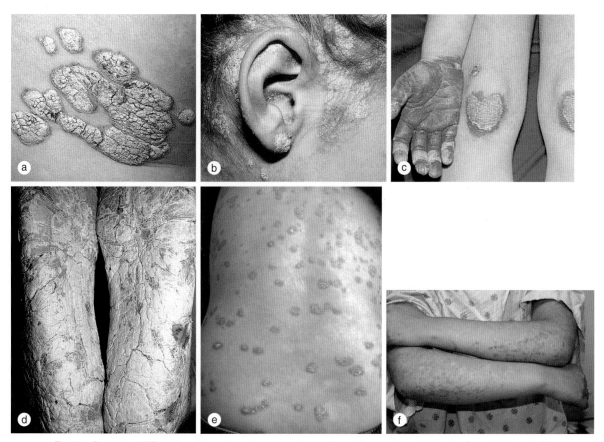

Fig. 3.1 Psoriasis. **(a)** Typical erythematous plaques are topped by a silver scale on the trunk of an adolescent. **(b)** Thick, tenacious scale extends from the forehead, neck, and ears onto the scalp of this 10-year-old girl. **(c)** Thick plaques on the palms, soles, elbows, and knees of this 8-year-old boy caused severe pain when he attempted to walk or use his hands. **(d)** Another boy with an impressive plantar keratoderma had difficulty walking. **(e)** Widespread guttate lesions erupted on the trunk and extremities of this healthy 9-year-old boy 1 week after a streptococcal pharyngitis. **(f)** Disseminated guttate lesions also developed on this 13-year-old girl after an upper respiratory infection.

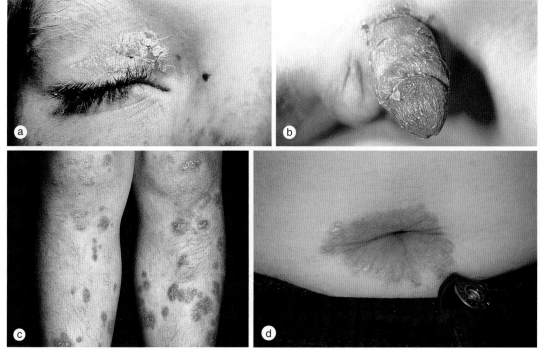

Fig. 3.2 These lesions were present on the **(a)** eyelids, **(b)** penis, and navel of this 8-year-old boy for 6 months before **(c)** he developed widespread papules and plaques on his arms and legs. **(d)** This 11-year-old girl had a persistent periumbilical plaque for over a year.

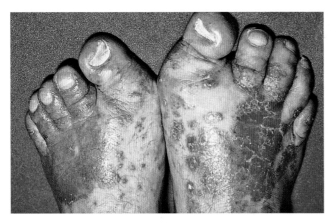

Fig. 3.3 Psoriasis and psoriatic arthritis were debilitating in this adolescent girl.

The diagnosis is usually made by identifying the typical morphology and by the distribution of skin lesions. Confirmatory skin biopsy findings include regular thickening of the epidermal rete ridges, elongation and edema of the dermal papillae, thinning of the epidermis overlying tortuous dermal capillaries, absence of the granular layer, parakeratosis, spongiform pustules of Kogoj, and Munro microabscesses. In children, skin biopsies may not always be diagnostic, particularly in early disease and certain anatomic sites such as the keratoderma of the palms and soles.

The course of psoriasis is chronic and unpredictable, marked by remissions and exacerbations. A number of different topical agents, which include lubricants, corticosteroids, tar, dithranol (anthralin), and keratolytics, are useful in managing cutaneous lesions. Topical calcipotriol (and other vitamin D3 analogs),

tazarotene (a member of the acetylenic class of retinoids), and topical corticosteroids with ultra-high potency may also play a role in the treatment of thick, localized plaques in some children. Occlusive dressings and pulsed-dye laser, which targets tortuous vessels at the base of psoriatic plaques, may be useful in localized disease. Disseminated, chronic or recalcitrant disease may require ultraviolet (UV) light therapy (broadband UVB 290–320 nm, narrowband UVB 311–313 nm, psoralen photosensitizer plus UVA [PUVA] 320–400 nm). Where available, narrowband UVB light therapy has replaced broadband UVB and PUVA in children because of improved safety and efficacy comparable with PUVA. Life-threatening erythrodermic and pustular psoriasis and psoriatic arthritis usually respond to oral retinoids (acitretin) and antimetabolites (methotrexate). Cyclosporine, an immunosuppressant that inhibits T-cell activation has been approved for use in adults with severe psoriasis and may be useful in children with severe, recalcitrant, disfiguring, incapacitating, or life-threatening disease. Recent studies with systemic tacrolimus and pimecrolimus have also shown these agents to be highly effective, but further data are needed on long-term safety. Both calcineurin inhibitors are also available in a topical formulation that may be effective for treating selective patients with facial and intertriginous (inverse) psoriasis. The use of systemic agents requires close laboratory and clinical monitoring.

A relatively new group of pathogenesis-based treatments capable of selective disruption of the psoriatic cascade show promise for management of severe disease in children. Apremilast is a small molecule inhibitor of phosphodiesterase 4, and the anti-tumor necrosis factor agents (adalimumab, etanercept, and infliximab), interleukin (IL)-17 signaling blockers (brodalumab, ixekizumab, and secukinumab), anti-IL-23 (guselkumab, risankizumab, and

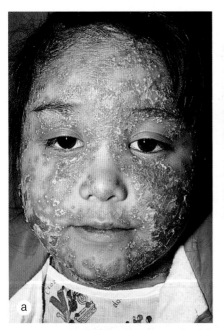
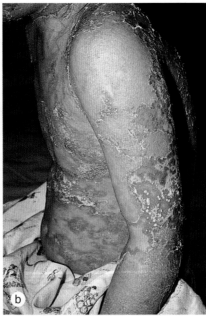
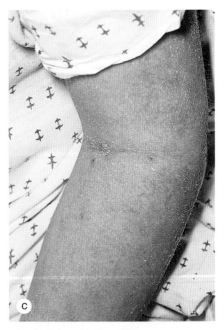

Fig. 3.4 Pustular and erythrodermic psoriasis. **(a,b)** Generalized pustulation developed suddenly within psoriatic plaques on this 8-year-old child. Skin lesions were associated with fever, chills, and arthralgias. **(c)** Erythroderma appeared in another 8-year-old girl with psoriasis. She also complained of chills, pruritus, and fatigue.

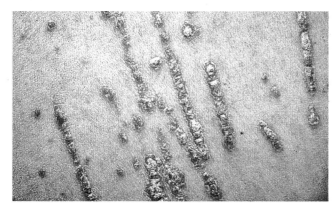

Fig. 3.5 Koebner phenomenon in psoriasis. Pruritus was severe in this child who developed linear plaques in excoriations.

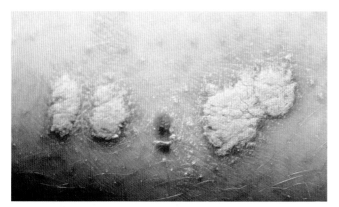

Fig. 3.6 Auspitz sign. Removal of the thick scale from a psoriatic plaque produces small points of bleeding from underlying tortuous capillaries.

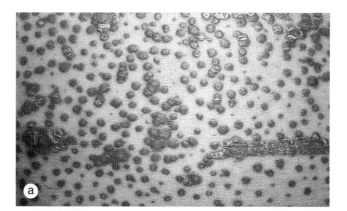

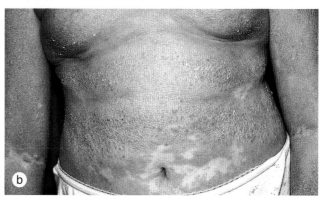

Fig. 3.7 Pityriasis rubra pilaris. **(a)** Discrete hyperkeratotic follicular papules on the trunk and extremities of this 10-year-old girl progressed over several weeks to give confluent plaques. **(b)** Note several discrete areas of sparing on the abdomen and arm flexures.

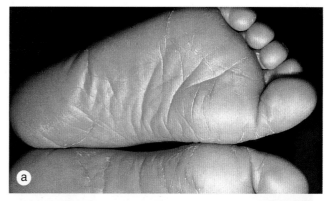

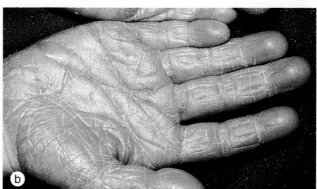

Fig. 3.8 Pityriasis rubra pilaris. This child developed a salmon-colored keratoderma of the **(a)** soles and **(b)** palms.

tildrakizumab), and the monoclonal antibodies directed against IL 12–23 pathway (ustekinumab) have been shown to be effective in adults. Because safety and efficacy data of these various classes are accumulating for the treatment of psoriasis in pediatric patients, the American Academy of Dermatology and the National Psoriasis Foundation issued joint recommendation guidelines for the management and treatment of psoriasis in this special cohort in late 2019. Etanercept and ustekinumab are U.S. Food and Drug Administration (FDA) approved for patients with psoriasis 4 years and older and 12 years and older, respectively. Recently, the manufacturers of ixekizumab received FDA approval for the treatment of the pediatric cohort from ages 6 to 18 with moderate to severe plaque psoriasis. In Europe, etanercept and ustekinumab along with adalimumab are also approved. Several other biologics are used off-label both here and abroad.

Pityriasis Rubra Pilaris

Pityriasis rubra pilaris (PRP) is an uncommon disorder of keratinization characterized by small follicular papules, widespread orange-red, scaly plaques surrounded by islands of spared skin, and marked thickening of the skin on the palms and soles (Fig. 3.7 and Fig. 3.8). Onset of disease occurs most commonly in prepubertal children and in adults over 50 years old, and it has been associated with trauma, acute, self-limited illness, and immunocompromised states such as HIV. Most cases are sporadic and acquired, but a familial variant has been reported. Overall, 75% of cases resolve spontaneously within 3–4 years, but in familial disease, persistence is the rule.

In childhood, the circumscribed variant, which accounts for a majority of the cases, begins with the development of coalescing hyperkeratotic papules on the elbows and knees and a palmoplantar keratoderma (Fig. 3.8). Superficial, red, scaly plaques occasionally appear on the face and trunk. Less commonly, children develop a pattern that mimics the classic adult variety. The eruption begins with follicular, hyperkeratotic patches on the back, chest, and abdomen, which expand to involve interfollicular skin. Lesions on the scalp and other sebaceous areas develop simultaneously or soon thereafter and may disseminate. Even in widespread disease, islands of normal appearing spared skin are characteristic. Discrete, hyperkeratotic papules may also remain present over the knuckles, wrists, elbows, and knees. In erythrodermic PRP, facial edema and scale may result in ectropion formation. Nail dystrophy with subungual hyperkeratoses may also be present.

The clinical presentation, particularly with keratoderma of the hands and feet and follicular papules, helps differentiate PRP from psoriasis, seborrheic dermatitis, atopic dermatitis, and pityriasis rosea. A skin biopsy that demonstrates interfollicular orthohyperkeratosis and perifollicular parakeratosis is typical, but not diagnostic.

Although PRP is usually self-limited in childhood, severe disabling disease may require systemic therapy with retinoids or methotrexate. Variable response to therapy has been reported with topical vitamin D analogs, phototherapy, and systemic immunosuppressive agents including steroids, cyclosporine, and azathioprine. Recently, there has been increasing clinical experience with the systemic biologic agents in adults and children with this disorder (see section on psoriasis).

Keratosis Follicularis (Darier Disease)

Keratosis follicularis is an autosomal-dominant disorder that typically presents in children from 8 to 15 years old and is characterized by hyperkeratotic follicular papules on the face, scalp, neck, and seborrheic areas of the trunk (Fig. 3.9). Although the onset is usually insidious, a rapidly progressive course may follow an inciting event, such as intense sun exposure or a viral infection. Red, scaly papules coalesce to form widespread, thick, odoriferous, greasy plaques, particularly on the scalp and forehead and around the ears, shoulders, mid-chest, and mid-back. Flexures may also be involved, with moist vegetative plaques.

Other characteristic lesions include flat-topped, warty papules on the dorsum of the hands and tiny hyperkeratotic papules and pits on the palms and soles. Subtle pebbly papules on the oral mucosa may simulate leukoplakia. Nail dystrophy, with thickening or thinning of the nail plate, fracture of the distal

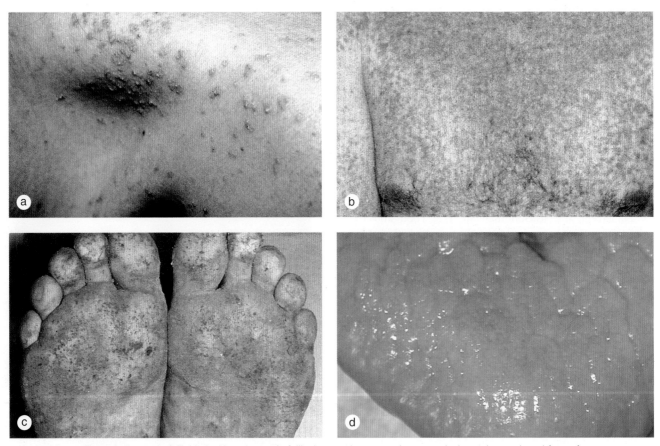

Fig. 3.9 Keratosis follicularis. Hyperkeratotic follicular papules erupted progressively on the trunk and face of this 9-year-old girl. **(a)** Some of the most prominent lesions are demonstrated on her shoulder. An adolescent demonstrates almost confluent papules on the **(b)** chest and an associated keratoderma on his **(c)** feet. **(d)** Asymptomatic confluent pebbly papules on the tongue of this 20-year-old man were noted with magnification.

nail plate, longitudinal white and red streaks, and subungual hyperkeratosis, may also be present.

The genetic defect in Darier disease has been mapped to chromosome 12q23–q24.1, which results in dysfunction of an endoplasmic reticulum Ca^{2+} ATPase (SERCA2) and subsequent disruption of intracellular Ca^{2+} signaling. Although the cause is unclear, there is also a predisposition to certain bacterial, viral, and fungal infections. The tendency of affected individuals to develop disseminated herpes simplex (Kaposi varicelliform eruption) and recurrent staphylococcal infections has been recognized for years.

The characteristic clinical picture permits easy differentiation of Darier disease from other papulosquamous disorders, such as seborrheic dermatitis, PRP, and psoriasis. Classic histologic changes from skin biopsy, which include dyskeratosis (with the formation of corps ronds and corps grains), suprabasal acantholysis (leading to the formation of suprabasal clefts), and the formation of villi by upward proliferating dermal papillae, confirm the diagnosis.

Although Darier disease tends to persist throughout life, many patients experience episodic flares and remissions in disease activity. Topical vitamin A acid may be helpful in managing early lesions. However, its use is limited by a high risk of irritation. Experience with oral retinoids has been promising, but prolonged use may be associated with unacceptable complications, which include hyperostosis, epiphyseal plate changes, increased skin fragility, and teratogenicity. Aggressive protection from the sun and treatment of secondary bacterial and viral infections also control exacerbations.

Ichthyoses

The ichthyoses are a heterogeneous group of scaling disorders characterized by retention hyperkeratosis (ichthyosis vulgaris, X-linked ichthyosis) or increased proliferation of epidermal cells (lamellar ichthyosis, epidermolytic hyperkeratosis). These diseases may be differentiated by clinical findings, histopathology, biochemical markers, and specific genetic mutations, as outlined in Chapter 2.

Palmoplantar Keratoderma

Keratoderma is a heterogeneous group of disorders of keratinization defined by the presence of focal or generalized thickening of the skin of the palms and/or soles. Although difficult to characterize, keratodermas can be classified based on whether they are acquired or inherited, isolated or associated with other cutaneous or systemic findings, and specific morphologic features and extent of involvement of lesions on the palms and soles (Table 3.1). Inherited keratodermas can be subdivided based on the mode of inheritance, presence of other ectodermal and non-ectodermal findings, and specific genetic and molecular markers. The astute clinician can often make a specific diagnosis by searching for key findings in the Online Mendelian Inheritance in Man database supported by the National Library of Medicine and the Johns Hopkins University School of Medicine.

Unna-Thost (non-epidermolytic type), the most common genetic variant, is inherited in an autosomal dominant pattern and is associated with a defect in type 1 and type 16 keratins. This keratoderma presents in the first year of life with diffuse

TABLE 3.1 Variants of Palmoplantar Keratoderma

Type	Disorder	Genetics	Onset	Involvement	Hyperhidrosis	Associated Findings
Diffuse palmoplantar keratoderma	Unna–Thost syndrome	Autosomal dominant (1:200–1:40 000); varies with ethnic group KRT1(keratin)1 chromosome 12q 13.13 KRT16 17q 21.2 chromosome	Infancy	Palms, soles	Severe	Occasional deafness, rarely total Anomalous pulmonary venous return
	Keratoma hereditarium mutilans (Vohwinkel syndrome)	Autosomal dominant (rare) Recessive variant with ectodermal dysplasia Mutation in connexin 26 and loricrin gene on chromosome 1q21.3	Infancy	Honeycomb keratoderma; star-shaped plaques on hands and feet, elbows, knees	±	Digital constriction band; deafness; alopecia May be associated with diffuse epidermolytic hyperkeratosis
	Mal de Meleda keratoderma	Autosomal recessive Mutation on chromosome 8q24.3 SLURP1 gene	Infancy	Palms, soles, elbows, knees, including dorsal surfaces (transgridiens)	±	Flexion contractures; constriction bands; koilonychia; diffuse ichthyosis
	Tylosis (Howel–Evans syndrome)	Autosomal dominant Linked to chromosome 17q25	Adolescence	Soles, sometimes palms	±	Esophageal carcinoma; epidermal cysts; thin lateral eyebrows, follicular papules

Continued

TABLE 3.1   Variants of Palmoplantar Keratoderma—cont'd

Type	Disorder	Genetics	Onset	Involvement	Hyperhidrosis	Associated Findings
	Papillon–Lefèvre syndrome	Autosomal recessive Mutation on 11q14.2	Birth to 2–3 years	Soles more severe than palms, intense erythema, wrists, ankles, elbows, knees; follicular hyperkeratoses	±	Nail dystrophy; periodontitis; calcification of falx cerebri; mental retardation; arachnodactyly
	Olmsted syndrome	Autosomal dominant? X-linked recessive? Defect in keratins 5,14	Infancy	Progressive, diffuse involvement of hands, feet, leads to flexion contractures, digital amputation	(Anhidrosis)	Periorificial hyperkeratosis Oral leukokeratosis
Focal palmoplantar keratoderma	Punctate palmoplantar keratoderma	Autosomal dominant (2–5% African Caribbean individuals)	Childhood, adolescence	Palms, soles	–	Variable
	Tyrosimia type II (oculo-cutaneous tyrisonosis, Richner–Hanhart syndrome)	Autosomal recessive 16q22.2	Infancy through adulthood	Fingertips, palms		Corneal ulcerations; mental retardation
	Porokeratosis palmar, plantar, and disseminated 1	Autosomal dominant (rare)	Childhood through adulthood	Extremities, trunk	–	Squamous cell carcinoma, increased with immuno-suppression

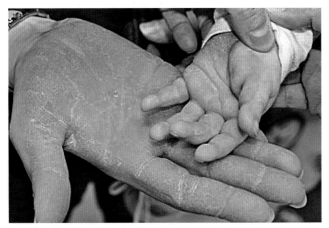

Fig. 3.10 Progressive hyperkeratosis began on the palms and soles of this father and toddler son by 3 months of age.

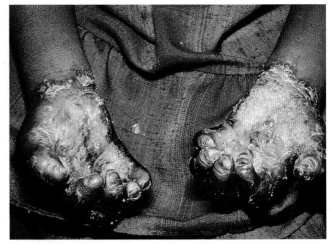

Fig. 3.11 Olmsted syndrome. Severe scarring keratoderma of the palms and soles was associated with perioral and perigenital hyperkeratosis, hyperhidrosis, recurrent cutaneous infections, and poor growth in this 5-year-old girl. Treatment with oral retinoids resulted in some decrease in the palmar and plantar lesions.

hyperkeratosis restricted to the palmar and plantar surfaces (Fig. 3.10). Although lesions may be asymptomatic, hyperhidrosis may lead to maceration and the formation of painful fissuring, blisters, and bacterial superinfection. Unna-Thost must be differentiated from a number of unusual keratodermas associated with hyperkeratoses that extend to the dorsal surfaces of the hands and feet, elbows, and knees and develop at distant sites (Fig. 3.11).

Focal keratoderma with discrete papules and plaques on the palms and soles also appears as an isolated phenomenon or in association with other cutaneous findings and systemic disease. A mild autosomal-dominant variant with pits and hyperkeratotic papules in the hand and foot creases occurs in 2–5% of black individuals (Fig. 3.12). Occasionally, this keratoderma is painful and requires surgical treatment.

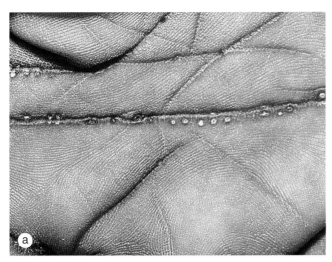 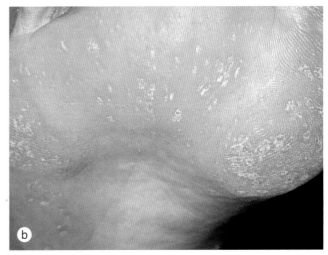

Fig. 3.12 Focal keratoderma. Asymptomatic hyperkeratotic papules and pits **(a)** developed on the hand creases of an African American teenager. Painful punctuate papules and pits began in adolescence on the palms and **(b)** soles of this young man similar to lesions on his father, uncle, grandfather, and several siblings.

Neurosensory deafness, carcinoma of the esophagus (Howel–Evans syndrome), and peripheral neuropathy (Charcot–Marie–Tooth disease) are rarely associated with palmoplantar keratoderma and may be excluded by auditory screening and a careful family history.

Hyperkeratosis of the palms and soles that presents as part of a diffuse disorder of keratinization, such as psoriasis or PRP, is differentiated by a thorough examination of the integument for other diagnostic clinical findings. Unfortunately, it may be difficult to make a specific diagnosis until other features of the underlying disorder manifest.

Porokeratosis

Porokeratosis is a disorder of keratinization characterized by annular, sharply demarcated plaques with raised hyperkeratotic borders (Fig. 3.13). Although many rare subtypes have been described, four distinctive variants are recognized, based on morphology and distribution of the lesions, time of onset, triggering factors, mode of inheritance, and, in some instances, specific genetic mutations.

Porokeratosis of Mibelli

Subtle, reddish-brown, scaly papules that slowly enlarge to form irregularly shaped plaques with hypopigmented atrophic centers and raised, grooved (double-edged) borders are typical of this condition, which invariably develops in childhood (Fig. 3.13a–c). Plaques are usually unilateral and vary in size from a few millimeters to several centimeters in diameter. One to three lesions are usually present. This rare, autosomal-dominant variant appears most commonly on the extremities, thighs, and perigenital skin, although any area that contains mucous membranes can be involved. Biopsies of the longitudinal furrow in the border demonstrate the diagnostic coronoid lamella, which consists of a parakeratotic column that fills a deep, epidermal invagination.

This variant has been associated with clonal chromosomal abnormalities in chromosome 3 in the region 3p14–p12. Chromosomal instability may rarely result in the development of squamous cell carcinoma within these slowly progressive lesions. Although excision or carbon dioxide laser surgery may be useful, recurrences have been reported.

Linear Porokeratosis

This variant presents much like the Mibelli variant. However, plaques are linearly arranged on the distal extremities and trunk, where they demonstrate a zosteriform pattern. Onset is also in early childhood, but the mode of inheritance has not been established.

Disseminated Superficial Actinic Porokeratosis

Disseminated superficial actinic porokeratosis (DSAP) is a common autosomal-dominant variant with delayed expression, found primarily in lightly pigmented individuals of Celtic extraction. Many small, 2–4 mm diameter, hyperkeratotic papules appear symmetrically on sun-exposed surfaces of the extremities during the second and third decades of life (Fig. 3.13d). These brown-, red-, or skin-colored lesions may coalesce to form irregular, circinate patterns. Progression of papules, which occurs particularly during the summer months, can be slowed by aggressive use of sun protection. A mutation in some families with DSAP has been identified at 12q23–24.1.

Punctate Porokeratosis

Punctate porokeratosis affects the palms and soles and has been described as a distinct entity. However, it usually presents in association with the Mibelli or linear variant. Punctate porokeratosis may also occur as a widely disseminated form reminiscent of disseminated superficial actinic porokeratosis, but with involvement of both sun-exposed and sun-protected areas. It is included in the differential diagnosis of punctate keratoderma.

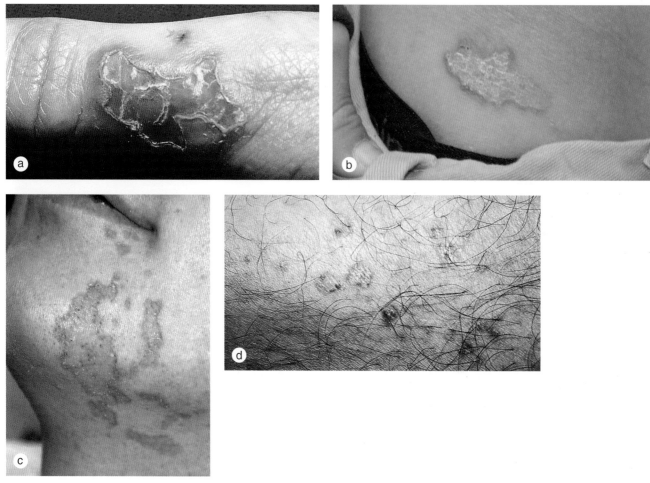

Fig. 3.13 Porokeratosis. Porokeratosis of Mibelli on **(a)** the thumb, **(b)** the right hip, and **(c)** the chin. **(d)** This adolescent with disseminated superficial actinic porokeratosis began to develop asymptomatic nummular patches on his legs after a sunburn when he was 16 years old. Note the hyperkeratotic borders in all of the patients, which demonstrated a coronoid lamella on skin biopsy. All lesions were slowly progressive.

INFLAMMATORY DERMATITIDES

Many of these disorders demonstrate changes of both acute (erythema, edema, vesiculation, crusts) and chronic (scaling, lichenification, hypopigmentation, hyperpigmentation) inflammation. Microscopically, dermatitis is recognized by the presence of intercellular edema (spongiosis), variable epidermal thickening (acanthosis), and the presence of dermal inflammatory cells, usually lymphocytes. Research and development of a number of new medications designed to selectively inhibit the dermatitic inflammatory cascade have led to more specific understanding of the molecular basis of these disorders. Various dermatitides may be differentiated by clinical features and specific histologic patterns.

A reasonable way to think of these conditions is as exogenous ("outside job") versus endogenous ("inside job") phenomena. Exogenous disorders include irritant and allergic contact dermatitis and photodermatitis. Endogenous dermatitides include atopic dermatitis, dyshidrotic eczema, nummular dermatitis, and seborrheic dermatitis. Juvenile palmar and plantar dermatosis and perioral dermatitis are triggered by a combination of inside and outside factors. Pityriasis rosea and parapsoriasis present with distinctive dermatitic patterns, but their causes are unclear.

Contact Dermatitis

Contact dermatitis refers to a group of conditions in which an inflammatory reaction in the skin is triggered by direct contact with environmental agents. In the most common form, irritant contact dermatitis, changes in the skin are induced by caustic agents such as acids, alkalis, hydrocarbons, and other primary irritants. Anyone exposed to these agents in a high enough concentration for a long enough period of time develops a reaction. The rash is usually acute (occurring within minutes), with itching or burning, well-demarcated erythema, edema, blister formation, and/or crust formation.

By contrast, allergic contact dermatitis is a T-cell–mediated immune reaction to an antigen that comes into contact with the skin. In the initial phase of the reaction, antigens are processed by Langerhans cells in the epidermis under the influence of keratinocyte-derived cytokines. T-cells subsequently migrate to regional lymph nodes where there is clonal expansion of the specifically sensitized lymphocytes. Elicitation of an allergic

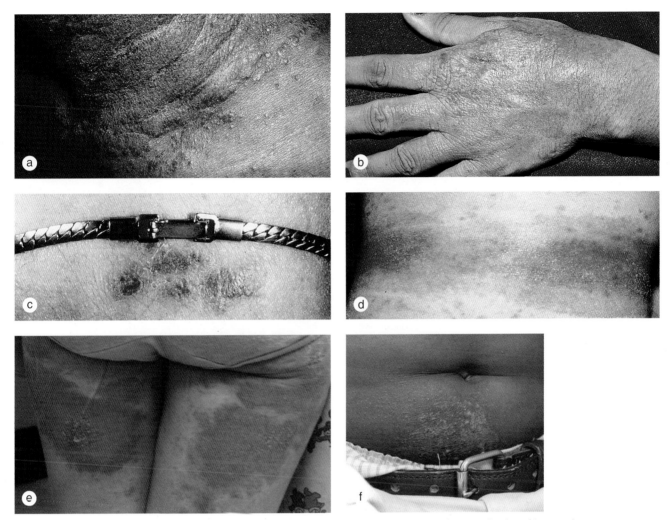

Fig. 3.14 Allergic contact dermatitis. Allergic contact dermatitis as a result of the application of benzocaine demonstrates sharply demarcated, hyperpigmented, lichenified patches on **(a)** the neck and **(b)** the top of the hands. **(c)** The location of the rash helps determine the cause of a contact dermatitis, such as in this girl with a nickel allergy. **(d)** This child became sensitized to the elastic waistbands of his underwear. **(e)** An 11-year-old girl had a persistent itchy dermatitis for 6 months, which resolved after she started using a paper toilet seat cover at school. **(f)** This 9-year-old boy with a history of atopic dermatitis developed a chronic nickel contact dermatitis, which cleared when his parents switched him to a metal buckle-free belt.

response occurs on subsequent exposure to the allergen with proliferation of T lymphocytes in the skin and regional lymph nodes.

Although contact dermatitis frequently presents with dramatic onset of erythema, vesiculation, and pruritus, the rash may become chronic with scaling, lichenification, and pigmentary changes (Fig. 3.14). At times the allergen is obvious, such as poison ivy or nickel-containing jewelry. Often, however, some detective work or formal patch testing is required to elicit the inciting agent (Fig. 3.14f). The initial reaction occurs after a period of sensitization of 7–14 days in susceptible individuals. Once sensitization has occurred, re-exposure to the allergen provides a more rapid reaction, sometimes within hours. This is a classic example of a type IV delayed-hypersensitivity response.

The most common allergic contact dermatitis in the United States is poison ivy or rhus dermatitis, which typically appears as linear streaks of erythematous papules and vesicles (Fig. 3.15).

However, with heavy exposure or in exquisitely sensitive individuals, the rash may appear in large patches. When lesions involve the skin of the face or genitals, impressive swelling can occur and obscure the primary eruption. Direct contact with the sap of the plant (poison ivy, poison oak, or poison sumac), whether from leaves, stems, or roots, produces the dermatitis (Fig. 3.16). Indirect contact, such as with clothing or pets that have brushed against the plant, with logs or railroad ties on which the vine has been growing, or with smoke from a fire in which the plant is being burned, is another means of exposure. Areas of skin exposed to the highest concentration of rhus antigen develop the changes first. Other sites that have received lower doses react in succession, which gives the illusion of spreading. However, once on the skin, the allergen becomes fixed to epithelial cells within about 20 min and cannot be spread further. Thorough washing within minutes of exposure may prevent or reduce the eruption. Barrier creams applied before exposure may afford some protection.

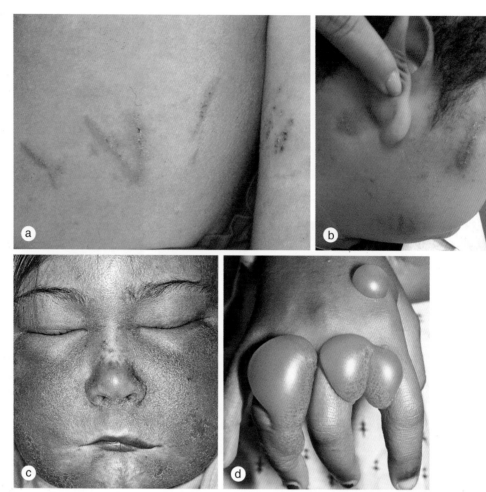

Fig. 3.15 Poison ivy or rhus dermatitis. **(a)** Crusted papules forming linear plaques were noted on the left side of the abdomen and left arm of this 11-year-old boy several days after a hike in the woods. **(b)** Similar lesions appeared on the face of this 7-year-old boy. **(c)** A 10-year-old girl developed intense facial edema after brushing against poison ivy. **(d)** In highly sensitized children, large blisters can develop. This child was swinging from vines in the woods.

Other common contact allergens include nickel, formaldehyde resin, wool alcohols, fragrance mix, and cobalt chloride. Several studies using standard patch-test techniques show that the prevalence of contact sensitivity to these allergens in children is similar to that of adults. Moreover, patch testing in children is safe and effective, and clinically significant findings may exceed 70% in carefully selected patients.

Some allergens, known as photosensitizers, require sunlight to become activated. Photocontact dermatitis caused by drugs (e.g. tetracyclines, sulfonylureas, and thiazides) characteristically erupts in a symmetric distribution on the face, the "V" of the neck, and the arms below the shirt sleeves. Topical photosensitizers (e.g. dyes, furocoumarins, halogenated salicylanilides, p-aminobenzoic acid) produce localized patches of dermatitis when applied to sun-exposed sites. These agents are found in cosmetics, sunscreens, dermatologic products, germicidal soaps, and woodland and house plants (see Chapter 7).

Occasionally, the local reaction in a contact dermatitis is so severe that the patient develops a widespread, immunologically mediated, secondary eczematous dermatitis. When the dermatitis appears at sites that have not been in contact with the offending agent, the reaction is referred to as "autoeczematization" or an "id" reaction (Fig. 3.17).

A careful history usually reveals the source of contact dermatitis. In some patients, patch testing with a standardized tray of common antigens or the suspected antigen and several controls is necessary to confirm the diagnosis.

Although small areas of contact dermatitis are best treated topically, widespread reactions require and respond within 48 h to a 2- to 3-week tapering course of systemic corticosteroid; these begin at 0.5–1.0 mg/kg per day. Patients may experience rebound of the rash when treated with a shorter course. Oral corticosteroids may also be indicated in severe local reactions that involve the eyelids, extensive parts of the face, the genitals, and/or the hands, where swelling and pruritus may become incapacitating.

Atopic Dermatitis

Also known as eczema, atopic dermatitis is a chronically recurrent, genetically influenced skin disorder of early infancy, childhood, and occasionally adult life. Although it was initially described in the nineteenth century, it was not until 1935 that Hill and Sultzberger first characterized the clinical entity. The term *atopy*, derived from the Greek word that means "not confined to a single place," was introduced in 1923 by Coca and Cooke to describe a cohort of patients with asthma and allergic rhinitis who demonstrated immediate wheal and flare reactions upon skin testing with a variety of environmental allergens. The sera of these patients contained skin-sensitizing antibodies that were subsequently characterized as IgE immunoglobulins. It

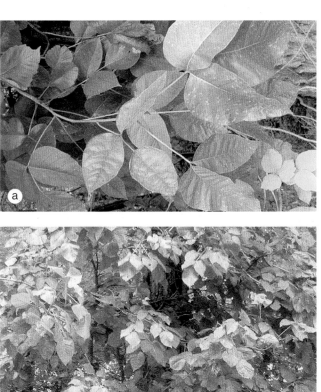

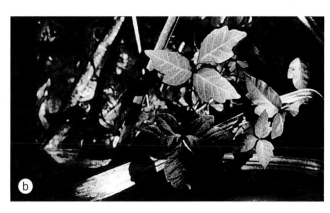

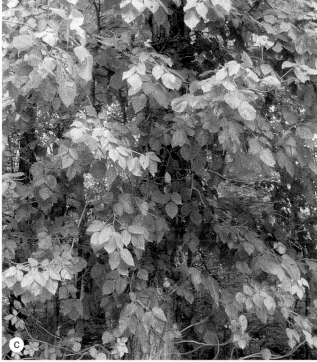

Fig. 3.16 Plants that provoke dermatitis after direct contact with the sap. **(a)** Poison ivy has characteristic shiny leaves in groups of three; it may grow as a vine or low shrub or bush. **(b)** Poison oak also has leaves in groups of three, although the edges tend to be more scalloped than those of poison ivy. (Courtesy Dr. Mary Jelks.) **(c)** Poison ivy vine climbing up a tree.

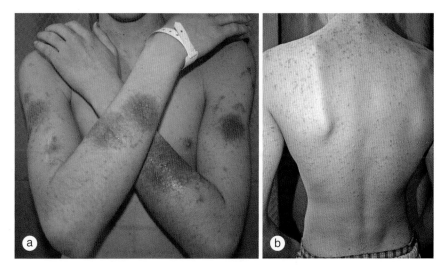

Fig. 3.17 (a) An adolescent boy developed severe poison ivy contact dermatitis on his arms the day after a hike in the woods. **(b)** The next day a widespread, itchy eczematous papular eruption appeared on his trunk and extremities.

was later recognized that these atopic individuals also frequently manifested the itchy, eczematous dermatitis that was labeled atopic dermatitis.

The term *eczema*, which means "boil over," is used by many physicians when referring to atopic dermatitis. However, most dermatologists use the word eczematous as a morphologic term to describe the clinical findings in various sorts of acute (erythema, scaling, vesicles, and crusts) and chronic (scaling, lichenification, and pigmentary changes) dermatitis. Both acute and chronic dermatitis may be present in atopic patients at different sites at the same time and the same site at different times during the course of the disease.

Although data are not precise, recent surveys reveal that atopic dermatitis is rather common with an incidence of 10% among Americans. The prevalence is highest among children, affecting 15–20% of all children between 6 months and 10 years of age. Subtle findings may be present during the first few months of life, and nearly 60% of patients have an initial outbreak by their first birthday. Another third develop disease between 1 and 5 years. The onset of eczema in adolescence and adulthood is unusual and should alert the clinician to the possibility of other diagnoses.

In families with a history of allergic rhinitis or asthma, nearly one-third of the children are expected to develop skin lesions of atopic dermatitis. Inversely, in patients with atopic dermatitis, one-third are expected to have a personal history of allergic rhinitis or asthma, with two-thirds showing a family history of these disorders. Half of those who manifest the dermatologic condition in infancy or childhood ultimately develop allergic respiratory symptoms. Atopic dermatitis appears to be linked to the histocompatibility locus antigen (HLA-DRB1), as has been described in allergic rhinitis. Still, it seems to be inherited as an autosomal trait with multifactorial influences.

Many external factors, which include dry skin, soaps, wool fabrics, foods, infectious agents, and environmental antigens, act in concert to produce pruritus in susceptible individuals. The resultant scratching leads to acute and chronic changes typical of atopic dermatitis.

The pathogenesis of inflammation is unclear, and no single factor has been implicated in the initiation of the inflammatory cascade. However, there is evidence that expansion of type 2 cytokine-secreting lymphocytes plays a major role in the acute phase of atopic dermatitis (Fig. 3.18). This results in increased levels of proinflammatory cytokines such as IL-4, -10, and -13, and of IgE and a corresponding decrease in interferon-gamma. Inflammatory dendritic cells have also been shown to increase in atopic skin, which further fuels inflammation and the itch–scratch cycle.

In a subset of atopics, defects in barrier function may play an initiating role. Mutations in the filaggrin gene are associated

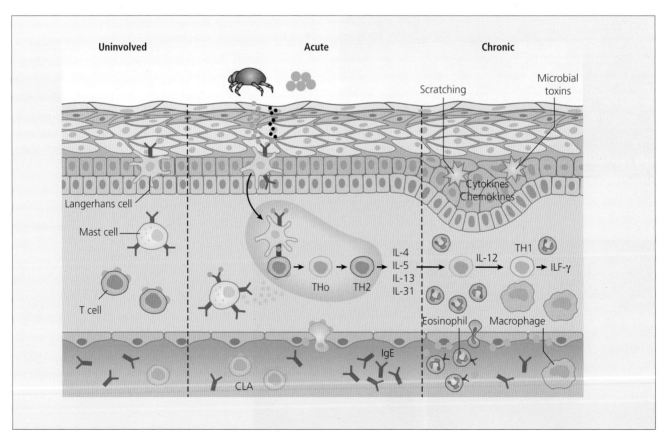

Fig. 3.18 In genetically predisposed individuals, external factors including environmental irritants and allergens, bacteria, fungi, viruses, and foods trigger the differentiation of Th2 lymphocytes from Th0 lymphocytes and the release of acute inflammatory mediators (interleukin (IL)-4, -5, -13, -31). In chronic disease, Th1 lymphocytes are activated and chronic inflammatory mediators are upregulated. *Ig,* Immunoglobulin.

TABLE 3.2 Diagnostic Criteria for Atopic Dermatitis

Major Criteria (All Required for Diagnosis)	Common Findings (At Least Two)	Associated Findings (At Least Four)
Pruritus	Personal or family history of atopy	Ichthyosis, xerosis, hyperlinear palms
Typical morphology and distribution of rash	Immediate skin-test reactivity	Pityriasis alba
	White dermographism	Facial pallor, infraorbital darkening
	Anterior subcapsular cataracts	Dennie–Morgan folds
		Keratoconus
		Hand dermatitis
		Repeated cutaneous infections

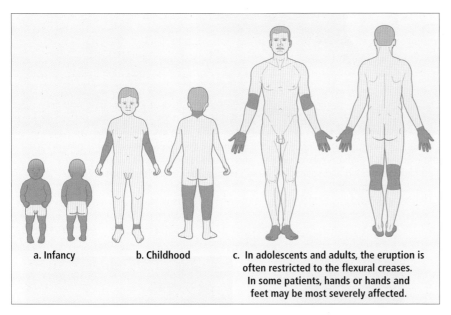

a. Infancy   **b. Childhood**   **c. In adolescents and adults, the eruption is often restricted to the flexural creases. In some patients, hands or hands and feet may be most severely affected.**

Fig. 3.19 Characteristic distribution of lesions of atopic dermatitis in infancy, childhood, and adulthood. **(a)** In infancy, widespread lesions may be generalized, sparing only the diaper area. The head and neck, as well as the flexural and extensor surfaces of the distal extremities, are often severely involved. **(b)** In older childhood, lesions tend to involve the flexural surfaces of the upper and lower extremities, as well as the neck. With severe flares of disease activity, the rash may become more generalized. **(c)** In adolescents and adults, the eruption is often restricted to the flexural creases. In some patients, hands or hands and feet, may be most severely affected.

with the development of ichthyosis vulgaris and barrier dysfunction and an increased risk of developing atopic dermatitis. Predisposition to atopic dermatitis has also been associated with alteration in ceramide content of stratum corneum and disturbed maturation of lamellar bodies, which serve as water-retaining molecules in the barrier.

Although there is no one specific laboratory study or clinical finding in atopic dermatitis, over the years, clinicians and investigators have developed a series of major and minor diagnostic criteria (Table 3.2). In addition to a history of pruritus, the distribution, morphology, and evolution of skin lesions in atopic dermatitis follow a characteristic pattern (Fig. 3.19). The infantile phase begins between shortly after birth and 6 months of age and lasts about 2–3 years. Typically, the rash is composed of red, itchy papules and plaques, many of which ooze and crust. Lesions are symmetrically distributed over the cheeks, forehead, scalp, trunk, and the extensor surfaces of the extremities (Fig. 3.20). The diaper area is usually spared.

The childhood phase of atopic dermatitis occurs between 4 and 10 years of age. Circumscribed, erythematous, scaly, lichenified plaques are symmetrically distributed on the wrists, ankles, and flexural surfaces of the arms and legs (Fig. 3.21). The ear creases and back of the neck are also commonly involved. These areas develop frequent secondary infections, probably as a result of the introduction of organisms by intense

scratching. Although the eruption may become chronic and rarely generalized, remissions may occur at any time. Most children experience improvement during the warm, humid summer months and exacerbations during the fall and winter.

Of children with atopic dermatitis, 75% improve by 10–14 years of age; the remaining individuals may go on to develop chronic adult disease. Major areas of involvement include the flexural creases of the arms, neck, and legs. Chronic dermatitis may be restricted to the hands or feet, but some patients develop recurrent, widespread lesions.

Nummular Eczematous Dermatitis

Although nummular eczematous dermatitis was initially described as distinct from atopic dermatitis, clinicians frequently use this term to describe the discrete, coin-shaped, red patches seen on many patients with atopic dermatitis (Fig. 3.22). Lesions typically appear as tiny papules and vesicles, which form confluent patches on the arms and legs. Nummular lesions may be extremely pruritic, and they are difficult to treat, particularly during the winter months, when the incidence seems to peak.

Prurigo Nodularis

Although chronic rubbing results in lichenification, and scratching in linear excoriations, individuals who pick and gouge at their itchy, irritated skin tend to produce markedly thickened

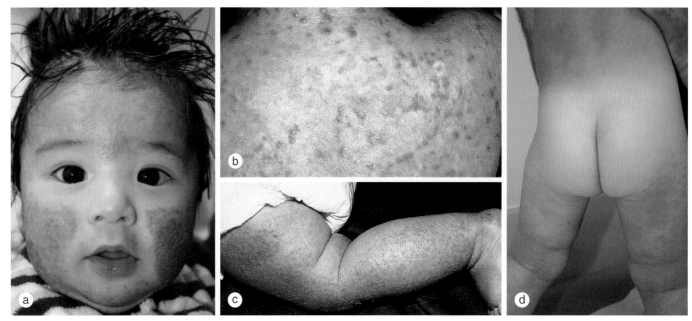

Fig. 3.20 Infantile eczema. **(a)** This infant has an acute, weeping dermatitis on the cheeks and forehead. Involvement of **(b)** the trunk and **(c)** the extremities with erythema, scaling, and crusting is evident. Note the severe involvement of the extensor surfaces of the leg and sparing of the leg crease. **(d)** Usually the diaper area is the only portion of the skin surface that is spared.

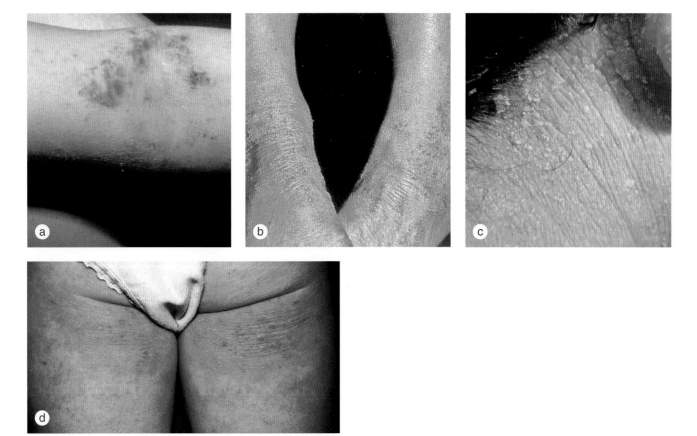

Fig. 3.21 Childhood eczema with lesions on **(a)** the arm, **(b)** the ankles, **(c)** the neck, and **(d)** the buttock creases.

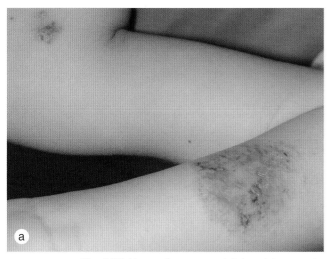
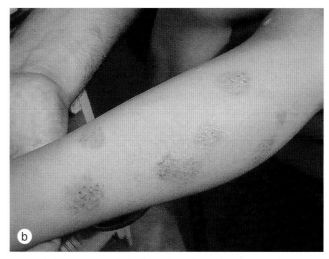

Fig. 3.22 Nummular eczema. **(a)** An adolescent demonstrated the acute exudative round patches of nummular eczema. **(b)** The term nummular eczema is also used to describe the chronic circular patches on the extremities and trunks of atopic patients, exemplified by the patches on another adolescent.

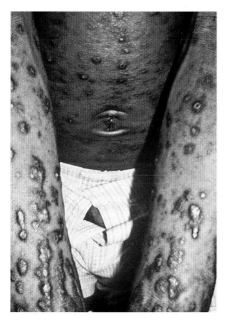

Fig. 3.23 Prurigo nodularis. Widespread lichenified nodules involve the trunk and extremities of an adolescent boy with severe atopic dermatitis. Nodules may be particularly resistant to therapy.

papules known as prurigo nodules (Fig. 3.23). Although prurigo nodularis is not specific to atopic dermatitis, many patients with these nodules also have an atopic diathesis, which manifests as allergic rhinitis, asthma, or food allergy. Frequently, other stigmata of atopic dermatitis are present as well. Prurigo lesions tend to localize to the extremities, although widespread cutaneous involvement is observed in some cases.

Follicular Eczema

Although a few atopic patients present initially with a predominance of follicular papules, virtually all patients develop these 2–4 mm diameter follicular lesions sometime during their clinical course (Fig. 3.24). Lesions are usually widespread on the

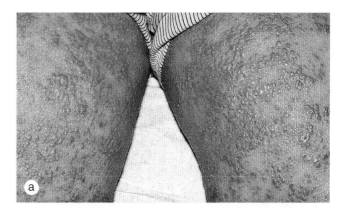
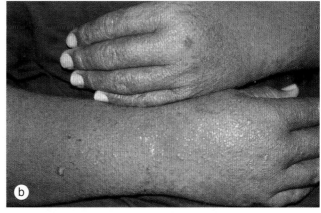

Fig. 3.24 Follicular eczema. In some patients, follicular papules may be the only manifestation of atopic dermatitis. These lesions also occur in many atopic patients during the course of their disease, as in **(a)** this adolescent with follicular papules on his thighs and legs and **(b)** a 10-year-old boy with lesions involving his hands and forearms.

trunk, but careful observation also reveals their presence on the extremities, particularly early in flares of disease activity. In children with chronic disease, discrete papules may be obscured by excoriations and lichenification, particularly in the flexural creases.

Ichthyosis Vulgaris

Although ichthyosis vulgaris (IV) is inherited independently of atopic dermatitis, hyperlinearity of the palms and soles typical of IV is a frequent finding in patients with atopic dermatitis. Moreover, discoveries of the filaggrin loss-of-function mutations causing IV and the prevalence of these defects in atopics have highlighted the potentiation of atopic dermatitis in IV-affected individuals (Fig. 3.25).

IV, which is inherited in an autosomal-dominant pattern with an incidence of 1:250, is associated with a defect in profilaggrin that is converted into filaggrin, the major protein comprising keratohyalin. The severity of IV increases with decreasing levels of functioning filaggrin. Retained polygonal scales are usually evident on the distal lower extremities (see Fig. 2.34), but they may also show a generalized distribution. Xerosis associated with ichthyosis may contribute to the pruritus present in atopic dermatitis.

Keratosis Pilaris

Although keratosis pilaris is often an isolated finding, it is commonly associated with atopic dermatitis and/or IV. Keratosis pilaris results from retention of scales in the follicular infundibulum, which clinically is characterized by horny follicular papules and erythema on the upper arms, medial thighs, and cheeks (Fig. 3.26). Occasionally, more widespread papules appear on the back, buttocks, and legs.

Infraorbital Folds

Often referred to as Dennie–Morgan lines, extra infraorbital folds are suggestive of atopy (Fig. 3.27). In many patients, these

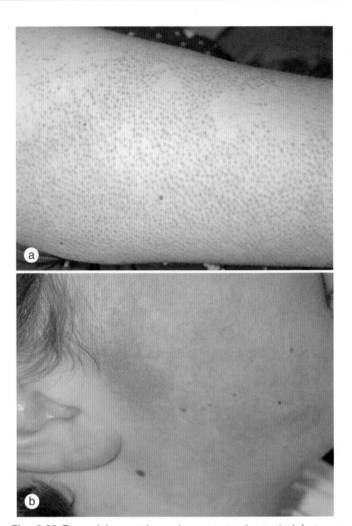

Fig. 3.26 Two adolescent boys demonstrate the typical features of keratosis pilaris with dramatic horny follicular papules on **(a)** the extensor surfaces of the thigh and **(b)** the lateral aspect of the cheek.

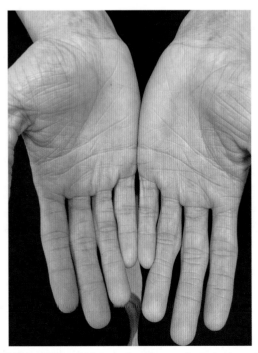

Fig. 3.25 This 14-year-old boy had a history of atopic dermatitis and ichthyosis vulgaris associated with hyperlinearity of the palms and soles and coarse non-inflammatory scale on his legs.

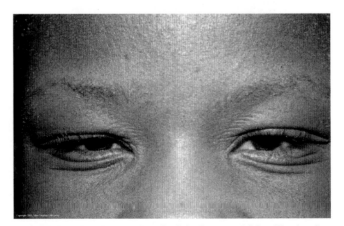

Fig. 3.27 Dennie–Morgan sign. Eyelid edema and lichenification from chronic rubbing resulted in the development of a double infraorbital fold. Although not specific to atopic dermatitis, this feature suggests such a diagnosis when seen in association with other, more pathognomonic findings.

represent current or past local inflammation produced by persistent scratching and rubbing of the tissues. Although not specific for atopic dermatitis, it may be a useful finding when seen in association with other typical physical signs.

Pigmentary Changes

Postinflammatory hypopigmentation and hyperpigmentation occur commonly in atopic patients, especially in the setting of chronic disease (Fig. 3.28). Although pigmentary changes may be quite prominent, this is not always the case; subtle and poorly demarcated areas of hypopigmentation in atopic subjects are referred to as pityriasis alba (Fig. 3.29). Changes are most marked in darkly pigmented individuals or lighter-skinned patients after tanning. The extremities and face are the areas most commonly involved. Although some postinflammatory pigmentary changes persist indefinitely, fading of hypopigmentation and repigmentation of lightened areas usually occur during prolonged remissions.

Hand (and Foot) Dermatitis

Involvement of the hands and feet is common at all ages and may be the only manifestation of atopic dermatitis in adolescents and adults. The rash is commonly triggered by contact irritants. However, in children with recalcitrant dermatitis, a contact allergen should be excluded. Clinical findings include dry, scaly patches

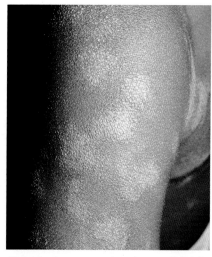

Fig. 3.29 Pityriasis alba. In some atopic patients, subtle inflammation may result in poorly demarcated areas of hypopigmentation, known as pityriasis alba. Lesions are most prominent in darkly pigmented individuals.

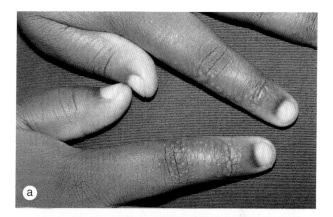

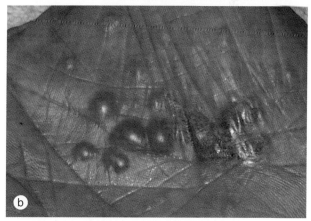

Fig. 3.30 Dyshidrosis. Chronic pruritic deep-seated papules and vesicles recurred on the fingers (a,b) of this atopic 12-year-old boy. He had typical flexural lesions on his arms and legs.

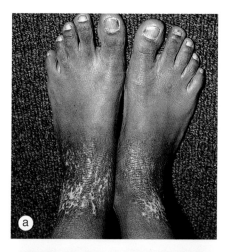

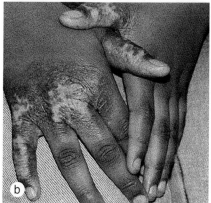

Fig. 3.28 Postinflammatory hypopigmentation and hyperpigmentation associated with lichenification are marked on the (a) ankles and (b) hands of this 9-year-old girl with severe, chronic atopic dermatitis.

on the palms and soles and frequent fissuring of the palms, soles, and digits. The term "dyshidrotic eczema" is reserved for patients with atopic dermatitis who develop intensely pruritic, deep-seated, inflammatory vesicles on the sides of the palms, soles, and/or digits (Fig. 3.30). This is actually an inaccurate name,

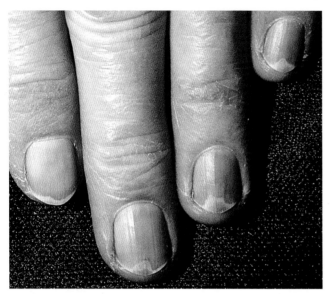

Fig. 3.31 Nail dystrophy. Nail changes, including onycholysis and pitting, can occur when chronic dermatitis affects the fingertips, as in this adolescent.

because histopathology of these lesions demonstrates spongiotic vesicles, typical of an acute dermatitis, and normal sweat glands. Involvement of the paronychial skin may result in separation of the nail from the underlying nail bed (onycholysis), as well as in yellowing and pitting of the nail plate (Fig. 3.31).

Secondary bacterial infection is the most frequent complication of atopic dermatitis. Because it may also trigger an acute exacerbation of clinical disease, early recognition and treatment are mandatory. Crusted, exudative patches suggest superinfection (Fig. 3.32). Although Group A β-hemolytic streptococci are occasionally found in these infected areas, investigators now report a predominance of *Staphylococcus aureus*.

Complications of Atopic Dermatitis

Primary herpes simplex may produce widespread cutaneous and, on rare occasions, disseminated visceral disease in patients with atopic dermatitis. The acute development of multiple, grouped, 2–3 mm diameter vesicles or crusts associated with high fever and worsening pruritus suggests the diagnosis of eczema herpeticum (Fig. 3.33). Tzanck smear, viral culture, double fluorescent antibody, and/or herpes-simplex–specific polymerase chain reaction confirm the diagnosis, and an antiviral agent such as acyclovir or valacyclovir is started immediately.

A number of other organisms, which include human papillomaviruses (warts), the poxvirus that causes molluscum contagiosum, and dermatophytes such as *Trichophyton rubrum*, may produce chronic, recalcitrant infections in atopic patients.

Differential diagnosis. Although the histopathology of affected skin is characteristic (hyperkeratosis, acanthosis, spongiosis, lymphocytic dermal inflammation), skin biopsies are not diagnostic. Atopic dermatitis is a clinical diagnosis. Characteristic pruritic cutaneous findings in a patient with a family history of atopy suggest the disorder.

A number of conditions may mimic the clinical findings of atopic dermatitis. It can be differentiated from infantile seborrheic dermatitis by the distribution of lesions, because atopic dermatitis spares moist, intertriginous areas such as the axilla and perineum, where seborrhea is prominent. Exposure history and distribution help differentiate contact dermatitis, as do the discreteness of lesions, pattern, and lack of symptoms in pityriasis rosea. Thick, silvery scale and the Koebner phenomenon help differentiate psoriasis, and central clearing with an active, scaly, vesiculopustular border helps differentiate tinea corporis. The eruption in Langerhans cell histiocytosis is usually hemorrhagic, often involves skin creases, and is accompanied by chronic draining ears, hepatosplenomegaly, and other systemic findings. An acral distribution of lesions, lack of pruritus, and associated viral symptoms suggest Gianotti–Crosti syndrome.

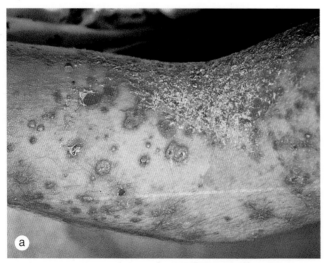
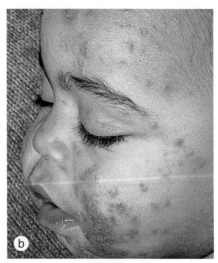

Fig. 3.32 Secondary bacterial infection in atopic dermatitis. **(a)** Bullous impetigo developed in the flexural creases of an 8-year-old child with severe atopic dermatitis. **(b)** This toddler with atopic dermatitis required multiple courses of oral antibiotics for recurrent impetigo of the face.

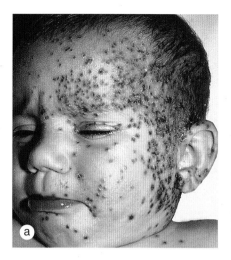
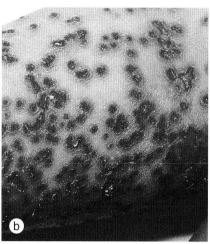

Fig. 3.33 Herpes simplex. Eczema herpeticum, the primary cutaneous manifestation of herpes simplex virus infection in atopic patients, spread rapidly over **(a)** the trunk and face and **(b)** the extremities of this 10-month-old girl. Note the uniform, clustered 2–3 mm diameter vesicles and punched-out vesicles and erosions. A Tzanck smear at the bedside showed multinucleated giant cells, and a positive viral culture confirmed the diagnosis 12 h later.

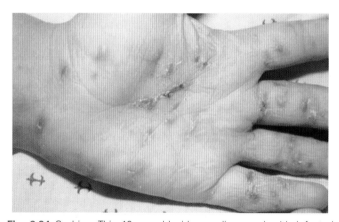

Fig. 3.34 Scabies. This 10-year-old girl was diagnosed with infected eczema. Although she did improve with oral antibiotics, the burrows were readily visible on her palms and wrists, and scrapings from several elongated papulopustules yielded female mites.

Many patients infested with scabies develop a widespread immunologically mediated autoeczematization, which may obscure the burrows. A careful search for the primary lesions on the genitals, wrists, finger web spaces, breasts, and axillae will aid in distinction of this easily treated, sometimes chronic pruritic eruption from atopic dermatitis (Fig. 3.34; see Table 3.2).

Treatment of atopic dermatitis. Therapeutic measures are individualized according to the morphology of the skin lesions, distribution of the rash, and age of the patient. Infants, for instance, may benefit from aggressive efforts to protect their skin from environmental irritants and scratching. Loose-fitting cotton clothing with long sleeves and foot coverings may be optimal.

Although bathing and the use of soaps was once believed to exacerbate atopic dermatitis, increasing evidence contradicts this view. Daily swimming or baths in the summer and on alternating days in winter, followed by liberal application of lubricants, help to cleanse and hydrate the skin. Emollients are tailored to the patient to increase compliance. In general, greasy, occlusive preparations are safest and most effective. However, some patients may prefer less occlusive agents. Mild cleansers may help to reduce bacterial colonization and the risk of secondary infection. Their use should be restricted to areas in which bacteria are most likely to thrive, such as the groin, axilla, and umbilicus. Bleach baths have become popularized for decolonization of the integument.

Low- and medium-potency topical corticosteroids are particularly useful during periods of increased disease activity. Twice-daily applications are restricted to the worst areas and tapered as soon as possible. The skin is monitored for signs of corticosteroid overuse, which include atrophy, loss of pigment, and telangiectasias. High-potency products are reserved for special instances in which severe disease is limited to small patches of thick skin, such as on the hands and feet or for brief courses over large areas as an alternative to oral corticosteroids.

The topical non-steroidal calcineurin inhibitors tacrolimus and pimecrolimus may be highly effective in many atopics. These agents can be used safely on the face, genital area, breasts, and axillae without risk of atrophy or pigmentary alteration. They are also compatible with emollients and topical steroids and are approved for daily short-term use (3 months), as well as long-term, intermittent use (for 1 year or longer). These agents are approved for use in children over 2 years of age, and pharmacologic studies in patients down to 3 months of age show these medications to be comparable in safety and efficacy in younger children. Data from two long-term safety studies sponsored by the manufacturer with the sanction of the FDA should be available within the next 5 years.

Another topical non-steroidal used to treat mild to moderate atopic dermatitis is the phosphodiesterase inhibitor, crisaborole, now approved for use in children as young as 3 months. For children with moderate to severe atopic dermatitis that is not well controlled with topical prescription therapies, systemics, such as methotrexate may often be needed. Dupilumab is the first biologic approved for the treatment of atopic dermatitis in patients 12 years and older. Dupilumab is a fully humanized monoclonal antibody that inhibits IL-4 and IL-13 signaling. These cytokines are the primary drivers of type 2 inflammation in atopic dermatitis. In 2020, the FDA approved dupilumab as an add-on maintenance treatment for children aged 6 to 11 years with moderate to severe atopic dermatitis whose disease is not adequately controlled with topical thera- pies alone. Positive safety and efficacy data in these younger patients will most likely expand its indications in the coming year. Studies for new molecular modulators and biologics are ongoing, and early data for topical and systemic janus kinase (jak) inhibitors are promising.

Although antihistamines may not generally be effective in managing the inflammatory process in atopic dermatitis, they may be useful at bedtime, when itching is the most severe, and their sedative effects may help. However, antihistamines must be used with caution in infants and toddlers, who may develop paradoxic excitation. Tachyphylaxis to a given agent may de- velop after prolonged therapy, and it may be necessary to change the class of antihistamine prescribed. Moreover, there is no evidence that long-active, non-sedating antihistamines are effective in suppressing pruritus.

Secondary bacterial infections are frequently associated with exacerbation and may cause an acute flare of atopic dermatitis. This complication requires prompt intervention. Oral antibiot- ics, such as cephalosporins and semisynthetic penicillins, or al- ternatively, clindamycin and erythromycin, are indicated when infection is evident. If the infection is widespread, parenteral antibiotics may be necessary. Localized patches of impetiginiza- tion may be managed with topical antibiotics, such as mupiro- cin. In severe disseminated infections, appropriate cultures are obtained before initiating antibiotic therapy.

Infection unresponsive to antibacterials raises the specter of eczema herpeticum. Patients with disseminated primary cutane- ous herpes simplex infection also present with acute worsening of their dermatitis and, frequently, mucous membrane involvement, fever, adenopathy, irritability, and decreased appetite. These chil- dren require aggressive, symptomatic treatment and immediate parenteral antiviral therapy (acyclovir 15 mg/kg per day in three divided doses). Unfortunately, oral acyclovir is not well absorbed in children. However, the antiviral medications, famciclovir and valacyclovir hydrochloride, are readily bioavailable when taken orally. A special syrup formulation of valacyclovir is available at many pharmacies:

Valacyclovir oral suspension (50 mg/ml). *Ingredients*: Vala- cyclovir caplets 500 mg #9, Ora-Plus 45 ml, Ora-Sweet qs 90 ml. *Directions*: (1) Crush caplets bring in a mortar, and add 5 ml sterile water. (2) Mix together into smooth paste. (3) Add Ora- Plus in small increments. (4) QS to 90 ml with Ora-Sweet. (5) Shake well, and refrigerate (expiration 21 days).

During acute flares with vesicle and crust formation, appli- cation of tepid tap water compresses three times a day for 15–20 min, topical lubricants, such as petrolatum, Eucerin cream, Aquaphor and Acid Mantle cream, and oral antibiotics should result in rapid improvement. In chronic disease, liberal use of emollients, judicious use of low- and medium-potency topical corticosteroid ointments twice daily, antihistamines, and avoid- ance of environmental irritants may bring symptomatic relief.

The soak and smear technique with bathing or compressing followed by the application of emollients, plastic wrap occlusion, and long underwear or other occlusive garments to strategic ar- eas, particularly at bedtime, may also help to shut down flares and heal chronic skin changes. In selected children with severe

recalcitrant long-standing disease, there may be a role for photo- therapy (e.g. UVB, PUVA) and oral immunosuppressive anti- inflammatory medications (e.g. cyclosporine, methotrexate).

Most patients with chronic atopic dermatitis are troubled by the effect of the rash on their physical appearance. Therefore, emotional support and psychologic counseling may be helpful adjuncts in the care of these patients. Behavioral feedback and counseling can also be used to help patients and their parents manage chronic pruritus.

Seborrheic Dermatitis

Seborrheic dermatitis is characterized by a symmetric, red, scal- ing eruption, which occurs predominantly on the hair-bearing, intertriginous areas. Affected sites include the scalp, eyebrows, eyelashes, perinasal, presternal, and postauricular areas, as well as the neck, axilla, and groin. In affected infants, scalp lesions consist of a greasy, salmon-colored, scaly dermatitis called cra- dle cap (see Fig. 2.38d). A severe type may be more generalized. In adolescents, the dermatitis may manifest as dandruff or flak- ing of the eyebrows, postauricular areas, nasolabial folds, and/ or flexural areas (Fig. 3.35). When the patches on the face are well defined, they may form a petaloid pattern (Fig. 3.35a). Occasionally, non-inflammatory scale reminiscent of infantile cradle cap develops in the scalp of older children and adoles- cents. Tinea (pityriasis) amiantacea probably represents a vari- ant of scalp seborrheic dermatitis in older children, consisting of thick tenacious localized plaques of sticky scale that bind down tufts of hair (Fig. 3.35b).

Although the pathogenesis of seborrheic dermatitis is un- known, *Malassezia (Pityrosporum)* and *Candida* species have been implicated as causative agents. A role for neurologic dys- function is suggested by the increased incidence and severity in neurologically impaired individuals. Immunodeficiency states, particularly acquired immunodeficiency syndrome, in which 20–80% of individuals are affected, may also be associated with severe atypical clinical manifestations.

The dermatitis of seborrhea is usually subtle and non- pruritic. Most cases respond to low-potency topical corticoste- roids, but it may also clear spontaneously. Antiseborrheic shampoos that contain pyrithione zinc, selenium, or salicylic acid may help. Ketoconazole and ciclopirox shampoo and cream have also been approved for the treatment of seborrhea. Secondary bacterial infection with Group A β-hemolytic strep- tococcus and/or *Staphylococcus aureus* occurs commonly in the neck, axillary, and groin creases in infants and should be cul- tured and treated with appropriate topical or oral antibiotics.

In infants and young children, atopic dermatitis, Langerhans cell histiocytosis, acrodermatitis enteropathica, or psoriasis may be confused with seborrheic dermatitis. However, atopic dermatitis in infants invariably spares protected moist sites, such as the diaper area and axilla, and produces intense pruri- tus. The distribution of rash in Langerhans cell histiocytosis may resemble seborrheic dermatitis. However, the presence of purpura, poor growth, diarrhea, and other systemic complaints would be unusual for uncomplicated seborrheic dermatitis. Erosive patches in a seborrheic distribution associated with poor growth, diarrhea, irritability, and hair loss suggest the

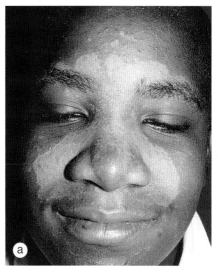
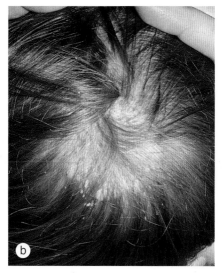
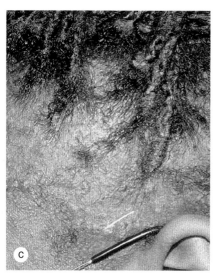

Fig. 3.35 Seborrheic dermatitis. **(a)** A 12-year-old boy developed scaly, pink, hypopigmented patches on the face in a petaloid pattern, while **(b)** a 10-year-old boy demonstrates the thick adherent scale typical of tinea amiantacea. **(c)** Note the confluent red scaly patches on the scalp and forehead of this 15-year-old girl.

diagnosis of acrodermatitis enteropathica or other nutritional deficiencies. Finally, persistent diaper dermatitis and cradle cap may be difficult to differentiate from psoriasis even with a skin biopsy because of overlapping histologic features.

Juvenile Palmar-Plantar Dermatosis

Also known as sweaty sock syndrome, juvenile palmar-plantar dermatosis is seen commonly in toddlers and children of school age. Chronic pink, scaly patches with cracking and fissuring begin in the fall or winter on the anterior plantar surfaces of the feet and great toes, resulting in a shiny, glazed appearance (Fig. 3.36). Occasionally, patches spread to the other toes and

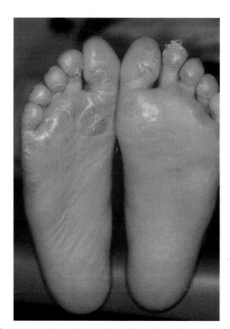

Fig. 3.36 Sweaty sock syndrome (juvenile palmar-plantar dermatosis) was evident on the weight-bearing surfaces of the toes and soles of this healthy 8-year-old boy. The rash resolved with aggressive use of lubricants alone.

hands. Although the cause is unknown, excessive sweating and/or the repeated cycle of wetting of the skin during the day while shoes are worn and drying of the skin at night may trigger the condition. Consequently, treatment consists of lubrication and covering the feet at night. Topical corticosteroids may be necessary in severe cases. The eruption tends to subside in the summer, and resolution in adolescence is common. Children with atopic dermatitis may be particularly prone to develop this dermatosis.

Allergic contact dermatitis differs from sweaty sock syndrome by the tendency for involvement of the dorsum of the hands and feet. Tinea pedis usually presents on the instep and interdigital web spaces. Chronic atopic dermatitis may be difficult to differentiate from sweaty sock syndrome unless other stigmata of atopy are present.

Perioral/Periorificial Dermatitis

In the simplest form, perioral dermatitis represents a contact dermatitis from repeated wetting and drying of the skin associated with persistent lip-licking or thumb-sucking, especially during the winter months. Elements of both acute and chronic dermatitis closely encircle the mouth and may involve the vermilion border (Fig. 3.37).

Some children develop asymptomatic red papules, pustules, and nodules on either a normal-appearing or red, scaly base on the chin and nasolabial folds, referred to as periorificial granulomatous dermatitis (Fig. 3.38a,b). Lesions may extend to the cheeks, eyelids, and forehead. Although initially reported in association with the use of fluorinated topical corticosteroids on the face, this type of perioral dermatitis occurs more frequently in children with no history of topical agents. It has also been described most commonly in black school-age boys (Fig. 3.38c). Some immunocompromised patients may develop a rosacea-like facial eruption indistinguishable from periorificial dermatitis and attributed to a hypersensitivity reaction to *Demodex* mites on the face.

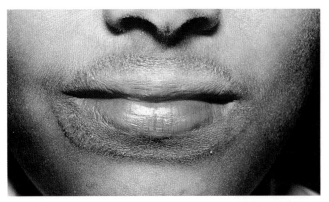

Fig. 3.37 Lip-licker's contact dermatitis recurred every winter in this teen-age boy. Involvement was always restricted to the lips and contiguous skin.

Interestingly, histopathology demonstrates features of dermatitis, folliculitis, and occasionally granulomatous inflammation consistent with rosacea or sarcoidosis. However, affected children are usually otherwise healthy, and the rash improves with oral antibiotics such as erythromycin and tetracycline (for children over 8 years old). Topical antibiotics, calcineurin

inhibitors, benzoyl peroxide, vitamin A acid, and other keratolytics may also be useful. Topical corticosteroids are used with extreme caution because of the risk of precipitating a superimposed folliculitis, telangiectasias, and atrophy, particularly with long-term exposure.

Pityriasis Rosea

Pityriasis rosea (PR) is an innocent, self-limited disorder that can occur at any age, but it is more common in school-age children and young adults. A prodrome of malaise, headache, and mild constitutional symptoms occasionally precedes the rash. In about half of the cases, the eruption begins with the appearance of a "herald patch" (Fig. 3.39a). This 3–5 cm diameter, isolated, oval, scaly, pink patch may appear anywhere on the body surface, although it occurs most commonly on the trunk and thighs. Central clearing produces a lesion that commonly simulates tinea corporis. Within 1–2 weeks, numerous smaller lesions appear on the body, usually concentrated on the trunk and proximal extremities (Fig. 3.39b–d). These begin as small, round papules, which enlarge to form 1–2 cm diameter oval patches with dusky centers and scaly borders. The long axes of the patches often run parallel to the skin lines over the thorax

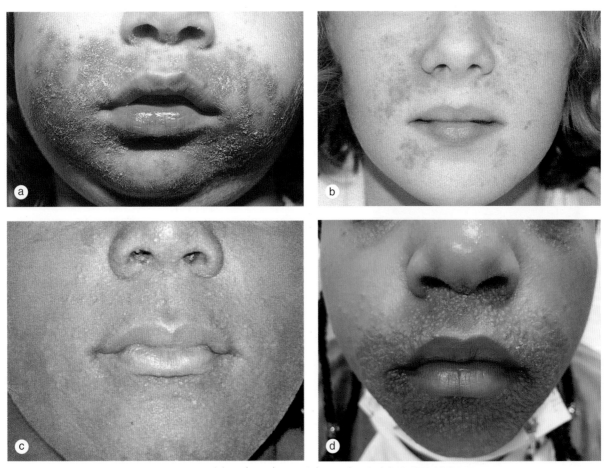

Fig. 3.38 Perioral dermatitis with bright-red papules, pustules, and scale **(a)** erupted on the cheeks, chin, upper lip, and nose of this 4-year-old boy. **(b)** Note the perioral sparing in this 10-year-old girl. The rash vanished after 4 weeks of treatment with oral erythromycin and non-comedogenic moisturizers. **(c)** The perioral dermatitis in this adolescent failed to respond to topical and oral agents but resolved after 6 weeks of oral tetracycline. **(d)** A 7-year-old girl developed uniform, red, edematous papules around the eyes, nose, and mouth with sparing of the vermillion border that failed to improve with topical and oral steroids. Lesions cleared with oral erythromycin.

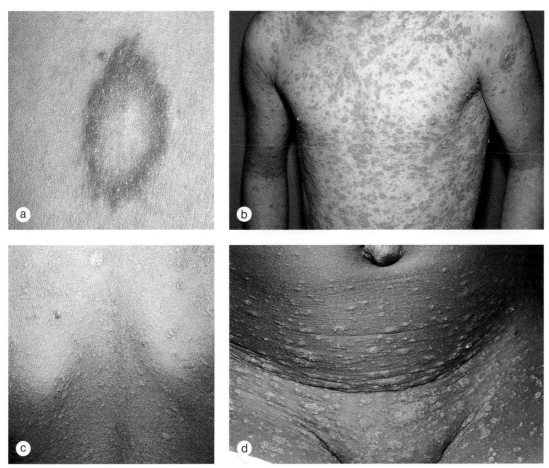

Fig. 3.39 Pityriasis rosea. **(a)** The large herald patch on the chest of this 10-year-old girl shows central clearing, which mimics tinea corporis. **(b)** Numerous oval lesions on the chest of a white teenager. **(c)** Note the Christmas-tree pattern on the back of a black adolescent. **(d)** Small, papular lesions, as well as larger scaly patches, were most prominent on the abdomen and thighs of this 5-year-old girl.

and back, to create a "Christmas-tree" pattern. Occasionally, PR spreads to involve much of the skin surface, including the face and distal extremities. Inflammation may be so intense that some blistering and hemorrhage become clinically apparent. The rash reaches a peak in several weeks and slowly fades over 6–12 weeks.

Although the cause of PR has not been established, the frequent reporting of a viral-like prodrome, clustering of cases, occasional occurrence among close contacts, and peak incidence in winter and early spring suggest a viral etiology. Several investigators have detected DNA sequences for human herpesvirus 6 and human herpesvirus 7 in patients with PR. PR-like eruptions have also been reported in association with acute infection with *Mycoplasma pneumoniae* and enteroviruses. However, in most case studies, no infectious agents have been identified.

UV light and oral erythromycin may hasten the disappearance of the eruption. However, postinflammatory hyperpigmentation, particularly in dark-complected individuals, may persist for months. Phototherapy can also be used to camouflage these distressing pigmentary changes.

Other eruptions that can resemble PR include guttate psoriasis, viral exanthems (particularly some cases of Gianotti–Crosti syndrome), secondary syphilis (Fig. 3.40), and drug reactions (gold salts, bismuth, clonidine, penicillamine, isotretinoin, metronidazole, ACE inhibitors). The herald patch may suggest tinea, but fungus can be excluded by a negative potassium hydroxide (KOH) preparation and fungal culture.

Pityriasis Lichenoides

Pityriasis lichenoides includes a group of self-limited disorders with a spectrum of clinical presentations from the acute, papulonecrotic eruption of pityriasis lichenoides et varioliformis acuta ([PLEVA], Mucha–Habermann disease) to the chronic dermatitic papules of pityriasis lichenoides chronica (PLC). Although most common in older children and young adults, pityriasis lichenoides may occasionally occur in infants and young children, with a slight predominance in boys.

Acute forms usually begin with the sudden onset of 2–4 mm diameter red macules and papules, which evolve over several days into vesicular, necrotic, and eroded lesions (Fig. 3.41). Healing occurs within several weeks with postinflammatory pigmentary changes and occasionally chickenpox-like scars. Although the rash is usually asymptomatic and has a predilection for the trunk, pruritus may be intense, and lesions may spread to involve the neck, face, and extremities, which include the palms and soles. Fever and other mild constitutional symptoms may

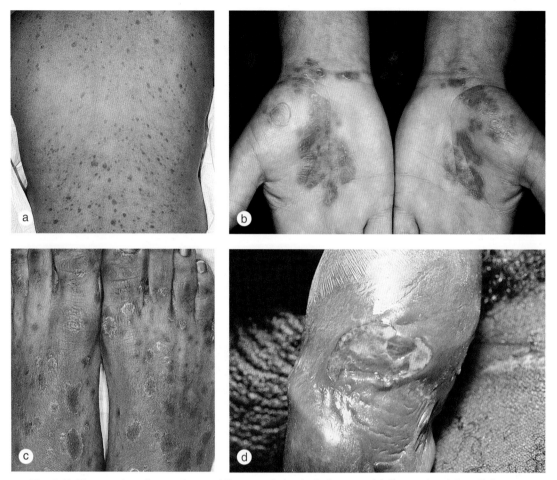

Fig. 3.40 The eruption of secondary syphilis may mimic pityriasis rosea. **(a)** A truncal rash in a Christmas-tree pattern on this adolescent resolved after treatment with intramuscular penicillin. Her Venereal Disease Research Laboratory titer was 1:2056. Hyperkeratotic "copper penny" papules, which are distinctive for syphilis, are seen on **(b)** the palms and **(c)** the tops of the feet of adolescents. These also resolved quickly with antibiotics. **(d)** A painless chancre developed on the penile shaft of a teenage boy with primary syphilis.

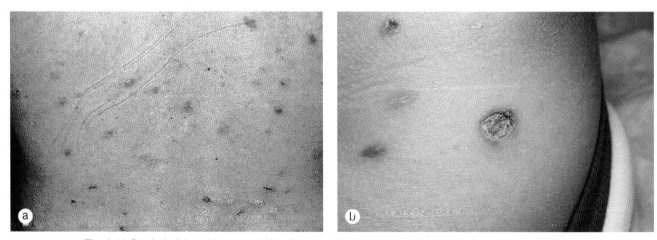

Fig. 3.41 Pityriasis lichenoides et varioliformis acuta. **(a)** Asymptomatic hemorrhagic papules erupted in a pityriasis rosea-like pattern on the trunk and proximal extremities of this 15-year-old boy. **(b)** Recurrent papulonecrotic lesions continued to evolve on the trunk of this 5-year-old for over a year.

precede or accompany the acute phase. The eruption appears in successive crops, which settle down over weeks to months. Relapses and remissions occur episodically, but after several months, most patients develop the more subtle lesions of PLC.

In PLC, which may also appear *de novo*, the typical rash consists of round 2–10 mm diameter, reddish-brown papules that develop a shiny brown scale adherent at the center (Fig. 3.42). Episodic crops of papules heal over several weeks, with pigmentary changes but no evidence of scarring. In fact, postinflammatory pigmentary changes may be the first findings to bring attention to the rash (Fig. 3.43). Although the eruption is self-limiting and usually heals without scarring, it may evolve for 5–10 years.

Although the cause is unknown, the detection of monoclonal T-cell populations in the inflammatory infiltrate in some cases of acute and chronic pityriasis lichenoides suggests a benign, self-limited lymphoproliferative process.

The histopathology of skin biopsies is distinctive, but not diagnostic. In the mild form, minimal dermatitic changes are seen, with spongiosis and parakeratosis. A mild, chronic, perivascular infiltrate is found in the dermis associated with some hemorrhage and pigment incontinence. In acute disease, the inflammation may be intense and extend down into the deep dermis and up into the epidermis. Dyskeratosis is usually marked, and necrosis of the epidermis may occur with the formation of erosions. Endothelial cell swelling is marked, and vascular necrosis may occur. Hemorrhage is seen in the dermis and epidermis.

Although most children do well without treatment, phototherapy with UVB, PUVA, or natural sunlight may be useful in persistently symptomatic individuals. There may also be a role for oral antibiotics, such as erythromycin or tetracyclines. However, the use of systemic corticosteroids and methotrexate does not seem warranted except in rare patients with destructive, painful, or scarring disease.

At the onset, PLEVA may be mistaken for varicella. However, the lack of symptoms or mucous membrane lesions and the subsequent chronic course help to exclude chicken pox. Lymphomatoid papulosis is a chronic, benign, self-limiting disorder that is often clinically indistinguishable from PLEVA. However, the histopathology is characterized by an atypical lymphohistiocytic infiltrate, suggestive of lymphoma. In some children and adults, a lymphomatoid papulosis-like eruption rarely occurs as a presenting picture for systemic lymphoma. Cutaneous vasculitis, impetigo, insect bites, and scabies are also considered during the acute phase.

The only differentiation between PLC and PR is the extremely protracted course. In pityriasis alba, the borders of the patches are indistinct and other stigmata of atopy are usually present. Patch-stage mycosis fungoides, a cutaneous T-cell lymphoma, may begin with subtle, scaly, hypopigmented or hyperpigmented patches that mimic PLC (Fig. 3.44). Consequently,

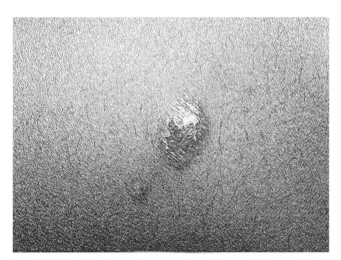

Fig. 3.42 Pityriasis lichenoides chronica. A few diffusely scattered, shiny, hyperpigmented papules continued to appear for years in this 11-year-old boy. Note the central adherent scale.

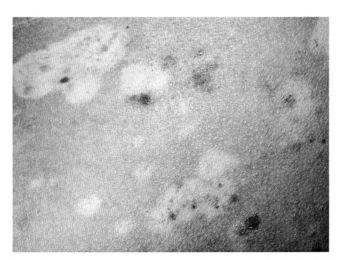

Fig. 3.43 Postinflammatory hyperpigmentation was severe in this child with generalized pityriasis lichenoides et varioliformis acuta. Fortunately, the pigmentary changes healed over several months as his disease evolved into the more indolent pityriasis lichenoides chronica.

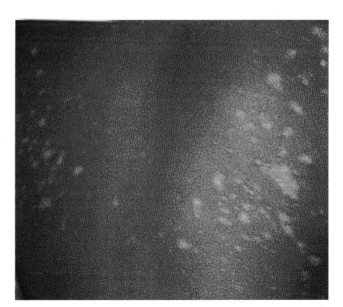

Fig. 3.44 A 10-year-old child had asymptomatic, hypopigmented, minimally scaly oval patches on his trunk for several years. A skin biopsy demonstrated atypical, dermal, lymphocytic inflammation with extension into the epidermis characteristic of cutaneous T-cell lymphoma.

any child with a long-standing rash suggestive of PLC must have a skin biopsy to exclude lymphoma. Parents are counseled regarding the chronic but innocent course of this disorder.

LICHENOID DERMATOSES

Lichen Planus

Lichen planus (LP) is a distinctive dermatosis characterized by pruritic, purple, polygonal papules (the "4-p sign") that involve the flexures of the arms and legs, mucous membranes, genitals, nails, and scalp (Fig. 3.45). The eruption in LP typically demonstrates the Koebner or isomorphic phenomenon, in which cutaneous lesions appear to extend in areas of trauma (scratches, excoriations, burns, scars). Only 2% of cases present before 20 years of age; however, patients with the familial variant develop LP in childhood. Some investigators have found an increased prevalence in African American children compared with Caucasian children. Although the cause of LP is unknown, complement and immunoglobulin depositions along the basement membrane zone suggest an immunologic mechanism.

Typically, itchy, violaceous 3–6 mm diameter papules appear abruptly on the wrists, ankles, and/or genitals. Lesions may spread over the forearms, shins, and lower back. Rarely, widespread rash covers much of the body surface. In areas of involvement, contiguous, shiny-topped papules may form a

white, lacy, reticulated network known as Wickham striae. Their visibility may be enhanced by the application of a small quantity of mineral oil and examination with side lighting and a hand lens. Confluent lesions may form annular or linear plaques. Intense, dermal inflammation may be associated with the development of vesiculobullous lesions, and hypertrophic, verrucous plaques may evolve, particularly on the shins, in chronic disease (Fig. 3.46). In some reported series, the incidence of thick hypertrophic pruritic plaques on the legs, particularly the shins, may approach 25%.

Wickham striae may also be present on the buccal mucosa, gingivae, lips, and tongue. Mucous membrane findings, which are present in two-thirds of patients with LP, also include erythema, white papules that resemble leukoplakia, vesicles, erosions, and deep, painful ulcerations.

Also, LP may present with follicular papules, particularly in the scalp where cicatricial alopecia may be progressive. Nail involvement, seen in about 10% of patients, includes brittleness, thinning, fragmentation, longitudinal ridging or striations, and partial or complete shedding of the nail. Pterygium formation, atrophy, subungual hyperkeratosis, and lifting of the distal nail plate may also occur (see Fig. 8.60). Rarely, nail disease appears without cutaneous involvement.

Skin biopsies characteristically demonstrate hyperkeratosis, focal thickening of the granular layer, irregular acanthosis, and

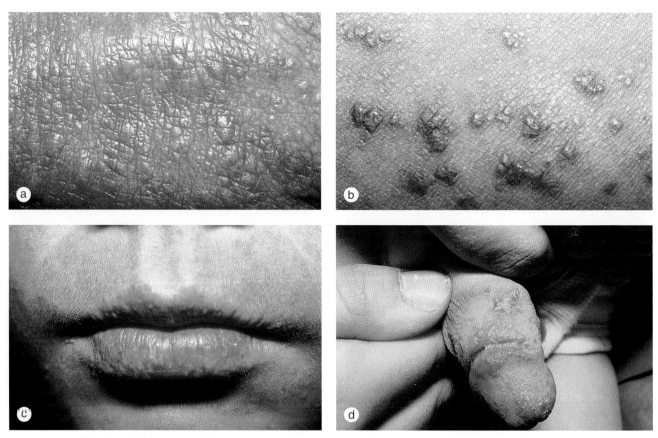

Fig. 3.45 Lichen planus. **(a)** Violaceous, polygonal papules almost to confluence appeared over several weeks on the dorsum of the hands and feet, ankles, and wrists of this 16-year-old boy. **(b)** Lesions are somewhat hyperpigmented on the forearm of this black adolescent. **(c, d)** White papules formed Wickham striae on the lips of this child, who also had typical papules on the penis.

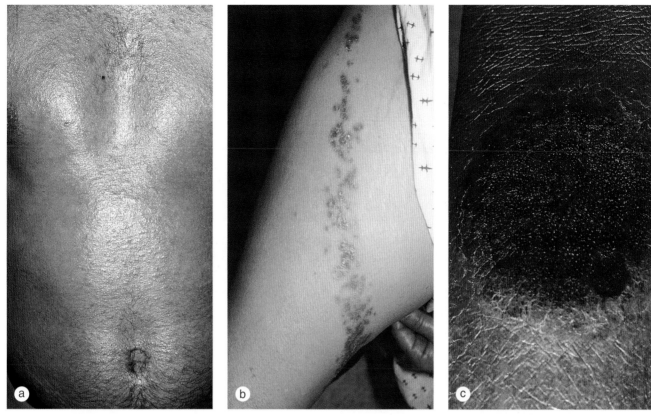

Fig. 3.46 Lichen planus variants. **(a)** Diffuse, eruptive lichen planus responded to treatment with psoralen ultraviolet A. Over 90% of this boy's body was involved with confluent papules on the trunk and extremities. **(b)** This asymptomatic, linear plaque progressed slowly for over a year. **(c)** Extremely pruritic, hypertrophic plaques were present on the shins of this 18-year-old girl.

a band-like or interface infiltrate of lymphocytes and histiocytes in the dermis, close to the epidermis, and associated with damage to the basal cell layer.

Although the cause is unknown, cell-mediated immunologic reactions are probably important in the pathogenesis of disease. This is supported by a predominance of CD4+ and CD8+ T-cells in the inflammatory infiltrate. Moreover, some patients with graft-vs-host disease and drug reactions associated with T-cell dysregulation have developed eruptions clinically indistinguishable from LP.

The presence of eosinophils in the dermal infiltrate suggests the possibility of a drug reaction. Prurigo nodules in eczema may be associated with other stigmata of atopic dermatitis, and the lesions of discoid lupus erythematosus usually demonstrate atrophy. Nail disease must be differentiated from other causes of nail dystrophy, and oral LP may mimic viral infection, primary blistering dermatoses, erythema multiforme, and leukoplakia.

Although many cases resolve within 1–2 years, some eruptions persist for 10–20 years. Localized lesions often respond well to topical corticosteroids. Oral LP may be resistant to treatment, and some success has been achieved with topical retinoic acid, topical tacrolimus ointment, intralesional corticosteroids, oral retinoids, oral corticosteroids, and swish-and-spit cyclosporine or tacrolimus. Although quite painful, intralesional corticosteroids are also useful in the treatment of nail disease.

Patients with generalized LP have been treated with systemic corticosteroids and retinoids. However, therapeutic benefits must be weighed against the long-term consequences of these medications. In fact, PUVA may provide a relatively safe alternative for disseminated disease.

Lichen Nitidus

Lichen nitidus, an uncommon, chronic, asymptomatic eruption, is characterized by flat-topped, flesh-colored 2–3 mm diameter monomorphic papules that demonstrate the isomorphic phenomenon (Fig. 3.47). Although many practitioners consider lichen nitidus to be a variant of LP, the peak incidence in children between 7 and 13 years, the uniformly tiny lesions (which do not have a tendency to coalesce), and the lack of pruritus establish this disorder as a distinct entity. The rash progresses slowly over months to years, with a predilection for the arms, abdomen, and genitals. The majority of patients are males with darker skin types (Fitzpatrick skin types IV–VI).

Skin biopsies demonstrate findings reminiscent of LP but are restricted to only one or a few papillae. The overlying horny layer exhibits parakeratosis, and at the lateral margin of the lesion, the rete ridges extend downward to form a claw around the underlying infiltrate.

Papular or follicular eczema may be differentiated from lichen nitidus by the presence of pruritus and other markers of atopy.

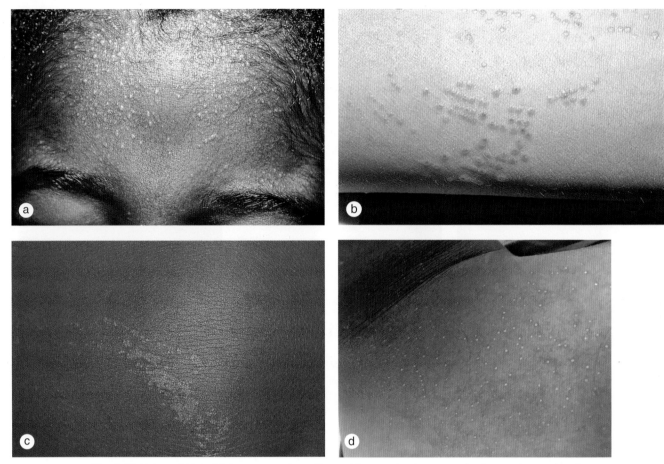

Fig. 3.47 Lichen nitidus. **(a)** Asymptomatic, uniform, shiny papules began on the face and spread to the trunk and extremities of this 6-year-old boy. **(b)** Note the Koebner phenomenon on the arm of this 6-year-old girl after incidental scratching. **(c)** Typical lesions developed on the knees of this healthy 4-year-old boy. **(d)** Asymptomatic lichenoid papules developed on the upper trunk of this 7-year-old boy and spread to the left arm.

Keratosis pilaris usually shows some scale and appears in characteristic locations and is inherited as an autosomal-dominant trait. Examination of flat warts with side lighting and magnification and dermoscopy usually reveals a rough surface, unlike the smooth, shiny surface of papules in lichen nitidus. However, both lichen nitidus and flat warts can develop a Koebner phenomenon, and a skin biopsy may be necessary to differentiate them.

Lichen Striatus

Lichen striatus is a linear, lichenoid eruption that appears most commonly in children of school age. Flat-topped papules arise suddenly in unilateral streaks and swirls conforming to the lines of Blaschko, usually on the extremities, upper back, or neck. However, any area, including the palms, soles, nails, genitals, and face, may become involved (Fig. 3.48). Lesions usually develop some overlying dusty scale and mild erythema. Hypopigmentation may bring attention to the eruption, especially in dark-skinned children.

Lichen striatus usually fades without treatment in 1–2 years. Lubricants and topical corticosteroids may be useful to decrease scale and inflammation in cosmetically important areas. There are also reports of successful treatment with topical tacrolimus ointment.

Although the cause is unclear, the development of lesions along the lines of Blaschko suggests that the cutaneous defect may result from a somatic mutation that arises embryologically. Expression of the aberrant clone may be triggered by an environmental insult such as a viral infection or trauma. The ensuing inflammation results in clinical lesions with a predominance of CD8+ T-cells, and resolution occurs with elimination of the abnormal keratinocyte clone. A similar process may explain linear LP and linear graft-vs-host disease.

This condition can also be mistaken for linear epidermal nevi, linear porokeratosis, flat warts, linear psoriasis, and linear ichthyotic eruptions. When the clinical course is confusing, a skin biopsy helps differentiate these disorders. Lichen striatus usually demonstrates dermatitic changes in the epidermis, with a lymphocytic perivascular infiltrate in the superficial and mid-dermis that frequently extends into the deep dermis.

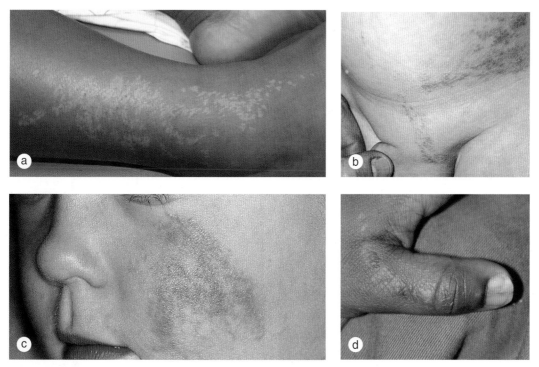

Fig. 3.48 Lichen striatus. Asymptomatic, scaly, hypopigmented to pink papules in a linear pattern appeared on the **(a)** leg, **(b)** abdomen and scrotum, **(c)** left cheek, **(d)** and right hand of healthy children. Histology revealed changes typical of lichen striatus, and all lesions healed without treatment in 6–24 months. Note the nail dystrophy on the involved thumbnail.

FUNGAL INFECTIONS

Tinea

Two types of fungal organisms, dermatophytes and yeasts, produce clinical cutaneous disease. Dermatophytes include tinea or ringworm fungi, which infect skin, nails, and hair (see Chapter 8). Although *Candida* and *Pityrosporum* yeast infections usually involve the skin, *Candida* can infect mucous membranes and rarely disseminates to viscera in vulnerable immunocompromised patients.

Tinea Corporis

This is a superficial fungal infection of non-hairy or glabrous skin. It has been called *tinea* (Latin for intestinal worm) or "ringworm" because of its characteristic configuration, which consists of pruritic annular plaques with central clearing or scale and an active, indurated, and/or vesiculopustular, worm-like border (Fig. 3.49). Lesions, which may be single or multiple, typically begin as red papules or pustules that expand over days to weeks to form 1–5 cm diameter plaques. Tinea corporis can be found in any age group and is usually acquired from an infected domestic animal (*Microsporum canis*) or through direct human contact (*Trichophyton*, *Microsporum*, and *Epidermophyton* species).

Clinically, tinea may be differentiated from atopic dermatitis by its propensity for autoinoculation from the primary patches to other sites on the patient's skin, by spread to close contacts, and by the central clearing noted in many lesions. Moreover, the rash of atopic dermatitis tends to be symmetric, chronic, and

recurrent in a flexural distribution. Unlike tinea, patches of nummular eczema are self-limited and do not clear centrally. The herald patch of PR is often mistaken for tinea. However, scrapings obtained for KOH preparation are negative, and subsequent development of the generalized rash with its characteristic truncal distribution is distinctive. The clinical patterns, associated findings, and chronicity help differentiate psoriasis and seborrhea from tinea. Granuloma annulare produces a characteristic ringed plaque. However, on palpation, the lesions are firm and do not have epidermal changes (scales, vesicles, pustules). Granuloma annulare is also asymptomatic.

The diagnosis of tinea is confirmed by sending scrapings of scale, nail, or hair for fungal culture. However, a bedside KOH examination of the skin (see Fig. 1.6) can be fun and may yield a rapid result. The first step is to obtain material by scraping the loose scales, vesicles, and pustules at the margin of a lesion. These are mounted on the center of a glass slide, and 1 or 2 drops of 20% KOH are added. Next, a glass coverslip is applied and gently pressed down with a fingertip or the eraser end of a pencil to crush the scales. The slide can then be heated gently, taking care not to boil the KOH solution, and, again, the coverslip is pressed down. The slide is placed under a microscope, with the condenser and light at low levels to maximize contrast, and with the objective at low power. On focusing up and down, true hyphae are seen as long, greenish, hyaline, branching, and often septate rods of uniform width that cross the borders of epidermal cells. Cotton fibers, cell borders, or other artifacts may be falsely interpreted as positive findings.

Tinea infections on glabrous skin respond readily to topical antifungal creams or lotions (imidazoles such as clotrimazole, econazole, miconazole, ketoconazole, sulconazole, oxiconazole; the allylamines naftifine and terbinafine; ciclopirox olamine; tolnaftate). When lesions are multiple and widespread, oral therapy with griseofulvin, itraconazole, terbinafine, or fluconazole is indicated.

Although topical steroids may be used in combination with topical or oral antifungal agents for short periods of time to suppress severe inflammation and resultant pruritus, prolonged use of steroids may delay proper diagnosis or result in premature discontinuation of antifungal therapy. Ringworm skin lesions suppressed by steroids are referred to as tinea incognito (Fig. 3.50).

Tinea Pedis

Commonly referred to as athlete's foot, tinea pedis is a fungal infection of the feet with a predilection for web space involvement (Fig. 3.51). It is common in adolescence, but somewhat less so in prepubertal children. The infecting organisms are probably acquired from contaminated showers, bathrooms, and locker room and gym floors, and their growth is fostered by the warm, moist environment of shoes.

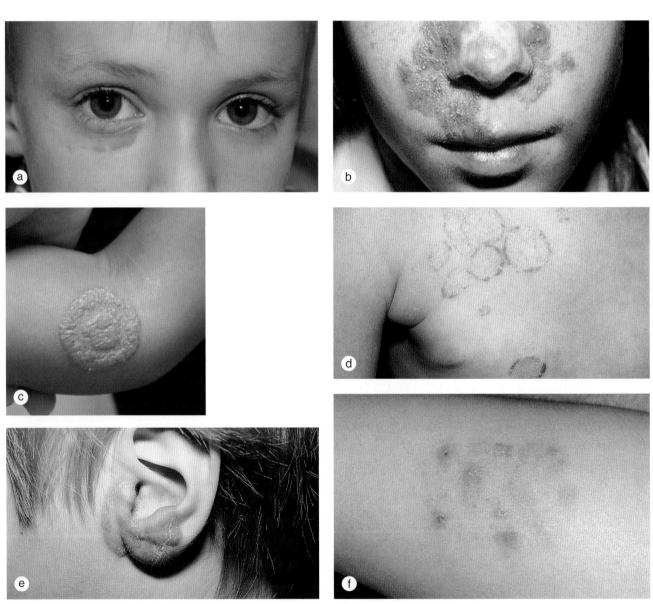

Fig. 3.49 Tinea corporis. The characteristic annular lesions show many variations in appearance. **(a)** This lesion has a raised active border and shows some central clearing and scale. **(b)** Sharply circumscribed tinea faciei demonstrates erythema, scale, and pustule formation throughout the expanding plaque. **(c)** Inflammatory tinea, or kerion, on the arm has marked edema and vesiculation. **(d)** Multiple expanding lesions spread quickly on a toddler who acquired infection from the family kitten. **(e)** This child had an itchy isolated expanding plaque on the ear. **(f)** An annular cluster of follicular papules and pustules on the leg of an adolescent girl failed to improve with 4 months of treatment with oral antibiotics. A skin biopsy showed granulomatous inflammation around hair follicles typical of Majocchi granuloma, and a culture grew *Trichophyton tonsurans*.

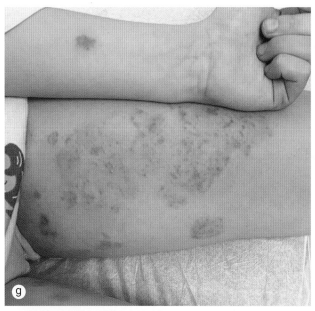

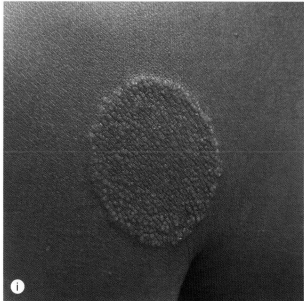

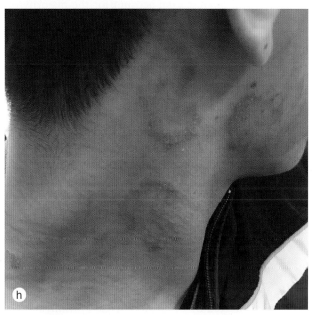

Fig. 3.49, cont'd (g) Majocchi granuloma developed on the thigh of this 5-year-old girl who also failed to respond to antibiotics, and then cleared with oral terbinafine. Fungal culture also grew *Trichophyton tonsurans*. **(h)** Tinea corporis spread on the neck and upper trunk of this wrestler and several of his teammates. **(i)** A healthy 9-year-old boy developed an itchy expanding plaque on the back of his left shoulder. The lesion cleared with topical antifungal cream that was applied twice daily for 3 weeks.

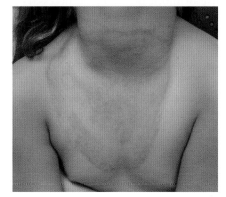

Fig. 3.50 Tinea incognito. This 9-year-old girl with tinea corporis was treated repeatedly for 6 months with topical steroids. Each time she improved, but the rash flared as soon as the treatment was discontinued. Note the multiple concentric annular and serpiginous plaques typical of tinea corporis within the larger well-demarcated border.

In some cases, scaling and fissuring predominate; in others, vesiculopustular lesions, erythema, and maceration are found. The infection starts and may remain between and along the sides of the toes. However, lesions can extend over the dorsum of the foot and can involve the plantar surface as well, particularly the instep and the ball of the foot. Patients complain of burning and itching, which are frequently intense. Although the rash occasionally involves both feet and the hands, asymmetric involvement with sparing of one hand or foot is typical of tinea.

Diagnosis is suspected on clinical grounds and confirmed by KOH preparation and/or fungal cultures of skin scrapings. The mainstays of treatment include topical antifungal creams or powders and measures to reduce foot moisture. Oral antifungal agents may be necessary for persistent, widespread tinea pedis.

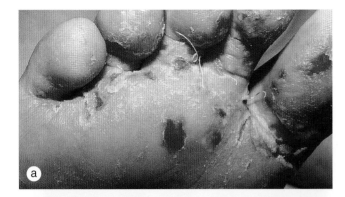

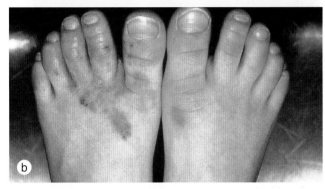

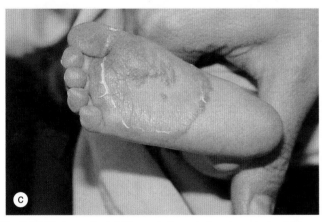

Fig. 3.51 Tinea pedis. **(a)** Macerated, eroded, and crusted patches extend from the toe web spaces to the plantar surfaces of the toes and foot in this 5-year-old boy. **(b)** Dry, scaly, red patches extend from the web spaces to the top of the toes and foot in a 4-year-old boy. **(c)** This 6-week-old girl had a 10-day history of an expanding annular plaque on the plantar surface of the right foot. All of these children had at least one parent with chronic or recurrent tinea pedis.

Onychomycosis or tinea unguium occurs when tinea pedis spreads to nails. Although onychomycosis is unusual in young children, the prevalence increases with increasing age and should be considered in any child with asymmetric nail dystrophy and contiguous skin involvement. Three months of daily oral therapy with oral terbinafine or griseofulvin may be curative in up to 50% of affected individuals and is approved for children over 2 years old. Many individuals do better during the summer months, while wearing sandals. For those with severe

inflammatory lesions, oral antifungal agents may be required, and secondary bacterial infections, particularly with Gram-negative organisms, may be a problem.

Tinea pedis is differentiated from contact dermatitis of the feet by the tendency of the latter to involve the dorsum of the feet and to spare the interdigital web spaces. In dyshidrotic eczema, KOH preparations and fungal cultures are negative. Psoriasis and PRP are differentiated from tinea by their symmetric moccasin-glove distribution and other characteristic stigmata. Cutaneous larva migrans, most commonly caused by a hookworm of dogs and cats, *Ancylostoma braziliense*, creates a narrow serpiginous erythematous plaque that may become vesicular, bullous, and crusted on the sole of the foot (Fig. 3.51c). The tunnel-like lesion should be distinguished from the asymmetric dermatitic lesions of tinea pedis, as well as the symmetric lesions of dyshidrotic eczema.

Yeast

Candida and *Pityrosporum* account for the majority of yeast-related cutaneous disease.

Candidiasis

Candida colonizes the gastrointestinal tract and skin shortly after birth and may produce localized infection (thrush and diaper dermatitis), as well as disseminated cutaneous and systemic infection in the newborn. Recurrent and persistent infection in infancy may be associated with the use of antibiotics. However, it should also raise the suspicion of heritable or acquired immunodeficiency (Fig. 3.52a,b). Candidal paronychia is also a common problem in otherwise healthy toddlers who suck on fingers and toes (Fig. 3.52c). Yellowing, pitting, and other signs of nail dystrophy associated with *Candida* in this setting usually resolve without therapy; however, patients may benefit from the application of topical antifungal creams. Perlèche, manifested as erythema, maceration, and fissuring of the corners of the mouth, occurs commonly in diabetics and lip-lickers and may become secondarily infected by *Candida*. Topical antifungals, as well as aggressive use of lubricants, may be necessary to eradicate the condition.

Candidiasis, resulting from the use of oral antibiotics in older children and adolescents or persistent infection in compromised hosts, will respond quickly to oral fluconazole when topical measures are difficult or ineffective. In some patients, intermittent oral antifungal prophylaxis may be necessary.

Tinea Versicolor

Tinea versicolor is a common dermatosis characterized by multiple, small, oval, scaly patches that measure 1–3 cm in diameter, usually located in a guttate or raindrop pattern on the upper chest, back, and proximal portions of the upper extremities of adolescents and young adults (Fig. 3.53a,b). However, all ages may be affected, including infants (Fig. 3.53c). Facial lesions are seen occasionally and may be the only area of

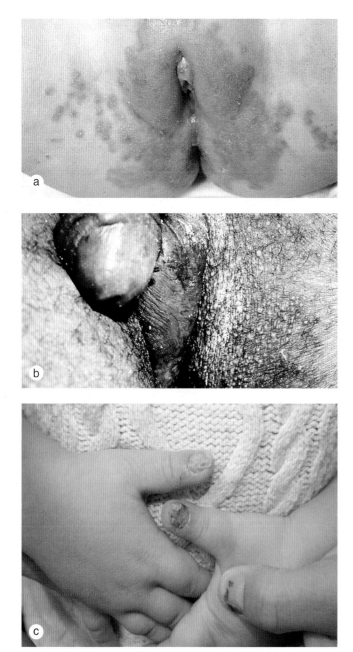

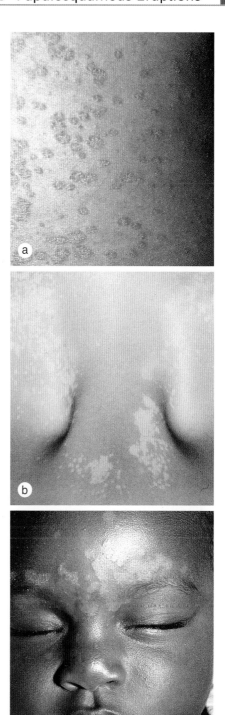

Fig. 3.52 Candidiasis. **(a)** A red, papular rash with pustules at the periphery erupted on the anogenital area of this child who was on chronic antibiotics for recurrent ear infections. **(b)** A teenage diabetic on antibiotics developed a painful, red, macerated eruption dotted with pustules on the scrotum, penis, and groin. **(c)** A chronic paronychia with erythema at the base of the nail, loss of the cuticle, and dystrophic changes of the nail developed in a 2-year-old thumb-sucker. Scrapings from all three patients grew *Candida* species.

Fig. 3.53 Tinea versicolor. **(a)** The well-demarcated, scaly papules appear darker than surrounding skin on the back of a white adolescent. **(b)** Sun-exposed papules on the back of this child failed to tan, resulting in a hypopigmented rash. **(c)** A 4-month-old black girl developed hypopigmented, scaly papules on her face. Her mother had widespread lesions on the chest and back.

involvement in breastfeeding babies, who acquire the organism from their mothers.

The rash is usually asymptomatic, although some patients complain of mild pruritus. Typically, the cosmetic appearance is more bothersome. Lesions may be light tan, reddish, or white in color, giving rise to the term versicolor. Patches tend

to appear hyperpigmented in light-pigmented patients and hypopigmented in dark-pigmented patients. In some individuals, a folliculitis, characterized by 2–3 mm diameter red papules and pustules, develops on the chest, the back, and occasionally the face.

Tinea versicolor is caused by a dimorphous form of *Pityrosporum* (*Malassezia*), which commonly colonizes the skin by 4–6 months of age. Warm, moist climates, pregnancy, immunodeficiency states, and genetic factors predispose to the development of clinical lesions.

The diagnosis of tinea versicolor can generally be made on the basis of the clinical appearance of lesions and their distribution. It can be confirmed by a KOH preparation of the surface scale, which demonstrates short pseudohyphae and yeast forms that resemble spaghetti and meatballs. Although the pathogenesis of the color change is not fully understood, the fungus is known to produce azelaic acid, a substance that interferes with tyrosinase activity and subsequent melanin synthesis.

The differential diagnosis of tinea versicolor includes postinflammatory hypopigmentation and vitiligo. The history, distribution, and distinct borders help to differentiate tinea versicolor from postinflammatory hypopigmentation, and the presence of fine, superficial scaling and some residual pigmentation helps exclude vitiligo.

Topical desquamating agents, such as selenium sulfide and propylene glycol, produce rapid clearing of tinea versicolor. Localized lesions may be treated effectively with topical antifungal creams, while recalcitrant cases may respond to oral itraconazole or fluconazole. Patients must be counseled about the high risk of recurrence and reminded that pigmentary changes may take months to clear, even after eradication of the fungus.

Confluent and Reticulated Papillomatosis of Gougerot and Carteaud

Gougerot–Carteaud syndrome is an uncommon eruption that comprises brown or slate-gray papules, which often become confluent on the seborrheic areas of the chest and back, particularly in black adolescents and young adults (Fig. 3.54). Although this eruption may be noted in healthy adolescents with a normal body mass index, the prevalence is increased in obesity. Reticulated patches may extend over much of the back, shoulders, chest, and abdomen. Although the cause is not known, many investigators attribute the rash to *Pityrosporum* infection, while others consider it to be a variant of acanthosis nigricans. Histological features from skin biopsy of confluent and reticulated papillomatosis show features similar to those seen in acanthosis nigricans.

Unfortunately, the rash is usually refractory to topical antifungal treatment. However, over a period of months to years, most patients improve without treatment, and others respond to traditional therapy for tinea versicolor. Several investigators have also demonstrated a response to oral minocycline, oral isotretinoin, and topical calcipotriol. In fact, the standard of care has shifted to oral tetracyclines and other oral antibiotics, when tetracyclines are contraindicated, for widespread and/or recalcitrant cases.

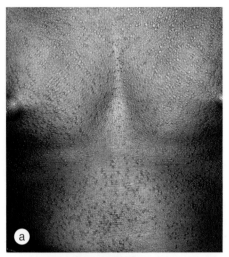

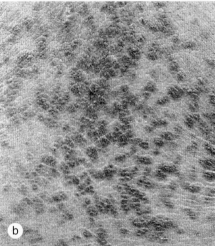

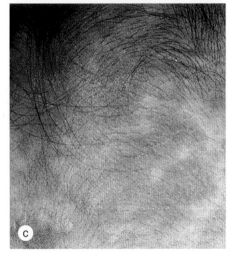

Fig. 3.54 Confluent and reticulated papillomatosis. **(a)** Asymptomatic, hyperpigmented papules disseminated over the trunk of this healthy African American adolescent. Multiple scrapings for tinea versicolor were negative, and he failed therapy with topical keratolytics. **(b)** At a visit several months later, the papules on his upper trunk were confluent and reticulated. The rash disappeared 2 years later without treatment. **(c)** A similar eruption developed on the neck of this healthy light-pigmented adolescent before disseminating over the back and chest.

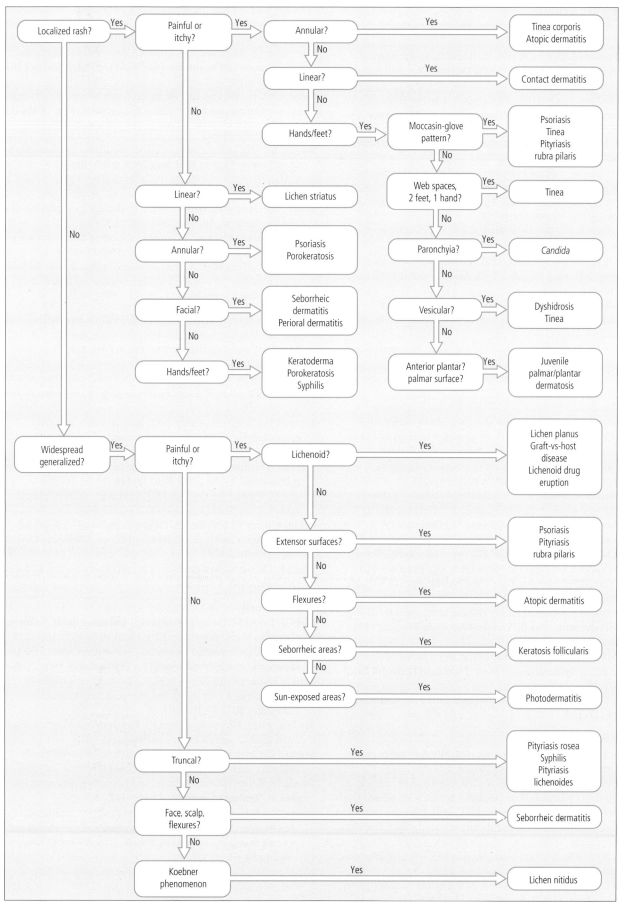

Fig. 3.55 Algorithm for evaluation of papulosquamous disorders.

FURTHER READING

Psoriasis

Beylot C, Puissant A, Bioulac P, et al. Particular clinical features of psoriasis in infants and children. Acta Dermatol Venereol Suppl (Stockh) 1979; 87:95–97.

Brecher AR, Orlow SJ. Oral retinoid therapy for dermatologic conditions in children and adolescents. J Am Acad Dermatol 2003; 49:171–182.

Farber EM, Nall ML. The natural history of psoriasis in 5600 patients. Dermatologica 1974; 148:1–18.

Holgate MC. The age-of-onset of psoriasis and the relationship to parental psoriasis. Br J Dermatol 1975; 92:443–448.

Judge MR, McDonald A, Bloit MM. Pustular psoriasis in childhood. Clin Exp Dermatol 1993; 189:97–99.

Karman B, Dhar S, Handa S, et al. Methotrexate in childhood psoriasis. Pediatr Dermatol 1994; 11:1271–1273.

Lansang P, Bergman JN, Fiorillo L, et al. Management of pediatric plaque psoriasis using biologics. J Am Acad Dermatol 2020; 82(1):213–221.

Lara-Corrales I, Xi N, Pope E. Childhood psoriasis treatment: evidence published over the last 5 years. Rev Recent Clin Trials 2011; 6(1):36–43.

Leman J, Burden D. Psoriasis in children: a guide to its diagnosis and management. Pediatr Drugs 2001; 3:673–680.

Marcoux D, Prost Y. Pediatric psoriasis revisited. J Cutan Med Surg 2002; 6(3 Suppl):22–28.

Marji JS, Marcus R, Moennich J, et al. Use of biologic agents in pediatric psoriasis. J Drugs Dermatol 2010; 9(8):975–986.

Menter A, Cordoro KM, Davis DMR, et al. Joint American Academy of Dermatology–National Psoriasis Foundation guidelines of care for the management and treatment of psoriasis in pediatric patients. J Am Acad Dermatol 2020; 82(1):161–201.

Morris A, Regers M, Fische G, et al. Childhood psoriasis: a clinical review of 1262 cases. Pediatr Dermatol 2001; 18:188–198.

Nyfors A, Lemholt K. Psoriasis in children. Br J Dermatol 1975; 92:437–442.

Oranje AP, Marcoux D, Svenson A, et al. Topical calcipotriol in childhood psoriasis. J Am Acad Dermatol 1997; 32(2 Pt 1):203–208.

Rogers M. Childhood psoriasis. Curr Opin Pediatr 2002; 14:404–409.

Stern RS, Nicholas T. Therapy with orally administered methoxsalen and ultraviolet A radiation during childhood increases the risk of basal cell carcinoma. The PUVA follow-up study. J Pediatr 1996; 129(6):915–917.

Tollefson MM, Crowson CS, McEvoy MT, et al. Incidence of psoriasis in children: a population-based study. J Am Acad Dermatol 2010; 62(6):979–987.

Trueb RM. Therapies for childhood psoriasis. Curr Probl Dermatol 2009; 38:137–159.

Pityriasis Rubra Pilaris

Allison DS, El-Azhary RA, Calobrisi SD, et al. Pityriasis rubra pilaris in children. J Am Acad Dermatol 2002; 47:386–389.

Boyd AH, Polcari IC. Methotrexate treatment in a case of juvenile pityriasis rubra pilaris. Pediatr Dermatol 2018; 35(1):e62–e63.

Braun-Falco O, Ryckmanns F, Schmoeckel C, et al. Pityriasis rubra pilaris: a clinicopathological and therapeutic study. Arch Dermatol Res 1983; 275:287–295.

Cohen PR, Prystowsky JH. Pityriasis rubra pilaris. A review of diagnosis and treatment. J Am Acad Dermatol 1989; 20:801–807.

Darmstadt GL, Tunnessen WW. Picture of the month. Juvenile pityriasis rubra pilaris. Arch Pediatr Adolesc Med 1995; 149:923–924.

Huntley CC. Pityriasis rubra pilaris. Am J Dis Child 1971; 122:22–23.

Klein A, Landthaler M, Karrer S. Pityriasis rubra pilaris: a review of diagnosis and treatment. Am J Clin Dermatol 2010; 11(3):157–170.

Roenneberg S, Biedermann T. Pityriasis rubra pilaris: algorithms for diagnosis and treatment. J Eur Acad Dermatol Venereol 2018; 32(6):889–898.

Snahidullah H, Aldridge RD. Changing forms of juvenile pityriasis rubra pilaris, a case report. Clin Exp Dermatol 1994; 19:354–356.

Keratosis Follicularis

Bale SJ, Toro JR. Genetic basis of Darier-White disease: bad pumps cause bumps. J Cutan Med Surg 2000; 4:103–106.

Beck AL Jr, Finochio AF, White JP. Darier disease: a kindred with a large number of cases. Br J Dermatol 1977; 97:335–339.

Cooper SM, Burge SM. Darier disease: epidemiology, pathophysiology, and management. Adv Dermatol 2002; 4:97–105.

Harris A, Burge SM, Dykes PJ, et al. Handicap in Darier disease and Hailey-Hailey disease. Br J Dermatol 1996; 35:685–694.

Svendsen IB, Albrechtseb B. The prevalence of dyskeratosis follicularis (Darier disease) in Denmark. An investigation of hereditary in 22 families. Acta Derm Venereol (Stockh) 1959; 39:356.

Keratoderma (Hyperkeratosis of the Palms and Soles)

Kimyai-Asadi A, Kotcher LB, Jih MH. The molecular basis of hereditary palmoplantar keratodermas. J Am Acad Dermatol 2002; 47:327–343.

Kress DW, Seraly MP, Falo L, et al. Olmsted syndrome, case report and identification of a keratin abnormality. Arch Dermatol 1996; 132:297–300.

Mascaro JM, Torros H. A child with unusual palms and soles, epidermolytic palmoplantar keratoderma of Vorner. Arch Dermatol 1996; 132:1509–1512.

McLean WH. Epithelial Genetics Group. Genetic disorders of palm, skin and nail. J Anat 2003; 202:133–141.

Ortega M, Quintana J, Camacho F. Keratosis punctata of the palmar creases. J Am Acad Dermatol 1985; 13:381–382.

Poulin Y, Perry HO, Muller SA. Olmsted syndrome – congenital palmoplantar and periorificial keratoderma. J Am Acad Dermatol 1984; 10:600–610.

Smith F. The Mendelian genetics of keratin disorders. Am J Clin Dermatol 2003; 4:347–364.

Porokeratosis

Cox GF, Jarratt M. Linear porokeratosis and other linear cutaneous eruptions of childhood. Am J Dis Child 1979; 133:1258–1259.

Ibbotson SH. Disseminated superficial porokeratosis: what is the association with ultraviolet radiation? Clin Exp Dermatol 1996; 21:48–50.

Kaur S, Thami GP, Mohan H, et al. Co-existence of variants of porokeratosis: a case report and report of the literature. J Dermatol 2002; 29:305–309.

Madojana RM, Katz R, Rodman OG. Porokeratosis plantaris discreta. J Am Acad Dermatol 1984; 10:679–682.

Mikhail GR, Wertheimer FW. Clinical variants of porokeratosis (Mibelli). Arch Dermatol 1968; 98:124–131.

Sasson M, Krain AD. Porokeratosis and cutaneous malignancy, a review. Dermatol Surg 1996; 22:339–342.

Scappaticci S, Lambiase S, Orecchia G, et al. Clonal chromosome abnormalities with preferential involvement of chromosome 3 in patients with porokeratosis of Mibelli. Cancer Genet Cytogenet 1989; 43:89–94.

Shamroth JM, Zlotogorski A, Gilead L. Porokeratosis of Mibelli. Overview and review of the literature. Acta Derm Venereol 1997; 77:207–213.

Contact Dermatitis

Beltrani VS, Beltrani VP. Contact dermatitis. Ann Allergy Asthma Immunol 1997; 78:160–173.

Bruckner AL, Weston WL. Beyond poison ivy, understanding allergic contact dermatitis in children. Pediatr Ann 2001; 30:203–206.

Jacob SE, Herro EM, Sullivan K, et al. Safety and efficacy evaluation of TRUE TEST panels 1.1, 2.1, and 3.1 in children and adolescents. Dermatitis 2011; 22(4):204–210.

Rudzki E, Rebandel P. Contact dermatitis in children. Contact Dermatitis 1996; 34:66–67.

Silverberg NB, Pelletier JL, Jacob SE, et al. Nickel allergic contact dermatitis: identification, treatment, and prevention. Pediatrics 2020; 145(5): e20200628.

Simonsen AB, Deleuran M, Johansen JD, et al. Contact allergy and allergic contact dermatitis in children – a review of current data. Contact Dermatitis 2011; 65(5):254–265.

Wantke F, Hemmer W, Jarisch R, et al. Patch test reactions in children, adults and the elderly, a comparative study in patients with suspected allergic contact dermatitis. Contact Dermatitis 1996; 34:316–319.

Weston WL, Bruckner A. Allergic contact dermatitis. Pediatr Clin North Am 2000; 17:897–907.

Wolf R, Wolf D. Contact dermatitis. Clinical Dermatol 2000; 18:661–666.

Atopic Dermatitis

Besnier E. Première note et observations préliminaires pour servir d'introduction a l'études des pruripos diathesiques. Ann Dermatol Syph 1892; 23:634–637.

Boguniewicz M, Leung DY. Recent insights into atopic dermatitis and implications for management of infectious complications. J Allergy Clin Immunol 2010; 125(1):4–15.

Coca AF, Cooke RA. On the classification of the phenomena of hypersensitiveness. J Immunol 1923; 8:163.

de la O-Escamilla NO, Sidbury R. Atopic dermatitis: update on pathogenesis and therapy. Pediatr Ann 2020; 49(3):e140–e146.

Dimson S, Nanayakkara C. Do oral antihistamines stop the itch of atopic dermatitis? Arch Dis Child 2003; 88:832–833.

Eichenfield LF, Tom WL, Berger TG, el al. Guidelines of care for the management of atopic dermatitis: section 2. Management and treatment of atopic dermatitis with topical therapies. J Am Acad Dermatol 2014; 71(1):116–132.

Gupta AK, Chow M. Pimecrolimus: a review. J Eur Acad Dermatol Venereol 2003; 17:493–503.

Hanifin JM. An overview of atopic dermatitis. Dermatol Nurs 2003; (Suppl):6–9.

Kalavala M, Dohil MA. Calcineurin inhibitors in pediatric atopic dermatitis: a review of current evidence. Am J Clin Dermatol 2011; 12(1):15–24.

Leung AK, Barber KA. Managing childhood atopic dermatitis. Adv Ther 2003; 200:129–137.

Leung DY. Infection in atopic dermatitis. Curr Opin Pediatr 2003; 15:399–404.

Mannschreck D, Feig J, Selph J, et al. Disseminated bullous impetigo and atopic dermatitis: case series and literature review. Pediatr Dermatol 2020; 37(1):103–108.

Novak N, Simon D. Atopic dermatitis – from new pathophysiologic insights to individualized therapy. Allergy 2011; 66(7):830–839.

Oranje AP. Development of childhood eczema and its classification. Pediatr Allergy Immunol 1995; 6(Suppl 7):31–35.

O'Regan GM, Irvine AD. The role of filaggrin loss-of-function mutations in atopic dermatitis. Curr Opin Allergy Clin Immunol 2008; 8(5):406–410.

Patel RR, VanderStraten MR, Korman NJ. The safety and efficacy of tacrolimus therapy in patients younger than 2 years with atopic dermatitis. Arch Dermatol 2003; 139:1184–1186.

Simon D. Systemic therapy of atopic dermatitis in children and adults. Curr Probl Dermatol 2011; 41:156–164.

Simpson EL. Atopic dermatitis: a review of topical treatment options. Curr Med Res Opin 2010; 26(3):633–640.

Stone KP. Atopic diseases of childhood. Curr Opin Pediatr 2003; 15:495–511.

Seborrheic Dermatitis

Abdel-Hamid IA, Agha SA, Moustafa YM, et al. Pityriasis amiantacea: a clinical and etiopathologic study of 85 patients. Int J Dermatol 2003; 42(4):260–264.

Broberg A. Pityrosporum ovale in healthy children, infantile seborrheic dermatitis and atopic dermatitis. Arch Dermatol Venereol (Stockh) 1995; 191(Suppl):1–47.

Faergemann I. Management of seborrheic dermatitis and pityriasis versicolor. Am J Clin Dermatol 2000; 1:75–80.

Gupta AK, Bluhm R, Cooper EA, et al. Seborrheic dermatitis. Dermatol Clin 2003; 21:401–412.

Gupta AK, Madzia SE, Batra R. Etiology and management of seborrheic dermatitis. Dermatology 2004; 208(2):89–93.

Mimouni K, Mukamel M, Zehaira A, et al. Progress of infantile seborrheic dermatitis. J Pediatr 1995; 127:744–746.

Poindexter GB, Burkhart CN, Morrell DS. Therapies for pediatric seborrheic dermatitis. Pediatr Ann 2009; 38(6):333–338.

Skinner RB, Noah PW, Taylor RM, et al. Doubleblind treatment of seborrheic dermatitis with 2% ketoconazole cream. J Am Acad Dermatol 1985; 12:852–856.

Yates VM, Kerr RE, Frier K, et al. Early diagnosis of infantile seborrheic dermatitis and atopic dermatitis: clinical features. Br J Dermatol 1983; 108:633–638.

Juvenile Palmar-Plantar Dermatosis

Moorthy TT, Rajan VS. Juvenile plantar dermatosis in Singapore. Int J Dermatol 1984; 23:476.

Steck WD. Juvenile plantar dermatosis: the 'wet and dry foot syndrome.' Cleve Clin Q 1983; 50:145–149.

Perioral Dermatitis

Hafeez AH. Perioral dermatitis: an update. Int J Dermatol 2003; 42:514–517.

Knautz MA, Lesher JL. Childhood granulomatous periorificial dermatitis. Pediatr Dermatol 1996; 13:131–134.

Kroshinsky D, Glick SA. Pediatric rosacea. Dermatol Ther 2006; 19(4):196–201.

Marks R, Black MM. Perioral dermatitis. A histopathological study of 26 cases. Br J Dermatol 1971; 84:242.

Miller SR, Shalita AR. Topical metronidazole gel (0.75%) for the treatment of perioral dermatitis in children. J Am Acad Dermatol 1994; 31(5 Pt 2):847–848.

Nguyen V, Eichenfield LF. Periorificial dermatitis in children and adolescents. J Am Acad Dermatol 2006; 55(5):781–785.

Takiwaki H, Tsuda H, Arase S, et al. Differences between intrafollicular microorganism profiles in perioral and seborrheic dermatitis. Clin Exp Dermatol 2003; 28:531–534.

Tepark T, Shwayder TA. Perioral dermatitis: a review of the condition with special attention to treatment options. Am J Clin Dermatol 2014; 15(2):101–113.

Urbatsch AJ, Frieden I, Williams ML, et al. Extrafacial and generalized granulomatous periorificial dermatitis. Arch Dermatol 2002; 138(10):1354–1358.

Yung A. Perioral dermatitis and inadvertent topical corticosteroid exposure. Br J Dermatol 2002; 147:1279–1280.

Pityriasis Rosea

Allen RA, Janniger CK, Schwartz RA. Pityriasis rosea. Cutis 1995; 56:198–202.

Blauvelt A. Skin diseases associated with human herpesviruses 6, 7, and 8. J Invest Dermatol Suppl Proc 2001; 6:197–202.

Browning JC. An update on pityriasis rosea and other similar childhood exanthems. Curr Opin Pediatr 2009; 21(4):481–485.

Cavanaugh RM. Pityriasis rosea in children. Clin Pediatr 1983; 22:200.

Chuang T-Y, Ilstrup DM, Perry HO, et al. Pityriasis rosea in Rochester, Minnesota 1969–1978. J Am Acad Dermatol 1982; 7:80–89.

DeAraujo T, Berman B, Weinstein A. Human herpesvirus 6 and 7. Dermatol Clin 2002; 20:301–306.

Drago F, Rebora A. Treatments for pityriasis rosea. Skin Therapy Lett 2009; 14(3):6–7.

Sharma PK, Yadav TP, Gautam RK, et al. Erythromycin in pityriasis rosea: a double-blind, placebo-controlled clinical trial. J Am Acad Dermatol 2000; 42(2 Pt 1):241–244.

Stulberg DL, Wolfrey J. Pityriasis rosea. Am Fam Physician 2004; 69(1):87–91.

Pityriasis Lichenoides

Ersoy-Evans S, Greco MF, Mancini AJ, et al. Pityriasis lichenoides in childhood: a retrospective review of 124 patients. J Am Acad Dermatol 2007; 56(2):205–210.

Fernandes NF, Rozdeba PJ, Schwartz RA, et al. Pityriasis lichenoides et varioliformis acuta: a disease spectrum. Int J Dermatol 2010; 49(3):257–261.

Lam J, Pope E. Pediatric pityriasis lichenoides and cutaneous T-cell lymphoma. Curr Opin Pediatr 2007; 19(4):441–445.

Patel DG, Kihiczak G, Schwartz RA, et al. Pityriasis lichenoides. Cutis 2002; 65:17–20.

Romani J, Puig L, Fernandez-Figueras MT, et al. Pityriasis lichenoides in children: a clinicopathologic review of 22 patients. Pediatr Dermatol 1998; 15:1–6.

Truhan AP, Hebert AA, Esterly NB. Pityriasis lichenoides in children: therapeutic response to erythromycin. J Am Acad Dermatol 1986; 15:66–70.

Tsuji T, Kasamatsu M, Yokota M, et al. Mucha-Habermann disease and its febrile ulceronecrotic variant. Cutis 1996; 58:123–131.

Lichen Planus

Handa S, Sahoo B. Childhood lichen planus: a study of 87 cases. Int J Dermatol 2002; 41(7):423–427.

Kanwar AJ, De D. Lichen planus in childhood: report of 100 cases. Clin Exp Dermatol 2010; 35(3):257–262.

Nurmohamed S, Hardin J, Haber RM. Lichen planus pigmentosus inversus in children: case report and updated review of the literature. Pediatr Dermatol 2018; 35(1):e49–e51.

Payette MJ, Weston G, Humphrey S, et al. Lichen planus and other lichenoid dermatoses: kids are not just little people. Clin Dermatol 2015; 33(6):631–643.

Ragaz A, Ackerman AB. Evolution maturation, and regression of lesions of lichen planus. Am J Dermatopathol 1981; 3:5–25.

Rivers JK, Jackson R, Orozaga M. Who was Wickham and what are his striae? Int J Dermatol 1986; 25:611–613.

Sanchez-Perez J, DeCastro M, Buezo G, et al. Lichen planus and hepatitis C virus: prevalence and clinical presentation of patients with lichen planus and hepatitis C virus infection. Br J Dermatol 1996; 343:715–719.

Sharma R, Maheshawari V. Childhood lichen planus: a report of fifty cases. Pediatr Dermatol 1999; 16:345–348.

Silverman RA, Rhodes AR. Twenty-nail dystrophy of childhood: a sign of localized lichen planus. Pediatr Dermatol 1984; 1:207.

Walton KE, Bowers EV, Drolet BA, et al. Childhood lichen planus: demographics of a U.S. population. Pediatr Dermatol 2010; 27(1):34–38.

Lichen Nitidus

Arizaya AT, Gaughan MD, Bang RH. Generalized lichen nitidus. Clin Exp Dermatol 2002; 27:115–117.

Kundak S, Cakir Y. Pediatric lichen nitidus: a single-center experience. Pediatr Dermatol 2019; 36(2):189–192.

Lapins NA, Willoughby C, Helwid EB. Lichen nitidus: a study of 43 cases. Cutis 1978; 21:634.

Soroush V, Gurevutch AW, Peng SK. Generalized lichen nitidus: a case report and review. Cutis 1999; 64:135–136.

Sysa-Jedrzejowska A, Wozniacka A, Robak E, et al. Generalized lichen nitidus, a case report. Cutis 1996; 58:170–172.

Tilly JJ, Drolet BA, Esterly NB. Lichenoid eruptions in children. J Am Acad Dermatol 2004; 51(4):606–624.

Lichen Striatus

Fujimato N, Tajima S, Ishibashi A. Facial lichen striatus: successful treatment with tacrolimus ointment. Br J Dermatol 2003; 148:587–590.

Gianotti R, Restano L, Grindt R, et al. Lichen striatus – a chameleon: an histopathological and immunohistochemical study of 41 cases. J Cutan Pathol 1995; 22:18–22.

Herd RM, McLaren KM, Aldridge RD. Linear lichen planus and lichen planus – opposite ends of a spectrum. Clin Exp Dermatol 1993; 18:335–337.

Kavak A, Kathuay L. Nail involvement in lichen striatus. Pediatr Dermatol 2002; 19:136–138.

Keegan BR, Kamino H, Fangman W, et al. 'Pediatric blaschkitis': expanding the spectrum of childhood acquired Blaschko-linear dermatoses. Pediatr Dermatol 2007; 24(6):621–627.

Müller CS, Schmaltz R, Vogt T, et al. Lichen striatus and blaschkitis: reappraisal of the concept of Blaschko linear dermatoses. Br J Dermatol 2011; 164(2):257–262.

Peramiquel L, Baselga E, Dalmau J, et al. Lichen striatus: clinical and epidemiological review of 23 cases. Eur J Pediatr 2006; 165(4):267–269.

Taieb A, Youbi AE, Grosshaus E, et al. Lichen striatus: a Blaschko linear acquired inflammatory skin eruption. J Am Acad Dermatol 1991; 25:637–642.

Fungal Infections

Adams BB. Tinea corporis gladiatorum. J Am Acad Dermatol 2002; 47:286–290.

Alston SJ, Cohen BA, Braun M. Persistent and recurrent tinea corporis in children treated with combination antifungal/corticosteroid agents. Pediatrics 2003; 111(1):201–203.

Andrews MD, Burns M. Common tinea infections in children. Am Fam Physician 2008; 77(10):1415–1420.

Bonifaz A, Gomez-Daza F, Paredes V, et al. Tinea versicolor, tinea nigra, white piedra, and black piedra. Clin Dermatol 2010; 28(2):140–145.

Bowman PH, Davis LS. Confluent and reticulated papillomatosis: response to tazarotene. J Am Acad Dermatol 2003; 48(5 Suppl):S80–S81.

Ferreira LM, Diniz LM, Ferreira CJ. [Confluent and reticulated papillomatosis of Gougerot and Carteaud: report of three cases]. An Bras Dermatol 2009; 84(1):78–81.

Greenberg HL, Shwayder TA, Bieszk N, et al. Clotrimazole/betamethasone dipropionate: a review of costs and complications in the treatment of common cutaneous fungal infections. Pediatr Dermatol 2002; 19(1):78–81.

Gupta AK, Cooper EA. Update in antifungal therapy of dermatophytosis. Mycopathologia 2008; 166(5–6):353–367.

Gupta AK, Cooper EA, Ryder JE, et al. Optimal management of fungal infections of the skin, hair, and nails. Am J Clin Dermatol 2004; 5(4):225–237.

Gupta AK, Chaudry M, Elewski B. Tinea corporis, tinea cruris, tinea nigra, and piedra. Dermatol Clin 2003; 21:395–400.

Hamilton D, Tavafoghi V, Shafer JC. Confluent and reticulated papillomatosis of Gougerot and Carteaud. Its relation to other papillomatoses. J Am Acad Dermatol 1980; 2:401.

Hawranek T. Cutaneous mycology. Clin Immunol 2002; 81:129–166.

Hu SW, Bigby M. Pityriasis versicolor: a systematic review of interventions. Arch Dermatol 2010; 146(10):1132–1140.

Jang HS, Oh CK, Cha JH, et al. Six cases of confluent and reticulated papillomatosis alleviated by various antibiotics. J Am Acad Dermatol 2001; 44:652–655.

McLean T, Levy H, Lue YA. Ecology of dermatophyte infections in South Bronx, New York, 1969–1981. J Am Acad Dermatol 1987; 16:336–340.

Mendez-Tovar LJ. Pathogenesis of dermatophytosis and tinea versicolor. Clin Dermatol 2010; 28(2):185–189.

Nordby CA, Mitchell AJ. Confluent and reticulated papillomatosis responsive to selenium sulfide. Int J Dermatol 1986; 25:194–199.

Parker J. Management of common fungal infections in primary care. Nurs Stand 2009; 23(43):42–46.

Scheinfeld N. Confluent and reticulated papillomatosis: a review of the literature. Am J Clin Dermatol 2006; 7(5):305–313.

Weistin A, Berman B. Topical treatment of common superficial tinea infections. Am Fam Physician 2002; 65:2095–2102.

Zampella JG, Kwatra SG, Blanck J, et al. Tinea in tots: cases and literature review of oral antifungal treatment of tinea capitis in children under 2 years of age. J Pediatr 2017; 183:12–18.

4

Vesiculopustular Eruptions

Nidhi Shah and A. Yasmine Kirkorian

INTRODUCTION

Vesiculopustular eruptions range from benign, self-limited conditions to life-threatening diseases. Early diagnosis, especially in the young or immunocompromised child, is mandatory. An algorithmic approach to diagnosis for vesiculopustular dermatoses is summarized at the end of the chapter (see Fig. 4.29).

An understanding of the structures that account for normal epidermal and basement membrane zone adhesion provides clues to the clinical diagnosis and pathogenesis of blistering diseases (Fig. 4.1). Epidermal cells are held together by desmosome–tonofilament complexes. Electron-dense tonofilaments insert into desmosomes in the keratinocyte plasma membrane and project toward the nucleus. Intercellular bridges extend between keratinocytes and are associated with a sticky, glycoprotein-rich, intercellular cement substance. In the basement membrane zone, tonofilaments insert into hemidesmosomes, which are attached to the lamina densa by anchoring filaments that traverse an electron-lucent layer known as the lamina lucida. The electron-dense lamina densa is, in turn, affixed to the dermis by anchoring fibrils. Elastic microfibril bundles, which arise in the upper dermis, also insert into the lamina densa.

A number of proteins that play a role in the structural integrity of the skin have been identified in the basement membrane zone, and hereditary-or autoantibody-induced defects in these proteins may lead to clinical disease. Bullous pemphigoid (BP) antigen appears on the bottom of the basal cell plasma membrane and within the lamina lucida. Laminin is present within the lamina lucida, and type IV collagen has been isolated to the lamina densa. In epidermolysis bullosa acquisita (EBA), antibodies against type VII collagen have been identified in the dermis, just beneath the lamina densa. Fluorescein-tagged antibodies directed against these proteins may be used to identify the site of blister formation in disorders that involve the dermal–epidermal junction. Salt-split skin can be used as a substrate to more specifically localize antibodies above or below the basal lamina region.

In general, flaccid bullae arise within the epidermis, and tense lesions involve the dermis. Specific diagnoses, however, rely on identification of clinical patterns, histopathology, and immunofluorescent findings. A few rapid diagnostic techniques also aid in developing a working diagnosis.

VIRAL INFECTIONS

Herpes Simplex Virus

Herpes simplex virus (HSV) is a common cause of oral lesions in toddlers and children of school age. Primary herpetic gingivostomatitis begins with extensive perioral vesicles and pustules and intraoral vesicles and erosions (Fig. 4.2). The gingivae become edematous, red, and friable and bleed easily. Epithelial debris and exudates may form a membrane on the mucosal surfaces. The eruption is usually accompanied by fever, irritability, and cervical adenopathy. Lesions may also be scattered on the face and upper trunk. In infants and toddlers, lesions are frequently auto-inoculated onto the hands. Patients are observed for dehydration as symptoms abate over 7–10 days.

Herpetic gingivostomatitis can be differentiated from enteroviral infections, which usually produce vesicles, ulcerations, and petechiae on the hard palate and spare the gingivae. Although aphthae may be very painful, they are usually isolated lesions that lack the diffuse inflammation associated with herpes.

Primary herpes simplex infections may involve any cutaneous or mucous membrane surface and generally result from direct inoculation of previously injured sites. Lesions consist of herpetiform or clustered red papules, which evolve into vesicles and pustules in 24–48 h (Figs. 4.2–4.5). During the following 5–7 days, vesicles rupture and crust over. Desquamation and healing are complete in 10–14 days. Primary herpes infection on the distal finger is called herpetic whitlow (Fig. 4.3b,c). Just as in herpetic gingivostomatitis, primary infections at other sites may be associated with painful local adenopathy and flu-like symptoms. When an HSV-1 and HSV-2 naive individual acquires either HSV type 1 or HSV type 2, a first-episode primary infection ensues. Likewise, when an individual with pre-existing HSV-1 antibody acquires an HSV-2 infection (or vice versa), a first-episode non-primary infection results.

In children, most infections are caused by HSV type 1, whereas HSV type 2 is most commonly found in genital infections in adolescents and adults (Fig. 4.4). However, HSV type 2 can also be found in non-genital areas, and type 1 virus may be spread from mouth to hand to genital sites. Although sexual contact must be considered in any child who develops genital herpes, non-venereal sources are probably most common. Confirmed genital HSV type 2 in children should prompt a referral to child abuse specialists and can put the child at risk for HSV

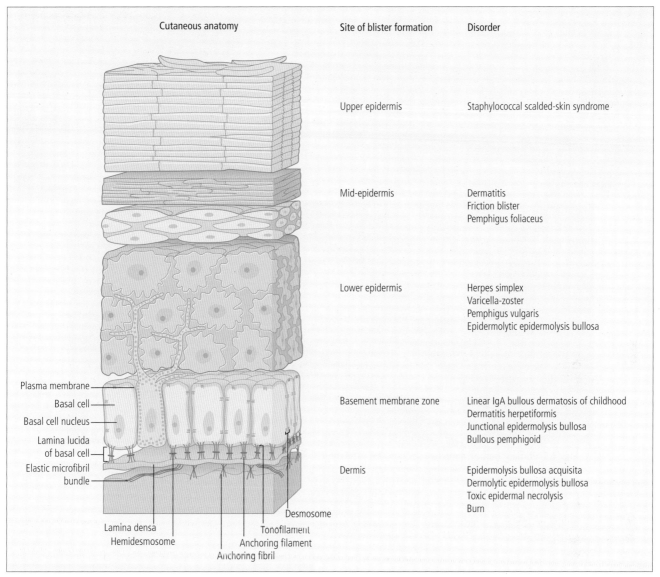

Cutaneous anatomy   Site of blister formation   Disorder

Upper epidermis   Staphylococcal scalded-skin syndrome

Mid-epidermis   Dermatitis
Friction blister
Pemphigus foliaceus

Lower epidermis   Herpes simplex
Varicella-zoster
Pemphigus vulgaris
Epidermolytic epidermolysis bullosa

Plasma membrane
Basal cell
Basal cell nucleus   Basement membrane zone   Linear IgA bullous dermatosis of childhood
Dermatitis herpetiformis
Junctional epidermolysis bullosa
Lamina lucida
of basal cell   Bullous pemphigoid

Elastic microfibril
bundle   Dermis   Epidermolysis bullosa acquisita
Dermolytic epidermolysis bullosa
Toxic epidermal necrolysis
Burn
Desmosome
Lamina densa   Tonofilament
Hemidesmosome   Anchoring filament
Anchoring fibril

Fig. 4.1 Anatomy of vesiculopustular dermatoses.

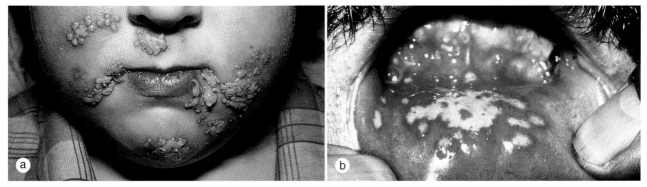

Fig. 4.2 Herpetic gingivostomatitis. **(a)** This 6-year-old boy developed extensive perioral vesicles and mucous membrane erosions with his first bout of herpes simplex. **(b)** A 19-year-old experienced severe pain from widespread gingival and buccal mucosal vesicles and erosions during the peak of his primary herpes infection.

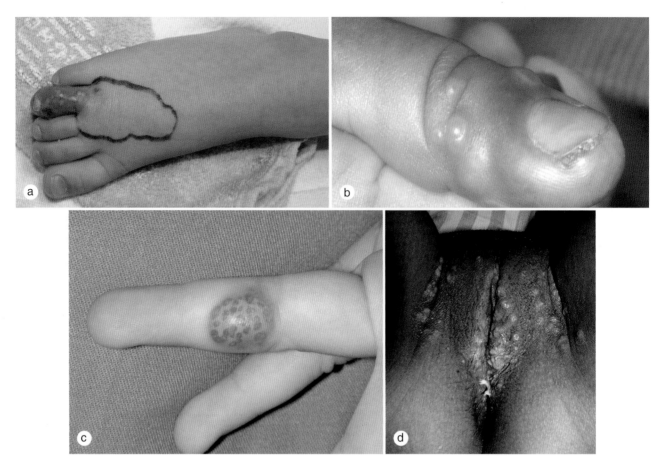

Fig. 4.3 Primary herpes simplex infection. **(a)** A healthy 3-year-old girl developed clustered uniform vesicles and pustules on her right fourth toe associated with painful erythema, edema, and a sterile lymphangitis on the top of her foot. **(b)** Herpetic whitlow developed by autoinoculation from oral lesions in this 4-year-old boy. Oral and finger lesions resolved without treatment in 2 weeks. **(c)** A multiloculated bulla was also noted on the finger of this child with herpetic whitlow. **(d)** A 16-year-old sexually active girl developed painful vesicles on the genital area, which cleared after 10 days of oral acyclovir.

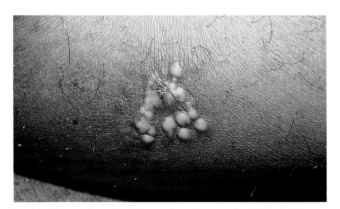

Fig. 4.4 Clustered pustules appeared on the posterior thigh of a teenager with recurrent herpes simplex type 2 infection.

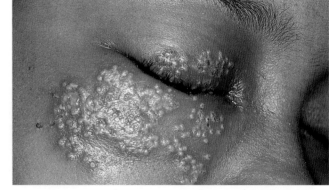

Fig. 4.5 Recurrent herpes simplex erupted around the eye of this 11-year-old boy. The cornea was not involved, and vesicles crusted over in less than a week.

type 2 meningitis. Both HSV type 1 and HSV type 2 can cause neonatal herpes, and higher risk of acquisition is associated with first-episode primary maternal infection, followed by non-primary infection, and finally recurrent infections. In the United States, neonatal herpes is estimated to affect 1500 neonates annually, with a 4% mortality rate. Vesicles are usually restricted to the

perineum and genital skin and quickly ulcerate. Erythema and edema may result in severe dysuria and urinary retention.

In immunocompromised children or patients with certain skin conditions, such as atopic dermatitis, seborrheic dermatitis, and immunologic blistering disorders, herpes simplex may disseminate over the entire skin surface (eczema herpeticum or

Kaposi varicelliform eruption; and to the lungs, viscera, and central nervous system (CNS). HSV may also produce sepsis and/or meningitis with neurologically disabling or life-threatening disease in the nursery. Early diagnosis and antiviral therapy can reduce morbidity and mortality in these clinical settings.

After the initial episode, HSV enters a dormant state. A number of endogenous and environmental factors may trigger reactivation of the virus, such as a *Streptococcus* infection of the throat, an upper respiratory infection, sunburn, and surgery (Fig. 4.5). Lesions usually occur near the site of the primary eruption, mucous membranes are not usually involved, systemic symptoms are absent, and the rash heals in less than a week. Although recurrences are unpredictable, disease-free periods tend to increase with time, even in individuals who initially experience frequent recurrences.

A clinical suspicion of herpes simplex can be confirmed quickly by performing a Tzanck smear at the bedside. Viral culture is rarely used and has been replaced by polymerase chain reaction (PCR) studies or direct immunofluorescence for rapid and reliable confirmation. PCR of the cerebrospinal fluid (CSF) has revolutionized diagnosis of CNS herpes disease by identifying patients who appear to have disease localized to skin, eye, and mouth and triaging appropriate treatment. If CSF PCR is found to be positive, patients are treated with a 21-day course of acyclovir as opposed to the 14-day course with disease localized to skin, eye, and mouth.

The Tzanck smear is obtained by removing the roof of a blister with a scalpel or scissors and scraping its base to obtain the moist, cloudy debris. This is spread onto a glass slide with the scalpel blade, desiccated with 95% ethanol, and stained with Giemsa or Wright stain. The diagnostic finding in viral blisters is the multinucleated giant cell, which is a syncytium of epidermal cells with multiple, overlapping nuclei; hence, it is much larger than other inflammatory cells. Unfortunately, a positive Tzanck smear cannot be used to differentiate between HSV and varicella, and a viral PCR should be obtained when the clinical situation dictates.

In general, management of herpes infections is symptomatic with cool compresses, lubricants, and oral analgesics. Topical antiviral agents are of little use in the treatment of uncomplicated infections in normal hosts. Immunocompromised children with primary or recurrent herpes simplex infections and patients with severe primary herpetic gingivostomatitis or genital herpes usually improve quickly with parenteral acyclovir. In some children, especially older patients without oral involvement, oral acyclovir may be administered. Several orally administered drugs, which include valaciclovir hydrochloride and famciclovir, achieve consistent blood levels. Valaciclovir is U.S Food and Drug Administration (FDA) approved for the treatment of herpes labialis in children 12 and older and genital HSV in adolescents. This medication is preferred to acyclovir given its better bioavailability and less frequent dosing. In recurrent disease, initiation of oral acyclovir with the prodromal tingling in the skin before the appearance of blisters may abort the episode. In selected children with frequent, multiple, widespread recurrent eruptions, long-term, suppressive therapy may be necessary.

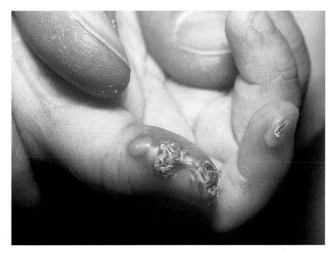

Fig. 4.6 Blistering distal dactylitis developed on the right thumb and index finger of a 5-year-old girl. Cultures from her throat and thumb grew Group A β-hemolytic streptococci. The infection responded quickly to oral amoxicillin.

Extended oral suppressive therapy for infants following parental treatment for neonatal HSV infection can reduce the risk of late neurologic sequelae.

Herpes simplex infections are usually differentiated from other blistering eruptions by the typical clustering of lesions, the clinical course, a positive Tzanck smear and viral PCR, and characteristic skin-biopsy findings. Impetigo may mimic herpes. However, bullae tend to be relatively large, with a central crust and peripheral extension, and a Gram stain demonstrates Gram-positive cocci. Blistering distal dactylitis, which is caused by Group A β-hemolytic streptococci or *Staphylococcus aureus*, may be mistaken for herpetic whitlow (Fig. 4.6). In staphylococcal or streptococcal infection, the lesions on the finger tips usually coalesce to form one or several 5–10 mm diameter blisters, and Gram stains and cultures demonstrate the causative bacterium. Unlike impetigo at other sites, blisters on the fingers tend to be tense because the stratum corneum is thick on acral surfaces. Occasionally, the eruption of herpes simplex may form a dermatomal pattern. In this situation, a viral PCR is required to exclude herpes zoster.

Varicella (Chickenpox)

Varicella is a mild, self-limited infection in most children. However, disseminated disease is a problem in the neonate and immunosuppressed child. Early administration of varicella zoster immune globulin to immunocompromised children exposed to varicella may be preventive, and antiviral therapy in patients with disseminated lesions may be life-saving. The introduction of the varicella vaccine in 1995 reduced varicella mortality and morbidity, with no reported pediatric deaths since 2010, as well as reduced the likelihood of herpes zoster in children. Congenital varicella syndrome can occur when women are infected with the varicella virus during pregnancy, causing multiple anomalies in the newborn. Treatment involves antivirals and varicella immunoglobulin irrespective of gestational age.

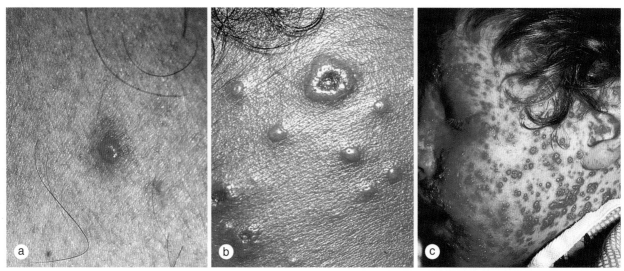

Fig. 4.7 Chickenpox. **(a)** A dew drop on a rose petal is the characteristic primary lesion in chickenpox. **(b)** Lesions in various stages of development, including red papules, vesicles, umbilicated vesicles, and crusts developed in close proximity on the forehead of a toddler with varicella. **(c)** Severe varicella with blisters almost to confluence erupted within 24 h over much of the skin surface of this 6-year-old boy who was on high-dose systemic corticosteroids for inflammatory bowel disease.

After exposure to varicella, the incubation period varies from 7 to 21 days. Fever, sore throat, decreased appetite, and malaise precede the skin lesions by several days. Early cutaneous findings vary from a few scattered, pruritic, red papules to generalized papules that evolve in 24 h to vesicles on a bright red base (dew drops on a rose petal, Fig. 4.7). Central umbilication of blisters follows rapidly, and crusting and desquamation occur within 10 days. New papules and vesicles continue to appear for 3–4 days. The rash often begins on the head and trunk, moving to the extremities but can involve any area including mucosal surfaces, particularly the buccal mucosa and gingivae. Although the blisters are intraepidermal and usually heal without scarring, some develop deep inflammation or become secondarily infected and heal with pitted or hypertrophic scars (Fig. 4.8a,b).

Oral or parenteral acyclovir is indicated for treatment of varicella in immunocompromised patients and normal hosts with severe disease. However, famciclovir and Valaciclovir provide better bioavailability and more convenient dosing. Valaciclovir is FDA approved for treatment of varicella in immunocompetent children 2 years and older. Unfortunately, the newer antiviral agents are not routinely available in liquid preparations. However, special formulating pharmacies may be able to prepare Valaciclovir syrup for children who cannot swallow capsules. Pruritus may be intense and responds to cool compresses, calamine lotion, and oral antihistamines. Topical products containing antihistamines should be avoided because of the risk of significant percutaneous absorption and systemic toxicity. Secondary infection is usually caused by staphylococci and is treated with oral antibiotics such as dicloxacillin, cefalexin, or erythromycin (Fig. 4.8c). When cellulitis or other deep, soft-tissue infection complicates chickenpox, hospitalization and parenteral therapy may be required (Fig. 4.8d). Rarely, progressive purpura and necrosis of large areas of skin herald the onset of disseminated intravascular coagulation (Fig. 4.8e).

This phenomenon, referred to as purpura fulminans, occurs in fewer than 1 in 20 000 cases of varicella.

Administration of systemic corticosteroids, even in normal children, during varicella infection may result in severe blistering, disseminated viral infection, and increased risk of complications. As a consequence, it is important to differentiate chickenpox from contact dermatitis, insect bites, or other viral infections. The Tzanck smear may be particularly useful early in the course of disease, when only a few skin lesions are present. PCR confirmation for varicella infection is useful in immunocompromised hosts or when the diagnosis is in question.

Although the world was declared officially free of smallpox (variola) in 1980, this virus has resurfaced as a potential biological warfare agent. Chickenpox can be distinguished from smallpox in which lesions develop on the face and distal extremities and spread centrally. Early red macules and papules become vesicular and pustular over several days, and adjacent lesions tend to be in the same stage of development. New lesions, which are firm and deep-seated, may appear for 1–2 weeks, become confluent, and often heal with scarring. Patients are usually ill-appearing, and the rapid diagnostic Tzanck smear is negative for multinucleated giant cells. Many medical centers have developed protocols for isolating and evaluating patients with suspected smallpox infection.

Herpes Zoster

Herpes zoster or shingles represents a reactivation of the dormant varicella virus from the sensory root ganglia. The most commonly involved sites include the head and neck and the thoracic sensory nerves (Fig. 4.9). After a variable prodrome, which may include mild constitutional symptoms and localized itching and burning, linear, clustered, red papulovesicles appear in a unilateral linear pattern in one or several dermatomes. In some children, the eruption may be completely asymptomatic.

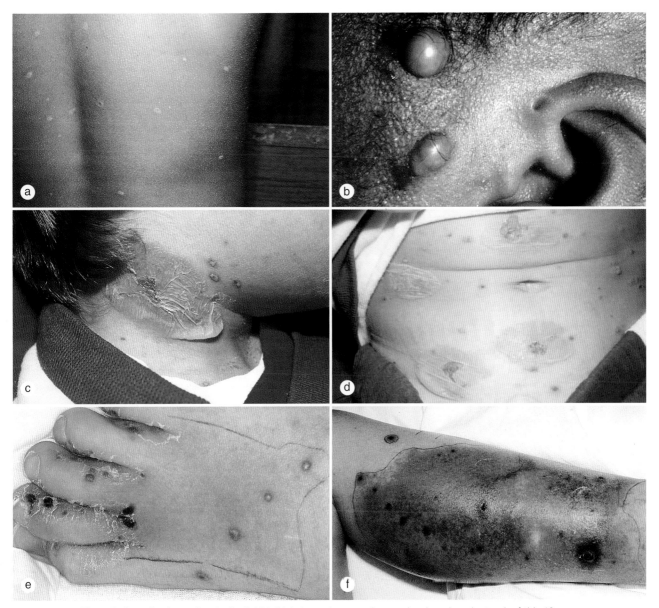

Fig. 4.8 Complications of varicella. **(a)** Multiple hypopigmented scars developed on the trunk of this 10-year-old boy several weeks after chickenpox. **(b)** Dome-shaped hypertrophic scars developed on the preauricular skin of this toddler. Note the small congenital pit at the anterior end of the superior helix. **(c,d)** Bullous impetigo spread quickly by scratching in a 4-year-old boy with chickenpox. Note the pus at the bottom of the large bulla **(c)** and infected lesions on the abdomen **(d)**. **(e)** While this child was recovering from varicella, several lesions on the top of her foot became infected with Group A β-hemolytic streptococci. The rapidly spreading area of erythema responded quickly to high-dose parenteral penicillin. **(f)** A 7-year-old girl with healing chickenpox developed purpura fulminans, with expanding bruises on her legs. Laboratory studies were consistent with disseminated intravascular coagulation, which resolved on heparin therapy. Note the resolving chickenpox vesicles on her leg.

Over 3–5 days, the rash reaches its full extent, and during the ensuing 1–2 weeks, vesicles and erosions develop umbilicated crusts and desquamate, much like in chickenpox.

Although 6–10 lesions may appear outside the primary dermatomes in normal individuals, the development of widespread cutaneous lesions suggests the possibility of an immunodeficiency state and an increased risk of visceral involvement. Herpes zoster is rare in healthy children but can occur and is not a sign of immunodeficiency in the setting of just one episode.; however,

immunocompromised children or children with cancer are at a greater risk for zoster. Varicella can also spread into cerebral and extracranial arteries, producing varicella zoster virus vasculopathy, manifesting as stroke, giant cell arteritis, aneurysms, and sinus thrombosis. In children, stroke can occur 4 months after varicella infection and is often monophasic.

The presence of a dermatomal bullous eruption is virtually diagnostic for herpes zoster. However, herpes simplex occasionally presents in a dermatomal pattern. Moreover, zoster may be

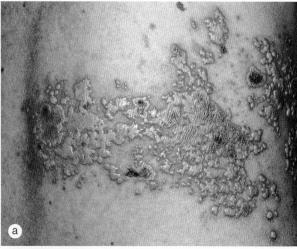

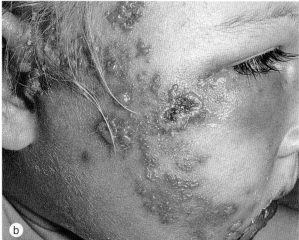

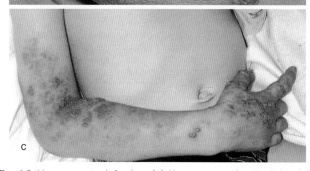

Fig. 4.9 Herpes zoster infection. **(a)** Herpes zoster involved the right, mid-thoracic dermatomes in an otherwise healthy 10-year-old girl with a history of chickenpox when 2 years old. **(b)** Periorbital cellulitis was initially considered in this toddler with impressive edema and erythema of the right eye. The diagnosis of shingles became apparent 1 day later, when the characteristic dermatomal vesiculopustular rash appeared. Both children had uneventful recoveries without treatment. **(c)** This 9-year-old boy complained of painful swelling for several days before dermatomal clustered vesicles erupted on his right arm and hand. He improved quickly with oral Valaciclovir.

confused with herpes simplex early in the course, when only a few clustered vesicles are present and the dermatomal organization is not yet apparent. In the event of diagnostic uncertainty, Varicella zoster virus (VZV) and HSV PCR should be obtained.

Management of shingles is usually limited to supportive measures similar to those for chickenpox. In disseminated disease,

administration of parenteral acyclovir may be life-saving. Oral acyclovir, Valaciclovir, or famciclovir can also be used in immunocompromised hosts and normal patients with symptomatic disease. Immunocompetent individuals who develop eye involvement also benefit from antiviral therapy and are followed closely by an ophthalmologist. The high risk of zoster in patients undergoing bone marrow transplantation or other elective immunosuppression may require antiviral prophylaxis in these children. Although there is no approved herpes zoster vaccine for children, and the risk of infection is generally low, zoster vaccines exist in the market for prophylaxis against zoster in adults over age 50. In 2008, the live attenuated zoster vaccine, ZOSTAVAX (Merck & Co. Inc.) was licensed in the United States; however, it only demonstrates effectiveness of 70% in adults aged 50–59, and less than 38% in adults aged 70 and older. In 2017, the FDA approved a recombinant zoster vaccine, Shingrix (GlaxoSmithKline), which demonstrates an overall efficacy of 97% without decline in efficacy with increasing age.

Although systemic corticosteroids may be administered to reduce the risk of postherpetic neuralgia in adults over 60 years of age, this treatment has not been shown to be beneficial in young adults or children. Children with shingles must be isolated from individuals who are susceptible to chickenpox because of the risk of acquiring infection from direct contact with skin lesions.

Hand-Foot-and-Mouth Disease

Hand-foot-and-mouth disease (HFMD) is a distinctive, self-limited viral eruption mostly occurring in children younger than 10 years old caused most frequently by Coxsackie virus A16 and enterovirus 71 (EV-71). The disease is highly infectious, and, like other enteroviruses, peak incidence occurs in the late summer and fall. After exposure, the incubation period is 4–6 days. A 1–2-day prodrome of fever, anorexia, and sore throat is followed by the development of 3–6 mm diameter elongated, gray, thin-walled vesicles on a red or non-inflamed base. As the name suggests, lesions appear most commonly on the palms, soles, and sides of the hands and feet, but red papules and vesicles may also erupt on the buttocks, trunk, face, arms, and legs (Fig. 4.10a,b). The enanthem is characterized by vesicles that rapidly ulcerate to leave sharply marginated erosions on a red base on the tongue, buccal mucosa, and posterior pharynx (Fig. 4.10c). Most cases do not involve internal findings and are limited to fever, malaise, and herpangina, ulcerations of oropharyngeal surface without papulovesicular eruptions on the skin. Although cutaneous and mucosal lesions may be completely asymptomatic, pruritus and burning can be severe. Systemic symptoms, which include fever, diarrhea, sore throat, and cervical adenopathy, may be absent or mild, and treatment is supportive. The eruption usually clears in less than a week. Inactivated monovalent vaccines against EV-A71 were introduced in China in 2016 in efforts to lower the burden of HFMD among children aged 6–71 months.

In late 2011 and spring 2012, a new clinical variant caused by Coxsackie A6 virus, previously reported in Asia and Africa, spread to North America. Although symptoms and the rash were also self-limited, high fever and more widespread skin

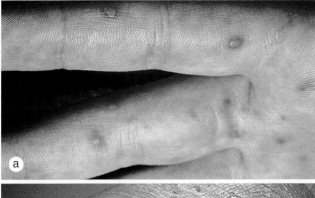

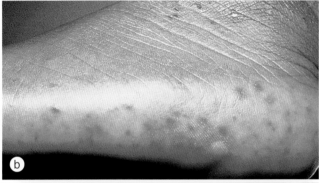

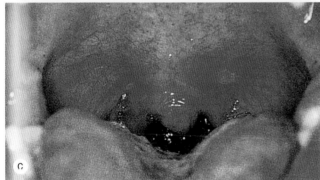

Fig. 4.10 Hand-foot-and-mouth disease. Characteristic elongated vesicles on a red base are shown on **(a)** the palmar surface of the fingers and **(b)** the plantar surface of the foot of children with Coxsackie hand-foot-and-mouth disease. **(c)** The enanthema, consisting of shallow yellow ulcers surrounded by red halos, which may be found on the labial or buccal mucosa, tongue, soft palate, uvula, and anterior tonsillar pillars. When the enanthema occurs in the absence of a rash, the disorder is known as herpangina.

lesions are characteristic. The skin eruption is reminiscent of disseminated herpes simplex infection, but identification of the typical lancet-shaped enteroviral vesicles on the hands and feet provides a clue to the diagnosis (Fig. 4.11). Typical HFMD may not require viral testing; however, atypical strains such as CVA6 may be subjected to enteroviral PCR to differentiate from herpes virus.

BACTERIAL INFECTIONS

Impetigo

Expanding, honey-colored, crusted patches or bullae with a central crust suggest the diagnosis of impetigo (Fig. 4.12). In older children in temperate climates, lesions appear most commonly on exposed skin during the summer months. Although Group A β-hemolytic streptococci were the predominant organisms 25–30 years ago, *Staphylococcus aureus* alone or in combination with streptococci is recovered from a majority of cultures. As a consequence, anti-staphylococcal antibiotics are now the drugs of choice for treatment.

Impetigo is often a self-limiting process, likely to resolve in 4 weeks; however, the lesions are highly contagious and subject to social stigma. Complications, which include cellulitis and disseminated infection, as well as spread to family members and classmates, can be limited by antibiotic therapy. Topical antibiotics, such as bacitracin, polymyxin B, neomycin, and mupirocin may be used in localized disease, but increasing resistance to traditional topical antibiotics makes retapamulin a better first-line agent. More recently, ozenoxacin 1% cream has demonstrated efficacy in treating impetigo with activity against methicillin-resistant *Staphylococcus aureus* (MRSA) and low probability of spontaneous mutants in quinolone-resistant and sensitive stains. Widespread lesions have been treated with oral agents such as cephalexin, amoxicillin-clavulanate, and erythromycin. Unfortunately, there is increased evidence for resistance against erythromycin, clindamycin, cephalexin, and cloxacillin. Previously, MRSA was confined to health care facilities; however, its prevalence is increasing in community settings. Consequently, the practitioner must select antibiotic coverage based on the resistance patterns in their respective communities (e.g. clindamycin, trimethoprim-sulfamethoxazole, tetracyclines) and consider resistance when patients fail to respond to appropriate doses of anti-staphylococcal antibiotics.

Impetigo should be contrasted from the rarer variant, bullous impetigo (BI), which is characterized by fragile fluid-filled vesicles caused by the staphylococcal exfoliative toxin. As opposed to the hematogenous spread of toxin in staphylococcal scalded-skin syndrome, the toxin in BI is restricted to the site of infection. Hence, wound culture is encouraged to guide treatment specific to antibiotic sensitivity. The first-line agent for localized BI is mupirocin, whereas the first-line agent for widespread BI is cephalosporins.

Staphylococcal Scalded-Skin Syndrome

Staphylococcal scalded-skin syndrome (SSSS), also known as Ritter disease, occurs almost exclusively in infants and toddlers (Fig. 4.13), with an incidence of about 7.5 per 100 000 infants <1 year old. It has, however, been reported with increasing frequency in older children and adults, particularly in debilitated patients with decreased renal function. The in-hospital mortality rate for SSSS in children is low (0.31%), whereas the mortality rate for SSSS in adults is 4.3%. This process is considered in any child who develops a generalized, tender erythema associated with a Nikolsky sign. When a Nikolsky sign is present, a minimal shearing force produced by finger pressure induces a skin slough or blister formation. The diagnosis is mainly clinical with the presence of tender erythroderma, positive Nikolsky sign, desquamation particularly at friction zones, perioral crust, and absence of mucosal involvement; however, cultures may be necessary to guide antibiotic choice.

SSSS occurs when exfoliative toxin produced by certain staphylococci binds to a desmosomal adhesion molecule desmoglein-1

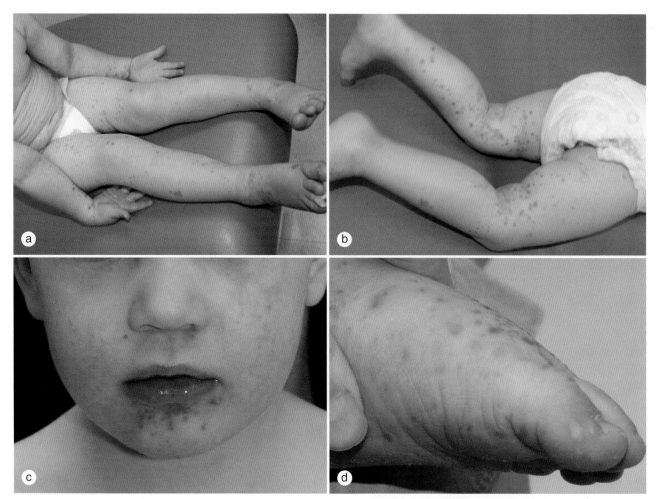

Fig. 4.11 Coxsackie A6 virus infection. A 2-year-old boy developed high fever and widely disseminated vesicles and crusts concentrated on the **(a)** arms, on the **(a,b)** legs, and around the **(c)** mouth. He had erosions on his palate and, on careful observation, lancet-shaped vesicles on a red base on his hands and **(d)** feet. The blisters began to dry in 2 days and resolved within 5 days without treatment.

in the subgranular region of the epidermis, resulting in cleavage at this site high in the epidermis. Interestingly, this is the same adhesion molecule that is targeted by autoantibodies in pemphigus foliaceus.

Although SSSS is usually self-limiting in healthy children who rapidly develop antibodies to the toxin, immunocompromised patients may develop complications related to their primary staphylococcal infection. Moreover, renal excretion of the toxin may be slowed in patients with impaired renal function (e.g. chronic renal failure) or renal clearance of the toxin (e.g. infants). Most SSSS is associated with a primary cutaneous infection. However, the soluble toxin that causes the rash may be produced by an occult infection, such as osteomyelitis, septic arthritis, pneumonia, or meningitis. Healthy children respond to oral anti-staphylococcal antibiotics, which eradicate the infection and subsequent toxin production; however, there is an increase in mupirocin and fusidic acid resistant strains. Infants, severely ill older children, and patients with occult infection require appropriate culturing and parenteral therapy. Consider MRSA in patients not clinically improving or critically ill, and use vancomycin. Parents are also counseled about the

generalized desquamation that develops 10–14 days after the acute infection.

Staphylococcal Folliculitis

Staphylococcal folliculitis is a common problem in older children and adults. Red papules and pustules on an inflamed base erupt in a follicular pattern, most frequently on the buttocks, thighs, back, and upper arms (Fig. 4.14). Occasionally, superficial follicular pustules evolve into painful, deep-seated furuncles or spread to neighboring follicles and soft tissue to create an abscess or carbuncle. Abscesses and resultant cellulitis may be associated with fever, malaise, and sepsis. The incidence of furunculosis and abscess formation has increased dramatically with the spread of MRSA and should not be mistaken for insect or spider bites.

Localized folliculitis may improve with topical antibiotics. However, widespread lesions respond best to topical benzoyl peroxide wash or systemic antibiotics. Additionally, abscesses are incised and drained, and cellulitis may require parenteral antibiotics.

Children with Down syndrome are particularly prone to follicular occlusion disorders such as folliculitis, acneiform

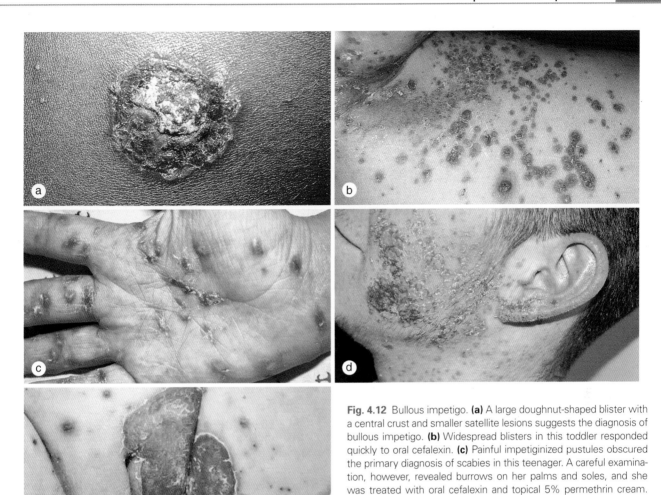

Fig. 4.12 Bullous impetigo. **(a)** A large doughnut-shaped blister with a central crust and smaller satellite lesions suggests the diagnosis of bullous impetigo. **(b)** Widespread blisters in this toddler responded quickly to oral cefalexin. **(c)** Painful impetiginized pustules obscured the primary diagnosis of scabies in this teenager. A careful examination, however, revealed burrows on her palms and soles, and she was treated with oral cefalexin and topical 5% permethrin cream. **(d)** A healthy adolescent with an irritant dermatitis from shaving developed expanding confluent crusted papules typical of secondary impetiginization from *Staphylococcus aureus*. **(e)** A 5-year-old girl who was recovering from varicella developed several confluent erosions with an expanding bulla at the periphery and central crusting.

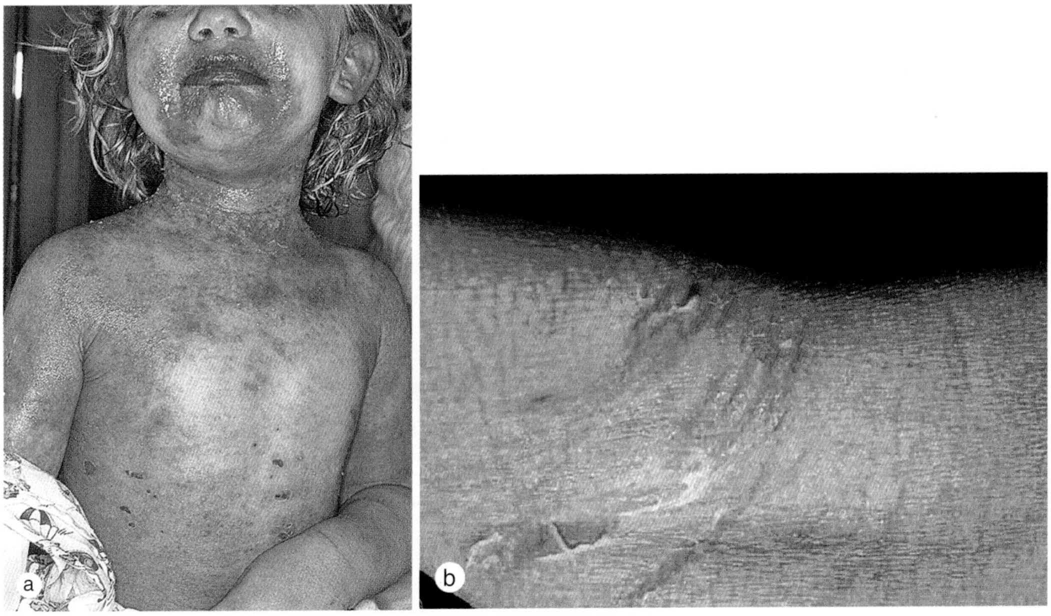

Fig. 4.13 Staphylococcal scalded-skin syndrome. **(a)** A healthy 3-year-old boy developed fever, periorificial periarticular crusting, and generalized, tender red skin. Nikolsky sign was present, and *Staphylococcus aureus* was cultured from the crust around the eyes. **(b)** Note the Nikolsky sign in the axilla as evidenced by superficial sloughing of the skin from movement of the arm.

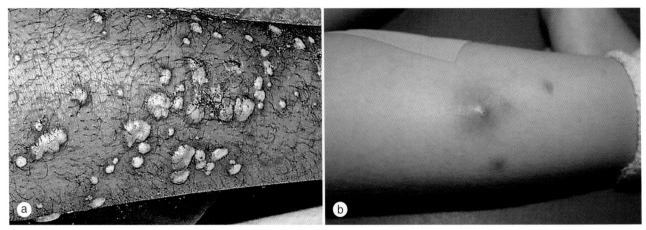

Fig. 4.14 (a) Staphylococcal folliculitis recurred chronically on the extremities of a healthy adolescent. He cleared with anti-staphylococcal antibiotics, and preventative antibiotics helped somewhat. **(b)** A 4-year-old boy developed recurrent pustules and deep-seated boils on his extremities. A bacterial culture revealed methicillin-resistant *Staphylococcus aureus* sensitive to clindamycin.

eruptions, and pilonidal cysts. Further, immunosuppressive states and isotretinoin use resulting in reduction of white blood cell count have been associated with an increased risk for staphylococcal folliculitis. Long-term use of antiseptic soaps, topical antibiotics (e.g. clindamycin, tetracycline, erythromycin), dilute bleach baths, and peeling agents (e.g. benzoyl peroxide, retinoic acid, salicylic acid) may reduce the risk of recurrent infection. Persistent or difficult-to-treat folliculitis, especially when associated with furunculosis, should prompt culturing for MRSA infection.

Regardless of the etiology, infectious or non-infectious, folliculitis responds well to normal warm saline compresses, followed by topical erythromycin or bacitracin ointment and sterile gauze dressing. Certain hydrating lotions and creams that are also designed to remove scale (e.g. Carmol and Ureacin with urea, LactiCare, AmLactin and Lac-Hydrin with lactic acid) may be beneficial. Patients are also instructed to avoid tight clothing and occlusive moisturizers. In toddlers, folliculitis may improve after toilet training. Older children with enuresis should also be encouraged to remove wet clothing as soon as possible.

IMMUNOBULLOUS DERMATOSES

Although there is clinical overlap among the various immunologically mediated vesiculobullous dermatoses, they can be differentiated on the basis of specific clinical patterns, histopathology, immunopathology, and response to therapy (Table 4.1). In pemphigus, blisters form within the epidermis. Chronic bullous dermatosis of childhood (CBDC), BP, dermatitis herpetiformis (DH), and EBA are characterized by subepidermal blisters.

Intraepidermal Disorders

Childhood pemphigus refers to a group of rare, chronic, potentially life-threatening immunobullous disorders characterized by flaccid intraepidermal bullae that erupt on normal-appearing or erythematous skin. Clinically and histologically, pemphigus can be divided into two types: pemphigus vulgaris (PV) and

pemphigus foliaceus (PF). Though observed around the world, the geographic distribution of PV is highest in Ashkenazi Jews of Mediterranean origin. In most countries, PV is more prevalent than PF except for Finland, Brazil, and Tunisia.

Although the pathogenesis of pemphigus is still not completely understood, immunoglobulin (Ig)G, IgA, IgM, and complement have been identified in blister fluid. In pemphigus, the target antigen was identified as a desmoglein, one of several cadherin-type adhesion molecules that comprises desmosomes. Disruption of desmosomes results in cleavage of the epidermis and blister formation. Desmoglein-1 is found throughout the epidermis and only minimally in the oral mucosa, whereas desmoglein-3 occurs primarily in the oral mucosa and the lower half of the epidermis. As a consequence, patients with autoantibodies directed against desmoglein-1 develop superficial lesions within the epidermis resulting in PF. In contrast, patients with autoantibodies directed against desmoglein-3 develop PV of the oral mucosa and limited or no lesions in the skin because of normally functioning desmoglein-1 in the upper half of the epidermis. Finally, individuals with autoantibodies directed against both desmoglein-3 and -1 develop deep epidermal skin blisters, as well as oral mucous membrane involvement.

Pemphigus Vulgaris

Childhood PV is highly uncommon and represents about 1.4–2.9% of all PV cases. In PV, intraoral erosions or scalp blisters precede more widespread lesions in half the patients for months. Eventually, vesicles and bullae develop on the trunk, scalp, face, and extremities in a seborrheic distribution (Fig. 4.15). Blisters heal insidiously without scarring, unless they become secondarily infected. Of these patients, 95% have intraoral involvement that may extend into the posterior pharynx and larynx. Pruritus, pain, and burning of the skin and mucous membranes may be severe, which results in decreased oral intake and marked weight loss. Nikolsky sign is usually present, and downward pressure on previously formed blisters may cause extension at the periphery (Asboe–Hansen sign). Pemphigus may also occur transiently in

TABLE 4.1   Immunobullous Dermatoses

	Immunoglobulin	Location in Skin	Target Antigen	Clinical Findings
Intraepidermal				
Pemphigus foliaceus	IgG	Intercellular, upper epidermis	Desmoglein-1	Seborrheic distribution
Pemphigus vulgaris	IgG	Intercellular Lower half or full-thickness epidermis	Desmoglein-3 Desmoglein-3, −1	Intraoral lesions Intraoral lesions, widespread skin-deep erosions
Subepidermal				
Linear IgA bullous dermatosis (CBDC)	IgA	Linear pattern in lamina lucida	97 kDa cleaved ectodimer of BP180 antigen	Vesicles, bullae, lower trunk, thighs, occasionally disseminated
Bullous pemphigoid (BP)	IgA C3	Epidermal side of lamina lucida	BP230 (BPA1) BP180 (BPA2)	Bullae tend to be >2.0 cm but can mimic CBDC
Dermatitis herpetiformis	IgA	Granular deposits in basement membrane zone at dermal papillary tips		Extremely pruritic papules, crusted vesicles on extensor surfaces of extremities, buttocks
Epidermolysis bullosa acquisita (EBA)	IgG IgA	Subbasement zone in lamina lucida	Collagen VII	May mimic dystrophic EB or CBDC, mucous membranes often involved

Ig, Immunoglobulin; *CBDC,* chronic bullous dermatosis of childhood

the newborn as a result of transplacental passage of the pemphigus IgG antibody from the mother to the baby.

In virtually 100% of patients, fluorescein-labeled IgG can be demonstrated to bind to the epidermal intercellular space in the patient's normal-appearing and perilesional skin, referred to as positive direct immunofluorescence (DIF) (Fig. 4.15c). Deposits of C3, IgA, or IgM are also identified in nearly half of the patients. Indirect immunofluorescence (IIF) involves application of fluorescence-labeled antihuman IgG at various dilutions to the patient's serum and test specimen. When the study is positive, fluorescence is seen in the intercellular spaces of the test specimen. Although DIF is very sensitive, even early in the course of disease,

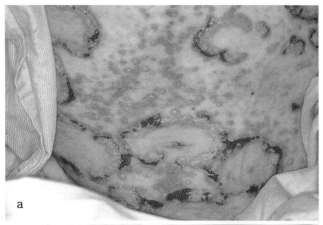

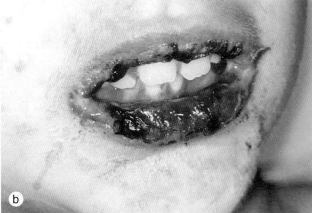

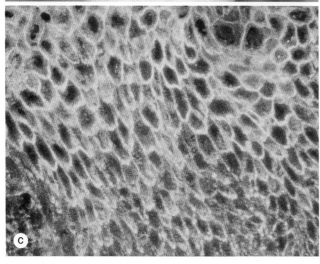

Fig. 4.15 Pemphigus vulgaris. **(a)** A 7-year-old boy developed widespread superficial vesicles, bullae, and erosions on his trunk, extremities, and scalp. **(b)** He also had mucosal involvement with erosions on the lips, buccal mucosa, and larynx, as well as the urethra and anus. **(c)** Anti-IgG antibody marks the epidermal intercellular cement substance on direct immunofluorescence.

IIF is less useful, particularly before lesions become widespread. Enzyme-linked immunosorbent assay (ELISA) is a very sensitive and specific assay for identifying IgG antibodies against desmoglein-1 and desmoglein-3, with a strong correlation for clinical severity, serving as a marker for patient progress.

Early PV restricted to the mouth must be differentiated histologically from other disorders that involve the oral mucosa,

such as erosive lichen planus and aphthosis. Once cutaneous lesions appear, the typical clinical pattern, histology, and immunofluorescence differentiate PV from other immunobullous disorders.

The introduction of corticosteroids resulted in a drop in mortality rate from 50%, largely caused by sepsis, to now 10%. Management of fluid and electrolyte losses and supportive skin care may require admission to a burn unit. High-dose prednisone may be life-saving. Recently, an anti-CD20 antibody, rituximab, directed against plasma cells has been used to achieve long-term remission of systemic corticosteroids, and studies have demonstrated rituximab plus short-term prednisone may be more effective than prednisone alone. Some patients may require other corticosteroid-sparing immunosuppressive agents such as cyclophosphamide, azathioprine, or mycophenolate depending on their response to the corticosteroid taper and rituximab. Adjunctive therapy might also include intravenous immunoglobulin (IVIG) and immunoablative therapy with cyclophosphamide and plasmapheresis. Currently, studies investigating the role of anti–B-cell drugs are underway. The clinical course of PV varies; however, very few patients reach complete remission. Compared with adults, children are reported to have better long-term outcomes given early initiation of treatment.

Pemphigus Foliaceus

PF is a more superficial and less aggressive immunobullous disorder. Although it occurs most commonly in middle age, in children, this variant is more common than PV. Although PF tends to be sporadic, and most cases have been reported in North America and Europe, an endemic variant known as fogo selvagem occurs primarily in children and adolescents in Brazil. Clinically and histologically, PF is indistinguishable from Brazilian pemphigus. Some medications, such as penicillamine, have also been reported to trigger a PF-like eruption.

Much like PV, PF begins with crops of vesicles, flaccid bullae, and erosions on an erythematous base in a seborrheic distribution. However, the blisters, which result from autoantibodies directed against desmoglein-1, arise high in the epidermis and quickly crust over. The Nikolsky sign is usually positive, but mucous membranes, which contain little desmoglein-1, are invariably spared. When lesions become generalized, vesicles may be obscured by crust and scale, which gives the patient the appearance of an exfoliative erythroderma (Fig. 4.16). Even with widespread rash, patients tend to appear clinically well, and the course is often self-limiting.

Histopathology demonstrates acantholysis and bullae formation, much like in PV. However, the action occurs in the upper half of the epidermis, sometimes restricted to the area immediately beneath the stratum corneum. The intercellular space in the upper half of the epidermis shows IgG staining with DIF, and the IIF is also usually positive. Chronic lesions typically show acanthosis, eosinophilic spongiosis, and eosinophilic dermal inflammation.

Patients with mild disease may respond to moderate- or highpotency topical corticosteroids. In many cases, systemic corticosteroids may be required for a while, and some investigators have reported success with antimalarials (hydroxychloroquine and

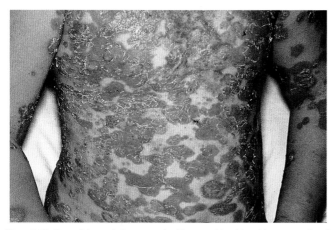

Fig. 4.16 Pemphigus foliaceus. A 10-year-old girl with generalized, slightly itchy, scaly, and crusted patches was referred for evaluation of possible pemphigus foliaceus. Although a skin biopsy was suggestive of pemphigus, a skin culture grew *Staphylococcus aureus*, and the rash resolved after 7 days of oral dicloxacillin. The recent understanding of the desmoglein story in pemphigus and SSSS explains the clinical and histological similarity of these two blistering disorders.

chloroquine) and sulfonamides (sulfapyridine and dapsone). In severe cases, similar to PV, rituximab has also been used to achieve long-term remission off corticosteroids.

Subepidermal Disorders
Chronic Bullous Dermatosis of Childhood

CBDC is a term used to describe a subepidermal immunobullous disorder with characteristic clinical features and linear IgA deposition at the basement membrane zone noted on direct immunofluorescent examination of perilesional skin. Recent data suggest that CBDC may represent a number of different disorders with similar and overlapping clinical findings but varying and specific immunofluorescent markers. Various inducing factors have been associated in CBDC such as autoimmune disease, malignancy, and gastrointestinal disease. In drug-induced CBDC, vancomycin is the most frequently implicated agent, whereas non-steroidal anti-inflammatory drugs (NSAIDs), cephalosporins, penicillin, and captopril are less commonly implicated. Further, drug-induced CBDC may be more severe and mimic toxic epidermal necrolysis.

Although tense, 1.0–2.0 cm diameter bullae typically appear in CBDC in preschool children on the lower trunk, buttocks, legs, and top of the feet, children of any age may be affected (Fig. 4.17). Widespread lesions may involve any site on the body surface including the face, scalp, upper trunk, hands, and arms. Lesions erupt on red, as well as normal-appearing skin, and they often form rings composed of sausage-shaped bullae around a central crust or healing blister. The "string of pearls" sign demonstrates the tendency of vesicles to form on an inflamed base (Fig. 4.18 and Fig. 4.19). Mucous membranes are not usually involved in linear IgA disease, a Nikolsky sign is not present, and burning and pruritus are variable. Some children are completely asymptomatic.

Histopathology of CBDC is indistinguishable from that of adult BP, which demonstrates a subepidermal blister with a

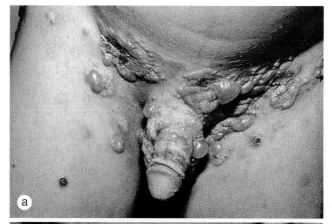

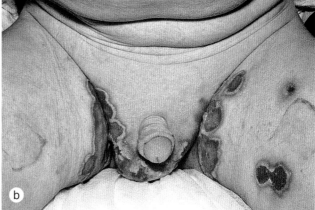

Fig. 4.17 Linear IgA bullous dermatosis. Two 3-year-old boys presented with chronic, recurrent blisters in the diaper area. **(a)** Fresh, tense bullae spread along the inguinal creases onto the thighs and penis. **(b)** Ruptured bullae left annular and scalloped erosions.

dermal infiltrate of neutrophils and eosinophils. Occasionally, eosinophils form microabscesses at the tips of the dermal papillae reminiscent of DH. However, DIF shows linear deposits of IgA at the dermal–epidermal junction and is diagnostic (Fig. 4.20). Investigators have also shown that the site of deposition is within the lamina lucida, with accentuation near the basal cell membrane around hemidesmosomes. Circulating IgA antibodies are present in 50–75% of patients.

Although CBDC is often self-limiting, with spontaneous resolution over 3–5 years, occasional cases persist after adolescence. Many children are exquisitely sensitive to small doses of dapsone. Resistant cases may require systemic corticosteroids, at least until the eruption comes under control. All patients on dapsone must be monitored for clinical and laboratory signs of hemolysis, methemoglobinemia, and neurologic complications.

Bullous Pemphigoid

In BP, bullae tend to be large (>2 cm), but vesiculobullous lesions and distribution may be indistinguishable from linear IgA dermatosis (Fig. 4.21). BP is the most common autoimmune blistering disorder in the elderly, and its occurrence in children is rare, with most cases occurring in early childhood. Skin biopsies in BP also demonstrate subepidermal bullae with

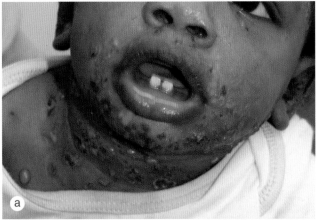

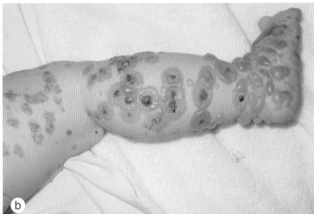

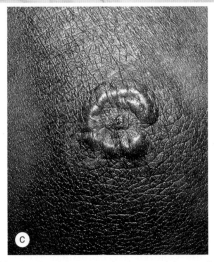

Fig. 4.18 Widespread vesicles erupted over several days on the face, trunk, and extremities of two toddlers with linear IgA dermatosis **(a,b)**. Blisters were densest on the face and trunk **(a)** of the 12-month-old boy and the lower extremities **(b)** of the 14-month-old girl. **(c)** Annular blisters spread over the trunk and extremities in this 4-year-old boy.

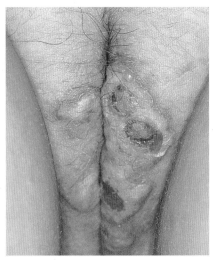

Fig. 4.19 This adolescent girl with a 9-month history of genital blisters and erosions failed to improve with topical antibiotics, antifungal creams, lubricants, or oral acyclovir. Sexual abuse was suspected until a skin biopsy, which demonstrated the classic findings of linear IgA bullous dermatosis, was performed.

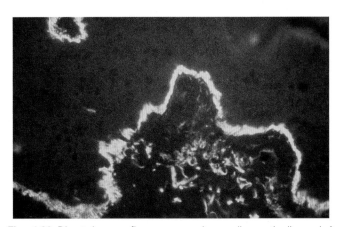

Fig. 4.20 Direct immunofluorescence shows diagnostic linear IgA deposition along the dermal–epidermal junction.

find BP230 and BP180 antigens. An unusual cicatricial variant of BP involves primarily the mucous membranes and occurs only rarely in childhood.

Studies have demonstrated tetracyclines to be non-inferior to corticosteroids in their anti-inflammatory effects against bullous pemphigoid and also are associated with a lower incidence of side effects. Further, nicotinamide, the water-soluble and active form of B3, has been used for blistering diseases as a result of its anti-inflammatory effects.

Dermatitis Herpetiformis

Symmetric, extremely pruritic, clustered, 3–4 mm diameter vesicles on extensor surfaces of the extremities, lower trunk, and buttocks may suggest DH (Fig. 4.22). In DH, the lesions arise on both red and normal-appearing skin and may occasionally exceed 1.0 cm in diameter. The skin biopsy of

an eosinophilic dermal infiltrate. However, linear depositions of IgG and C3 at the dermal–epidermal junction in the lamina lucida are diagnostic for BP. When salt-split skin is used as a substrate for immunofluorescent studies, staining occurs on the epidermal side of the cleavage where one would expect to

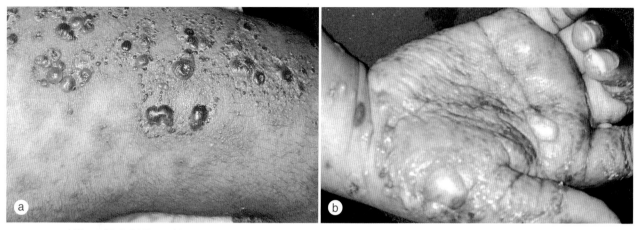

Fig. 4.21 (a,b) Tense blisters on an urticarial base developed insidiously on the extremities and trunk of an adolescent with bullous pemphigoid.

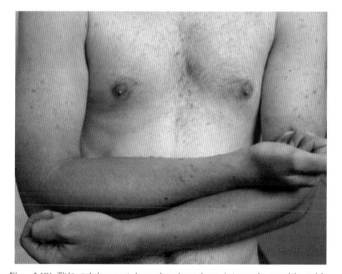

Fig. 4.22 This adolescent boy developed an intensely pruritic widespread blistering eruption most densely distributed on the extensor surfaces of his arms and legs, back, and buttocks. Histologic and immunofluorescent findings were typical of dermatitis herpetiformis.

perilesional skin reveals characteristic, granular IgA deposits in the basement membrane zone and prominent neurophilic microabscesses at the dermal papillary tips. The high incidence of human leukocyte antigen (HLA) B8 antigens also defines DH, as does a gluten-sensitive enteropathy and a rapid response to dapsone. Treatment involves compliance with gluten-free diet, which also reduces the risk of lymphoma. In severe cases, dapsone or topical clobetasol may be utilized for rapid control.

Epidermolysis Bullosa Acquisita

Although initially thought to be rare in childhood, the use of salt-split skin as a substrate for immunofluorescent studies has often resulted in a diagnosis of EBA in children who would have previously been grouped with CBDC or BP (Fig. 4.23). EBA shares some clinical features with hereditary dystrophic epidermolysis bullosa, and in both disorders, blisters result

from disruption of type VII collagen. Clinically, patients with EBA may be indistinguishable from CBDC or BP. However, they have a higher incidence of mucous membrane involvement and may be more resistant to therapy. Although EBA probably occurs most commonly as an isolated autoimmune disorder, until recently, it has been reported primarily in association with other immunologically mediated conditions such as systemic lupus erythematosus and inflammatory bowel disease.

Histology reveals a subepidermal blister with a neutrophil-rich infiltrate, but eosinophils may also be present. DIF typically shows deposition of linear IgG at the basement membrane zone. IIF with salt-split skin demonstrates IgG on the dermal side of the split, whereas immune deposits are on the epidermal side of the split in BP. Recently, a group of patients with IgA EBA have been reported. Clinicians should consider the addition of prednisone-sparing medications early in the management of these patients, particularly if mucous membrane involvement is widespread and severe.

The IIF findings in cicatricial pemphigoid are similar to EBA. However, cutaneous lesions are usually limited. In some cases, these disorders can only be distinguished with immunofluorescent electron microscopy, in which type VII collagen is identified as the autoantibody target on an ultrastructural level.

The target lesions of classic erythema multiforme (EM), particularly when blistering is present, may be confused with those of CBDC. However, the acute clinical course, histopathology, and negative immunofluorescence readily differentiate EM. Early in its course, CBDC is often misdiagnosed as BI. Moreover, bullae of CBDC that are secondarily infected respond to antibiotic therapy. However, the persistence of blistering despite antibiotic therapy, the widespread distribution of the eruption, and negative Gram-stains and cultures suggest a non-infectious etiology.

Recurrent HSV infection and the possibility of sexual abuse can also be excluded by the characteristic skin biopsy findings (Fig. 4.23). Though treatment of EBA is difficult, both IVIG and rituximab have been associated with complete remission in some patients.

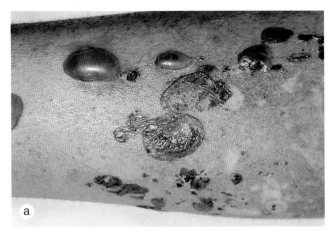

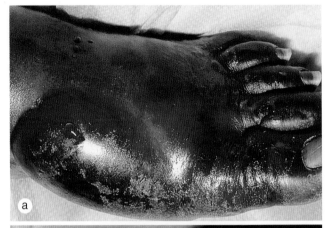

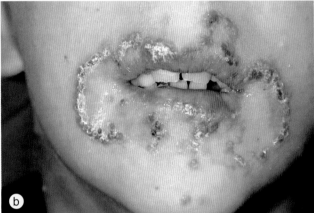

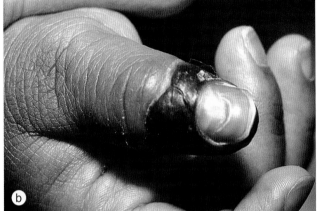

Fig. 4.24 (a) Friction blisters. Large, hemorrhagic blisters developed in areas of minor trauma on the trunk and extremities of a cachectic, chronically ill child during an episode of acute renal failure. Blistering healed as renal function returned to normal and cutaneous edema resolved. A skin biopsy demonstrated intraepidermal blisters without inflammation. **(b)** Sucking blisters. Recurrent hemorrhagic blisters appeared on the thumb of a 10-year-old thumb-sucker. These blisters can arise within the epidermis or basement membrane zone.

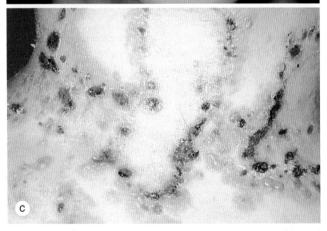

Fig. 4.23 Epidermolysis bullosa acquisita. **(a)** An adolescent with poorly controlled systemic lupus erythematosus developed a diffuse painful blistering eruption composed of large bullae, which on biopsy and immunofluorescent studies showed changes typical of (IgG) epidermolysis bullosa acquisita. This disorder is indistinguishable from bullous lupus erythematosus. **(b,c)** A 9-year-old boy without underlying connective tissue disease developed annular urticarial plaques with vesicles and bullae on his face **(b)**, neck **(c)**, and upper trunk. Laboratory findings were diagnostic for IgA epidermolysis bullosa acquisita.

MECHANOBULLOUS DISORDERS

Friction Blisters

Friction blisters occur frequently on the soles, palms, and palmar surfaces of the fingers after vigorous exercise or other repetitive activities, causing shearing of thick areas of epidermis that are firmly attached to underlying tissue (Fig. 4.24a). In patients with chronic localized or generalized edema, particularly in the setting of malnutrition, minor trauma may result in blister formation. Similar blisters can result from rubbing and sucking (Fig. 4.24b). Neonatal sucking blisters occur in about 1 in every 240 live births and can often be confused for more serious conditions such as HSV, neonatal lupus erythematous, or EB. These blisters occur as a result of a strong intrauterine sucking reflex and are commonly located on distal upper extremities. Further, hydration of the skin surface has been associated with an increased the risk of blister formation. Histologically, these lesions may be identified as non-inflammatory, intraepidermal blisters, which are usually located just beneath the granular layer. Although blisters heal quickly in healthy individuals, impetiginization and cellulitis are frequent complications in compromised hosts. The use of barriers, such as socks and antiperspirants have shown efficacy in prevention of friction blisters.

Epidermolysis Bullosa

Hereditary epidermolysis bullosa is a heterogeneous group of skin fragility disorders differentiated by clinical findings, depth of blister formation, biochemical markers, inheritance patterns, and specific genetic mutations (see Table 2.4). In most of these conditions, vesiculobullous lesions appear at birth or in early infancy, with an incidence of 20 per 1 million live births. Several variants, however, do not present until adolescence or adult life.

In epidermolysis bullosa simplex, localized variant (EBS localized, previously Weber–Cockayne syndrome), blisters may first appear on the soles during rigorous physical activity such as track-and-field sports and military boot camp. Localized EBS is due to autosomal dominant mutations in keratins 5 and 14 and integrin beta 4. Vesicles and bullae are usually restricted to the distal extremities, and particularly the palms and soles. Healing occurs without scar formation, and the nails and mucous membranes are not affected. Histopathology demonstrates a suprabasilar split in the epidermis, and electron microscopy shows cytolysis within the basal cell layer. Although these findings are also typical of friction blisters in normal individuals, clumping of tonofilaments in basal cell keratinocytes is specific for EBS.

Recurrent blistering of the palms and soles, particularly during warm weather when blistering is more common, suggests the disorder. A positive family history clinches the diagnosis, although novel spontaneous mutations can occur in the absence of family history. The hallmark of the disorder is blistering triggered by minor trauma consequently resulting in erosions, ulcers, scarring, and sometimes aggressive squamous cell carcinoma. Blistering may be reduced by using extra cushioning in shoes and avoiding unnecessary trauma to the hands and feet, particularly during warm weather.

A multidisciplinary approach is needed for the management of epidermolysis bullosa. Cool tap water compresses may help symptomatically, and topical antibiotics reduce the risk of secondary infection; however, the increased use of antibiotics in this population has led to a rise in mupirocin-resistant bacteria. Recently, evidence for the use of vitamin D and phenytoin has emerged to modulate the inflammation in chronic wound healing. The use of topical antiperspirants, such as 10–20% aluminum hydroxide, 10% formaldehyde, or 10% glutaraldehyde, may decrease the blistering, as well as associated hyperhidrosis of the palms and soles. Some patients have also benefited from applications of tincture of benzoin or Mastisol. As a result of the increased risk of melanoma and non-melanoma type cancer in patients with epidermolysis bullosa, patients should be encouraged for regular screenings starting in their 20s or 30s.

DERMATITIS

In acute dermatitides, inflammation and associated edema may be so intense that vesiculation occurs. Blisters erupt frequently in acute contact irritant and allergic dermatitis, as well as in atopic dermatitis, seborrhea, and insect bite reactions (Fig. 4.25). Whenever blistering develops in this setting, secondary infection with *Staphylococcus* or HSV is also considered.

Bacterial culture and viral PCR as indicated exclude infections. Skin biopsies demonstrate variable acanthosis or thickening of the epidermis, exocytosis or an influx of lymphocytes into the epidermis, and spongiosis or intercellular edema. It is the intense edema that eventually breaks apart desmosomal attachments and results in spongiotic blister formation. Immunofluorescence studies are negative. Blistering from dermatitic reactions can usually be differentiated clinically from thermal burns, cold injury, and ischemic insults to the skin that result in subepidermal blisters.

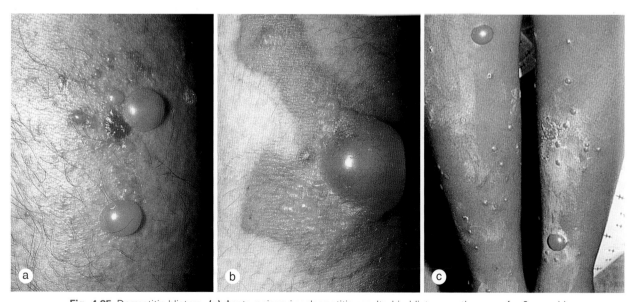

Fig. 4.25 Dermatitic blisters. **(a)** Acute poison ivy dermatitis resulted in blisters on the arm of a 9-year-old boy. Note the surrounding erythema, edema, and papules typical of an allergic contact dermatitis. **(b)** Vesicles and a large bulla erupted on an extremely well-demarcated red base on the arm of a teenager who admitted to applying acid to create the lesions. **(c)** This child's lower legs are studded with numerous, thick-walled vesicles and bullae, which formed in response to flea bites.

ERYTHEMA MULTIFORME, STEVENS–JOHNSON SYNDROME, TOXIC EPIDERMAL NECROLYSIS, MYCOPLASMA-INDUCED RASH AND MUCOSITIS

In the past, clinicians have considered EM and Stevens–Johnson syndrome (SJS) and toxic epidermal necrolysis (TEN), as related disorders with clinical and histologic overlap. Although they may share some clinical and histologic features, EM and mycoplasma-induced rash and mucositis should be viewed separately, as a usually benign, self-limiting disorder with rare complications, while SJS and TEN represent the variable expression of a distinct syndrome with a significant risk of morbidity and mortality. SJS and TEN are most commonly triggered by medications, while EM and mycoplasma-induced rash and mucositis usually follow an infection.

Erythema Multiforme

In the classic eruption, originally described by Ferdinand von Hebra in 1860, the rash is symmetric and may occur on any part of the body, although it usually appears on the dorsum of the hands and feet and the extensor surfaces of the arms and legs (Fig. 4.26). Involvement of the palms and soles is common. The initial lesions are dusky, red macules or edematous papules that evolve into target lesions with multiple, concentric rings of color change. The annular configuration occurs as the central inflammatory process spreads peripherally and leaves behind a depressed, damaged epidermis. When epidermal injury is severe, full-thickness necrosis results in central bulla formation. The eruption continues in crops that last 1–3 weeks. In most children with this so-called minor variant, mucous membrane involvement is minimal and restricted to the mouth, the disease is self-limiting, and systemic manifestations are limited to low-grade fever, malaise, and myalgia. Rarely, oral involvement is severe enough to interfere with oral intake and require parenteral rehydration. Recurrent EM occurs in association with recurrent HSV infection; however, there is little utilization of continuous acyclovir treatment. Agents such as dapsone, Janus Kinase (JAK) inhibitors, Phosphodiesterase (PDE)-4 inhibitors, and thalidomide may be considered for recurrent or acyclovir resistant EM.

Stevens–Johnson Syndrome and Toxic Epidermal Necrolysis

SJS is a severe mucocutaneous syndrome with epidermal involvement and large areas of mucous membrane necrosis and

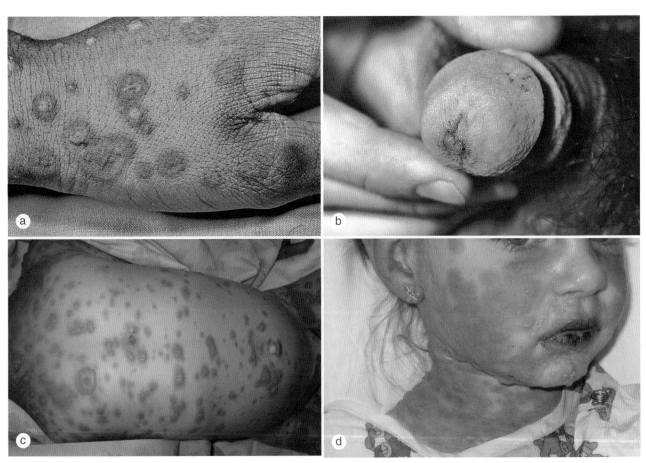

Fig. 4.26 Erythema multiforme. **(a)** Typical target lesions erupted on the arms and legs of this 9-year-old boy with recurrent erythema multiforme associated with herpes simplex infection. He had only minimal mucous membrane involvement. **(b)** An adolescent with erythema multiforme minor developed painful erosions around the urethra. **(c,d)** A healthy 5-year-old girl developed widespread bullous erythema multiforme with sparing of the mucous membranes. She cleared with 10 days of tapering oral prednisolone.

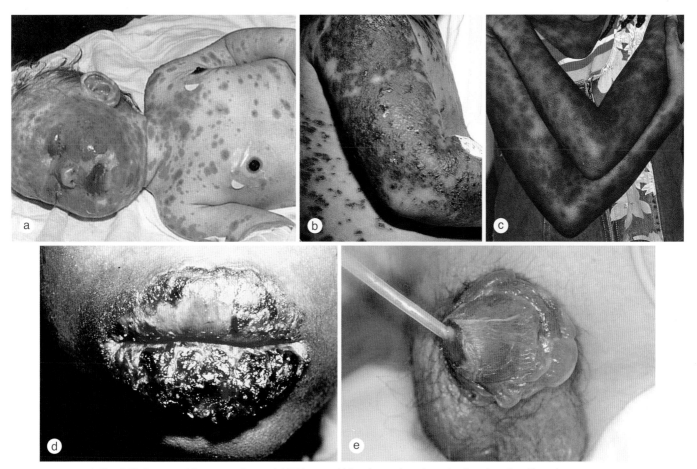

Fig. 4.27 Stevens–Johnson syndrome. **(a)** Widespread blistering and erosions developed on the skin and mucous membranes of this 3-year-old girl with Stevens–Johnson syndrome. **(b)** Widespread areas of necrotic blisters and ulcerations can heal **(c)** with marked permanent hyperpigmentation in dark-pigmented individuals. **(d,e)** Hemorrhagic crusts on the lips are characteristic of Stevens–Johnson syndrome.

sloughing. TEN represents the most severe end of the spectrum with widespread cutaneous and mucous membrane involvement. SJS and TEN are differentiated by the degree of skin involvement: SJS involves <10% of the skin, SJS/TEN overlap involves 10–30% of the skin, and TEN involves >30% of the skin. In SJS, constitutional symptoms are severe and include high fever, cough, sore throat, vomiting, diarrhea, chest pain, and arthralgias. After a prodrome lasting 1–14 days, but usually 1–3 days, abrupt onset of symmetric erythematous macules occurs on the head and neck and spreads to the trunk and extremities (Fig. 4.27). Blister formation occurs within hours and is often hemorrhagic, extensive, and confluent. Mucous membrane involvement, particularly of the eyes, nose, and mouth, is widespread and severe. SJS consists of the formation of fragile, thin-walled bullae that rupture with minimal trauma, to leave ulcerations that are rapidly covered by exudate. Keratitis may result in ocular infection and synechiae formation. The urogenital and perirectal areas may also become involved. Loss of the epidermal barrier results in fluid and electrolyte imbalances and a high risk of secondary bacterial infection. Mortality ranges between 5% and 25%, and in the acute phase, septicemia is the leading cause of mortality.

Toxic Epidermal Necrolysis

With TEN, patients usually begin with fever, sore throat, malaise, and a generalized, sunburn-like erythema, followed by sloughing of large areas of skin (Fig. 4.28). The entire skin surface, as well as conjunctivae, urethra, rectum, oral and nasal mucosa, larynx, and tracheobronchial mucosa, may become involved. Although a Nikolsky sign is present and the erythema is reminiscent of SSSS, the site of cleavage in TEN as in SJS is at the dermal–epidermal junction, which results in full-thickness epidermal necrosis.

Frozen sections of sloughed epidermis can be used for rapid differentiation of TEN from SSSS while the practitioner awaits the definitive results of a skin biopsy. However, clinical distinction of these disorders is usually possible because erosions and sloughing of the mucous membranes do not develop in SSSS. Intensive supportive measures are required to avoid fluid and electrolyte losses and secondary bacterial infection. Respiratory distress syndrome has been reported in severe cases.

Morbidity and mortality risks may be higher than those in patients with SJS. In uncomplicated cases, re-epithelialization of the skin occurs within several weeks and full recovery in 4–6 weeks. Scarring may develop in areas of secondary infection. As in SJS,

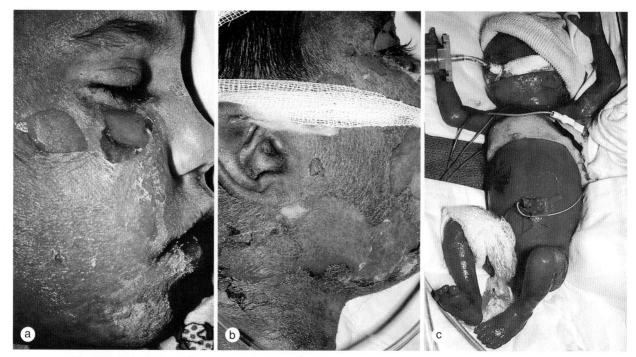

Fig. 4.28 Toxic epidermal necrolysis. **(a)** After 7 days of a course of oral co-trimoxazole for otitis media, this 8-year-old girl developed high fever and generalized erythema and edema, followed by sloughing of large sheets of skin. Mucous membranes were severely involved. Note Nikolsky sign on her upper cheek, induced by accidental minor trauma. **(b)** At 3 weeks after starting an anticonvulsant, this 10-year-old boy developed generalized erythema, followed by diffuse blistering and sloughing of the skin and mucous membranes. **(c)** At 10 days of age, this tiny premature infant developed toxic epidermal necrolysis while on multiple anti-biotics. Denuded areas of skin occurred over bony prominences and around tape and monitor sites. Stevens–Johnson syndrome.

careful ongoing ophthalmologic evaluation is necessary to reduce the complications of severe conjunctival and corneal involvement.

Skin biopsy findings in EM, SJS, and TEN show a perivascular mononuclear cell infiltrate with some eosinophils in the papillary dermis. Variable hydropic degeneration of the basal cell layer is associated with the formation of colloid bodies and subepidermal blister formation. In SJS and certainly TEN, widespread dyskeratosis and epidermal necrosis are present.

In the event of drug-induced SJS and TEN, it is imperative that the clinician identifies the inciting agent. Failure to do so may result in a persistent reaction, higher risk of complications and mortality, and severe recurrent disease on re-exposure to the medication. During acute episodes, careful cleaning and protection of bullous lesions is imperative to reduce the risk of infection. Patients with severe SJS and TEN may require intensive supportive care in a burn unit. Although systemic corticosteroids were previously associated with increased risk of bacterial infection in SJS/TEN and slower rate of re-epithelization, studies demonstrate that an early pulse of dexamethasone does not cause these complications and in fact can reduce ocular complications. Recently, some studies have demonstrated the efficacy of cyclosporine A and etanercept in both children and adults for SJS and TEN. The use of immunoglobulins remains controversial, whereas previously utilized cyclophosphamide and thalidomide are no longer used.

Mycoplasma-Induced Rash and Mucositis

Mycoplasma pneumonia infection can be associated with extrapulmonary complications including mycoplasma-induced rash and mucositis (MIRM). MIRM is a term that was coined to differentiate the presentation of this disorder from SJS triggered by medications. Specifically, patients with MIRM invariable have mucositis involving two or more mucous membranes but have variable and sometimes no skin involvement. Furthermore, skin lesions are reminiscent of bullous EM in that there is little to no sloughing of skin compared with SJS/TEN where extensive sloughing is the rule. Previously, reports of SJS-like mucositis without skin involvement were referred to as "incomplete SJS" and "Fuchs syndrome." Many authors suspect these cases were actually undiagnosed cases of MIRM or another infection-induced mucositis. Factors distinguishing MIRM from SJS/TEN and EM include predominant mucosal involvement with sparse or no cutaneous eruptions and excellent prognosis. Further, unlike delayed hypersensitivity reaction and Fas-ligand-mediated toxicity in SJS/TEN and EM, MIRM is thought to involve polyclonal B cells causing immune complex deposition and compliment activation.

Many genetically distinct variants of *M. pneumonia* have been implicated in MIRM, which may explain the variability in presentation from no cutaneous involvement to mild to moderate involvement. Recent cases have reported oral and genital erosions

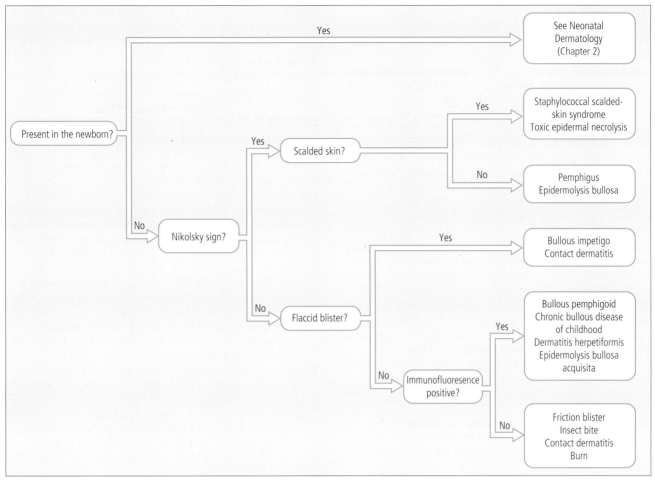

Fig. 4.29 Algorithm for evaluation of vesiculopustular dermatoses.

similar to that of MIRM but caused secondary to *Chlamydia pneumoniae* infection. The spectrum of MIRM is still evolving and should expand to include *Chlamydia*-induced mucositis. Most commonly, MIRM has been reported in children and young male adolescents. Often prodromal symptoms of fever, cough, and malaise will occur before the onset of mucosal and cutaneous lesions. Cutaneous rash presents as vesiculobullous target-like eruptions in a sparse distribution. Patients with MIRM may recover with mucosal synechiae and pigmentary changes; however, systemic complications are rare. Though no guidelines for treatment currently exist, antibiotics, immunosuppression, IVIG, cyclosporine, and etanercept have demonstrated efficacy in some patients.

FURTHER READING

Herpes Simplex Infection

Aronson PL, Yan AC, Mittal MK, et al. Delayed acyclovir and outcomes of children hospitalized with eczema herpeticum. Pediatrics 2011; 128(6):1161–1167.

Bessner JM, Crouch NA, Sullivan M. Laboratory diagnosis to differentiate smallpox, vaccinia, and other vesicular/pustular illnesses. J Lab Clin Med 2003; 5:1221–1230.

Chayavichitsilp P, Buckwalter JV, Krakowski AC, et al. Herpes simplex. Pediatr Rev 2009; 30(4):119–129.

Douglas JM, Critchlow C, Benedetti J, et al. A double-blind study of oral acyclovir for suppression of recurrences of genital herpes simplex virus infection. N Engl J Med 1984; 310:1551–1556.

Enright AM, Prober C. Antiviral therapy in children with varicella-zoster and herpes simplex infections. Herpes 2003; 10:32–37.

Erlich KS. Management of herpes simplex and varicella-zoster virus infection. West J Med 1997; 166:211–215.

Jen M, Chang MW. Eczema herpeticum and eczema vaccinatum in children. Pediatr Ann 2010; 39(10):658–664.

Kimberlin D, Powell D, Gruber W, et al. Administration of oral acyclovir suppressive therapy after neonatal herpes simplex virus disease limited to the skin, eyes and mouth: results of a Phase I/II trial. Pediatr Infect Dis J 1996; 15:247–254.

Kimberlin DW, Whitley RJ, Wan W, et al. National Institute of Allergy and Infectious Diseases Collaborative Antiviral Study Group. Oral acyclovir suppression and neurodevelopment after neonatal herpes. N Engl J Med 2011; 365(14):1284–1292.

Pinninti SG, Kimberlin DW. Neonatal herpes simplex virus infections. Semin Perinatol 2018; 42(3):168–175. doi:10.1053/j.semperi.2018.02.004.

Waggoner-Fountain LA, Grossman LB. Herpes simplex virus. Pediatr Rev 2004; 25:86–93.

Whitley RJ. Therapy of herpes virus infections in children. Adv Exp Med Biol 2008; 609:216–232.

Whitley R, Baines J. Clinical management of herpes simplex virus infections: past, present, and future. F1000Res 2018; 7:F1000. doi:10.12688/f1000research.16157.1.

Varicella-Zoster Infection

Ahn KH, Park YJ, Hong SC, et al. Congenital varicella syndrome: a systematic review. J Obstet Gynaecol 2016; 36(5):563–566. doi: 10.3109/01443615.2015.1127905.

Baba K, Yabuuchi H, Takahashi M, et al. Immunologic and epidemiologic aspects of varicella infection acquired during infancy and early childhood. J Pediatr 1982; 100:881–888.

Blair RJ. Varicella zoster virus. Pediatr Rev 2019; 40(7):375–377. doi:10.1542/pir.2017-0242.

Christian CW, Singer ML, Crawford JE, et al. Perianal herpes zoster presenting as suspected child abuse. Pediatrics 1997; 99:608–610.

Committee on Infectious Disease. The use of acyclovir in otherwise healthy children with varicella. Pediatrics 1993; 91:674–676.

Dunkle LM, Arvin AM, Whitley RJ, et al. A controlled trial of acyclovir for chickenpox in normal children. N Engl J Med 1991; 325: 1539–1544.

Harpaz R. Do varicella vaccination programs change the epidemiology of herpes zoster? A comprehensive review, with focus on the United States. Expert Rev Vaccines 2019; 18:793–811. doi:10.1080/14760584.2019.1646129.

Javed S, Javed SA, Tyring SK. Varicella vaccines. Curr Opin Infect Dis 2012; 25(2):135–140.

Krause PR, Klinman DM. Efficacy, immunogenicity, safety and use of attenuated chickenpox vaccine. J Pediatr 1995; 127:518–525.

Kurlan JG, Connelly BL, Lucky AW. Herpes zoster in the first year of life following postnatal exposure to varicella-zoster virus: four case reports and a review of infantile herpes zoster. Arch Dermatol 2004; 140(10):1268–1272.

Lin HC, Chao YH, Wu KH, et al. Increased risk of herpes zoster in children with cancer: a nationwide population-based cohort study. Medicine (Baltimore) 2016; 95(30):e4037. doi:10.1097/MD.0000000000004037.

Marin M, Meissner HC, Seward JF. Varicella prevention in the United States: a review of successes and challenges. Pediatrics 2008; 122(3):e744–e751.

Maltz F, Fidler B. Shingrix: a new herpes zoster vaccine. P T 2019; 44(7):406–433. http://www.ncbi.nlm.nih.gov/pubmed/31258310. Accessed August 4, 2019.

Merlo HC, Vaid SK, Meyer A, et al. Clinical inquiry: is it safe to vaccinate children against varicella while they're in close contact with a pregnant woman? J Fam Pract 2011; 60(7):432–433.

Nagel MA, Jones D, Wyborny A. Varicella zoster virus vasculopathy: the expanding clinical spectrum and pathogenesis. J Neuroimmunol 2017; 308:112–117. doi:10.1016/j.jneuroim.2017.03.014.

Nikkels AF, Nikkels-Tassoudji N, Pierard GE. Revisiting childhood herpes zoster. Pediatr Dermatol 2004; 21:18–23.

Preblud SR, Orenstein WA, Bart KJ. Varicella: clinical manifestations, epidemiology and health impact in children. Pediatr Infect Dis 1984; 3:505–509.

Rodríguez-Fanjul X, Noguera A, Vicente A, et al. Herpes zoster in healthy infants and toddlers after perinatal exposure to varicella-zoster virus: a case series and review of the literature. Pediatr Infect Dis J 2010; 29(6):574–576.

Rozenbaum MH, van Hoek AJ, Vegter S, et al. Cost-effectiveness of varicella vaccination programs: an update of the literature. Expert Rev Vaccines 2008; 7(6):753–782.

Shah RA, Limmer AL, Nwannunu CE, et al. Shingrix for herpes zoster: a review. Skin Therapy Lett 2019; 24:5–7.

Weibel RE, Neff BJ, Kuter BJ, et al. Live attenuated varicella virus vaccine: efficacy trial in healthy children. N Engl J Med 1984; 310:1409–1415.

Wu CT, Tsai SC, Lin JJ, et al. Disseminated varicella infection in a child receiving short-term steroids for asthma. Pediatr Dermatol 2008; 25(4):484–486. doi:10.1111/j.1525-1470.2008.00720.x.

Hand-Foot-and-Mouth Disease

B'arlean L, Avram G, Pavlov E, et al. Investigation of five cases of vesicular enteroviral stomatitis with exanthema induced by Coxsackie A5 virus. Rev Roum Virol 1994; 45:3–9.

Bendig JW, Fleming DM. Epidemiologic, virological and clinical features of an epidemic of hand, foot and mouth disease in England and Wales. Comm Dis Rep CDR Rev 1996; 6:R81–R86.

Frydenberg A, Starr M. Hand, foot, and mouth disease. Am Fam Physician 2003; 32:594–595.

Li Y, Zhou Y, Cheng Y, et al. Effectiveness of EV-A71 vaccination in prevention of paediatric hand, foot, and mouth disease associated with EV-A71 virus infection requiring hospitalisation in Henan, China, 2017–18: a test-negative case-control study. Lancet Child Adolesc Heal 2019; 3:697–704. doi:10.1016/S2352-4642(19)30185-3.

Shah VA, Chong CY, Chan KP, et al. Clinical characteristics of an outbreak of hand, foot, and mouth disease in Singapore. Ann Acad Med Singapore 2003; 32:381–387.

Solomon T, Lewthwaite P, Perera D, et al. Virology, epidemiology, pathogenesis, and control of enterovirus 71. Lancet Infect Dis 2010; 10(11):778–790.

Ventarola D, Bordone L, Silverberg N. Update on hand-foot-and-mouth disease. Clin Dermatol 2015; 33(3):340–346. doi:10.1016/j.clindermatol.2014.12.011.

Yang T, Xu G, Dong H, et al. A case-control study of risk factors for severe hand-foot-mouth disease among children in Ningbo, China, 2010–2011. Eur J Pediatr 2012; 171(9):1359–1364.

Bacterial Infections

Arnold JD, Hoek SN, Kirkorian AY. Epidemiology of staphylococcal scalded skin syndrome in the United States: a cross-sectional study, 2010-2014. J Am Acad Dermatol 2018; 78(2):404–406. doi:10.1016/j.jaad.2017.09.023.

D'Cunha NM, Peterson GM, Baby KE, et al. Impetigo: a need for new therapies in a world of increasing antimicrobial resistance. J Clin Pharm Ther 2018; 43:150–153. doi:10.1111/jcpt.12639.

Doudoulakakis A, Spiliopoulou I, Syridou G, et al. Emergence of staphylococcal scalded skin syndrome associated with a new toxinogenic, methicillin-susceptible Staphylococcus aureus clone. J Med Microbiol 2019; 68(1):48–51. doi:10.1099/jmm.0.000871.

Johnston GA. Treatment of bullous impetigo and the staphylococcal scalded skin syndrome in infants. Expert Rev Anti Infect Ther 2004; 2(3):439–446. http://www.ncbi.nlm.nih.gov/pubmed/15482208. Accessed September 24, 2019.

Firsowicz M, Boyd M, Jacks SK. Follicular occlusion disorders in Down syndrome patients. Pediatr Dermatol 2020; 37:219–221. doi:10.1111/pde.14012.

Laureano AC, Schwartz RA, Cohen PJ. Facial bacterial infections: folliculitis. Clin Dermatol 2014; 32(6):711–714. doi:10.1016/j.clindermatol.2014.02.009.

Leung AKC, Barankin B, Leong F. Staphylococcal-scalded skin syndrome: evaluation, diagnosis, and management. World J Pediatr 2010; 14(2):116–120. doi:10.1007/s12519-010-0150-x.

Martinez N, Jordan KS. Staphylococcal scalded skin syndrome: a pediatric dermatological emergency. Adv Emerg Nurs J 2019; 41:129–134. doi:10.1097/TME.0000000000000235.

Pereira LB. Impetigo - review. An Bras Dermatol 2014; 89(2):293–299. doi:10.1590/abd1806-4841.20142283.

Schachner L, Andriessen A, Bhatia N, et al. Topical ozenoxacin cream 1% for impetigo: a review. J Drugs Dermatol 2019; 18(7):655–661. http://www.ncbi.nlm.nih.gov/pubmed/31334625. Accessed August 4, 2019.

Simkin DJ, Grossberg AL, Cohen BA. Bullous impetigo rapid diagnostic and therapeutic quiz: a model for assessing basic dermatology knowledge of primary care providers. Pediatr Dermatol 2016; 33(6):627–631. doi:10.1111/pde.12974.

Vila J, Hebert AA, Torrelo A, et al. Ozenoxacin: a review of preclinical and clinical efficacy. Expert Rev Anti Infect Ther 2019; 17:159–168. doi:10.1080/14787210.2019.1573671.

Pemphigus

Anhalt GJ, Labib RS, Vorhees JJ, et al. Induction of pemphigus in neonatal mice by passive transfer of IgG from patients with the disease. N Engl J Med 1982; 306:1189–1196.

Bernett CN, Fong M, Rosario-Collazo JA. Linear IGA Dermatosis. In: *StatPearls*. Treasure Island (FL): StatPearls Publishing; January 15, 2021.

Casuriaga Lamboglia AL, Gubitosi AM, Bakerdjian CG, et al. Pemphigus vulgaris in pediatrics: a case report. Rev Chil Pediatr 2018; 89(5):650–654. doi:10.4067/S0370-41062018005000708.

Chen DM, Odueyungbo A, Csinady E, et al. Rituximab is an effective treatment in patients with pemphigus vulgaris and demonstrates a steroid-sparing effect. Br J Dermatol 2019; 182:1111–1119. doi:10.1111/bjd.18482.

Fuertes I, Guilabert A, Mascaró JM Jr, et al. Rituximab in childhood pemphigus vulgaris: a long-term follow-up case and review of the literature. Dermatology 2010; 221(1):13–16.

Grunwald MH, Zaninu E, Avinoach I, et al. Pemphigus neonatorum. Pediatr Dermatol 1993; 10:169–170.

Gürcan H, Mabrouk D, Razzaque Ahmed A. Management of pemphigus in pediatric patients. Minerva Pediatr 2011; 63(4):279–291.

Lara-Corrales I, Pope E. Autoimmune blistering diseases in children. Semin Cutan Med Surg 2010; 29(2):85–91.

Lyde CB, Cox SE, Cruz PD Jr. Pemphigus erythematous in a five year old child. J Am Acad Dermatol 1994; 31(5 Pt 2):906–909.

Mabrouk D, Ahmed AR. Analysis of current therapy and clinical outcome in childhood pemphigus vulgaris. Pediatr Dermatol 2011; 28(5):485–493.

Porro AM, Seque CA, Ferreira MCC, et al. Pemphigus vulgaris. An Bras Dermatol 2019; 94:264–278. doi:10.1590/abd1806-4841.20199011.

Smitt JH. Pemphigus vulgaris in childhood: clinical features, treatment and prognosis. Pediatr Dermatol 1985; 2:185–190.

Bullous Pemphigoid and Chronic Bullous Dermatosis of Childhood

Antiga E, Maglie R, Quintarelli L, et al. Dermatitis herpetiformis: novel perspectives. Front Immunol 2019; 10:1290. doi:10.3389/fimmu.2019.01290.

Aydin M, Hakan N, Zenciroglu A, et al. A rare location of sucking blister in newborn: the lips. Eur J Pediatr 2013; 172(10):1423–1424. doi:10.1007/s00431-013-2055-y.

Edwards S, Wakelin SH, Wojnarowska F, et al. Bullous pemphigoid and epidermolysis bullosa acquisita. Presentation, prognosis, and immunopathology in children. Pediatr Dermatol 1998; 15:184–190.

Gajic-Veljic M, Nikolic M, Medenica L. Juvenile bullous pemphigoid: the presentation and follow-up of six cases. J Eur Acad Dermatol Venereol 2010; 24(1):69–72.

Gereige RS, Washington KR. Pathologic case of the month. Linear IgA dermatosis of childhood (benign chronic bullous dermatosis of childhood). Arch Pediatr Adolesc Med 1997; 15:320–321.

Kayani M, Aslam AM. Bullous pemphigoid and pemphigus vulgaris. BMJ 2017; 357:j2169. doi:10.1136/bmj.j2169.

Khanna N, Pandhi RK, Gupta S, et al. Response of chronic bullous dermatosis of childhood to combination dapsone and nicotinamide. J Eur Acad Dermatol Venereol 2002; 15:368.

Lara-Corrales I, Pope E. Autoimmune blistering diseases in children. Semin Cutan Med Surg 2010; 29(2):85–91.

Mammen C, White CT, Prendiville J. Childhood bullous pemphigoid: a rare manifestation of chronic renal allograft rejection. J Am Acad Dermatol 2011; 65(1):217–219.

Mintz EM, Morel KD. Clinical features, diagnosis, and pathogenesis of chronic bullous disease of childhood. Dermatol Clin 2011; 29(3):459–462, ix.

Mintz EM, Morel KD. Treatment of chronic bullous disease of childhood. Dermatol Clin 2011; 29(4):699–700.

Rye B, Webb JM. Autoimmune bullous disease. Am Fam Physician 1997; 55:2709–2718.

Wojnarowska F, Marsden RA, Bhogal B, et al. Chronic bullous dermatosis of childhood, childhood cicatricial pemphigoid and linear IgA disease of adults. J Am Acad Dermatol 1988; 19:792–805.

Salmi TT. Dermatitis herpetiformis. Clin Exp Dermatol 2019; 44:728–731. doi:10.1111/ced.13992.

Tate C, Christian W, Newell L. Chronic bullous dermatosis of childhood and the string of pearls sign. J Pediatr 2018; 202:325–325.e1. doi:10.1016/j.jpeds.2018.07.070.

Wojnarowska F. Mixed immunobullous disease of childhood: a good response to antimicrobials. Br J Dermatol 2001; 144:769–774.

Zone JJ, Taylor TB, Kadunce DP, et al. IgA antibodies in chronic bullous disease of childhood react with 97 kDa basement membrane zone protein. J Invest Dermatol 1996; 106:1277–1280.

Epidermolysis Bullosa Acquisita

Amagai M. Desmoglein as a target for autoimmunity and infection. J Am Acad Dermatol 2003; 48:244–252.

Borok M, Heng MCY, Ahmed AR. Epidermolysis bullosa acquisita in an 8-year-old girl. Pediatr Dermatol 1986; 3:315–322.

Cohn HI, Teng JMC. Advancement in management of epidermolysis bullosa. Curr Opin Pediatr 2016; 28(4):507–516. doi:10.1097/MOP.0000000000000380.

Fine JD. Epidemiology of inherited epidermolysis bullosa based on incidence and prevalence estimates from the national epidermolysis bullosa registry. JAMA Dermatology 2016; 152(11):1231–1238. doi:10.1001/jamadermatol.2016.2473.

Iwata H, Vorobyev A, Koga H, et al. Meta-analysis of the clinical and immunopathological characteristics and treatment outcomes in epidermolysis bullosa acquisita patients. Orphanet J Rare Dis 2018; 13(1):153. doi:10.1186/s13023-018-0896-1.

Kawachi Y, Ikegami M, Tanaka T, et al. Autoantibodies to bullous pemphigoid and epidermolysis bullosa acquisita antigen in an infant. Br J Dermatol 1996; 135:443–447.

Kirkham S, Lam S, Nester C, et al. The effect of hydration on the risk of friction blister formation on the heel of the foot. Skin Res Technol 2014; 20(2):246–253. doi:10.1111/srt.12136.

Schmidt E, Hopfner B, Kuhn C, et al. Childhood epidermolysis bullosa acquisita: a novel variant with reactivity to all 3 structural domains of type VII collagen. Br J Dermatol 2002; 147:592–597.

Wu JJ, Wagner AM. Epidermolysis bullosa acquisita in an 8-year-old girl. Pediatr Dermatol 2002; 19:368–371.

Worthing RM, Percy RL, Joslin JD. Prevention of friction blisters in outdoor pursuits: a systematic review. Wilderness Environ Med 2017; 28(2):139–149. doi:10.1016/j.wem.2017.03.007.

Erythema Multiforme

Lerch M, Mainetti C, Terziroli Beretta-Piccoli B, et al. Current perspectives on erythema multiforme. Clin Rev Allergy Immunol 2018; 54(1):177–184. doi:10.1007/s12016-017-8667-7.

Leaute-Labreze C, Lamireau T, Chauki D, et al. Diagnosis, classification, and management of erythema multiforme and Stevens–Johnson syndrome. Arch Dis Child 2000; 83:347–352.

Ng PP, Sun YJ, Tan HH, et al. Detection of herpes simplex virus genomic DNA in various subsets of erythema multiforme by polymerase chain reaction. 2003; 207:349–353.

Stevens–Johnson Syndrome and Toxic Epidermal Necrolysis

Amon RB, Dimond RL. Toxic epidermal necrolysis: rapid differentiation between staphylococcal and drug-induced disease. Arch Dermatol 1975; 111:1433–1437.

Forman R, Koren G, Shear NH. Erythema multiforme, Stevens–Johnson syndrome, and toxic epidermal necrolysis in children: a review of 10 years experience. Drug Saf 2002; 25:965–972.

Hawk RJ, Storer JS, Danon RS. Toxic epidermal necrolysis in a 6-week-old infant. Pediatr Dermatol 1985; 2:197–200.

Jones WG, Halebian P, Madden M, et al. Drug-induced toxic epidermal necrolysis in children. J Pediatr Surg 1989; 24:167–170.

Kakourou T, Klontza D, Soteropoulou F, et al. Corticosteroid treatment of erythema multiforme major (Stevens–Johnson syndrome) in children. Eur J Pediatr 1997; 156:90–93.

Lerch M, Mainetti C, Terziroli Beretta-Piccoli B, et al. Current perspectives on Stevens-Johnson syndrome and toxic epidermal necrolysis. Clin Rev Allergy Immunol 2018; 54(1):147–176. doi:10.1007/s12016-017-8654-z.

Morici MV, Galen WK, Shetty AK, et al. Intravenous immunoglobulin therapy for children with Stevens–Johnson syndrome. J Rheumatol 2000; 27:294–297.

Noskin GA, Patterson R. Outpatient management of Stevens–Johnson syndrome: a report of four cases and management strategy. Allergy Asthma Proc 1997; 18:29–32.

Prendiville J. Stevens–Johnson syndrome and toxic epidermal necrolysis. Adv Dermatol 2002; 18:151–173.

Shin HT, Chang MW. Drug eruptions in children. Curr Prob Pediatr 2001; 31:207–234.

Tay YK, Huff JC, Weston WL. Mycoplasma pneumoniae infection is associated with Stevens–Johnson syndrome, not erythema multiforme (von Hebra). J Am Acad Dermatol 1996; 35:757–760.

Weighton W. Toxic epidermal necrolysis. Aust J Dermatol 1996; 37:167–175.

Mycoplasma-Induced Rash and Mucositis

Canavan TN, Mathes EF, Frieden I, et al. Mycoplasma pneumoniae-induced rash and mucositis as a syndrome distinct from Stevens-Johnson syndrome and erythema multiforme: a systematic review. J Am Acad Dermatol 2015; 72(2):239–245. doi:10.1016/j.jaad.2014.06.026.

Frantz GF, McAninch SA. Mycoplasma Mucositis. In: StatPearls. Treasure Island (FL): *StatPearls* Publishing; August 13, 2020.

Mayor-Ibarguren A, Feito-Rodriguez M, González-Ramos J, et al. Mucositis secondary to chlamydia pneumoniae infection: expanding the mycoplasma pneumoniae-induced rash and mucositis concept. Pediatr Dermatol 2017; 34(4):465–472. doi:10.1111/pde.13140.

Umapathi KK, Tuli J, Menon S. Chlamydia pneumonia - induced mucositis. Pediatr Neonatol 2019; 60:697–698. doi:10.1016/j.pedneo.2019.06.005.

5

Nodules and Tumors

Kaiane Anoush Habeshian and Bernard A. Cohen

INTRODUCTION

Nodules and tumors in the skin often raise fears of skin cancer. Fortunately, primary skin cancer is extremely rare in childhood, and most infiltrated plaques and tumors are benign (Table 5.1). Hemangiomas, congenital nevi, and tumors of the newborn are reviewed in Chapter 2, while pigmented nevi and melanomas are discussed in Chapter 6. The focus in this chapter is disorders of childhood and adolescence.

Several clinical clues, including the depth and color of lesions, aid in developing a differential diagnosis. Superficial growths are readily moved back and forth over the underlying dermis, whereas the overlying epidermis and superficial dermis may slide over deep-seated tumors. Some dermal and subcutaneous lesions characteristically produce tethering of the overlying skin. Epidermal tumors include warts, molluscum, and seborrheic keratoses. Milia, neurofibromas, granuloma annulare, mastocytomas, scars, keloids, xanthomas, xanthogranulomas, melanocytic nevi, and adnexal tumors involve the superficial and mid-dermis. Leukemia, lymphoma, melanoma, lipomas, and metastatic solid tumors involve the dermis and/or fat and may extend deep into subcutaneous structures.

Color may suggest the specific cell types that comprise various cutaneous nodules and tumors. For instance, yellow tumors might include large quantities of fat in a lipoma or lipid-laden histiocytes in xanthomas or xanthogranulomas. Melanocytic nevi, epidermal nevi, mastocytomas, and seborrheic keratosis contain varying amounts of the brown pigment melanin in melanocytes or keratinocytes. Vascular tumors are usually red or blue, and primary or metastatic nodules may appear in various shades of red, purple, and blue, depending on their depth and degree of vascularity.

Finally, the diagnosis of certain genodermatoses associated with cutaneous and/or internal malignancies allows the clinician to develop strategies for close monitoring. Early recognition of malignancy in this setting may be life-saving (Table 5.2). An algorithmic approach to diagnosis for nodules and tumors is summarized at the end of the chapter (Fig. 5.39).

SUPERFICIAL NODULES AND TUMORS

Warts

Warts are benign epidermal tumors produced by human papillomavirus (HPV) infection of the skin and mucous membranes.

In children they are seen most commonly on the fingers, hands, and feet. The face and lips are often involved. However, they can infect any area on the skin or mucous membranes (Fig. 5.1–Fig. 5.8). The incubation period for warts varies from 1 to 3 months and possibly up to several years, and the majority of lesions disappear within 3–5 years. Local trauma promotes inoculation of the virus. Thus, periungual warts are common in children who bite their nails or pick at hangnails (Fig. 5.3), which may lead to oral inoculation as well.

Investigators have identified over 100 HPV types capable of producing warts, and many of these strains produce characteristic lesions in specific locations. For instance, the discrete, round, skin-colored papillomatous papules typical of verruca vulgaris (common warts) are produced by HPV-1, HPV-2, and HPV-4 (Figs. 5.1 and 5.4). The subtle, minimally hypo- or hyperpigmented flat warts (verruca plana), which are caused by HPV-3 and HPV-10, are frequently spread by deliberate or accidental scratching, shaving, or picking and may become widespread on the face, arms, and legs (Fig. 5.5).

Plantar warts are most commonly caused by HPV-1 (Fig. 5.2). Although not proved, the transmission of these warts probably occurs by contact with contaminated, desquamated skin in showers, pool decks, and bathrooms. Although often subtle on the surface, their large size may be hidden by a collarette of skin of normal appearance, and the overlying or surrounding calluses often cause pain when the patient walks. Although plantar warts may be confused with corns, calluses, or scars, they can be differentiated by their disruption of the normal dermatoglyphics. Characteristic black dots in the warts are thrombosed capillaries.

Warts can also be found on the trunk, oral mucosa, and conjunctivae. Condyloma acuminatum and flat warts in the anogenital area are usually caused by non-carcinogenic HPV-6 and HPV-11 (Fig. 5.6). However, a number of HPV types including 16 and 18 have been associated with cervical carcinoma and oropharyngeal carcinoma. The 9-valent HPV vaccine (9vHPV) (Gardasil-9) is U.S. Food and Drug Administration (FDA)-approved for patients aged 9–45 (expanded in October 2018 to include patients aged 27–45) and protects against oncogenic HPV types 16, 18, 31, 33, 45, 52, and 58 and non-oncogenic types 6 and 11 that cause genital warts. The quadrivalent (Gardasil) vaccine (HPV types 6, 11, 16, 18) and bivalent (Cervarix) vaccine (HPV types 6, 11) are approved for patients aged 9–26 years and females aged 9–25, respectively. These vaccinations may prove to be a useful treatment for common warts. In a 2019 prospective

TABLE 5.1 Histologic Diagnosis of 775 Superficial Lumps Excised in Children

Type	n	(%)
Epidermal inclusion cysts	459	59
Congenital malformations (pilomatrixoma, lymphangioma, brachial cleft cyst)	117	15
Benign neoplasms (neural tumors, lipoma, adnexal tumors)	56	7
Benign lesions of undetermined origin (xanthomas, xantho-granulomas, fibromatosis, fibroma)	50	6
Self-limited processes (granuloma annulare, urticaria pigmentosa, insect-bite reaction)	47	6
Malignant tumors	11	1.4
Miscellaneous	35	4

Modified from Knight PJ, Reiner CB. Superficial lumps in children: what, when, and why? Pediatrics. 1983;72(2):147–153

study by Nofal et al. of 44 adult patients with multiple recalcitrant common warts, the bivalent HPV vaccine administered intramuscularly either as per the FDA-approved protocol (0, 1, 6 months) or until clearance, or intralesionally to the largest wart in 2-week intervals, led to complete resolution in 63.3% and 81.8% of the patients, respectively. The benefit for treating common warts caused by strains not formulated in those specific vaccines is thought to arise from cross-reaction of the viral capsid proteins.

Anogenital warts may be found in children and always raises the question of sexual abuse. However, in young children, most anogenital warts are transmitted in a non-venereal fashion. This includes vertical transmission before and during pregnancy or delivery and horizontal transmission via heteroinoculation by direct contact with affected parents or caretakers with

TABLE 5.2 Cancer-Associated Genodermatoses

Disease	Associated Cancer	Clinical Manifestations	Genetics
Basal cell nevus syndrome (Gorlin syndrome)	Many basal cell carcinomas (mean age of onset 15 years) on sun-exposed and non-sun-exposed areas; medulloblastoma; astrocytoma	Many basal cell nevi, palmar and plantar pits, jaw cysts, calcification of the falx cerebri, ovarian fibromas, fused ribs	Autosomal dominant; *PTCH1* gene on chromosome 9q22.32
Hidrotic ectodermal dysplasia (Clouston syndrome)	Squamous cell carcinoma of palms, soles, nail bed	Normal sweating, total alopecia, severe nail dystrophy, palmar and plantar hyperkeratosis	Autosomal-dominant *GJB6* gene
Acrokeratosis paraneoplastica (Bazex syndrome)	Basal cell carcinomas of the face (second to third decade)	Follicular atrophoderma, localized anhidrosis, and/or generalized hypohidrosis	Autosomal-dominant Xq24–q27
Dysplastic nevus syndrome (familial, atypical, multiple-mole syndrome)	Cutaneous and intraocular melanoma, lymphoreticular malignancy, sarcomas	Multiple, large reddish-brown moles with irregular borders and non-uniform colors, usually on trunk and arms; familial occurrence of melanoma	Autosomal-dominant genetic heterogeneity
PTEN hamartoma tumor syndrome (formerly Cowden disease)	Carcinoma of the breast, colon, thyroid	Storiform collagenoma. Coexistence of multiple, ectodermal, mesodermal, and endodermal nevoid neoplasms; punctate keratoderma of the palms; multiple angiomas, lipomas	Autosomal dominant; *PTEN* gene on chromosome 10q23.31
Neurofibromatosis type 1 (von Recklinghausen disease)	Optic pathway gliomas / Malignant peripheral nerve sheath tumors / Fibrosarcomas / Squamous cell carcinomas / Non-lymphocytic leukemia / Pheochromocytoma / Carcinoid meningiomas	Café-au-lait spots / Skeletal anomalies / Neurofibromas / Lisch nodules / Axillary freckling / Xanthogranulomas (rare "triple association" with juvenile myelomonocytic leukemia)	Autosomal-dominant *NF1* gene / Sporadic mutations in 50% of cases
Neurofibromatosis type 2	Acoustic neuromas / Schwannomas / Meningiomas / Astrocytomas	Neurofibromas / ± Café-au-lait macules / Cataracts	Autosomal-dominant *NF2* gene / SCH gene on 22q11–13.1 / Sporadic mutations in 50% of cases
Multiple mucosal neuroma syndrome (multiple endocrine neoplasia type IIB)	Pheochromocytoma, medullary thyroid carcinoma	Pedunculated nodules on eyelid margins, lip; tongue with true neuromas	Autosomal dominant; gene locus 10q11.2; sporadic mutation in 50% *RET* gene
Intestinal polyposis II (Peutz–Jeghers syndrome)	Adenocarcinoma of the colon, duodenum; granulosa cell ovarian tumors	Pigmented macules on oral mucosa, lips, conjunctivae, digits; intestinal polyps	Autosomal dominant; *STK11/LKB1* gene on chromosome 19p13.3; sporadic mutation in 40%

TABLE 5.2   Cancer-Associated Genodermatoses—cont'd

Disease	Associated Cancer	Clinical Manifestations	Genetics
Intestinal polyposis III (Gardner syndrome)	Malignant degeneration of colon, adenomatous polyps; sarcomas, thyroid carcinoma	Polyps of the colon, small intestine; globoid osteoma of mandible with overlying fibromas; epidermoid cysts; desmoids	5q21–q22 *APC* gene
Tuberous sclerosis	Rhabdomyoma of myocardium, gliomas, mixed tumor of kidney	Triad of angiofibromas, epilepsy, intellectual delay; ash-leaf macules; shagreen patches; subungual fibromas; intracranial calcification in 50%	Spontaneous mutation in 75%; autosomal dominant in 25%; heterogeneous loci, 9q34 (*TSC1*), 16p13 (*TSC2*)
Epidermolysis bullosa dystrophica dominant	Squamous cell carcinoma in chronic lesions	Lifelong history of bullae; phenotype not as severe as in recessive forms	Autosomal recessive, chromosome 3p21 (collagen type VII gene)
Epidermolysis bullosa dystrophica recessive	Basal, squamous cell carcinoma in skin, mucous membranes (especially esophagus)	Bullae develop at sites of trauma; present at birth or early infancy; may involve mucous membranes, esophagus, conjunctivae, cornea	Autosomal recessive, chromosome 3p (collagen type VII gene)
Albinism	Increased incidence of cutaneous malignancies	Lack skin pigment, incomplete hypopigmentation of ocular fundi, horizontal congenital nystagmus, myopia	Tyrosinase positive: autosomal recessive, gene locus 15q11.2–q12 Tyrosinase negative: autosomal recessive, gene locus 11q14q21
Congenital telangiectasia erythema (Bloom syndrome)	High incidence of leukemia, lymphoma; squamous cell cancers of esophagus; adenocarcinoma of colon, often by 20 years of age	Small stature; cutaneous photosensitivity presenting as telangiectatic, facial (malar) erythema	Autosomal recessive; gene locus 15q26.1 *RECQL3* gene
Chédiak–Higashi syndrome	Malignant lymphoma	Decreased pigmentation of hair, eyes; photophobia; nystagmus; abnormal susceptibility to infection	Autosomal recessive *CHS1* gene
Poikiloderma congenitale (Rothmund–Thomson syndrome)	Cutaneous malignancies Osteosarcoma	Poikiloderma, short stature, cataracts, photosensitivity, nail defects, alopecia, bony defects	Autosomal recessive; gene locus 8q24.3 *RECQL4* gene
Xeroderma pigmentosum	Basal and squamous cell carcinoma of skin, malignant melanoma	Marked photosensitivity, early freckling, telangiectasia, keratoses, papillomas, photophobia, keratitis, corneal opacities	Autosomal recessive; gene loci— complementation group A—9q22.33 *XPA* gene group B—2q14.3 *ERCC3* gene group D— 19q13.32 *ERCC2* gene group F 13p13.12 *ERCC4* gene
Wiskott–Aldrich syndrome (eczema thrombocytopenia-immunodeficiency syndrome)	Lymphoreticular malignancies, malignant lymphoma, myelogenous leukemia, astrocytoma	Eczema, thrombocytopenia, bleeding problems (i.e. melena, purpura, epistaxis), increased susceptibility to skin infections, otitis, pneumonia, meningitis	X-linked recessive; gene locus Xp11.2–11.3 *WAS* gene
Dyskeratosis congenita	Squamous cell carcinoma of oral cavity, esophagus, nasopharynx, skin, anus	Reticulated hypo- and hyperpigmentation of skin, nail dystrophy, leukoplakia of oral mucosa, thrombocytopenia, testicular atrophy	X-linked recessive (most common); gene locus Xq28 *DKCI* gene

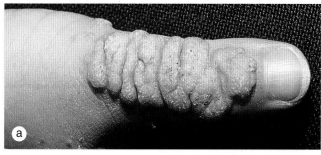
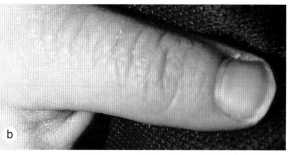

Fig. 5.1 Warts. **(a)** Multiple common warts grew to confluence on the thumb of a 4-year-old boy. **(b)** Shortly before surgery was scheduled, the warts began to regress without treatment.

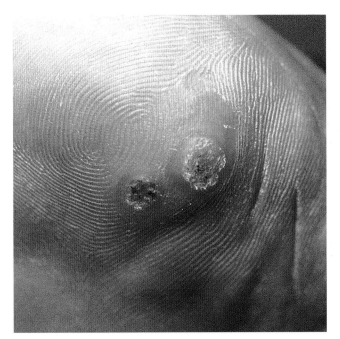

Fig. 5.2 Plantar warts. Two painful papules are seen over the ball of the foot. Note how they interrupt the normal skin lines.

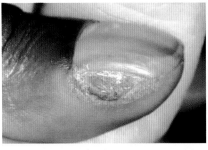

Fig. 5.3 Subungual common wart. This wart persisted despite repeated painful treatments with liquid nitrogen. A year later it resolved after therapy was discontinued.

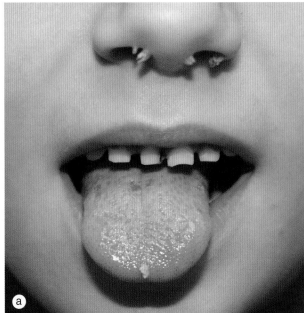

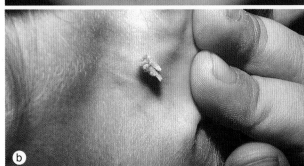

Fig. 5.4 Verruca vulgaris. Filiform warts developed on **(a)** the nose and tongue and **(b)** the ear of these children of school age.

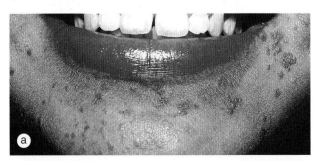

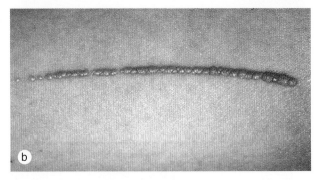

Fig. 5.5 Verruca plana. **(a)** The tiny, light-brown warts on the chin of a 12-year-old girl were spread by scratching. These asymptomatic warts were initially diagnosed as acne. **(b)** Flat warts were inoculated in a line on the flank of a 5-year-old girl.

common warts, as well as autoinoculation of common warts from hands to the anogenital region, with a latency period of 2–3 years leading to a delayed presentation. Some authors note increased concern for sexual abuse in children greater than 4 years of age. However, there is no established absolute age-cut off. Suspicion for abuse increases with age and with consideration to the patient's social history and presence of sexually transmitted diseases (including herpes simplex, gonorrhea, chlamydia, syphilis, or human immunodeficiency virus). HPV genotyping has not proven to be a reliable method for determining mode of transmission and is not widely utilized in the context of evaluation for sexual abuse. In addition, there are no clear malignancy screening guidelines in pediatric patients with anogenital warts. Warts are self-limited in most children, but persistent, widespread lesions suggest the possibility of congenital or acquired immunodeficiency (Fig. 5.7). In fact, warts may become a serious management problem in oncology and transplant patients who are chronically immunosuppressed.

Topical keratolytics, which nowork essentially by peeling off thickened skin from warts and callosities, include salicylic acid

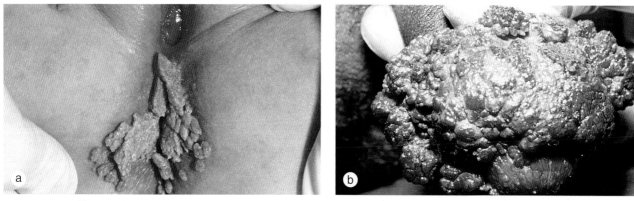

Fig. 5.6 Anogenital warts and condyloma. **(a)** The warts developed at 8 months of age in this infant whose mother had extensive vaginal and cervical papillomavirus infection at delivery. These lesions resolved after treatment with podophyllotoxin. **(b)** Large condyloma enveloped the glans penis of this adolescent boy.

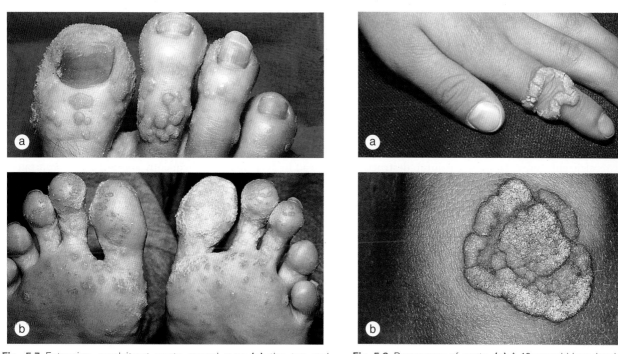

Fig. 5.7 Extensive, recalcitrant warts spread over **(a)** the top and **(b)** the bottom of the feet of a teenager with severe combined immunodeficiency.

Fig. 5.8 Recurrence of warts. **(a)** A 10-year-old boy developed a recurrent ring wart after liquid nitrogen treatment of a large common wart on the index finger. **(b)** A 10-year-old girl had a similar complication after treatment of a wart on her knee.

(SA) and lactic acid in occlusive vehicles such as collodion or under tape occlusion. These are safe, effective, and relatively painless preparations with which to treat warts that are not in sensitive areas such as the eyelids and perineum.

Recalcitrant lesions may respond to destructive measures, which include liquid nitrogen, electrocautery, and carbon dioxide laser surgery. Pulsed-dye laser is also used in recalcitrant cases and may exert its effect gradually over time via destruction of the blood supply to the wart, as well as heat destruction of the tissue and induction of immunity. However, patients and parents must be cautioned about the risk of recurrence and scarring with destructive methods (Figs. 5.8 and 5.9). Cryotherapy is used most commonly in general practice. There is limited positive evidence regarding the efficacy of either SA or cryotherapy

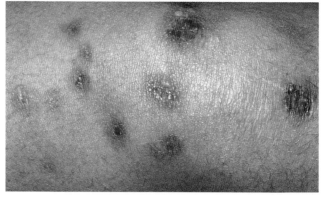

Fig. 5.9 A 10-year-old boy developed multiple scars after liquid nitrogen therapy of warts on his knee.

compared with placebo. There is also limited positive evidence for the efficacy of cryotherapy compared with placebo or SA on the hands and in combination with SA versus SA alone. Cantharidin, both alone and in combination with podophyllotoxin and SA for plantar warts, may be beneficial but also has a risk of blistering, pain, dyspigmentation, and even scarring. Topical imiquimod and topical fluorouracil are sometimes used in recalcitrant cases, though sufficient evidence is lacking. Candida antigen injections are also safe and effective wart treatments for some patients in whom it induces an "immunity" to HPV with side effects including pruritus, erythema, oozing and crusting, and rarely the "painful purple digit." Immunotherapy with topical contact sensitizers, such as squaric acid, diphenylcyclopropenone, and rhus extract, is still considered experimental, and parents are counseled accordingly. Sinecatechins (green tea derivative) ointment may be a promising, relatively novel, and safe treatment for extragenital and genital warts in children, though more studies are needed. Remember, most warts resolve without treatment in 3–5 years, and children should play a role in deciding on therapy for these benign lesions.

Large warts in the diaper area may cause itching, burning, bleeding, and secondary bacterial infection. Although not approved for use in children, judicious home application of topical imiquimod cream and podophyllotoxin gel or solution are safe and effective in symptomatic cases. Scissors excision with electrocautery and carbon dioxide laser ablation may be effective in recalcitrant cases. However, painful destructive measures can only be performed with deep sedation or general anesthetic. As with common warts, most anogenital warts in normal hosts will regress without treatment over 3–5 years.

Several innocent epidermal growths are often confused with warts. Epidermal nevi can have a verrucous appearance but are distinguished from viral warts by their linear configuration and lack of punctate hemorrhages. Heel-stick calcinosis can be mistaken for warts but have a chalky-white chalky appearance and classic location along the posterolateral aspect of the heel of the foot. Dermatosis papulosa nigra (DPN) describes a variant of seborrheic keratosis that appears in about a third of black individuals (Fig. 5.10). Although seborrheic keratoses usually do

not erupt until middle age, small, brown, warty DPN typically begins to develop during adolescence in a symmetric, malar distribution on the face. The neck and upper trunk may also be involved. Although DPN is of no medical consequence, irritated or unsightly lesions may be snipped, frozen, cauterized, or gently lasered after the application of a topical anesthetic. Patients must be warned about the risk of postinflammatory pigmentary changes after treatment. Another type of innocent epidermal lesion, pearly penile papule, is often diagnosed as warts. Uniform, 1–3 mm diameter papules ring the corona at the base of the glans penis. Pearly penile papules, which appear in up to one-third of men by adolescence, and vulvar vestibular papules are asymptomatic and probably represent a normal variant. No treatment is required.

Molluscum Contagiosum

Molluscum contagiosum, caused by a large DNA poxvirus, is characterized by sharply circumscribed single or multiple, superficial, pearly, dome-shaped papules (Fig. 5.11). They usually start as grouped, pinpoint papules and increase in size to 3–5 mm in diameter. Many lesions have umbilicated centers, which are best seen with a hand lens (dermatoscope, otoscope). Older lesions often appear crusted and lose their classic shiny, creamy appearance. Molluscum may leave behind subtle atrophic scars. Molluscum is endemic in young children, in whom involvement of the trunk, axillae, face, and diaper area is common. Lesions are spread by scratching and frequently appear in a linear arrangement (Fig. 5.11c). In teenagers and adults, molluscum occurs frequently in the genital area as a sexually transmitted disease (Fig. 5.12) and diffusely in immunocompromised hosts.

A white, cheesy core can be expressed from the center of the papule for microscopic examination, which reveals the typical molluscum bodies. Curettage and destruction of lesions by curetting their cores or by application of a blistering agent (cantharidin) and plastic tape may be curative of individual lesions. However, recurrences and the development of new papules are common, and most cases in normal hosts undergo spontaneous remission within 6 months to 2 years of diagnosis. Consequently, treatment is usually directed against symptomatic lesions only. Moreover, meta-analyses have not shown that any treatment is superior to placebo.

Bacterial superinfection may be treated with appropriate topical or oral antibiotics. The development of scaly, red eczematous rings around old papules, sometimes termed molluscum dermatitis, may herald the onset of a delayed hypersensitivity or "id" reaction and resolution of the infection (Fig. 5.11e). As in children with warts, patients with widespread, recalcitrant molluscum should be screened for congenital and acquired immunodeficiency.

Basal Cell Carcinoma

Basal cell carcinoma (BCC) presents as a non-healing, pearly, reddish-gray to brown papule or plaque with a central dell or crust and peripheral telangiectasias (Fig. 5.13). Although BCC occurs primarily in middle age and the elderly, the tumor is being recognized with increasing frequency in adolescents and young adults, particularly in fair-skinned individuals in sunny

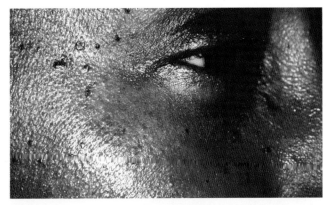

Fig. 5.10 Small, brown papules typical of dermatosis papulosa nigra slowly increased in number and size on the face of this black adolescent. Her parents had similar lesions, which began to appear in late childhood.

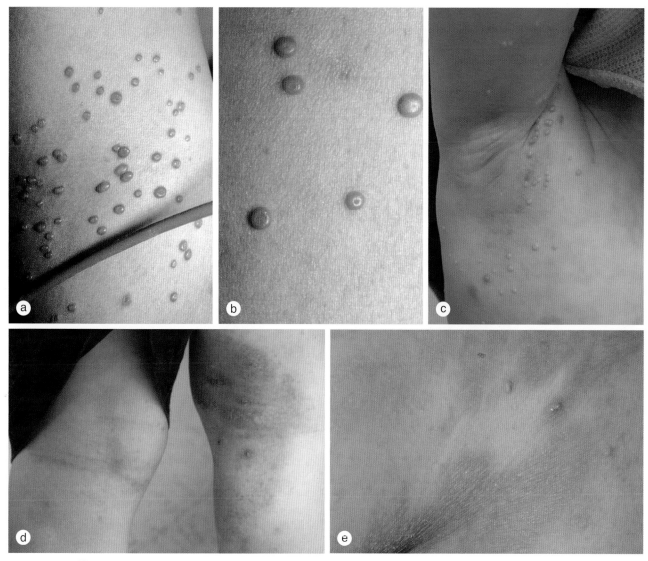

Fig. 5.11 Molluscum contagiosum. **(a)** Multiple, pearly papules dot the arm of this 8-year-old girl with widespread molluscum. **(b)** A close-up view demonstrates the central umbilication present on mature molluscum lesions. **(c)** Note the linear spread of papules on the right axilla, arm, and chest of this child which followed scratching and autoinoculation. **(d)** Molluscum on the eyelid margin and conjunctivae are particularly irritating and difficult to treat. **(e)** Red scaly dermatitic patches encircled this toddler's molluscum shortly before their resolution.

climates and with increased tanning bed use. The risk of developing BCC has been clearly linked to ultraviolet light exposure, and most lesions appear on sun-exposed sites, such as the face, ears, neck, and upper trunk. An indolent, superficial malignancy, uncomplicated BCC responds readily to electrodesiccation and curettage or simple excision. However, neglected lesions may become locally destructive and invade deep soft tissues, bone, and dura. Protection from excessive sun exposure, aggressive use of sunscreens, and careful skin surveillance should reduce the risk from BCC.

When BCC is diagnosed in sun-protected areas or in children, the practitioner must search for predisposing factors, such as radiation or arsenic exposure, a pre-existing nevus sebaceous or scar, or a hereditary condition such as xeroderma pigmentosum and basal cell nevus syndrome. In basal cell nevus syndrome, an autosomal-dominant disorder, numerous basal cell nevi are noted on the trunk, scalp, face, and extremities during the first decade (Fig. 5.14). Unlike classic BCCs, they often resemble milia or melanocytic nevi early in presentation. In time, many of these lesions begin to enlarge and ulcerate and develop into progressive BCCs. Other stigmata include macrocephaly, frontal bossing, coarse facial features, palmar and plantar pits, jaw cysts, calcification of the falx cerebri, ovarian fibromas, and fused ribs. Early diagnosis and removal of enlarging BCCs reduces the need for more extensive and disfiguring surgery.

In children, BCC may be confused with warts, molluscum contagiosum, seborrheic keratoses, pigmented nevi, and other epidermal and superficial dermal growths. It should be considered in any slowly progressive, crusted, or ulcerated plaque, particularly if risk factors are present.

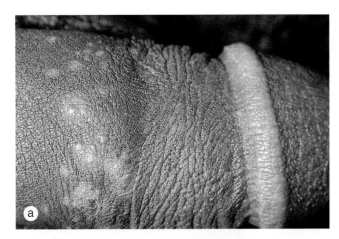

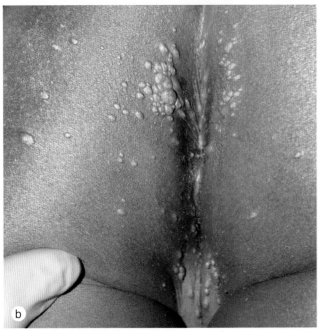

Fig. 5.12 Anogenital molluscum. **(a)** Molluscum developed on the penile shaft of this sexually active adolescent. **(b)** A healthy 6-year-old girl with molluscum on the chest and right arm accidentally inoculated lesions onto the anogenital skin.

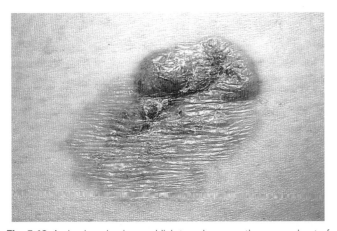

Fig. 5.13 A slowly enlarging, reddish-tan plaque on the upper chest of an 18-year-old boy developed a nodular component with overlying telangiectasias. A skin biopsy demonstrated basaloid budding typical of basal cell carcinoma. The child had red hair, blue eyes, light complexion, and a history of frequent sunburns since early childhood.

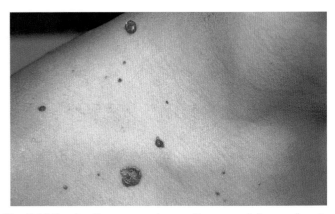

Fig. 5.14 Basal cell nevus syndrome. Numerous 1–3 mm diameter papules composed of proliferating basaloid cells and two larger nodules, which demonstrated changes typical of basal cell carcinoma, are on the shoulder and neck of a 15-year-old girl with basal cell nevus syndrome. In addition to the widespread cutaneous tumors, she had subtle palmar and plantar pits and a history of jaw cysts. Her father, uncle, and grandmother had similar cutaneous lesions.

DERMAL NODULES AND TUMORS

Granuloma Annulare

When fully evolved, granuloma annulare is an annular eruption histologically characterized by dermal infiltration of lymphocytes and histiocytes around altered collagen (Fig. 5.15a–d). The lesion begins as a firm papule or nodule, which gradually expands peripherally to form a ring 1–4 cm in diameter. Multiple rings may overlap to form large, annular plaques. In some cases, the rings are broken up into segments. The overlying epidermis is usually intact and has the same color as adjacent skin. However, it may be slightly red or hyperpigmented. Most lesions are asymptomatic, although a few are reported to be mildly pruritic. Granuloma annulare most commonly erupts on the extensor surfaces of the lower legs, feet, fingers, and hands, but other areas may be involved.

Over months to years, old plaques and papules regress while new lesions appear. Eventually, granuloma annulare resolves without treatment. The origin is unclear, but some lesions may be associated with insect-bite reactions or other antecedent trauma. The presence of an infectious trigger and/or aberrant immune regulation has been suggested as well. In adults, granuloma annulare, especially multiple eruptive lesions, have appeared in association with hyperlipidemia and diabetes mellitus (Fig. 5.15e). This is not the case in children.

Granuloma annulare is most commonly confused with tinea corporis or ringworm. However, the thickened, indurated character of the ring and lack of epidermal changes, such as scale, vesicles, or pustules, enable clinical distinction. A deep dermal or subcutaneous variant of granuloma annulare may be mistaken for rheumatoid nodules seen in rheumatic fever and other connective tissue disorders (Fig. 5.16). These lesions are referred to as subcutaneous granuloma annulare and pseudorheumatoid nodules. Practitioners should avoid the latter term because the subcutaneous variant is not associated with local symptoms or systemic disease. Subcutaneous nodules occur

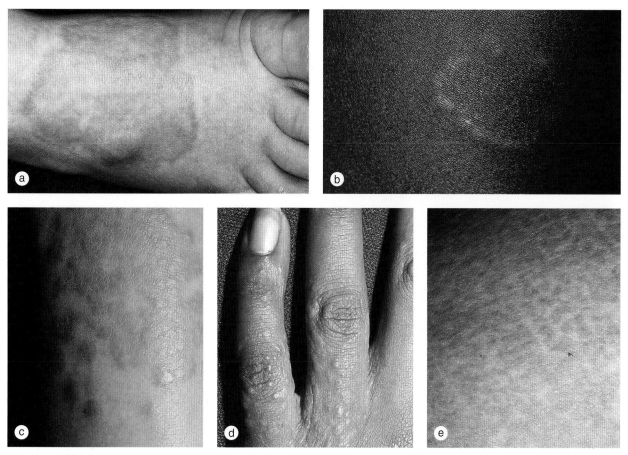

Fig. 5.15 Granuloma annulare. Characteristic, doughnut-shaped, dermal plaques on **(a)** the foot of a light-pigmented boy and **(b)** the thigh of a dark-pigmented girl. In both children the epidermal markings are preserved. **(c)** A large, confluent plaque is developing from merging papules on the arm of a 9-year-old boy. **(d)** Multiple, asymptomatic 2–4 mm diameter papules erupted on the hand of a teenager. **(e)** Disseminated granuloma annulare developed in a 20-year-old individual with insulin-dependent diabetes mellitus.

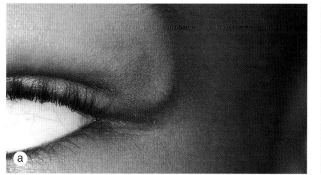
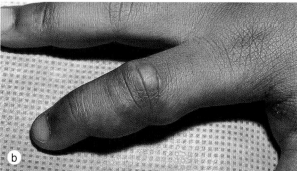

Fig. 5.16 Subcutaneous granuloma annulare. Asymptomatic subcutaneous nodules persisted for over a year **(a)** on the upper eyelid of a 7-year-old boy and **(b)** on several fingers of a 10-year-old girl.

most commonly on the extremities and scalp, where they are often fixed to the underlying periosteum. The diagnosis is often suggested by the presence of typical annular dermal plaques. When necessary, skin biopsies reveal changes similar to the more superficial lesions. Though treatment is often unsuccessful, options include topical corticosteroids, topical calcineurin inhibitors, intralesional corticosteroid injections, and cryotherapy. Skin biopsy may hasten resolution.

Adnexal Tumors

Neoplasms (benign and malignant) may arise from any structure in the skin. Although many tumors of the adnexal structures can only be differentiated by specific histopathology, some demonstrate distinctive clinical patterns.

Epidermoid Cysts

Epidermal inclusion cysts (EICs) are slow-growing dermal or subcutaneous tumors that usually reach a size of 1–3 cm diameter and

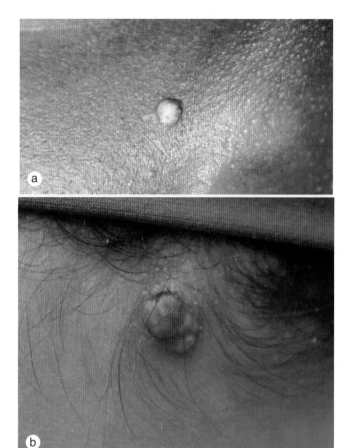

Fig. 5.17 Epidermal inclusion cyst. **(a)** A 6-mm epidermal inclusion cyst developed on the cheek of a 5-year-old boy after an insect bite. **(b)** An 11-year-old girl developed a 1.5-cm multiloculated epidermal inclusion cyst on the left side of her forehead after scratching scale associated with seborrheic dermatitis in her scalp.

occur most commonly on the face, scalp, neck, and trunk (Fig. 5.17). An overlying punctum may develop, and the lesions may drain a malodorous white to yellow keratinaceous material. In neonates, infants, and young children, they often present as a small shiny superficial white version of an EIC termed milia (see Fig. 2.18a,b), most commonly on the face of neonates. They may be acquired after acute and chronic cutaneous injury, such as abrasions, surgery, and recurrent blistering in epidermolysis bullosa (see Fig. 2.52). Although milia often resolve without treatment, some remain indefinitely. Curettage or gentle puncture and expression with a comedone extractor or 22-gauge needle is usually curative.

Small EICs can arise in neonates as median raphe cysts on the ventral surface of the penis and scrotum. EICs also occasionally develop on the palms and soles. These cysts account for a majority of cutaneous nodules found in children and may be present at birth or appear anytime in childhood. Although they are usually associated with hair follicles, EICs may arise from the epithelium of any adnexal structure. Primary lesions represent a keratinizing type of benign tumor. Other cysts occur as a response to trauma or inflammation such as in nodulocystic acne (see Fig. 8.23c).

Histologically, EICs consist of epidermal-lined sacs, which arise most commonly from the infundibular portion of the hair follicle. Rupture of the cyst and spillage of the epithelial debris contained within results in acute and chronic dermal inflammation. These lesions may become red and painful. Noninflamed cysts can be readily excised. However, inflamed lesions may be settled down first with intralesional injections of corticosteroids and oral antibiotics before surgery is attempted.

Most ECs are solitary. When multiple lesions are present, the preceding injury or inflammatory process is usually apparent. In other cases, the development of multiple cysts suggests the diagnosis of Gardner syndrome or intestinal polyposis type III. In this autosomal-dominant syndrome, increasing numbers of cysts, especially on the face and scalp, are associated with large-bowel polyposis and a ~100% risk of malignant degeneration, osteomatosis that involves the bones of the head, and desmoid tumors, particularly of the abdominal wall, as well as congenital hypertrophy of the retinal pigment epithelium that can be detected early in life on ophthalmologic examination. Members of affected families may be screened for mutations in the APC gene.

A number of other cystic tumors in the skin, including trichilemmal cysts, pilomatrixomas, vellus hair cysts, steatocystoma, and dermoid cysts, may be confused clinically with ECs.

Pilar Cysts

Pilar or trichilemmal cysts may be clinically indistinguishable from ECs. However, they are less common than ECs, occur almost exclusively on the scalp, and appear as multiple lesions in a majority of patients. They may have a distinct shiny pink appearance on the scalp and are less likely to drain than EICs. Trichilemmal cysts tend to be inherited in an autosomal-dominant pattern. Histologically, these lesions can be differentiated from epidermal cysts by the absence of a granular layer and homogeneous, pink keratinous material with calcification, unlike the laminated, horny material seen in ECs.

Pilomatrixoma

Pilomatrixoma, or calcifying epithelioma of Malherbe, presents as a sharply demarcated, firm, deep-seated nodule covered by normal or tethered overlying skin (Fig. 5.18). Superficial tumors develop a bluish-gray hue, and occasionally protuberant, red nodules are present. The "teeter totter" sign refers to elevation of the contralateral edge of the lesion upon application of pressure to one end. The "tent sign" refers to angular protrusion of the lesion above the skin. Lesions range in size from <1 cm to >3 cm diameter. Although pilomatrixomas may arise at any age, 40% appear before 10 years of age and over 50% by adolescence. These tumors often come to the attention of anxious patients or parents when rapid enlargement follows hematoma formation after trauma. They may intermittently become inflamed, which presents as pain and sudden increase in redness and size.

Pilomatrixomas occur most commonly on the face, scalp, upper arms, and upper trunk. They are usually solitary, but multiple lesions develop occasionally. Although most pilomatrixomas do not appear to be inherited, there are several reports of familial cases in an autosomal-dominant pattern and may be associated with certain genetic disorders including Gardner

Although pilomatrixomas are usually asymptomatic, rapid enlargement, ulceration, recurrent inflammation, or gradual progression to a large size may prompt surgical removal. They can usually be excised easily with local anesthetic.

Vellus Hair Cysts

Vellus hair cysts erupt as multiple, 1–2 mm diameter, follicular papules on the axillae, neck, chest, abdomen, and arm flexures of children and young adults (Fig. 5.19). Some of the papules have an umbilicated center, suggestive of molluscum contagiosum, and impacted, lightly pigmented vellus hairs may poke out of the center. These asymptomatic lesions resolve over months to years without treatment. Familial cases with autosomal-dominant inheritance have been described. Topical retinoids may hasten the resolution of these innocent cysts, but irritation may limit therapy.

Steatocystoma

Steatocystoma may appear sporadically as a solitary tumor or in an autosomal-dominant pattern with numerous, non-tender,

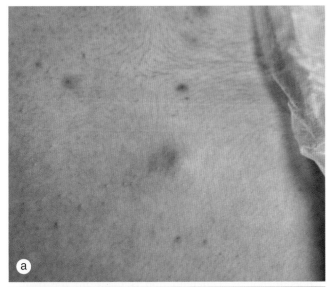

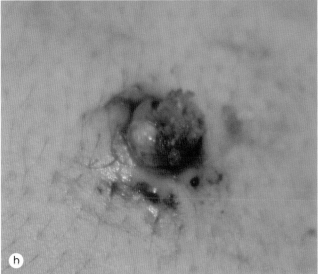

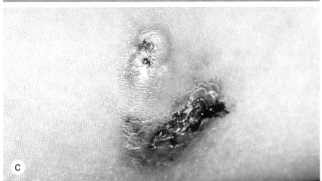

Fig. 5.18 Pilomatrixoma. **(a)** A pilomatrixoma caused intermittent itching and pain on the chest of this adolescent boy. **(b)** It was excised uneventfully with complete removal of the cyst lining. **(c)** This rock-hard nodule on the upper arm of a 5-year-old girl developed a central ulceration.

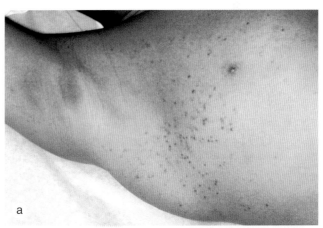

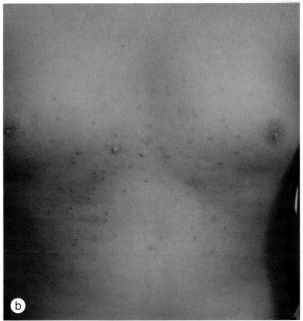

Fig. 5.19 Multiple asymptomatic 1–3 mm vellus hair cysts on the **(a)** axillae of a 7-year-old boy and **(b)** the chest of an 11-year-old boy.

syndrome (usually EIC with pilomatrical differentiation), Turner syndrome, Myotonic dystrophy, and Rubinstein–Taybi.

Histologically, this well-demarcated, encapsulated tumor demonstrates a distinctive pattern with islands of basophilic and shadow epithelial cells. Eosinophilic foci of keratinization and basophilic deposits of calcification are scattered throughout.

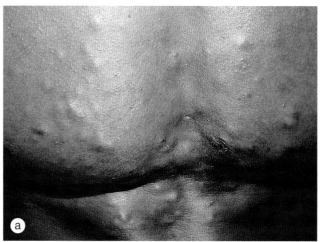

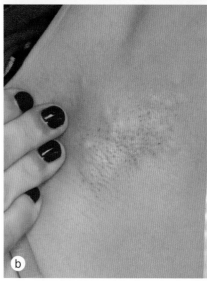

Fig. 5.20 **(a)** Numerous steatocystomas began to appear on the chest, neck, and face of this adolescent when he was 8 years old. His father and brother had similar nodulocystic lesions. **(b)** This 21-year-old woman has also had progressive nodules on her chest and axillae since adolescence, similar to her father and brother.

1–3 cm diameter, firm, rounded, cystic skin-colored to yellow papules or nodules tethered to the overlying skin (Fig. 5.20). Cysts usually begin to develop on the chest, arms, and face in childhood or adolescence. When ruptured, cysts exude an oily or milky fluid, and in some cases small hairs. Multiple steatocystomas may be associated with germline keratin 17 mutations either in isolation or within the genetic syndrome pachyonychia congenital type 2. The walls of the cyst characteristically contain flattened, sebaceous gland lobules or abortive hair follicles. A few bothersome cysts may be removed by simple excision. In some patients with hundreds of lesions, 13-cis-retinoid acid (isotretinoin) has been shown to shrink existing tumors and shut off the development of new ones at least temporarily.

Dermoid Cysts

Dermoid cysts are congenital, firm, subcutaneous cysts 1–4 cm in diameter, that occur within the suture lines and are found most commonly around the eyes, classically along the supraorbital

ridge at the lateral eyebrows, and on the head and neck (see Fig. 2.22). A dermoid cyst on midline nasal location has a differential diagnosis that includes heterotopic brain tissue and raises concern for an intracranial connection and requires imaging with magnetic resonance imaging (MRI) or computed tomography (CT) scan before surgical removal. On the head, most dermoids are non-mobile because they are often fixed to the periosteum. Retroauricular dermoid cysts may be softer. Dermoid cysts grow slowly and may cause thinning of the underlying bone. Unlike epidermal cysts, the epithelial lining of dermoid cysts contains multiple adnexal structures, which include hair follicles, eccrine glands, sebaceous glands, and apocrine glands. Surgical removal is required for cure if desired.

Multiple Facial Papules and Nodules

Multiple facial papules and nodules suggest the diagnosis of syringomas, angiofibromas (see section on fibrous tumors), or trichoepitheliomas. Differentiation is made on the basis of clinical and histologic findings.

Syringomas. Syringomas appear as multiple, 1–2 mm diameter, skin-colored to yellow-brown papules on the lower eyelids and cheeks (Fig. 5.21). Occasionally, they occur as isolated lesions or in a widely disseminated, eruptive form with hundreds of papules on the face, axillae, chest, abdomen, and genitals (Fig. 5.22). Although they develop most commonly in adolescent girls and young

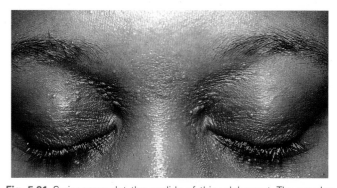

Fig. 5.21 Syringomas dot the eyelids of this adolescent. The papules responded quickly to gentle vaporization with carbon dioxide laser.

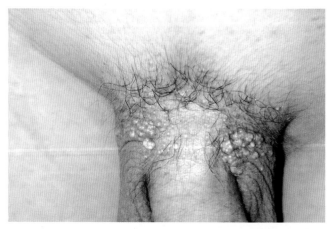

Fig. 5.22 Syringomas. Multiple 2–3 mm glistening whitish-yellow papules gradually increased in number on the genitals of a healthy 12-year-old boy.

women, they may appear at any age in males and females. They also develop more commonly in children with Down syndrome.

Histologic findings demonstrate characteristic, multiple small ducts lined by two rows of flattened epithelial cells in the superficial dermis. The lumina of the ducts contains amorphous debris, and some ducts possess comma-like tails that give the appearance of tadpoles.

Although occasionally disfiguring, lesions are usually asymptomatic. Syringomas may be effectively removed by a number of methods, including carbon dioxide laser, electrocautery, cryosurgery, and surgical excision.

Trichoepitheliomas. Trichoepitheliomas occur most commonly as solitary, skin-colored tumors <2 cm in diameter on the face of children or young adults. They cluster around the nose. Multiple lesions are inherited as an autosomal-dominant trait either in isolation in multiple familial trichoepithelioma or as part of Brooke–Spiegler syndrome, which is associated with spiradenomas and cylindromas (other benign tumors on the head and neck), as well as an increased risk of BCC and salivary gland tumors (Fig. 5.23). In this setting, trichoepitheliomas appear first in childhood and increase slowly in number and size. Numerous papules and nodules between 2 and 8 mm in diameter occur on the cheeks, nasolabial folds, nose, and upper lip. Histopathology shows a typical dermal tumor that consists of horn cysts of varying sizes and formations, resembling BCCs. Histologic differentiation from basal cell tumors is occasionally difficult.

Unfortunately, tumors may increase indefinitely and cause severe disfigurement. Surgical excision, electrocautery, and laser ablation have been used to deal with the most problematic lesions.

Xanthomas

Xanthomas are yellow dermal tumors that consist of lipid-laden histiocytes. In children, they are usually associated with an abnormality of lipid metabolism, and their presence may provide a clue to an underlying systemic disease.

Poorly soluble lipids are transported in serum by lipoproteins. Abnormalities in lipid transport and metabolism may result in elevations of serum triglycerides and/or cholesterol. The deposition of these lipids in skin and soft tissue results in the development of xanthomas.

Although conditions such as fulminant hepatic necrosis and poorly controlled diabetes mellitus may trigger hyperlipidemia, a number of primary inherited dyslipoproteinemias have been defined (Table 5.3). Medications such as antiretroviral agents used in the management of human immunodeficiency virus infection can also elevate lipids and trigger the formation of xanthomas.

The recognition of a number of clinical variants may help to define a particular systemic disorder (Fig. 5.24). Planar xanthomas present as soft, slightly infiltrated, yellow plaques at any site, but with a predilection for previously injured skin such as old lacerations and acne scars. Xanthelasma, an example of planar lesions on the eyelids, is associated with hypercholesteremia in about half of the cases. Diffuse lesions may involve the extremities, trunk, face, and neck. In childhood, planar xanthomas occur in diabetes mellitus, liver disease, and histiocytosis syndromes.

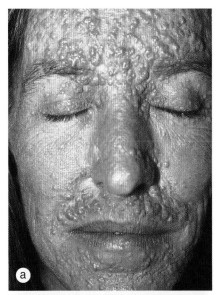

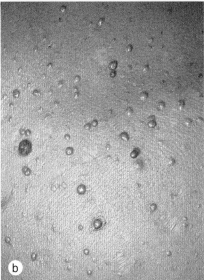

Fig. 5.23 Trichoepitheliomas slowly increased in size and number on **(a)** the face and **(b)** the back of this 17-year-old boy. Note the involvement of the nasolabial folds and the upper lip. At least five individuals in three generations of his family were affected.

Tuberous xanthomas arise as reddish-yellow nodules on the extensor surfaces of the extremities and buttocks. Although they may coalesce to cover a large area, tuberous lesions do not become adherent to the underlying soft-tissue structures, as do tendinous xanthomas. They may occur with elevations of cholesterol or triglycerides.

Tendinous xanthomas present as smooth, asymptomatic nodules on ligaments, tendons, and other deep, soft-tissue structures. They are usually several centimeters in size and occur most commonly on the ankles, knees, and elbows.

Eruptive xanthomas develop suddenly as 1–4 mm diameter, yellowish-red papules over the extensor surfaces of the extremities, buttocks, and bony prominences (Fig. 5.24c). Their appearance is usually associated with marked elevation in triglycerides, especially in poorly controlled diabetics or in patients with types I, III, IV, and V hyperlipidemias.

TABLE 5.3 Hyperlipidemias and Electrophoretic Patterns

Type (Prevalence)	Pattern	Chol	TG	Inheritance	Defect	Clinical Presentation	Age of Detection	Secondary Diseases
Type I a. Buerger–Gruetz syndrome or Familial hyperchylomicronemia	Chyl	+	+ + +	AR	Decreased lipoprotein lipase (LPL)	Eruptive xanthomata Abdominal colic Steatosis and organomegaly Lipemia retinalis	Early childhood	Pancreatitis, diabetes
b. Familial apoprotein CII deficiency					Altered ApoC2	Retinal vein occlusion Acute pancreatitis		
c.					LPL inhibitor in blood			
Type II a. Familial hypercholesterolemia	LDL	+ + +	+ or Nl	AD	LDL receptor non-functional or deficient	Xanthelasma Tendinous xanthomas Corneal arcus Tuberous xanthomas Atherosclerosis	Early childhood in homozygote	Hypothyroidism nephrotic syndrome
b. Familial combined hyperlipidemia (common)					Decreased LDL receptor and increased ApoB results in increase VLDL	Same, abnormal GTT		Hepatic disease
Type III Familial combined hyperlipidemia (relatively common)	IDL	+ + (variable)	+ (variable)	AR	Homozygous apolipoprotein E2, decreased remnant clearance, overproduction of VLDL	Xanthomas tuberous, palmar, tendinous, eruptive, abnormal GTT, hyperuricemia, atherosclerosis, obesity	Adult	Hepatic disease dys-globulinemia uncontrolled diabetes
Type IV Familial hypertriglyceridemia (most common)	VLDL and Chyl	+	+ +	AD	Increased VLDL production and Decreased LPL	Atherosclerosis, abnormal GTT, eruptive or tuberous xanthomas High TG levels can cause pancreatitis	Adult	Hypothyroidism, diabetes, pancreatitis glycogen storage disease, nephrotic syndrome, multiple myeloma
Type V (uncommon)	Chyl, VLDL	+	+ +	AR	Overproduction of VLDL, defect in catabolism of VLDL	Abnormal pain, obesity, xanthomas (eruptive), hepato-splenomegaly	Early adult	Diabetes, insulin dependent, pancreatitis, alcoholism

Chol, Cholesterol; *TG,* triglycerides; *Chyl,* chylomicrons; *LDL,* low density lipoproteins; *VLDL,* very low density lipoproteins; *IDL,* intermediate density lipoproteins; *AR,* autosomal recessive; *AD,* autosomal dominant; *GTT,* glucose tolerance test; *Nl,* normal.

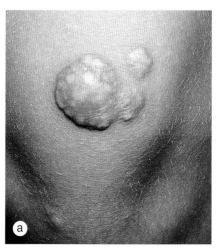
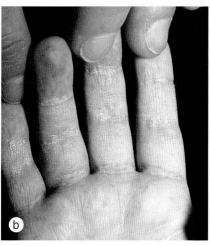
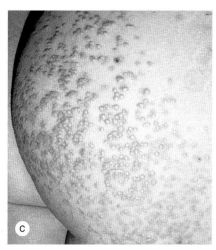

Fig. 5.24 Xanthomas erupted in two children **(a, b)** with congenital biliary atresia and chronic liver failure. **(b)** Note the involvement of the hand and finger creases. The infiltrated nodules and plaques resolved after liver transplantation. **(c)** Widespread xanthomas erupted in this 19-year-old woman with primary biliary cirrhosis.

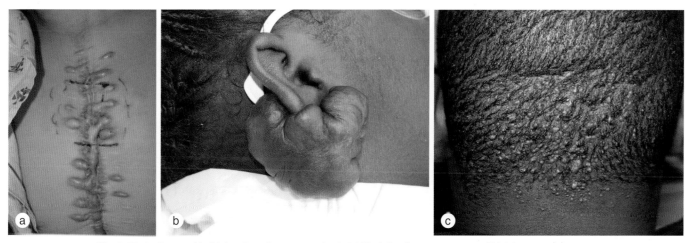

Fig. 5.25 A 10-year-old girl developed a progressive keloid in **(a)** a thoracotomy scar. **(b)** A large nodule grew on the ear lobe of this adolescent after ear piercing. **(c)** Acne keloidalis nuchae erupted on the back of the scalp of this 11-year-old boy. The appearance of the multiple small keloids was preceded by pseudofolliculitis.

Xanthomas must be differentiated from xanthogranulomas, which are not usually associated with systemic disease or elevated serum lipids (see Fig. 2.86). Xanthogranulomas rarely appear in large numbers; they are single in about 50% of the cases, and fewer than five nodules are present in most of the rest.

Fibrous Tumors
Keloids

A number of benign dermal tumors result from the proliferation of fibroblasts in the dermis. During the healing process that follows an injury to the skin, loss of normal structures and the laying down of collagen by fibroblasts may result in the formation of a scar. In certain predisposed individuals the collagen may become particularly thick, which results in a hypertrophic scar. Over the ensuing 6–9 months many of these scars flatten. However, some may persist or develop into keloids that continue to thicken and extend beyond the margins of the initial injury (Fig. 5.25). These rubbery nodules or plaques can be pruritic or tender, especially during the active growing phase. Keloids may arise sporadically or occur in a familial form. Isolated or atypical "keloids" with spontaneous onset may warrant biopsy to rule out other entities. They are most common in dark-pigmented individuals and have a predilection for the ear lobes, upper trunk, and shoulders. Fortunately, they are not seen on the mid-face. If treated early, hypertrophic scars and keloids may regress with intralesional corticosteroid injections alone or in combination with surgery. However, recurrences are common.

Dermatofibromas

Dermatofibromas present as firm, indolent, 0.3–1.0 cm diameter, reddish-brown dermal nodules (Fig. 5.26). Although dermatofibromas are most common in adults, they are occasionally found in children. Tumors may arise as single or multiple lesions (usually fewer than five) on any site, including the palms and soles. However, they appear most commonly on the arms

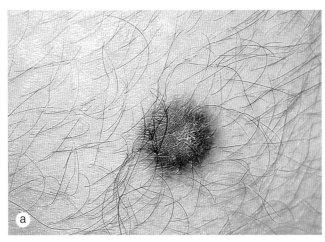
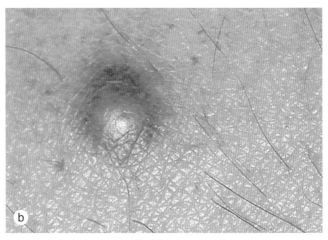

Fig. 5.26 Dermatofibroma. **(a)** An indolent, 1 cm diameter, firm, brown nodule appeared 2 years previously on the leg of this 17-year-old boy. The overlying epidermis was thickened and hyperpigmented. **(b)** A pink smooth-topped 1 cm papule with slight hyperpigmentation developed on the leg of a healthy adolescent girl. The asymptomatic nodule had changed little since it appeared 6 months earlier.

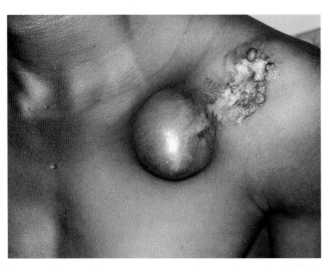

Fig. 5.27 Dermatofibroma sarcoma protuberans. A young adult had a large tumor excised from his left shoulder a year ago. He subsequently developed a new tumor on the left chest and recurrent nodules in the scar of the original lesion.

and legs. Many lesions are thought to follow minor trauma, such as insect bites or folliculitis.

On examination, dermatofibromas often demonstrate dimpling with lateral pressure because of attachment of the dermal nodule to an overlying, thickened, and hyperpigmented epidermis. Dermatofibromas may come to the attention of the patient after sudden enlargement following trauma and resultant hemorrhage, though most often they are asymptomatic. Histology, which reveals proliferating fibroblasts and histiocytes, permits differentiation from melanocytic tumors such as nevi and melanomas.

The early papules and nodules of dermatofibroma sarcoma protuberans (DFSP) may be mistaken for dermatofibroma (Fig. 5.27). However, the persistent slow or occasional accelerated growth of DFSP, multinodular appearance, and predilection for

the trunk and proximal extremities should suggest the diagnosis. Although these locally aggressive tumors are rare in children, congenital and early childhood cases have been reported. Treatment with wide local excision or Mohs micrographic surgery is indicated.

Angiofibromas

Although angiofibromas may develop as solitary papules in healthy individuals, their presence alerts the clinician to the diagnosis of tuberous sclerosis (Figs. 5.28 and 5.29). In children with tuberous sclerosis (TS), these dermal tumors gradually increase in size and number during childhood; involve the scalp, cheeks, and nasolabial folds; and spare the upper cutaneous lip (a sun-protected area). Subtle angiofibromas may be mistaken for periorificial dermatitis, flat warts, comedones, or seborrheic keratoses. Histopathology demonstrates a fibrous tumor with an increase in numbers of fibroblasts and amount of collagen, as well as capillary dilatation. The presence of acne-like papules beginning well before puberty suggests the diagnosis, even in otherwise healthy children of normal intelligence, and may warrant examination for other cutaneous and systemic signs of the syndrome. Topical rapamycin has proven to be an efficacious treatment for facial angiofibromas in TS.

In children without evidence of TS, the presence of progressive angiofibromas should prompt a search for multiple endocrine neoplasia type 1 (MEN1), which is also associated with angiofibromas. Multiple angiofibromas may occasionally be found in patients without other markers of systemic disease and may represent examples of mosaicism for TS or MEN1.

Vascular Tumor
Pyogenic Granuloma

Pyogenic granulomas, also known as lobular capillary hemangiomas, are common in children (especially toddlers) (Fig. 5.30). These benign, soft, bright red, usually solitary vascular neoplasms

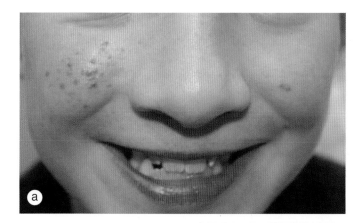

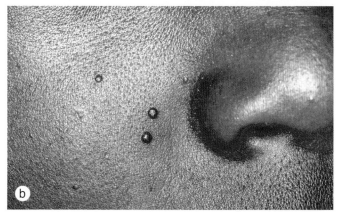

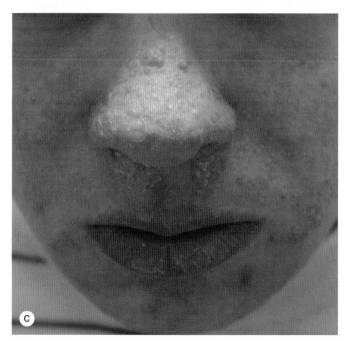

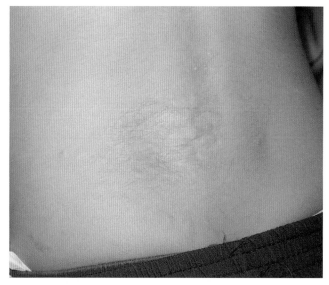

Fig. 5.29 A teenager with tuberous sclerosis demonstrated multiple discrete and confluent connective tissue nevi on his back in addition to facial angiofibromas and scattered truncal hypopigmented macules.

Fig. 5.28 Angiofibromas. (a) Small red facial papules were treated as acne. (b) Subtle brown papules were diagnosed as pigmented nevi. Both children were of normal intelligence and had no history of seizures. Skin biopsies demonstrated findings typical of angiofibromas. (c) This profoundly developmentally delayed boy with tuberous sclerosis developed progressive angiofibromas over much of his face. Note the involvement of the nasolabial folds and relative sparing of the upper lip.

range in size from 2 mm to 2 cm and are often preceded by trauma to the involved area. Pyogenic granulomas typically exhibit rapid growth and bleed readily with minor trauma. Bleeding can be dramatic and require sustained pressure to control. In children, 77% occur on the face or neck. They often develop a positive Band-Aid sign, or contact irritant dermatitis in the shape of the dressing and surrounding adhesive needed to keep pressure on the hemorrhagic papule. Mean age of presentation is around 6 years of age, and 14% occur in the first year of life. It rarely occurs before 4 months of age. There is a slight male predisposition of 1.5:1, and Caucasian patients make up 84% of cases. They are also associated with medications and may be seen in adolescents on isotretinoin treatment for acne vulgaris.

Pyogenic granulomas also tend to erupt on the buccal mucosa and gingivae of up to 2% of pregnant people during the first 5 months of pregnancy perhaps as a result of hormonal influences. In this setting they are referred to as granuloma gravidarum or pregnancy tumor. Pyogenic granulomas may also occur with increased frequency over vascular malformations such as port-wine stains, particularly after treatment with pulse-dye laser or during pregnancy.

Historically, the name "granuloma pyogenicum" was used because the lesion was presumed to be infectious and granulomatous, but it is actually neither. Although most clinicians still refer to these lesions as pyogenic granulomas, in 1980 the name lobular capillary hemangioma was introduced to reflect the pathophysiology of the benign vascular tumor.

Biopsy of the lesions shows a loose fibrous tissue matrix with proliferating capillaries similar to that of granulation tissue.

In children, pyogenic granulomas are most commonly confused with infantile hemangiomas. However, hemangiomas usually appear within the first few weeks of life, grow for 3–4 months, and then go on to regress. Fortunately, bleeding and ulceration do not occur in most lesions. This is in contrast to pyogenic

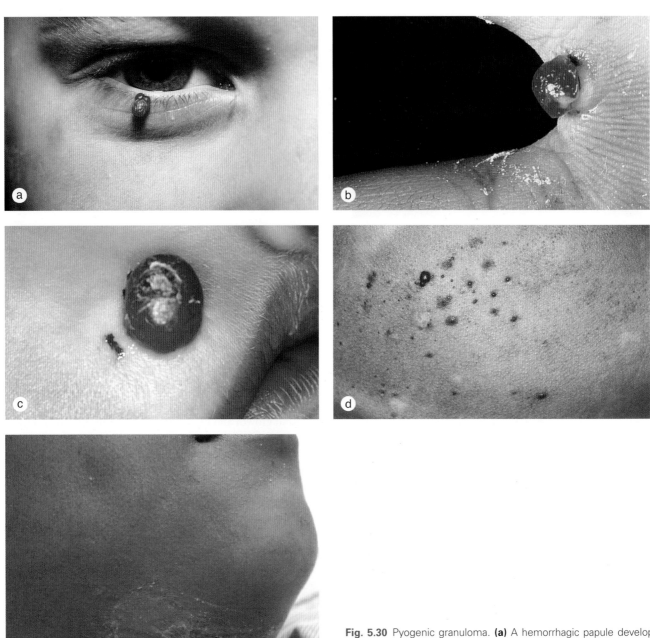

Fig. 5.30 Pyogenic granuloma. **(a)** A hemorrhagic papule developed on the lower eyelid of this 8-year-old boy. **(b)** Another rapidly growing, friable lesion is present between the fingers of a 5-year-old boy. **(c)** This 8 mm diameter nodule with a central crust bled profusely several times before surgical removal. **(d)** Multiple satellite lesions erupted on the back of a 10-year-old boy several months after the appearance of a single pyogenic granuloma. **(e)** This multiloculated pyogenic granuloma developed on the underside of the chin on this 3-year-old boy. Note the positive band-aid sign from irritation from the adhesive.

granulomas, which are only rarely present in the first few months of life and typically present with bleeding after minor trauma. The differential diagnosis for non-vascular solid red tumors includes spindle and epithelial cell nevi (Spitz nevus), amelanotic melanoma, and angiolymphoid hyperplasia with eosinophilia. These tumors have distinctive clinical findings, natural histories, and histologic findings.

Shave excision and electrocautery can be completed safely and effectively with minimal risk of scarring in less than a minute without sedation in most children. However, it is important to wait 5–7 min after anesthetic infiltration to allow the epinephrine to take effect and lower the risk of bleeding at the time of removal. Topical treatment with silver nitrate is often associated with rapid recurrence of lesions. Although pulsed-dye laser ablation may be used, it often requires repeated treatments over a period of weeks. Large lesions (>10 mm) may be treated with carbon dioxide laser or surgical excision.

Neural Tumors

Neurofibromas

Neurofibromas are the most common tumors of neural origin for which a patient might seek dermatologic consultation (Fig. 5.31). These soft, compressible, skin-colored to pink, 0.5–3 cm diameter tumors arise in the dermis and occasionally in the subcutaneous fat. Neurofibromas occur sporadically as solitary lesions or progressively in large numbers in patients with neurofibromatosis type 1 (NF1) starting in late childhood or adolescence (see Fig. 6.1) or in a segmental distribution in mosaic NF1. Occasionally in NF1 they appear as atrophic or red-blue macules. They may be pruritic with variable response to oral antihistamines.

Neuromas

Neuromas arise in three settings. Traumatic neuromas are solitary, painful nodules that develop in scars after surgery or

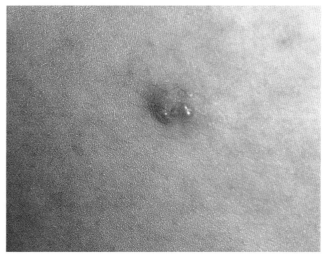

Fig. 5.32 Neuromas. Over 50 small, yellow, dermal nodules erupted on the face, neck, trunk, and extremities of a 3-year-old girl. She has no signs of multiple endocrine neoplasia, and the family history is negative.

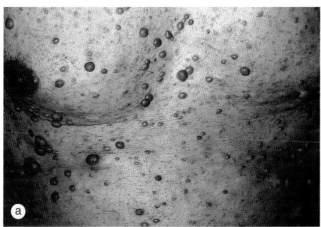

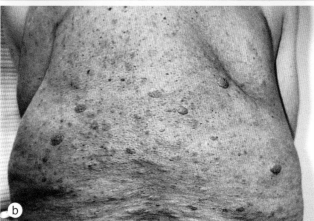

Fig. 5.31 Neurofibromas. **(a)** Widespread, compressible tumors developed over much of the body surface of this young man with neurofibromatosis type I. The neurofibromas began to appear when he was 10 years old. His 4-year-old son had multiple café-au-lait spots, but no cutaneous tumors. **(b)** A giant, plexiform neurofibroma slowly grew to involve most of this teenager's back. Note the multiple, overlying, cutaneous neurofibromas and café-au-lait spots.

trauma. Pain resolves quickly after surgical excision. Traumatic neuromas also include amputation neuromas and congenital, rudimentary, supernumerary digits, which occur most commonly on the ulnar side of the base of the fifth finger (see Fig. 2.23). Idiopathic neuromas are rare lesions that develop in early childhood through adult life as solitary or multiple 0.2–1 cm diameter dermal nodules on the skin and oral mucosa (Fig. 5.32). They are not associated with multiple endocrine neoplasia. Finally, multiple, mucosal neuromas are part of an autosomal-dominant syndrome (MEN type IIB) in which numerous small tumors begin to appear on the lips, oral mucosa, and face in early childhood. Recognition of this syndrome is important because of the associations with medullary thyroid carcinoma, which can develop in young children and adults, and pheochromocytoma in adolescents and adults.

In multiple mucosal neuroma syndrome, facial lesions may be confused with angiofibromas, trichoepitheliomas, multiple trichilemmomas in Cowden disease, and extensive papillomavirus infection. However, the large numbers of nerve bundles seen on skin biopsy are distinctive. Nodules on the trunk and extremities cannot be differentiated from other dermal tumors without a biopsy.

Lymphocytoma Cutis

Lymphocytoma cutis presents as asymptomatic nodules and plaques most commonly on the face, but any site may be involved. Although multiple lesions may erupt, solitary nodules ranging from less than 1 cm to several centimeters in diameter are the rule (Fig. 5.33). Most tumors develop in adolescents and young adults.

The differentiation from a non-Hodgkin lymphoma, which also presents as a single nodule, may be challenging, both clinically and histologically. Histologic findings demonstrate a mixed dermal infiltrate of large and small lymphocytes separated from the epidermis by a small band of normal collagen.

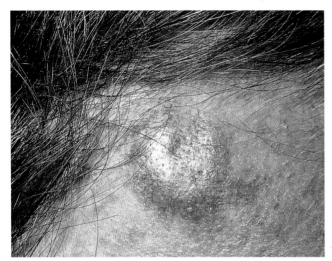

Fig. 5.33 Lymphocytoma cutis. A 1 cm diameter, painless nodule persisted for over a year on the forehead of a teenage boy. A skin biopsy from the center of the lesion demonstrated a lymphocytic infiltrate in the dermis that formed lymphoid, follicle-like structures. Intralesional corticosteroids resulted in some improvement.

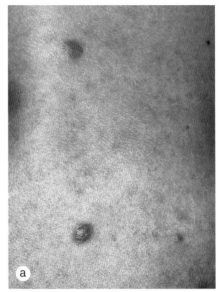

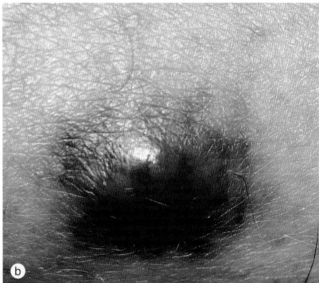

Fig. 5.35 Leukemia cutis. An adolescent with myelogenous leukemia developed **(a)** small, cutaneous nodules on his scalp and **(b)** several larger tumors on his trunk and extremities, associated with a recurrence of disease in his bone marrow.

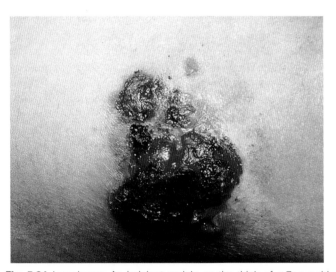

Fig. 5.34 Lymphoma. An indolent nodule on the thigh of a 7-year-old boy was initially diagnosed as a persistent insect-bite reaction. During the following year, several new nodules appeared on his legs and buttocks and regressed without treatment. Biopsy of the initial lesion shown here, which persisted throughout the period, demonstrated a lymphoma positive to Ki-1 marker.

The infiltrate may become organized into structures that resemble lymph follicles. The frequent presence of an admixture of plasma cells and/or eosinophils indicates no malignancy. Unfortunately, the histology is not specific, and the usual innocent nature of the eruption in children is defined by the clinical course. Nodules heal without treatment over months to years. Some patients may benefit from intralesional corticosteroids.

Clinically, lymphocytoma cutis may be indistinguishable from cutaneous nodules found in a secondary lymphoma (Fig 5.34) or metastatic leukemia (Fig 5.35), and all children deserve a careful history and complete physical examination to exclude signs and symptoms of systemic disease. Other infiltrative processes, such as Langerhans cell histiocytosis, non-Langerhans cell histiocytosis, idiopathic facial aseptic granulomas, follicular mucinosis (Fig. 5.36), and mastocytomas, as well as insect-bite reactions, sarcoidosis, deep fungal infections (Fig. 5.37), mycobacterial infections (Fig. 5.38), and dermatofibromas, may resemble lymphocytoma cutis. The clinical course, histologic findings, and culture results help define these entities. Rarely, other malignancies, such as leukemia, rhabdomyosarcoma, neuroblastoma, and renal carcinoma, present initially with cutaneous nodules. Their rapid growth and histologic pattern differentiate these malignancies from benign lymphocytoma cutis.

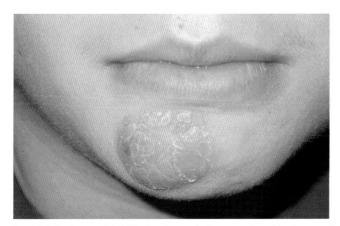

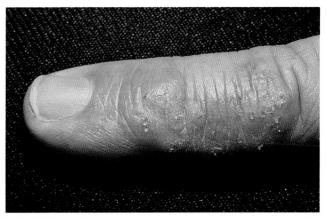

Fig. 5.36 A 13-year-old girl had a firm red plaque on her chin for over 6 months. A skin biopsy showed changes typical of alopecia mucinosa. Her mother applied a topical steroid, and the lesion resolved in several months.

Fig. 5.37 Sporotrichosis. A teenage boy developed a slowly expanding, painless, violaceous, indurated plaque on his left fifth finger. Sporotrichosis was diagnosed on a skin biopsy and confirmed by fungal culture. The lesion healed in 3 months with oral administration of a saturated solution of potassium iodide.

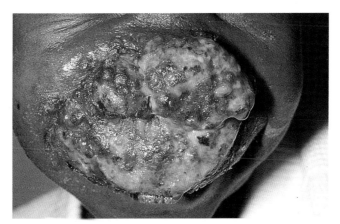

Fig. 5.38 Cutaneous tuberculosis. This infection began as a small nodule on the nose and grew into a large, infiltrative tumor that involved the center of her face. The diagnosis was confirmed by skin biopsy and mycobacterial culture. She responded to antibiotics with almost complete clearing of the tumor in 4 months.

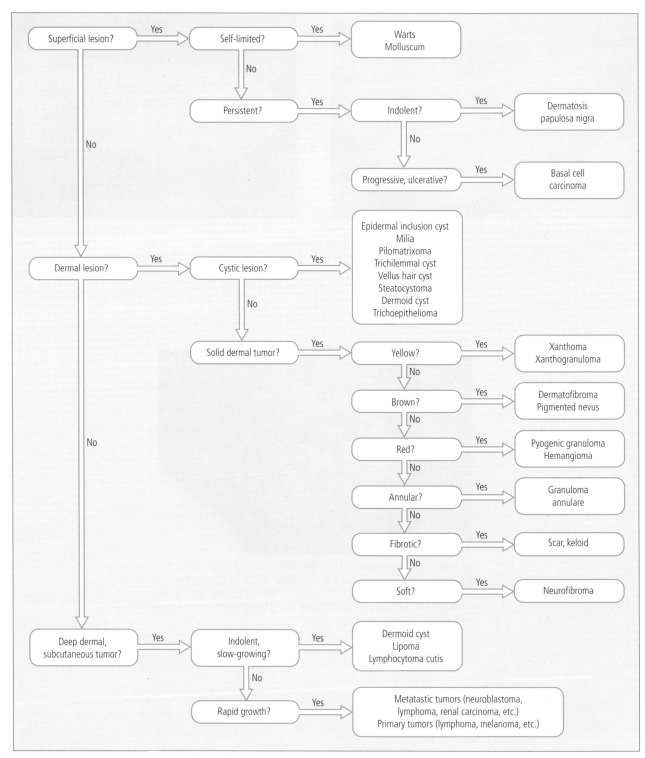

Fig. 5.39 Algorithm for evaluation of nodules and tumors.

FURTHER READING

Warts

Barnett N, Mark H, Winkelstein JA. Extensive verrucosis in primary immunodeficiency diseases. Arch Dermatol 1983; 119:5–7.

Berman B, Hengge U, Barton S. Successful management of viral infection and other dermatoses with imiquimod 5% cream. Acta Derm Venereol Suppl (Stockh) 2003; 214:12–17.

Borovoy MA, Borovoy M, Elson LM, et al. Flashlamp pulsed dye laser (585 nm). Treatment of resistant verrucae. J Am Pediatr Med Assoc 1996; 86:547–550.

Boull C, Groth D. Update: treatment of cutaneous viral warts in children. Pediatr Dermatol 2011; 28(3):217–229.

Cohen BA. Warts and children: can they be separated? Contemp Pediatr 1997; 14:128–149.

Cohen BA, Honig PG, Androphy E. Anogenital warts in children. Arch Dermatol 1990; 126:1575–1580.

Costa-Silva M, Fernandes I, Rodrigues AG, et al. Anogenital warts in pediatric population. An Bras Dermatol 2017; 92(5):675–681.

Deeb M, Levy R, Pope E, et al. Sinecatechins ointment for the treatment of warts in children. Pediatr Dermatol 2019; 36(1):121–124.

Frasier LD. Human papillomavirus infection in children (Review). Pediatr Ann 1994; 23:354–357.

Garnock-Jones KP, Giuliano AR. Quadrivalent human papillomavirus (HPV) types 6, 11, 16, 18 vaccine: for the prevention of genital warts in males. Drugs 2011; 71(5):591–602.

Glass AT, Solomon BA. Cimetidine for recalcitrant warts in adults. Arch Dermatol 1996; 132:680–682.

Higgins E, du Vivier A. Topical immunotherapy: unapproved uses, dosages, or indications. Clin Dermatol 2002; 20:515–521.

Ingelfinger JR, Grupe WE, Topor M, et al. Warts in a pediatric renal transplant population. Dermatologica 1977; 155:7–12.

Kwok CS, Gibbs S, Bennett C, et al. Topical treatments for cutaneous warts. Cochrane Database Syst Rev 2012; (9):CD001781.

Kwok CS, Holland R, Gibbs S. Efficacy of topical treatments for cutaneous warts: a meta-analysis and pooled analysis of randomized controlled trials. Br J Dermatol 2011; 165(2):233–246.

Messing AM, Epstein WL. Natural history of warts. Arch Dermatol 1963; 87:306–310.

Moresi JM, Herbert CR, Cohen BA. Treatment of anogenital warts in children with topical 0. 05% podofilox gel and 5% imiquimod cream. Pediatr Dermatol 2001; 18:448–450.

Muñoz Garza FZ, Roé Crespo E, Torres Pradilla M, et al. Intralesional candida antigen immunotherapy for the treatment of recalcitrant and multiple warts in children. Pediatr Dermatol 2015; 32(6):797–801.

Nofal A, Marei A, Ibrahim AM, et al. Intralesional versus intramuscular bivalent human papillomavirus vaccine in the treatment of recalcitrant common warts. J Am Acad Dermatol 2020; 82:94–100.

Obalek S, Jablonska S, Favre M, et al. Condylomata acuminata in children: frequent association with human papillomavirus responsible for cutaneous warts. J Am Acad Dermatol 1990; 23:205 213.

Ordoukhanian E, Lane A. Warts and molluscum: beware of treatments worse than the disease. Postgrad Med 1997; 101:223–226, 229 235.

Perman M, Sterling JB, Gaspari A. The painful purple digit: an alarming complication of Candida albicans antigen treatment of recalcitrant warts. Dermatitis 2005; 16(1):38–40.

Sarrin C. Human papillomavirus in children. Adv Nurse Pract 2001; 9:99–102.

Syrjänen S. Current concepts on human papillomavirus infections in children. APMIS 2010; 118(6–7):494–509.

Syrijänen S, Puranen M. Human papillomavirus infection in children: the potential role of maternal transmission. Crit Rev Oral Biol Med 2000; 11:259–274.

Torello A. What's new in the treatment of viral warts in children. Pediatr Dermatol 2002; 19:191–199.

Vakharia PP, Chopra R, Silverberg NB, et al. Efficacy and safety of topical cantharidin treatment for molluscum contagiosum and warts: a systematic review. Am J Clin Dermatol 2018; 19(6):791–803.

Veitch D, Kravvas G, Al-Niaimi F. Pulsed dye laser therapy in the treatment of warts: a review of the literature. Dermatol Surg 2017; 43(4):485–493.

Molluscum Contagiosum

Coloe J, Burkhart CN, Morrell DS. Molluscum contagiosum: what's new and true? Pediatr Ann 2009; 38(6):321–325.

Gottlieb SL, Myskowski PL. Molluscum contagiosum. Int J Dermatol 1994; 33:453–461.

Gur I. The epidemiology of Molluscum contagiosum in HIV-seropositive patients: a unique entity or insignificant finding? Int J STD AIDS 2008; 19(8):503–506.

Lee R, Schwartz RA. Pediatric molluscum contagiosum: reflections on the last challenging poxvirus infection, Part 1. Cutis 2010; 86(5):230–236.

Lee R, Schwartz RA. Pediatric molluscum contagiosum: reflections on the last challenging poxvirus infection, Part 2. Cutis 2010; 86(6):287–292.

Pauly CR, Artis WM, Jones HE. Atopic dermatitis, impaired cellular immunity, and molluscum contagiosum. Arch Dermatol 1978; 114:391–393.

Pierard-Franchimont C, Legrain A, Pierard GE. Growth and regression of molluscum contagiosum. J Am Acad Dermatol 1983; 9:669–672.

Silverberg N. Pediatric molluscum: optimal treatment strategies. Paediatr Drugs 2003; 5:505–512.

Smith KJ, Skelton H. Molluscum contagiosum: recent advances in the pathogenic mechanism and new therapies. Am J Clin Dermatol 2002; 3:535–545.

Steffen C, Markman JA. Spontaneous disappearance of molluscum contagiosum. Arch Dermatol 1980; 116:923–924.

van der Wouden JC, van der Sande R, Kruithof EJ, et al. Interventions for cutaneous molluscum contagiosum. Cochrane Database Syst Rev 2017; 5:CD004767.

Weston WL, Lane AT. Should molluscum be treated? Pediatrics 1980; 65:865–866.

Basal Cell Carcinoma and Genodermatoses Associated With Neoplasia

Cohen PR. Genodermatoses with malignant potential. Am Fam Physician 1992; 46(5):1479–1486.

Council on Environmental Health, Section on Dermatology, Balk SJ. Ultraviolet radiation: a hazard to children and adolescents. Pediatrics 2011; 127(3):588–597.

Gerstenblith MR, Goldstein AM, Tucker MA. Hereditary genodermatoses with cancer predisposition. Hematol Oncol Clin North Am 2010; 24(5):885–906.

Landau JM, Moody MN, Goldberg LH, et al. An unusual presentation of idiopathic basal cell carcinoma in an 8-year-old child. Pediatr Dermatol 2012; 29(3):379–381.

Milstone E, Helwig E. Basal cell carcinoma in children. Arch Dermatol 1978; 108:523.

Sasson M, Mallory SB. Malignant primary skin tumors in children. Curr Opin Pediatr 1996; 8:372–377.

Spitz JL. Genodermatoses: a full-color clinical guide to genetic skin disorders, 2nd edn. Williams and Wilkins, Baltimore, 2005.

Granuloma Annulare

Barron DF, Cootauco MH, Cohen BA. Granuloma annulare, a clinical review. Lippincott's Primary Care Practice 1997; 1:33–39.

Calista D, Landi G. Disseminated granuloma annulare in acquired immunodeficiency syndrome: case report and review of the literature. Cutis 1995; 55:158–160.

Cronquist SD, Stashower ME, Benson PM. Deep granuloma annulare presenting as an eyelid tumor in a child, with review of pediatric eyelid lesions. Pediatr Dermatol 1999; 16:377–380.

Dicken CH, Carrington SG, Winkelmann RK. Generalized granuloma annulare. Arch Dermatol 1969; 99:556–563.

Gregg KL, Nascimento AG. Subcutaneous granuloma annulare in childhood: clinicopathologic features in 34 cases. Pediatrics 2001; 107:E42.

Wells RS, Smith MA. The natural history of granuloma annulare. Br J Dermatol 1963; 75:199–206.

Adnexal Tumors

Berk DR, Bayliss SJ. Milia: a review and classification. J Am Acad Dermatol 2008; 59(6):1050–1063.

Brownstein MH, Helwig EB. Subcutaneous dermoid cysts. Arch Dermatol 1973; 107:237–239.

Cho S, Chang SE, Choi JH, et al. Clinical and histologic features of 64 cases of steatocystoma multiplex. J Dermatol 2002; 29(3): 152–156.

Esterly NB, Fretxin DF, Pinkus H. Eruptive vellus hair cysts. Arch Dermatol 1977; 113:500–503.

Friedman SJ, Butler DF. Syringoma presenting as milia. J Am Acad Dermatol 1987; 16:310–314.

Grimalt R, Gelmetti C. Eruptive vellus hair cysts: a case report and review of the literature. Pediatrics 1992, 9:98–102.

Knight PJ, Reiner CB. Superficial lumps in children. What, when, and why. Pediatrics 1983; 72:147–153.

Marrogi AJ, Wick MR, Dehner LP. Benign cutaneous adnexal tumors in childhood and young adults, excluding pilomatrixoma: review of 28 cases and literature. J Cutan Pathol 1991; 18:20–27.

Marrogi AJ, Wick MR, Dehner LP. Pilomatrical neoplasms in children and young adults. Am J Dermatopathol 1992; 14:87–94.

Pariser RJ. Multiple hereditary trichoepitheliomas and basal cell carcinomas. J Cutan Pathol 1986; 13:111–117.

Pollard ZF, Robinson HD, Calhoun J. Dermoid cysts in children. Pediatrics 1976; 57:379–382.

Roberts CM, Birnie AJ, Kaye P, et al. Papules on the trunk. Eruptive vellus hair cysts. Clin Exp Dermatol 2010; 35(3):e74–e75.

Soler-Carrillo J, Estrab T, Mascaro JM. Eruptive syringomas: 27 cases and review of the literature. J Eur Acad Dermatol Venereol 2001; 15:242–246.

Storm CA, Seykora JT. Cutaneous adnexal neoplasms. Am J Clin Pathol 2002; 118(Suppl):S33–S49.

Vidal A, Iglesias MJ, Fernández B, et al. Cutaneous lesions associated to multiple endocrine neoplasia syndrome type 1. J Eur Acad Dermatol Venereol 2008; 22(7):835–838.

Xanthomas

Babl FE, Regan AM, Pelton SI. Xanthomas and hyperlipidemia in a human immunodeficiency virus-infected child receiving highly active antiretroviral therapy. Pediatr Infect Dis J 2002; 21:259–260.

Blom DJ, Byrnes P, Jans S, et al. Dysbetalipoproteinemia: clinical and pathophysiological features. S Afr Med J 2002; 92:892–897.

Parker F. Xanthomas and hyperlipidemias. J Am Acad Dermatol 1985; 13:1–30.

Fibrous Tumors

Koenig MK, Bell CS, Hebert AA, et al. Efficacy and safety of topical rapamycin in patients with facial angiofibromas secondary to tuberous sclerosis complex: the TREATMENT randomized clinical trial. JAMA Dermatol 2018; 154(7):773–780.

Murray JC, Pollack SV, Pinnell SR. Keloids: a review. J Am Acad Dermatol 1981; 4:461–470.

Niemi KM. The rare benign fibrocystic tumors of the skin. Acta Derm Venereol (Stockh) 1970; 50(Suppl):43–66.

Pyogenic Granuloma

Amerigo J, Gonzales-Camara R, Galera H, et al. Recurrent pyogenic granuloma with multiple satellites. Dermatologica 1983; 166: 117–121.

Baselga E, Wassef M, Lopez S, et al. Agminated, eruptive pyogenic granuloma-like lesions developing over congenital vascular stains. Pediatr Dermatol 2012; 29(2):186–190.

Pagliai KA, Cohen BA. Pyogenic granuloma in children. Pediatr Dermatol 2004; 21(1):10–13.

Patrice SJ, Wiss K, Mulliken JB. Pyogenic granuloma (lobular capillary hemangioma): a clinicopathologic study of 178 cases. Pediatr Dermatol 1991; 8:267–276.

Winton GB. Dermatoses of pregnancy. J Am Acad Dermatol 1982; 6:977–998.

Neural Tumors

Holm TW, Prawer SE, Sahl WJ Jr, et al. Multiple cutaneous neuromas. Arch Dermatol 1973; 107:608–610.

Khairi MRA, Dexter RN, Burzynski NJ, et al. Mucosal neuroma, pheochromocytoma and medullary thyroid carcinoma: multiple endocrine neoplasia type 3 (review). Medicine (Baltimore) 1975; 54:89–112.

Lee MW, Lee DK, Choi JH, et al. Clinicopathologic study of cutaneous pseudolymphomas. J Dermatol 2005; 32(7): 594–601.

Schaffer JV, Kamino H, Witkiewicz A, et al. Mucocutaneous neuromas: an under-recognized manifestation of PTEN hamartoma-tumor syndrome. Arch Dermatol 2006; 142(5):625–632.

Lymphocytoma, Lymphoma Cutis

Burg G, Kerl H, Schmoekel C. Differentiation between malignant B-cell lymphomas and pseudolymphomas of the skin. J Dermatol Surg Oncol 1984; 10:271–275.

Iwatsuki K, Ohtsuki M, Harada H, et al. Clinicopathologic manifestations of Epstein Barr virus-associated lymphoproliferative disorder. Arch Dermatol 1997; 133:1081–1086.

VanHale HM, Winkelmann RK. Nodular lymphoid disease of the head and neck: lymphocytoma cutis, benign lymphocytic infiltrate of Jessner, and their distinction from malignant lymphoma. J Am Acad Dermatol 1985; 12:455–461.

6

Pigmentary Disorders

Daren J. Simkin, John C. Mavropoulos, and Bernard A. Cohen

INTRODUCTION

Although most disorders of pigmentation in infancy and childhood are of cosmetic concern only, some provide clues to an underlying multisystem disease. Disorders of pigmentation may be differentiated clinically by the presence of either increased or decreased pigmentation (and sometimes both in the same patient!) occurring in a localized or diffuse distribution. An algorithmic approach to diagnosis for disorders of pigmentation is summarized at the end of the chapter (see Fig. 6.28).

HYPERPIGMENTATION

Pigmented lesions are localized areas of hyperpigmentation that are frequently caused by developmental or hereditary factors, and often appear early in childhood. Pigmented lesions may also be acquired during childhood after inflammatory rashes or exposure to actinic, traumatic, chemical, or thermal injury. A useful way to classify pigmented lesions is by identifying whether they occur in the epidermis or dermis. Epidermal melanosis occurs when increased numbers of epidermal melanocytes are present in the basal cell layer or when increased quantities of melanin are present in epidermal keratinocytes. Dermal melanosis results from increased melanin in dermal melanocytes or melanophages. Although epidermal melanosis may result in dark-brown or black lesions, most appear tan or light brown. In contrast, dermal melanosis usually produces slate-gray, dark-brown, and bluish-green lesions.

Epidermal Melanosis
Café-Au-Lait Spots

Café-au-lait spots are discrete, tan macules that appear at birth or during childhood in 10–20% of normal individuals. Lesion sizes vary from freckles to patches greater than 20 cm in diameter and may involve any site on the skin (Fig. 6.1a,d–f).

Most children with café-au-lait spots are healthy. However, the presence of six or more lesions, each >5 mm in diameter in someone <15 years old (and lesions >1.5 cm in diameter for older individuals) is a diagnostic marker for classic neurofibromatosis (i.e. von Recklinghausen disease or National Institutes of Health classification NF-1), and 90% of individuals with neurofibromatosis have at least one café-au-lait spot. Often present at birth, café-au-lait spots usually increase in size and number throughout childhood, particularly during the first few years of life in children with neurofibromatosis. Other lesions in neurofibromatosis such as axillary freckling (Crowe's sign) (Fig. 6.1a), neurofibromas (Fig. 6.1b,c), and iris hamartomas (i.e. Lisch nodules) may not appear until later childhood or adolescence.

Histologic findings include increased numbers of melanocytes and increased melanin in epidermal melanocytes and keratinocytes. Giant pigment granules have been identified in café-au-lait spots of neurofibromatosis, but they may also be seen in sporadic café-au-lait spots, nevi, freckles, and lentigines.

Pigmented-lesion lasers (Q-switched ruby, neodymium: yttrium-aluminum-garnet, and alexandrite lasers) provide a safe, effective, and relatively painless therapeutic alternative for removing café-au-lait spots, particularly those with jagged or ill-defined borders. Unfortunately, they may recur after laser therapy.

Café-au-lait spots are not specific for neurofibromatosis and have also been associated with other disorders including tuberous sclerosis, McCune–Albright syndrome, epidermal nevus syndrome, Bloom syndrome, multiple endocrine neoplasia type 1 (MEN1), Fanconi syndrome, ataxia-telangiectasia, Silver–Russell syndrome, and other neuro-cardio-facio-cutaneous syndromes, such as Noonan syndrome, LEOPARD syndrome, and Legius syndrome (Table 6.1).

Freckles (Ephelides)

Freckles or ephelides are usually 2–3 mm in diameter, reddish-tan and brown macules that appear on sun-exposed surfaces, particularly the face, neck, upper chest, and forearms (Fig. 6.2). They typically arise in early childhood on lightly pigmented individuals. Lesions tend to fade in the winter and increase in number and pigmentation during spring and summer months. Photoprotection with clothing, sunblocks, and sunscreens may decrease the summer recurrence of freckles, which are generally of cosmetic importance only, although a large number of freckles in healthy children is an independent risk factor for development of melanoma in adulthood. Although it is common for freckles to increase in number during adolescence and partially fade thereafter, the development of progressive, widespread freckling in sun-exposed sites may suggest an underlying disorder of photosensitivity such as xeroderma pigmentosum (Fig. 6.3) (see p.196, Chapter 7).

Histologically, freckles demonstrate excess pigment at the basal cell layer of the epidermis. The number of melanocytes may be decreased, but those that remain are larger and show increased and more prominent dendritic processes.

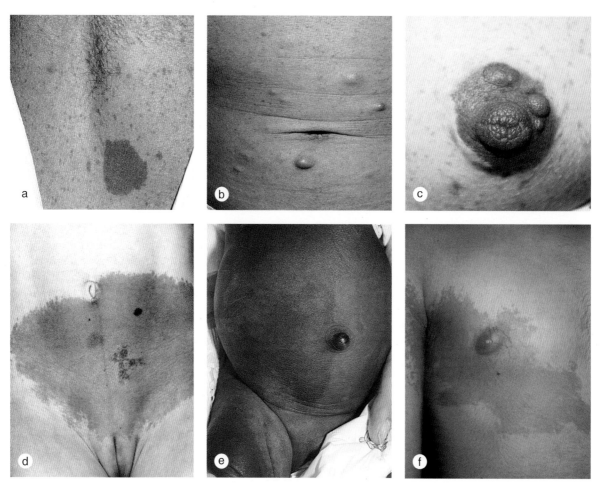

Fig. 6.1 Café-au-lait spots. **(a–c)** This 16-year-old girl with neurofibromatosis had multiple café-au-lait spots since early childhood. **(a)** Her axilla demonstrates a 4 cm diameter café-au-lait spot and diffuse freckling. **(b)** At puberty she began to develop widespread neurofibromas. Note the variable size of the dermal tumors on her abdomen. **(c)** Cutaneous neurofibromas also erupted on her nipples. Note the extensive freckling on her breasts. **(d)** In the center of a large café-au-lait spot, which was present at birth, this 6-year-old girl developed a spongy tumor. Skin biopsy of the mass demonstrated a neurofibroma. Note the dark-brown, pigmented nevus within the café-au-lait spot. **(e)** A large, unilateral café-au-lait spot was noted at birth on this infant's abdomen. She subsequently developed other findings typical of Albright syndrome. **(f)** This healthy 13-year-old boy had a large segmental café-au-lait macule that was unchanged from birth.

TABLE 6.1   Café-Au-Lait Spots

Disorder	Other Skin Findings	Systemic Involvement
Neurofibromatosis	Axillary freckling, Lisch nodules (iris), neurofibromas	Skeletal abnormalities, neurologic involvement
Albright syndrome	Few large café-au-lait spots	Precocious puberty in girls, polyostotic fibrous dysplasia
Watson syndrome	Axillary freckling	Pulmonary stenosis, intellectual disability, short stature
Silver–Russell syndrome	Hypohidrosis in infancy	Small stature, skeletal asymmetry, clinodactyly of fifth finger
Ataxia-telangiectasia	Telangiectasia in bulbar conjunctivae and on face, sclerodermatous changes	Growth retardation, ataxia and other neurological involvement, lymphopenia, IgA, IgE, lymphoid tissue, respiratory infections
Tuberous sclerosis	Hypopigmented macules, shagreen patch, adenoma sebaceum, subungual fibromas	Central nervous system, kidneys, heart, lungs
Turner syndrome	Loose skin, especially around the neck, lymphedema in infancy, hemangiomas	Short stature, gonadal dysgenesis, skeletal anomalies, renal anomalies, cardiac defects
Bloom syndrome	Telangiectatic erythema of cheeks, photosensitivity, ichthyosis	Short stature, malar hypoplasia, risk of malignancy
Multiple lentigines (LEOPARD) syndrome	Lentigines, axillary freckling	Electrocardiogram abnormalities, ocular hypertelorism, pulmonic stenosis, genital abnormalities, growth retardation, sensorineural deafness
Westerhof syndrome	Hypopigmented macules	Short stature with micromelia, intellectual disability

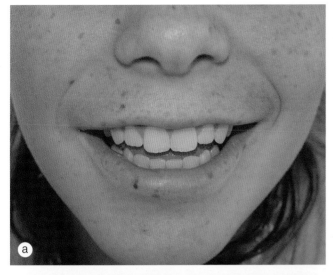

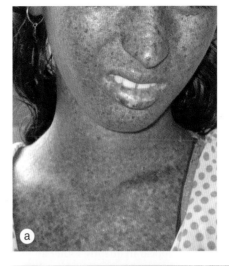

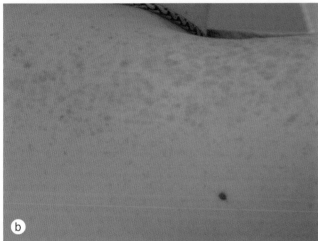

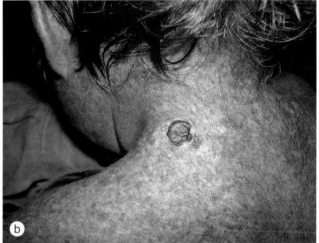

Fig. 6.2 Freckles and lentigines. **(a)** This fair adolescent girl with a history of extensive sun exposure developed widespread freckles in sun-exposed areas of her face, upper trunk, and extremities. Note the darker macules on her lower vermillion border and right upper lip, which persisted in the winter and were typical of solar lentigines. She also had a few small acquired pigmented nevi scattered in sun-exposed areas. **(b)** A 13-year-old boy had similar lesions on his shoulders.

Lentigo Simplex

In contrast to a freckle, a lentigo is a darker macule with more uniform color that does not demonstrate seasonal variation and becomes more prominent with age. A lentigo may be 2–5 mm in diameter and arise on any site on the skin or mucous membranes. Because it is rare to observe the presence of merely one lentigo, the plural term "lentigines" is often used in clinical practice (Figs. 6.2, 6.4, and 6.6).

Lentigo simplex commonly occurs during childhood and does not show a predilection for sun-exposed surfaces. The lentigines of lentigo simplex range from brown to black and may be indistinguishable clinically from junctional pigmented nevi.

Microscopically, lentigo simplex shows elongation of the rete ridges, an increase in concentration of melanocytes in the basal

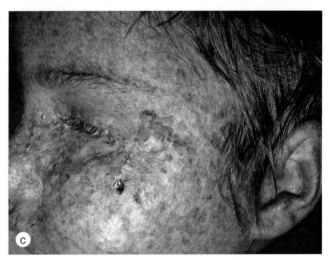

Fig. 6.3 Xeroderma pigmentosum. **(a)** This adolescent was exquisitely sensitive to sunlight and developed widespread solar lentigines in sun-exposed areas. Note the actinic cheilitis on her lower lip. **(b)** An 8-year-old boy with developed almost confluent solar lentigines, actinic keratoses, and squamous cell carcinomas such as the crusted plaques on his upper back and **(c)** face. He also had a persistent keratitis with scarring.

layer, an increase in melanin in both melanocytes and basal keratinocytes, and melanophages in the upper dermis.

Several special variants of lentigo simplex are recognized, which include lentiginosis profusa, LEOPARD syndrome (multiple lentigines syndrome), and speckled lentiginous nevus.

Lentiginosis profusa. Also known as generalized lentiginosis, Lentiginosis profusa is characterized by the presence of diffuse, multiple, small, darkly pigmented macules from birth or infancy. Occurrence is usually sporadic, and children are otherwise healthy and develop normally. This entity must be differentiated from LEOPARD syndrome, in which diffuse lentigines are associated with multisystem disease.

LEOPARD syndrome. In LEOPARD syndrome, the lentigines (L) are tan or brown, appear in the first few years of life and increase in number throughout childhood (Fig. 6.4). Axillary freckling and café-au-lait spots appear frequently. Other anomalies, which are suggested by the LEOPARD mnemonic and occur to a variable degree, include electrocardiographic conduction abnormalities (E), ocular hypertelorism (O), pulmonic stenosis (P), abnormal genitalia (A), growth retardation (R), and neural deafness (D). This disorder is inherited as an autosomal-dominant trait. LEOPARD syndrome is most commonly caused by a mutation in the *PTPN11* gene, which encodes for SHP-2, a protein tyrosinase phosphatase. In both lentiginosis profusa and LEOPARD syndrome the mucous membranes are spared, although scleral lentigines have been reported. In a related disorder called LAMB syndrome, multiple lentigines are associated with atrial myxoma (A), cutaneous papular myxomas (M), and blue nevi (B).

Speckled lentiginous nevus. Speckled lentiginous nevus, or nevus spilus, presents at birth or during the first year of life as a discrete tan or brown macule, which becomes dotted with darker, pigmented macules during childhood (Fig. 6.5). The light-brown patch demonstrates histologic changes typical of lentigo simplex,

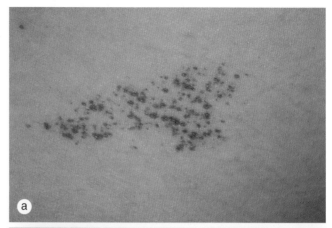

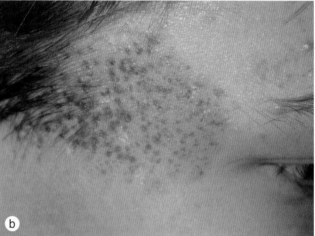

Fig. 6.5 Nevus spilus. These speckled nevi were unchanged since they were noted at birth. Note the subtle tan background studded with dark macules on the **(a)** leg and **(b)** temple of these school-age children.

while the dark, pigmented macules show nests of nevus cells at the dermal–epidermal junction. The risk of malignant change is very low, as in small congenital pigmented nevi. There are reports of the less common papular variant arising in association with ipsilateral neurological and musculoskeletal abnormalities, together termed speckled lentiginous nevus syndrome.

Peutz–Jeghers Syndrome

Peutz–Jeghers syndrome is an autosomal dominant disorder characterized by diffuse, small, slate-gray to black macules on the skin and mucous membranes that present at birth or during early childhood. Lesions increase in number throughout childhood. The face is most commonly involved, in particular the vermilion border of the lips and buccal mucosa, but macules may appear on the hands, arms, trunk, and perianal and genital skin (Fig. 6.6). Axillary freckling may also occur. Cutaneous lesions may either occur alone or be associated with intestinal polyposis usually of the small bowel, which can act as a lead point for intussusception and results in bleeding or obstruction in half of patients before age 20. The risk of malignant change in the gastrointestinal tract is markedly elevated as well and warrants close surveillance.

Although the pigmented lesions in Peutz–Jeghers syndrome are clinically indistinguishable from lentigines, the

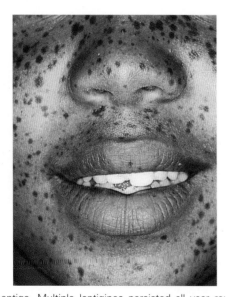

Fig. 6.4 Lentigo. Multiple lentigines persisted all year round on the face, upper trunk, and extremities of this 13-year-old boy with LEOPARD syndrome. The mucous membranes were spared, but he had lip involvement, axillary freckling, and multiple café-au-lait spots. His sister, father, and grandfather had similar cutaneous findings.

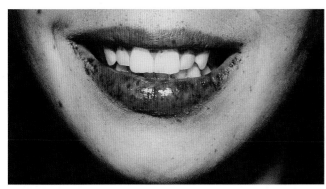

Fig. 6.6 Peutz–Jeghers syndrome. This smiling, 12-year-old girl developed progressive lentigines on her face, particularly her lips, in early childhood. She also has involvement of the extremities, trunk, and mucous membranes.

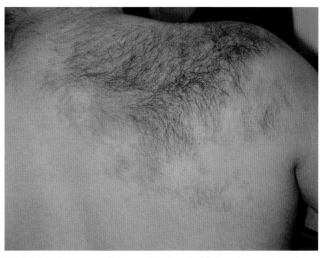

Fig. 6.7 Becker nevus. Progressive, mottled hyperpigmentation began at 13 years of age and was followed by the development of dark, coarse hair on the back of this 17-year-old boy.

histology reveals increased pigmentation only in the basal cell layer. Some investigators have found increased numbers of melanocytes, which suggests that this disorder may represent a distinct form of epidermal melanosis. Peutz–Jeghers syndrome is most often associated with mutations in the *STK11/LKB1* gene on chromosome 19p13.3, which encodes a serine-threonine protein kinase that serves a tumor suppressive role in cell cycle regulation.

Cutaneous macules may become disfiguring and typically respond well to destructive measures, such as gentle liquid nitrogen freezing or carbon dioxide laser ablation. Pigmented-lesion lasers are a safe, effective, and relatively painless therapeutic alternative.

Solar Lentigines

Solar lentigines usually do not become apparent until the fourth and fifth decades of life, although they may appear in later childhood or adolescence, particularly in lightly pigmented individuals who spend extensive time outdoors. These irregularly shaped, darkly pigmented macules range from a few millimeters to a few centimeters in diameter and appear on sun-exposed skin. Although the risk of malignant degeneration is minimal, they provide a marker of significant sun exposure. Children and parents should be counseled regarding the cumulative risk of actinic damage and use of protective clothing and sunscreens.

Becker Nevus

Becker nevus (hairy epidermal nevus) typically develops around puberty as a unilateral patch of hyperpigmentation on the shoulder, chest, or back, although any skin site may be involved. This common lesion is usually followed by overlying hypertrichosis within 2 years and occurs most frequently in boys (Fig. 6.7). Pigmentation is usually uniform and well demarcated, but reticulated patches may be present. The coarse, long hairs may extend beyond the area of hyperpigmentation.

Histologically, the epidermis demonstrates acanthosis and rete ridge elongation in association with increased pigment in the basal cell layer and melanophages in the upper dermis.

Smooth muscle bundles in the dermis may be increased in some cases, reminiscent of changes observed in congenital smooth muscle hamartomas.

As in other epidermal melanoses, gentle destructive measures may result in improvement of hyperpigmentation. Use of photoprotection decreases darkening from sun exposure during the summer months. A wide variety of lasers, most commonly pigmented-lesion lasers, have proven effective for eradication of excess pigment in Becker nevus, but recurrence may occur within 1–2 years. Bleaching agents containing hydroquinone or azelaic acid may be effective, however patients should be made aware that inadvertent contact of these drugs with normal contiguous skin may result in hypopigmentation. Other topicals, including glycolic acid and flutamide, may be beneficial as well. Shaving, depilatories, and electrolysis may be helpful for nevi with prominent hair.

Acanthosis Nigricans

Acanthosis nigricans is marked by brown-to-black hyperpigmentation within distinctive velvety or warty skin in intertriginous areas. A number of clinical variants are recognized. An inherited form usually erupts during infancy or childhood but may also occur at puberty (Fig. 6.8a). In this subtype, lesions tend to intensify in adolescence and may fade somewhat during adulthood. Inheritance is usually autosomal dominant, and cutaneous findings may be associated with insulin resistance. An endocrine variant is usually associated with a pituitary tumor or polycystic ovary syndrome and insulin resistance. Obesity is a variable feature. A paraneoplastic variant can often be differentiated from other variants of acanthosis nigricans by its extensive and more florid lesions, rapid progression, and onset usually in middle age and rarely in childhood. Gastrointestinal carcinoma is most commonly implicated, but other associated tumors include carcinomas of the lung, kidney, bladder, ovary, or pancreas, as well as lymphoma and osteogenic sarcoma. Idiopathic acanthosis nigricans is the most common variant (Fig. 6.8b–e). Although not associated with a specific

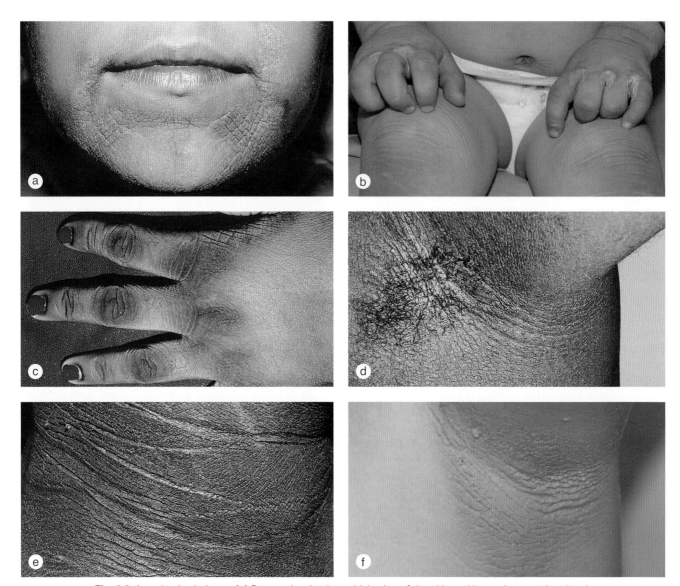

Fig. 6.8 Acanthosis nigricans. **(a)** Progressive, leathery thickening of the skin and hyperpigmentation developed on the face, neck, chest, back, and flexures of this healthy 9-year-old boy with familial acanthosis nigricans. Note the symmetric patches on his chin and cheeks. **(b)** This healthy toddler also with benign familial acanthosis nigricans developed progressive generalized thickening of the skin noted here on the abdomen, arms, and legs. **(c–e)** Symmetric, velvety patches appeared over the bony prominences and flexures of this obese, dark-pigmented adolescent with "benign" acanthosis nigricans. Lesions were most prominent over **(c)** the knuckles, **(d)** axilla, and **(e)** neck. A light-pigmented obese adolescent developed similar lesions most prominent on her **(f)** axillae and neck.

endocrine disorder, this variant often occurs in obese individuals with insulin resistance who are at significant risk for type II diabetes. Pigmentation may decrease after puberty, particularly in patients who undergo weight reduction. Drug-induced acanthosis nigricans may occur with nicotinic acid, diethylstilbestrol, oral contraceptives, and exogenous glucocorticoids. Acanthosis nigricans has also been reported in a subset of patients with Crouzon craniosynostosis resulting from a mutation in the *FGFR3* gene encoding for fibroblastic growth factor receptor 3 protein.

Although acanthosis nigricans is most intense in skin creases of the neck, axilla, and groin, it may also be present on skin over bony prominences, including the knuckles, elbows, knees, and ankles. In cases of paraneoplastic acanthosis nigricans, mucous membranes may be involved.

Histopathology demonstrates hyperkeratosis, minimal acanthosis, and marked papillomatosis. Although there may be a slight increase in melanin in the basal cell layer, hyperpigmentation is likely caused by compact hyperkeratosis.

Melasma

Melasma occurs as brown to brown-gray patches typically on the face but may also occur on the forearms and chest. The distribution is often symmetric and occurs primarily in pubertal girls and women (Fig. 6.9), although adolescent boys may also be affected. Although melasma is usually idiopathic,

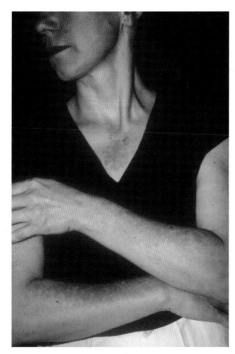

Fig. 6.9 Melasma. This healthy young woman developed diffuse mottled hyperpigmentation on her forehead, cheeks, neck, upper mid-chest, and forearms shortly after starting oral contraceptives.

it can be associated with pregnancy or the ingestion of oral contraceptives. Lesions tend to increase in size and degree of hyperpigmentation after sun exposure.

Histologically, epidermal and dermal melanization may occur, with many patients demonstrating pigment in both sites. An increased number of epidermal melanocytes is observed, and increased pigment is found in epidermal keratinocytes and dermal melanophages.

Clinically, melasma must be differentiated from postinflammatory hyperpigmentation and phytophoto contact (berloque) dermatitis. Berloque dermatitis frequently appears after sun exposure of skin with inadvertent application of a photosensitizer such as musk ambrette, a common component of perfumes.

Pigmentation often wanes after pregnancy or discontinuation of oral contraceptives. However, treatment is difficult: potent physical blocking topical sunscreens are mainstays to prevent further exacerbation, while bleaching agents or pigmented-lesion lasers may be helpful. Triple combination cream of hydroquinone, tretinoin, and a mild corticosteroid has proven significantly more effective than hydroquinone alone.

Dermal Melanocytosis/Melanosis

Dermal melanocytosis (formerly known as Mongolian spots) are poorly circumscribed, slate-gray to blue-green congenital macules or patches (Fig. 6.10a,b). Lesions range from a few millimeters to over 20 cm in diameter and are typically found on the trunk and proximal extremities of 80–90% of black infants, 75% of Asians, and 10% of white infants. Nearly 75% of all dermal melanocytosis spots appear on the lumbosacral region. They do not require therapy and usually fade or are camouflaged by normal pigment by 3–5 years of age. Rarely, persistent

and extensive dermal melanocytosis has been associated with genetic disorders, such as lysosomal storage diseases. When lesions are clinically confused with a pigmented nevus, skin biopsy reveals characteristic melanocytes in the dermis.

Special variants of dermal melanocytosis include the nevus of Ota and nevus of Ito, which tend to persist into adult life.

Nevus of Ota. Nevus of Ota (nevus fuscoceruleus ophthalmomaxillaris) represents a unilateral, patchy, dermal melanosis of the face in the distribution of the first and second branches of the trigeminal nerve (Fig. 6.10c,d). Although most cases are sporadic, rare family clusters have been reported. Lesions tend to be slate-gray to brown in color with a "powder-blast burn" appearance. The forehead, temple, periorbital area, cheek, and nose are commonly involved. Rarely, pigmentation is bilateral and large areas of the face and oral mucous membranes are affected. Melanin pigment involves the eye in about half the cases. About 50% of lesions are present at birth, and the remainder appear during puberty. Although lesions are most common on Asian and black people, all races are affected, and the majority of patients are female.

Nevus of Ito. Nevus of Ito (nevus fuscoceruleus acromiodeltoideus) is a similar pathologic process to nevus of Ota in which unilateral pigmentation is located over the supraclavicular, deltoid, and scapular regions. Although a nevus of Ito usually occurs as an isolated lesion, it may be accompanied by a nevus of Ota.

Although nevus of Ito and nevus of Ota are benign dermal melanoses, rare cases of malignant degeneration have been reported. Extensive lesions are amenable to corrective therapy, usually by cosmetic camouflage. Treatment with Q-switched ruby and other Q-switched pigmented lesion lasers results in safe, effective destruction of abnormal pigment with little risk of scarring or recurrence.

Incontinentia Pigmenti

Incontinentia pigmenti is an inherited, multisystem disorder with a sequence of cutaneous manifestations that follow embryonic cleavage lines known as the lines of Blaschko. Classically, the dermatologic lesions progress through four stages: (1) vesicles that develop within the first month of life; (2) verrucous papules over several weeks to two years of age; (3) hyperpigmented macules, often in a "splashy" pattern (see Fig. 2.62) that can persist into adolescence; and (4) hypopigmented macules. Not all of these phases are always seen clinically, however, and age ranges are not always respected. Incontinentia pigmenti is an X-linked dominant disease so is more commonly seen in females and is caused by a post-zygotic mutation when seen in males.

Nevoid Hyperpigmentation (Hypopigmentation)

Nevoid hyperpigmentation (and hypopigmentation) should be distinguished from incontinentia pigmenti and presents with localized or diffuse whorled hyperpigmentation *without* antecedent inflammation (Fig. 6.11). These children may demonstrate variable genetic mosaicism in the skin and occasional involvement of multiple organ systems. Localized lesions are

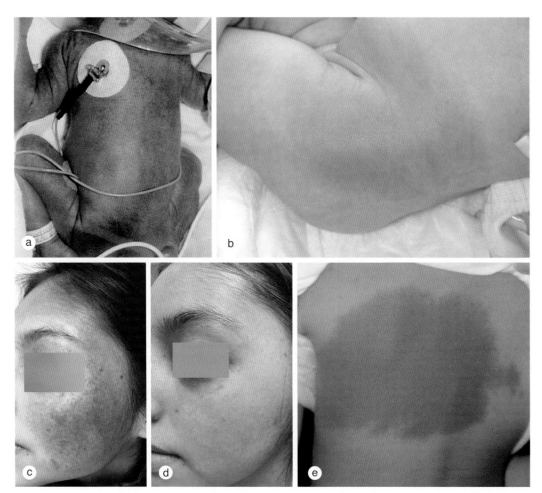

Fig. 6.10 Dermal melanocytosis. **(a)** Widespread and confluent dermal melanocytosis were noted at birth on this premature black infant. The pigment was slate-gray in color. **(b)** Note the large dermal melanocytosis on the left hip and abdomen of this light-pigmented infant. **(c)** A nevus of Ota involved the left side of the face extending into the scalp and left conjunctiva of this healthy adolescent. **(d)** The congenital lesion virtually cleared after four treatments with the Q-switched alexandrite laser. **(e)** This healthy toddler shows a nevus of Ito on the back.

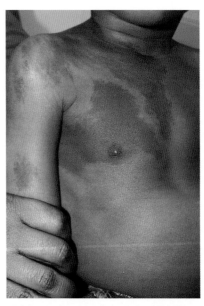

Fig. 6.11 Nevoid hyperpigmentation. A healthy 3-year-old boy was noted to have congenital hyperpigmented patches with segmental and Blaschkoid feature.

quite common and only rarely associated with systemic disease or genetic transmission. These skin lesions may be segmental or follow the lines of Blaschko and likely represent somatic mutations, which occur late in embryologic development. Widespread nevoid pigmentation probably occurs early in development and is more likely to be associated with systemic involvement and genetic transmission. Consequently, affected children, particularly those with disseminated cutaneous lesions, require a careful evaluation for neurocutaneous, skeletal, dental, cardiac, and other anomalies.

Postinflammatory Hyperpigmentation

The most common cause of increased pigmentation is postinflammatory hyperpigmentation. This alteration in normal pigmentation follows many inflammatory processes in the skin, such as a diaper dermatitis, insect bites, drug reactions, and traumatic injury. Lesions are usually localized and typically follow the distribution of the resolving disorder (Fig. 6.12). Although epidermal melanocytes appear normal, aberrant delivery of melanin to the surrounding keratinocytes results in deposition of pigment in dermal melanophages.

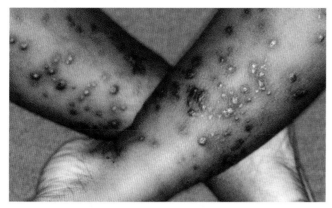

Fig. 6.12 Postinflammatory hyperpigmentation. Marked hyperpigmentation developed in this 5-year-old boy from recurrent insect bites. Although the pigment faded somewhat, it was still noticeable 2 years later.

Areas of hyperpigmentation are more marked in darkly pigmented children. No therapy is necessary, and lesions usually fade over several months.

Fixed Drug Eruption

A special subset of drug reactions known as a fixed drug eruption produces unusual persistent hyperpigmentation, particularly on the face, genitals, and scattered lesions on the trunk and extremities (see Fig. 7.4). From several hours to days after exposure to certain medications, such as minocycline, ibuprofen (and other non-steroidal anti-inflammatory drugs), phenobarbital, and phenolphthalein (in laxatives), patients develop acutely inflamed, dusky-red, edematous, round to oval, 1–3 cm diameter plaques, which may develop central bullae. These target lesions are clinically and histologically indistinguishable from those found in erythema multiforme minor (von Hebra). When the drug is discontinued the reaction subsides to leave residual postinflammatory pigmentation. On re-exposure to the inciting agent, new lesions may appear, but the old lesions recur in the same "fixed" spots. The reactivity of the skin seems to reside in the dermis. This notion is based on the observation that normal epidermis grafted over affected dermis becomes reactive, whereas involved epidermis loses its sensitivity once grafted onto normal dermis. Although the pathogenesis is not understood, investigators have proposed that the inciting drug triggers keratinocytes to release cytokines that ultimately activate epidermal T-lymphocytes.

Acquired Nevomelanocytic Nevi

Acquired nevomelanocytic nevi, also referred to as pigmented nevi and pigmented moles, begin to develop in early childhood as small, pigmented macules 1–2 mm in diameter. In early, flat lesions, nevus cells are located at the dermal–epidermal junction and are called junctional nevi (Fig. 6.13a). As nevi slowly enlarge and become papular, nevus cells migrate into the dermis to become compound nevi (Fig. 6.13b). Many nevi become fleshy or pedunculated over a period of years, particularly those on the upper trunk, head, and neck. Histopathology of these nevi demonstrates nevus cells restricted to the dermis, hence the so-called intradermal nevus.

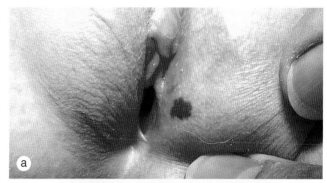

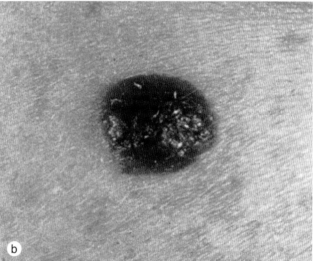

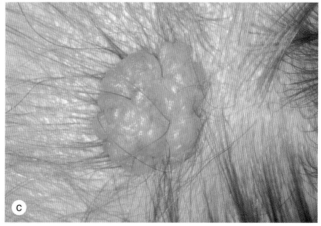

Fig. 6.13 Acquired nevomelanocytic nevus. **(a)** This brown macule on the labia of a 3-year-old girl was flat on palpation. Darkening and increase in size of the macule prompted a biopsy, which revealed a benign junctional nevus. **(b)** A shave excision of this facial nodule showed a compound nevomelanocytic nevus. **(c)** This young adult had a brown papule in adolescence, which became fleshy and lost most of the pigment. Biopsy showed an intradermal nevus.

During puberty, nevi increase in darkness, size, and number. However, most normal acquired nevomelanocytic nevi do not exceed 5 mm in diameter and retain their regularity in color, contour, texture, and symmetry. The majority of nevi appear on sun-exposed areas, but lesions may involve the palms, soles, buttocks, genitals, scalp, mucous membranes, and eyes. Generally, nevi change slowly over months to years and warrant observation only.

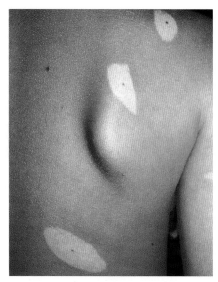

Fig. 6.14 Halo nevus. Large, depigmented halos surround innocent-looking nevi on the back of a 9-year-old boy.

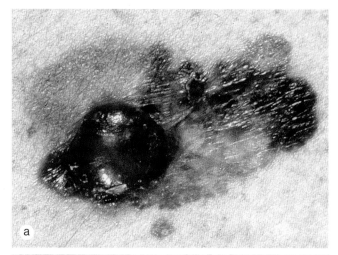

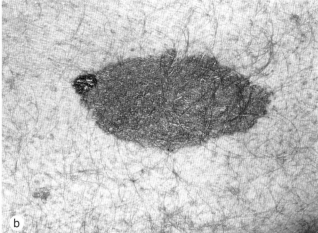

Fig. 6.15 Melanoma. **(a)** This lesion shows the irregularity of outline, color, and thickness typical of a melanoma. **(b)** A black papule developed in the border of a 3.5 × 1.5 cm congenital pigmented nevus. Biopsy showed a thin melanoma, and the lesion was excised with a 1 cm margin.

Sudden enlargement of a nevus, with redness and tenderness, may occur because of an irritant reaction or folliculitis. Trauma from clothing or scratching may produce hemorrhage or crust formation that heals uneventfully. Another more gradual change that causes concern in patients and parents is the appearance of a hypopigmented ring and mild local pruritus around a benign nevus (Fig. 6.14). This so-called halo nevus is caused by a cytotoxic T-lymphocyte reaction against both nevus cells and contiguous melanocytes. As a result, the nevus tends first to lighten and then disappear completely, and the halo eventually repigments. Occasionally, halo nevi are associated with vitiligo or the loss of pigmentation in areas of normal skin that have no nevi.

As long as the clinical appearance of a nevus is unremarkable, excision is unnecessary. However, a number of changes in pigmented lesions may portend the development of melanoma, including the following:

- Change in size, shape, or contours with scalloped, irregular borders
- Change in the surface characteristics, such as flaking, scaling, ulceration, or bleeding or the development of a small, dark, elevated papule or nodule within an otherwise flat plaque
- Change in color, with the appearance of black, brown, or an admixture of red, white, or blue
- Burning, itching, or tenderness, which may be an indication of an immunologic reaction to malignancy

Melanomas

Fortunately, melanomas are rare in children. However, the incidence is increasing, and curative treatment is contingent on early diagnosis and prompt excision. A keen awareness of diagnostic features is important.

Melanomas in children may occur *de novo* or within acquired or congenital nevi (Fig. 6.15a,b; see Fig. 2.85 and discussion in Chapter 2 for melanoma in congenital nevi). Family history of malignant melanoma and the presence of multiple, unusually large and irregularly pigmented, bordered, and textured nevi carries a high lifetime risk of melanoma, which may approach 100%. Malignant melanoma in this hereditary setting is referred to as familial atypical multiple mole melanoma syndrome (FAMMM; Fig. 6.16) and is most commonly associated with a mutation in the *CDKN2A* gene. During early life, children in such families may develop only innocent-looking nevi. However, regular screening should begin in late adolescence as carriers of this mutation have a much lower median age of melanoma onset than those with sporadic melanoma. Patients with FAMMM also have a markedly higher 5-year risk of developing a second melanoma. The presence of a large number of nevi, particularly on the scalp and sun-protected sites in prepubertal children, may be an early marker for this syndrome.

In general, changing nevi of unusual appearance must be biopsied to exclude malignant degeneration. As many as 5% of light-pigmented individuals with a negative family history of melanoma may develop at least one atypical mole in a lifetime.

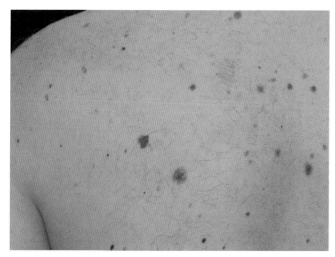

Fig. 6.16 Atypical pigmented nevi. This adolescent with a family history of malignant melanoma, and multiple individuals with atypical moles demonstrates numerous nevi with variable size, shape, and pigmentation in sun-exposed areas.

Patients with sporadic atypical mole syndrome (i.e. without a family history of melanoma) should also be observed for malignant changes, although the risk of melanoma is lower than in patients with a positive family history of melanoma.

A rare cause of melanoma in the pediatric age group is transplacental spread of maternal melanoma. Neonates born to mothers with a history of melanoma must be examined and followed carefully. Conversely, mothers of infants born with melanoma must be examined thoroughly for signs of malignancy.

Differential diagnosis of childhood melanoma includes congenital and acquired nevomelanocytic nevi, blue nevus (a small, firm, blue papule that consists of deep nevus cells; Fig. 6.17a,b), traumatic hemorrhage (especially under nails, on heels, or on mucous membranes), and a number of innocent vascular lesions such as pyogenic granuloma or hemangioma.

Spindle and Epithelial Cell Nevus

Spindle and epithelial cell nevus is an innocent nevomelanocytic nevus that may be clinically and histologically confused with malignant melanoma (Fig. 6.18a–e). This type of nevus is more commonly known as a Spitz nevus, named after Dr. Sophie Spitz, who first described this nevus histologically in 1948. Initially, Spitz nevus was also referred to as "benign juvenile melanoma." However, this term should be discarded because "melanoma" is misleading, and these lesions have also been described in adults. Spitz nevi frequently appear as rapidly growing, dome-shaped, red papules or nodules on the face or extremities. Occasionally they contain large quantities of melanin and may appear brown or black. If the lesion has clinical features of an innocent acquired nevus, it can be observed. However, early rapid growth may prompt the clinician to obtain a complete biopsy. In most histopathologic specimens, malignant melanoma can readily be excluded. If atypia is present on histology, expert consensus indicates that re-excision with 1–2 mm margins is appropriate.

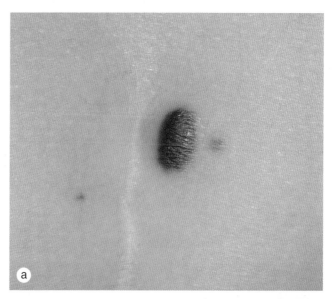

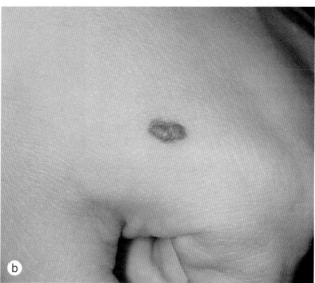

Fig. 6.17 Blue nevus. The blue papules are made up of deep nevus cells. **(a)** This 3-year-old girl had a blue nevus appear at 1 year of age above the gluteal cleft followed by a new smaller nevus 6 months later. She had a small sinus tract just below the nevus, which was removed shortly after birth. **(b)** An adolescent boy had a blue papule on the left hand for a year. After a few months of growth the nevus stabilized.

Diffuse Hyperpigmentation

Diffuse hyperpigmentation has rarely been reported as progressive familial hyperpigmentation. Affected infants are born with splotches of macular hyperpigmentation that slowly increase in size and number to involve much of the skin surface. This can usually be differentiated from the normal pigmentary darkening that occurs during the first year of life in many infants, particularly dark-skinned infants. Generalized bronze pigmentation may develop after phototherapy for hyperbilirubinemia, particularly in infants with a high conjugated bilirubin component. Most cases have resolved uneventfully after discontinuation of phototherapy, but occasional hepatic abnormalities and deaths have been reported.

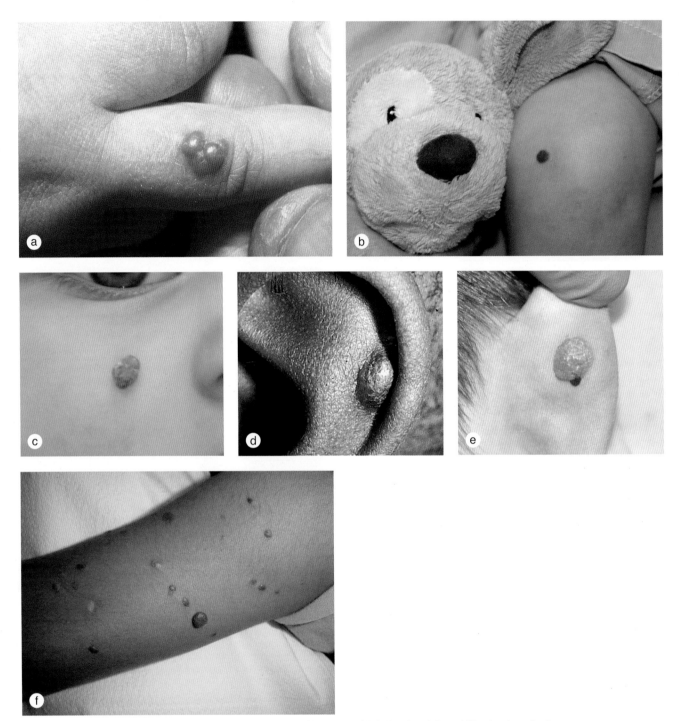

Fig. 6.18 Spindle and epithelial cell nevus. **(a)** This red multilobulated nodule stabilized at 1 cm in diameter a month after it first appeared. **(b)** This rapidly growing brown papule on the knee of a 5-year-old girl showed histologic findings typical of a pigmented Spitz nevus. Stable lesions in healthy children were biopsy proven Spitz nevi on the **(c)** right cheek, **(d)** left ear, and **(e)** right ear. **(f)** Multiple aggregated Spitz nevi erupted on the left arm of this healthy 6-year-old girl.

Generalized hyperpigmentation may also occur after exposure to certain drugs (e.g. heavy metals, phenothiazines, antimalarials) and in association with a number of systemic endocrine and inflammatory disorders. In adrenocortical insufficiency, Cushing syndrome, and acromegaly, melanotropin-stimulating hormone or other hormones capable of stimulating pigment production may cause generalized hyperpigmentation. Pigmentation may be particularly marked in skin creases on the palms and soles, as well as mucous membranes. Increased epidermal and dermal melanin also occurs in hemochromatosis, chronic renal and hepatic disease, and extensive cutaneous fibrosis associated with dermatomyositis and scleroderma.

HYPOPIGMENTATION AND DEPIGMENTATION

Partial or complete pigmentary loss may be congenital or acquired and may occur in a localized or diffuse pattern. Localized disorders of pigmentation include hypopigmented macules of the newborn, nevoid hypopigmentation (incontinentia pigmenti achromians), piebaldism, postinflammatory hypopigmentation, and vitiligo. Generalized pigmentary disturbances occur in albinism and progressive vitiligo.

Localized Hypopigmentation
Hypopigmented Macules

Localized hypopigmentation is characteristic of several nevoid phenomena, which include hypopigmented macules, nevoid hypopigmented anomaly (incontinentia pigmenti achromians), and piebaldism.

Although as few as 0.1% of normal newborns have a single hypopigmented or depigmented macule (see Nevus Depigmentosus), these findings may be a marker for tuberous sclerosis (Fig. 6.19a,b). These macules typically appear at birth as 0.2–3 cm diameter lesions on the trunk of 70–90% of individuals with tuberous sclerosis. Only a small minority of lesions are actually lancet- or ash leaf-shaped. They may be round, oval, dermatomal, segmental, or irregularly shaped and vary from pinpoint confetti spots to large patches over 10 cm in diameter. Although any site can be involved, truncal involvement is most common.

The identification of hypopigmented macules may be enhanced in lightly pigmented children by the use of a Wood lamp. The visible purple light that passes through the Wood filter is absorbed by melanin. In a darkened room, subtle areas of depigmentation or hypopigmentation appear bright violet, whereas normally pigmented skin absorbs most of the light and appears dull purple or black.

Although the majority of children with hypopigmented macules have no associated abnormalities, there is no reliable study to exclude systemic disease. Tuberous sclerosis is transmitted as an autosomal-dominant trait, but around 70% of affected children represent sporadic cases with new mutations in tuberous sclerosis complex genes, *TSC1* and *TSC2*. As mutational analysis of these genes is expensive and labor-intensive, affected children usually require close observation for the onset of other cutaneous findings (adenoma sebaceum, angiofibromas, or subungual fibromas) and systemic symptoms (seizures, intracranial tumors), which may be delayed for years (see Figs. 5.28 and 5.29). A careful family history and cutaneous examination of other family members may demonstrate subtle findings of tuberous sclerosis. The presence of asymptomatic rhabdomyomas, calcified intracranial tubers, renal angiomyolipomas, and cystic lesions in the kidneys and lungs also support the diagnosis in otherwise healthy-appearing individuals.

Nevus Depigmentosus

The term nevus depigmentosus (achromic nevus) should probably be used to describe the majority of children with one or two hypopigmented macules and no other signs of neurocutaneous disease (Fig. 6.20). However, nevus depigmentosus has been reported in rare cases in association with hemi-hypertrophy and intellectual disability without findings of tuberous sclerosis. Although the number of melanocytes present in nevi depigmentosus is often normal, pathogenesis is related to inefficient transfer of melanosomes into keratinocytes. Hypopigmented macules on cosmetically important areas are readily camouflaged by rehabilitative cosmetics.

Nevus Anemicus

Nevus anemicus is often misdiagnosed as an ash leaf macule. This congenital patch, usually located on the trunk, appears pale compared with surrounding normal skin (Fig. 6.21). However, a Wood lamp examination demonstrates the presence of

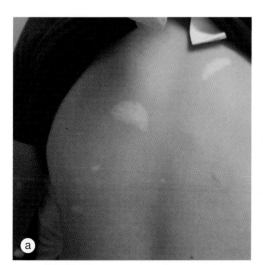
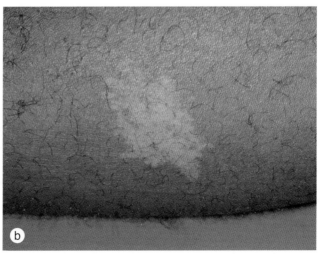

Fig. 6.19 Ash leaf macules. **(a)** Multiple hypopigmented macules were noted at birth on the back and left arm of this 10-year-old boy with tuberous sclerosis. **(b)** A congenital hypopigmented macule was present on the thigh of an 18-year-old boy with tuberous sclerosis.

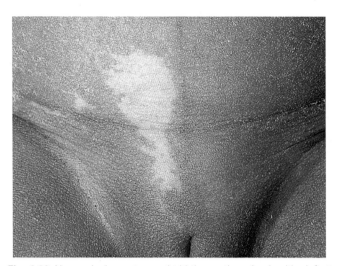

Fig. 6.20 Nevus depigmentosus. At birth an otherwise healthy infant was noted to have a hypopigmented patch on the suprapubic area.

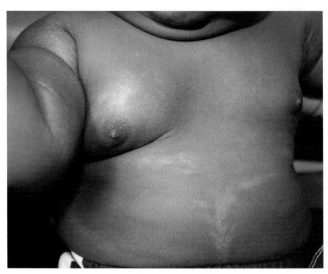

Fig. 6.22 Nevoid hypopigmentation. This healthy 6-month-old boy had congenital hypopigmented patches on the right arm, chest, and both sides of the abdomen which followed the lines of Blaschko.

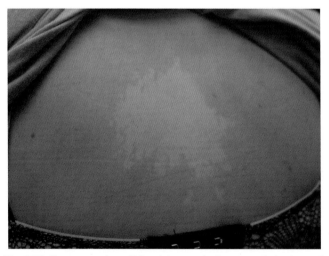

Fig. 6.21 Nevus anemicus. This adolescent had a congenital pale patch on her back, which was initially diagnosed as nevus depigmentosus. The patch becomes better defined after rubbing the surrounding skin as seen in this image. The patch tans normally in the summer and does not enhance with Wood light.

normal pigment. Rubbing the area results in erythema from vasodilatation in surrounding normal skin, while the lesion remains unchanged. A persistent increase in vascular tone, which results in maximal vasoconstriction in the nevus, seems to account for this phenomenon.

Nevoid Hypopigmentation (Incontinentia Pigmenti Achromians)

Nevoid hypopigmentation (incontinentia pigmenti achromians, also known as hypomelanosis of Ito) is characterized by congenital hypopigmentation with a marble-cake pattern. This Blaschkoid distribution of dyspigmentation resembles the pattern found in incontinentia pigmenti (Fig. 6.22).

Genetic mosaicism has been demonstrated in some patients when gene markers from hypopigmented skin are compared with those of normal skin and peripheral lymphocytes. The genetic mutations are quite varied and unrelated to incontinentia pigmenti. As a consequence, nevoid hypopigmentation is probably a better term for these skin lesions.

Although most children with nevoid hypopigmentation are healthy and develop normally, some patients manifest associated neurologic, developmental, dental, skeletal, and ophthalmologic anomalies. Affected children require a careful medical, neurologic, and ocular examination, as well as close neurodevelopmental observation with further in-depth studies tailored to clinical findings. As with nevoid hyperpigmentation, the extent of cutaneous lesions may correlate with the onset of mutations during embryologic development; more extensive cutaneous lesions may be a marker for earlier embryologic defects and a higher risk of systemic involvement and genetic transmission.

Piebaldism

Piebaldism is a rare, autosomal-dominant disorder characterized by a white forelock (poliosis) and circumscribed congenital leukoderma (Fig. 6.23a–c).

The typical lesions include a triangular patch of depigmentation and white hair on the frontal scalp, with the apex of the patch pointing toward the nasal bridge as well as hypopigmented or depigmented macules on the face, neck, ventral trunk, and extremities. However, depigmented patches may involve any part of the skin surface. Within areas of decreased pigmentation, scattered patches of normal pigment or hyperpigmentation may occur. The lesions are stable throughout life, although some variability in pigmentation may occur with sun exposure. Syndromes that present with cutaneous findings similar to piebaldism include Waardenburg

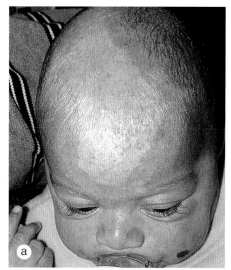

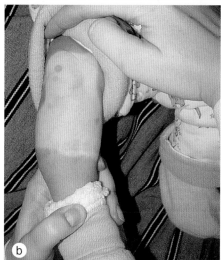

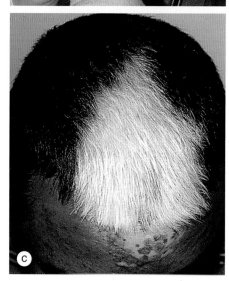

Fig. 6.23 **(a)** This healthy infant had a large patch of white skin and hair on the mid scalp extending to the forehead. **(b)** He also had a depigmented patch on his right leg, which was studded with normally pigmented and hyperpigmented macules. **(c)** His father, grandfather, and uncle had similar lesions on the scalp and scattered lesions on the trunk and extremities.

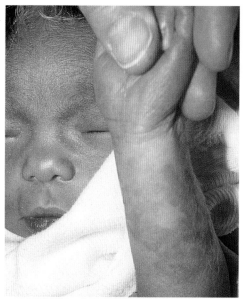

Fig. 6.24 At birth a patch of mottled hypopigmentation was discovered on this infant's forearm. Also note the white forelock characteristic of piebaldism. There was a family history of similar skin lesions associated with hearing loss and eye findings characteristic of Waardenburg syndrome.

syndrome (Fig. 6.24), an autosomal-dominant disease in which leukoderma is associated with lateral displacement of the inner canthi and inferior lacrimal ducts, a flattened nasal bridge, and sensorineural deafness, and Wolf syndrome, an autosomal-recessive disorder associated with multiple neurologic defects.

Piebaldism is caused by a mutation in the *KIT* proto-oncogene, which is required for the proliferation and migration of melanoblasts from the neural crest in murine embryogenesis. Waardenburg syndrome has been divided into several variants based on mutations in different but related genes, including *PAX3, MITF, and SOX10.*

Postinflammatory Hypopigmentation

Postinflammatory hypopigmentation may appear after any inflammatory skin condition. Patches are usually variable in size and irregularly shaped, although they may be remarkably symmetric in disorders such as seborrheic and atopic dermatitis (see Figs. 3.27–3.29). Areas of pigmentary alteration are usually seen in association with the primary lesions of the underlying disorder. Concomitant hyperpigmentation is also a frequent finding.

Postinflammatory hypopigmentation may be differentiated from vitiligo (Fig. 6.25a), which demonstrates well-demarcated depigmentation, and nevus depigmentosus, which appears at birth. In addition, postinflammatory hypopigmentation may be differentiated from tinea versicolor (see Fig. 3.51), which typically forms lesions that are uniform in size and shape, minimally scaly, and prominent in seborrheic areas on the trunk.

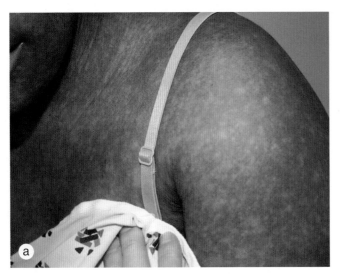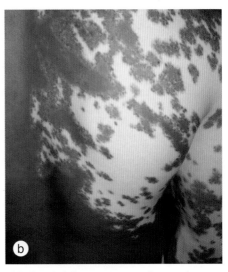

Fig. 6.25 **(a)** This 12-year-old girl had pityriasis lichenoides chronica with chronic inflammatory papules resulting in postinflammatory hypopigmentation. Note the indistinct borders of the hypopigmentation and few scattered subtle light red papules. **(b)** This adolescent boy with vitiligo had sharply demarcated depigmented macules without signs of inflammation.

Vitiligo

Vitiligo is an acquired disorder of pigmentation in which there is complete loss of pigment in involved areas. Lesions are macular, well circumscribed, and usually appear progressively in a characteristic distribution around the eyes, mouth, genitals, elbows, hands, and feet (Figs. 6.25b and 6.26a–e). Spontaneous but slow repigmentation, particularly after exposure to the summer sun, may occur from the edges of active lesions and within hair follicles, which results in a speckled appearance. Transient hyperpigmentation of the contiguous normal skin or hypopigmentation at the advancing edge may produce a trichrome, with depigmentation centrally and normal pigmentation around an area of hyper- or hypopigmentation. Rarely, the pigment in the eye may become involved. Consequently, a thorough eye examination is performed for all patients with vitiligo. Histologically, melanocytes are absent in areas of vitiligo. The pathogenesis is still controversial but has been attributed to a variety of factors, including autoimmunity, cell adhesion defect, oxidative stress, and sympathetic neurogenic disturbance.

Early in the course of vitiligo, some children respond to twice-daily applications of medium- to high-potency topical corticosteroids or the topical non-steroidal immunomodulator tacrolimus. Topical therapy may stabilize lesions in the winter until sunlight is readily available in the spring and summer. Some adolescents are pleased with the temporary camouflage provided by rehabilitative cosmetics and topical dyes. Most patients with progressive vitiligo that fails to respond to sunlight or topical corticosteroids will repigment at least partially with phototherapy. Narrow-band ultraviolet (UV)B light therapy has largely supplanted UVA-based treatments as a result of superior outcomes and safety profile. It is important to note, however, that systemic light therapy is rarely associated with cataract formation and requires diligent use of protective goggles and regular ophthalmologic follow-up. For treatment refractory cases, additional rarely used therapeutic options include punch grafting, epidermal cellular grafting, and autologous melanocyte suspension transplant. Although some investigators recommend autoimmune screening (antithyroid, antiadrenal, antigastrin antibodies, etc.) in patients with vitiligo, the results of studies comparing children with vitiligo with age-matched controls have been equivocal.

Vitiligo can be readily differentiated from nevoid pigmentary disorders, which are stable and usually congenital. Vitiligo is rare in infancy but appears before 20 years of age in about 50% of affected individuals. In postinflammatory hypopigmentation, the edges are not usually crisp and careful observation reveals residual pigmentation. Tinea versicolor can also be differentiated from vitiligo by the presence of pigment and fine scale, which reveals spores and pseudohyphae on potassium hydroxide preparation (see Fig. 1.6).

Diffuse Hypopigmentation
Albinism

Albinism is a heterogeneous group of inherited disorders manifested by generalized hypopigmentation or depigmentation of the skin, eyes, and hair (Fig. 6.27a–c). It occurs as an autosomal-recessive, oculocutaneous form and as an X-linked ocular variant form (Table 6.2).

In oculocutaneous albinism (OCA), both sexes and all races are equally involved. On the basis of clinical findings and biochemical markers, OCA may be divided into a number of variants. Tyrosinase-negative and tyrosinase-positive forms have been established based on the ability of plucked hairs to produce pigment when incubated in tyrosine-containing media. In tyrosinase-negative albinism, the tyrosinase enzyme is either absent or non-functional whereas tyrosinase-positive albinism is caused by a number of different defects in pigment synthesis and transport. The discovery of gene markers in some variants

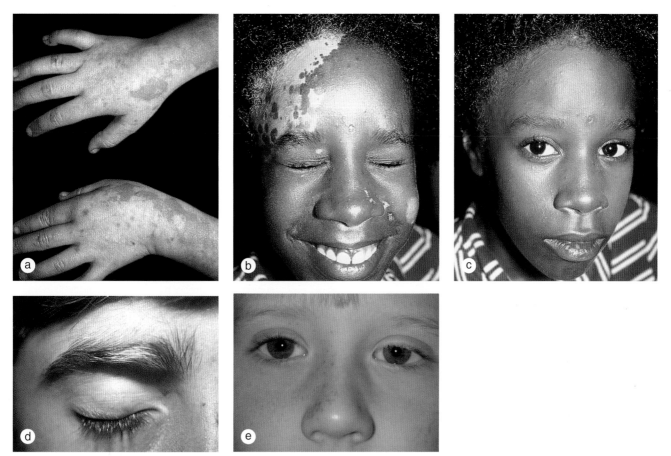

Fig. 6.26 Vitiligo. **(a)** Extensive depigmented patches developed on the backs of the hands of a 10-year-old girl. These patches were difficult to detect in the winter when her tan faded. **(b)** A progressive, disfiguring patch of vitiligo on the forehead of a 9-year-old girl was **(c)** well camouflaged with a corrective cosmetic. **(d)** A light-pigmented child with vitiligo developed white eyebrow hairs. **(e)** A light-pigmented 10-year-old girl with vitiligo developed white eye lashes. Note the vitiligo on her face manifested as lack of freckling on the left side of her nose and cheek.

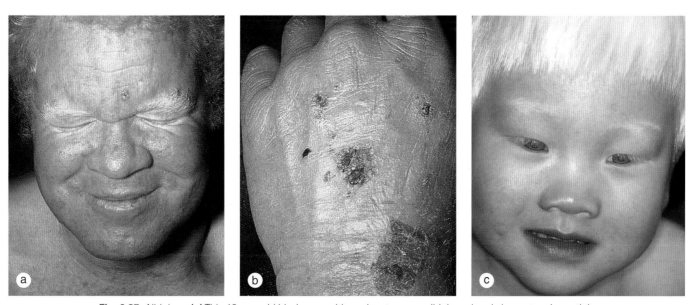

Fig. 6.27 Albinism. **(a)** This 19-year-old black man with oculocutaneous albinism already has extensive actinic damage. He works outdoors by the waterfront and has not used sunscreens. **(b)** Numerous actinic keratoses were removed from his face, upper back, and hands. The crusted plaque on the middle of his hand was a squamous cell carcinoma. **(c)** This 18-month-old boy had no detectable pigment. He had white hair, pale skin, nystagmus, and poor visual acuity.

TABLE 6.2 Oculocutaneous Albinism

Disorder	Incidence	Genetics	Pathogenesis	Clinical Findings	Comments
Tyrosinase-negative (OCA type 1A)	1:28000 African Caribbean individuals 1:39000 Caucasian individuals Male = female	Autosomal recessive; tyrosinase gene on chromosome 11q14.3	No tyrosinase activity	White hair and skin; blue-gray irides; no retinal pigment; nystagmus; poor visual acuity	Hair bulb test negative; DNA analysis available for prenatal diagnosis; no improvement with age
Reduced tyrosinase (OCA type 1B)	Rare, initially described in the ethnicities, now found in numerous races	Autosomal recessive; slicing of tyrosinase gene 11q14.3	Melanocytes produce pigment, but hair-bulb test negative Hairs produce pheomelanin when incubated with L-tyrosine and cysteine	White-to-light tan skin darkens somewhat with sun and age; white hair at birth turns yellow with age; blue eyes at birth may darken with age; some retinal pigment; poor visual acuity may improve with age	
Tyrosinase-positive (OCA type 2)	1:15000 African Caribbean individuals 1:37000 Caucasian individuals Male = female	Autosomal recessive; gene locus 15q12–q13	Some causes due to mutations in transport gene p with locus on chromosome 15q	White-to-cream color skin, light hair at birth darkening with age; blue, tan, hazel irides; minimal retinal pigment; nystagmus; photophobia; poor-to-fair visual acuity	Hair bulb test positive; DNA linkage analysis and mutation detection available for prenatal diagnosis; pigment may improve with age
Albinoidism	Unknown	Autosomal dominant		Marked pigment dilution of the skin may mimic tyrosinase-positive albinism, but only minimal involvement of the eyes; normal visual acuity	
Hermansky–Pudlak syndrome	Over 200 cases reported Male = female	Autosomal recessive	Tyrosinase-positive Bleeding secondary to platelet storage pool defect Lysosomal membrane defect results in accumulation of ceroid lipofuscin in macrophages in lung and gastrointestinal tract	Creamy white to almost normal skin varying with race; cream-to-red-brown hair; blue-to-brown irides; reduced retinal pigment; nystagmus; photophobia; poor visual acuity Increased bleeding with dental procedures, surgery, childbirth; epistaxis, menorrhagia, gingival bleeding Pulmonary fibrosis, granulomatous colitis, cardiomyopathy from ceroid deposition in viscera	
Chédiak–Higashi syndrome	Rare, fewer than 100 cases reported Male = female	Autosomal recessive, high consanguinity; LYST gene on chromosome 1q42.3	Lysosomal storage disease involving neutrophils, melanocytes, neurons, platelets, lymphocytes	White skin; blond-to-silver hair; blue-to-brown eyes with variable retinal pigment; photophobia; strabismus Recurrent sinusitis, pneumonia Progressive neurologic dysfunction with ataxia, muscle weakness, sensory loss, seizures Pancytopenia resulting in bleeding diathesis, anemia, sepsis	Fetoscopy at 18–21 weeks reveals fetal blood cells with characteristic neutrophilic granules
Cross syndrome	Rare	Autosomal recessive		White skin; white-to-blond hair; blue-to-gray irides; poor visual acuity; microphthalmia; cataracts Spastic diplegia, intellectual disability	
Griscelli syndrome	Rare	Autosomal recessive; gene maps to 15q21 in types 1 and 2; gene maps to 2q37 in type 3		Silver color hair in all types; neurologic deficits in type 1; severe combined immunodeficiency in type 2	Microscopic examination of hairs shows clumping of pigment in hair shafts, normal melanosomes, but reduced melanocyte dendritic processes

TABLE 6.2 Oculocutaneous Albinism—cont'd

Disorder	Incidence	Genetics	Pathogenesis	Clinical Findings	Comments
Prader–Willi syndrome	Unknown	Chromosomal and molecular changes of chromosome 15 at q11.2	Chromosomal and molecular changes of chromosome 15 at q11–q13 region	Light skin compared with relatives; normal-to-light hair; blue-to-brown irides; variable retinal pigment, normal to slightly reduced visual acuity Neonatal hypotonic hyperphagia; obesity; developmental delay, intellectual disability	
Angelman syndrome	Unknown	Sporadic autosomal recessive?	Chromosomal and molecular changes of the proximal region of chromosome 15 similar to those of Prader–Willi syndrome	Light skin compared with relatives; normal-to-light hair; blue-to-brown eyes; variable retinal pigment; normal to slightly reduced visual acuity Growth retardation, developmental delay, intellectual disability, ataxia, jerky gait, seizures Dysmorphic facies (microcephaly, flat occiput, protuberant tongue)	

of albinism has allowed for specific DNA diagnosis in patients and carriers. In classic tyrosinase-negative OCA, children are born without any trace of pigment. Affected individuals have snow-white hair, pinkish-white skin, and blue eyes. Nystagmus is common, as is moderate-to-severe strabismus and poor visual acuity. Although tyrosinase-positive OCA may be clinically indistinguishable from tyrosinase-negative OCA during infancy, children with tyrosinase-positive OCA usually develop variable amounts of pigment with increasing age. Eye color may vary from gray to light brown, and hair may change to blond or light brown. Most black patients acquire as much pigment as light-skinned white patients.

In both tyrosinase-positive and -negative variants of albinism, "clear cells" are noted in the basal cell layer of the epidermis, which may represent depigmented melanocytes. Electron microscopy demonstrates the presence of small amounts of melanin and mature melanosomes in tyrosinase-positive cases, but no melanin and only early stages of melanosome development in tyrosinase-negative patients.

Patients with OCA require aggressive sun protection to prevent actinic damage and early development of basal cell and squamous cell skin cancers. Strabismus and macular degeneration may also be associated with a progressive decrease in visual acuity. Consequently, regular eye examinations are important.

Although the skin and hair appear clinically normal in ocular albinism, characteristic macromelanosomes have been demonstrated by electron microscopy. This finding is a reliable marker and may be used to confirm the diagnosis and identify asymptomatic female carriers. When available, DNA analysis can also establish a specific diagnosis.

Other Disorders Associated With Diffuse Hypopigmentation

Diffuse hypopigmentation may suggest a number of systemic disorders associated with defects in melanin synthesis in the skin, hair, and eyes. Children with inborn errors of amino acid metabolism (e.g. phenylketonuria, histidinemia, and homocystinuria) often demonstrate widespread pigment dilution. Hypopigmentation of skin and hair in Menkes syndrome (also known as kinky hair disease) results from a defect in copper metabolism that interferes with the normal activity of copper-dependent tyrosinase (see Fig. 8.10). Hypohidrotic ectodermal dysplasia and deletion of the short arm of chromosome 18 are also associated with diffuse hypopigmentation and light hair color. Finally, children with malnutrition, particularly kwashiorkor, may develop hypopigmentation, which resolves when adequate calorie and protein intake resume.

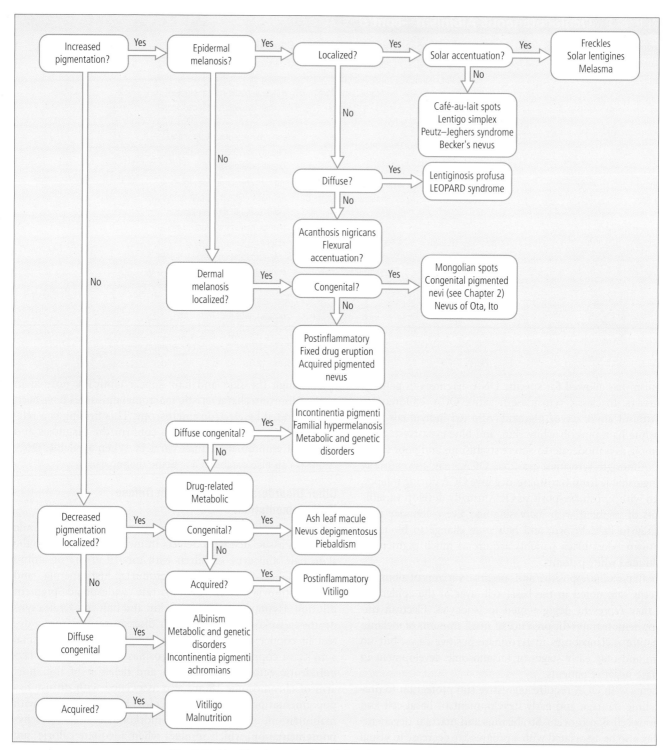

Fig. 6.28 Algorithm for evaluation of disorders of pigmentation.

FURTHER READING

Café-Au-Lait Spot

Belkin DA, Neckman JP, Jeon H, et al. Response to laser treatment of café au lait macules based on morphologic features. JAMA Dermatol 2017; 53:1158–1161.

Bernier A, Larbrisseau A, Perreault S. Café-au-lait macules and neurofibromatosis type 1: a review of the literature. Pediatr Neurol 2016; 60:24–29.e1.

Friedman JM. Neurofibromatosis 1: clinical manifestations and diagnostic criteria. J Child Neurol 2002; 17:548–554.

Goldberg Y, Dibbern K, Klein J, et al. Neurofibromatosis type 1—an update and review for the primary pediatrician. Clin Pediatr (Phila) 1996; 35:545–561.

Jett K, Friedman JM. Clinical and genetic aspects of neurofibromatosis 1. Genet Med 2010; 12(1):1–11.

Johnson BL, Charneco DR. Café-au-lait spots in neurofibromatosis and in normal individuals. Arch Dermatol 1970; 102:442–446.

Langenbach N, Pfau A, Landthaler M, et al. Naevi spili, café-au-lait spots and melanocytic naevi aggregated alongside Blaschko lines, with a review of segmental melanocytic lesions. Acta Derm Venereol 1998; 78:378–380.

North KW. Neurofibromatosis 1 in children. Semin Pediatr Neurol 1998; 5:231–242.

Riccardi VM. Neurofibromatosis and Albright syndrome. In: Alper JA (ed.), Genetic disorders of the skin. Mosby Year Book, St Louis, 1991:163–169.

Shah KN. The diagnostic and clinical significance of café-au-lait macules. Pediatr Clin North Am 2010; 57(5):1131–1153.

Tekin M, Bodurtha JN, Riccardi WM. Café-au-lait spots: the pediatrician's perspective. Pediatr Rev 2001; 22:82–90.

Lentigo

Atherton DJA, Pitcher DW, Wells RS, et al. A syndrome of various cutaneous pigmented lesions, myxoid neurofibromata and atrial myxoma; the NAME syndrome. Br J Dermatol 1980; 103:421–429.

Choi WW, Yoo JY, Park KC, et al. LEOPARD syndrome with a new association of congenital corneal tumor, choristoma. Pediatr Dermatol 2003; 20:158–160.

Chong WS, Klanwarin W, Fiam YC. Generalized lentiginosis in 2 children lacking systemic associations: case report and review of the literature. Pediatr Dermatol 2004; 21:39–45.

Cohen HJ, Minkin W, Frank SB. Nevus spilus. Arch Dermatol 1970; 102:433–437.

Digilio MC, Sarkozy A, de Zorzi A, et al. LEOPARD syndrome: clinical diagnosis in the first year of life. Am J Med Genet A 2006; 140(7):740–746.

Entius MM, Keller JJ, Westerman AM, et al. Molecular genetic alterations in hamartomatous polyps and carcinomas of patients with Peutz-Jeghers syndrome. J Clin Pathol 2001; 54:126–131.

Happle R. Speckled lentiginous nevus syndrome: delineation of a new distinct neurocutaneous phenotype. Eur J Dermatol 2002; 12(2):133–135.

Martínez-Quintana E, Rodríguez-González F. LEOPARD syndrome: clinical features and gene mutations. Mol Syndromol 2012; 3(4):145–157.

O'Neill JF, James WD. Inherited patterned lentiginosis in blacks. Arch. Derm. 125: 1231–1235, 1989.

Praetorius C, Sturm RA, Steingrimsson E. Sun-induced freckling: ephelides and solar lentigines. Pigment Cell Melanoma Res 2014; 27(3):339–350.

Sarkozy A, Digilio MC, Dallapiccola B. Leopard syndrome. Orphanet J Rare Dis 2008; 3:13.

Tovar JA, Eizaguirre I, Albert A, et al. Peutz-Jeghers in children: report of two cases and review of the literature. J Pediatr Surg 1983; 18:1–6.

van Lier MG, Westerman AM, Wagner A, et al. High cancer risk and increased mortality in patients with Peutz-Jeghers syndrome. Gut 2011; 60(2):141–147.

Xing Q, Chen X, Wang M, et al. locus for familial generalized lentiginosis without systemic involvement maps to chromosome 4q21.1-q22.3. Hum Genet. 117: 154–159, 2005.

Becker Nevus

Becker SW. Concurrent melanosis and hypertrichosis in distribution of nevus unius lateris. Arch Dermatol Syph 1949; 60:155–160.

Cordisco MR. An update on lasers in children. Curr Opin Pediatr 2009; 21(4):499–504.

Happle R, Koopman RJ. Becker nevus syndrome. Am J Med Genet 1997; 68:357–361.

Kopera D, Hohenlentner U, Landthaler M. Quality-switched ruby laser treatment of solar lentigines and Becker's nevus: a histopathologic and immunohistochemical study. Dermatology 1997; 194:338–343.

Polder KD, Landau JM, Vergilis-Kalner IJ, et al. Laser eradication of pigmented lesions: a review. Dermatol Surg 2011; 37(5):572–595.

Taheri A, Mansoori P, Sandoval LF, et al. Treatment of Becker nevus with topical flutamide. J Am Acad Dermatol 2013; 69(3):e147–148.

Urbanek RW, Johnson WC. Smooth muscle hamartoma associated with Becker nevus. Arch Dermatol 1978; 114:98–99.

Zhong Y, Yang B, Huang L, et al. Lasers for Becker's nevus. Lasers Med Sci 2019; 34(6):1071–1079.

Zhong Y, Yang B, Huang L, et al. Lightening Becker nevus with topical glycolic acid. J Am Acad Dermatol 2019; 80(1):e3.

Acanthosis Nigricans

Brockow K, Steinkraus V, Rinninger F, et al. Acanthosis nigricans: a marker for hyperinsulinemia. Pediatr Dermatol 1995; 12:323–326.

Garcia Hidalgo L. Dermatologic complications of obesity. Am J Clin Dermatol 2002; 3:496–506.

Higgins SP, Freemark M, Prose NS. Acanthosis nigricans: a practical approach to evaluation and management. Dermatol Online J 2008; 14(9):2.

Jabbour SA. Cutaneous manifestations of endocrine disorders: a guide for dermatologists. Am J Clin Dermatol 2003; 4:315–331.

Panidis D, Skiadopoulos S, Rousso D, et al. Association of acanthosis nigricans with insulin resistance in patients with polycystic ovary syndrome. Br J Dermatol 1995; 132:936–941.

Stuart CA, Gilkison CR, Keenan BS, et al. Hyperinsulinemia and acanthosis nigricans in African Americans. J Natl Med Assoc 1997; 89:523–527.

Torley D, Bellus GA, Munro CS. Genes, growth factors and acanthosis nigricans. Br J Dermatol 2002; 147:1096–1101.

Melasma

Farshi S. Comparative study of therapeutic effects of 20% azelaic acid and hydroquinone 4% cream in the treatment of melasma. J Cosmet Dermatol 2011; 10(4):282–287.

Ferreira Cestari T, Hassun K, Sittart A, et al. A comparison of triple combination cream and hydroquinone 4% cream for the treatment of moderate to severe facial melasma. J Cosmet Dermatol 2007; 6(1):36–39.

Grimes PE. Melasma. Etiologic and therapeutic considerations. Arch Dermatol 1995; 131:1453–1457.

Guevara IL, Pandya AF. Safety and efficacy of 4% hydroquinone combined with 10% glycolic acid, antioxidants, and sunscreen in the treatment of melasma. Int J Dermatol 2003; 42:966–972.

Sanchez NP, Pathak MA, Sato S, et al. Melasma: a clinical, light microscopic, ultrastructural, and immunofluorescence study. J Am Acad Dermatol 1981; 4:698–710.

Dermal Melanocytosis

Alimi Y, Iwanaga J, Loukas M, et al. A comprehensive review of Mongolian spots with an update on atypical presentations. Childs Nerv Syst 2018; 34(12):2371–2376.

Cordova A. The Mongolian spot. Clin Pediatr 1981; 20:714–722.

Hidano A, Kajima H, Ikeda S, et al. Natural history of nevus of Ota. Arch Dermatol 1967; 95:187–195.

Kopf AW, Weidman AJ. Nevus of Ota. Arch Dermatol 1962; 85:195–208.

Mevorah B, Frenk E, Delacretaz J. Dermal melanocytosis. Dermatologica 1977; 154:107–114.

Polder KD, Landau JM, Vergilis-Kalner IJ, et al. Laser eradication of pigmented lesions: a review. Dermatol Surg 2011; 37(5):572–595.

Reza AM, Farahnaz GZ, Hamideh S, et al. Incidence of Mongolian spots and its common sites at two university hospitals in Tehran, Iran. Pediatr Dermatol 2010; 27(4):397–398.

Sapadin AN, Friedman IS. Extensive Mongolian spots associated with Hunter syndrome. J Am Acad Dermatol 1998; 39:1013–1015.

Smalek JE. Significance of Mongolian spots. J Pediatr 1980; 97:504–505.

Stanford DG, Georgourajk E. Dermal melanocytosis: a clinical spectrum. Aust J Dermatol 1996; 37:19–25.

Fixed Drug Eruption

Brahimi N, Routier E, Raison-Peyron N, et al. A three-year-analysis of fixed drug eruptions in hospital settings in France. Eur J Dermatol 2010; 20(4):461–464.

Lee AG. Fixed drug eruption: incidence, recognition, and avoidance. Am J Clin Dermatol 2003; 5:277–285.

Masu S, Seiji M. Pigmentary incontinence in fixed drug eruptions. J Am Acad Dermatol 1983; 8:525–532.

Sharma VK, Dhas S, Gill AN. Drug related involvement of specific sites in fixed eruption: a statistical evaluation. J Dermatol 1996; 23:530–534.

Shiohara T. Fixed drug eruption: pathogenesis and diagnostic tests. Curr Opin Allergy Clin Immunol 2009; 9(4):316–321.

Pigmented Nevi

Baner J, Garbe C. Acquired melanocytic nevi as a risk factor for melanoma development. A comprehensive review of epidemiologic data. Pigment Cell Res 2003; 16:297–306.

Casso EM, Grin-Jorgensen CM, Grant-Kels JM. Spitz nevi. J Am Acad Dermatol 1992; 27:901–913.

English DR, Armstrong BK. Melanocytic nevi in children. I. Anatomic sites and demographic and host factors. Am J Epidemiol 1994; 139:390–401.

Gallagher RP, McLean DI. The epidemiology of acquired melanocytic nevi. A brief review. Dermatol Clin 1995; 13:595–603.

Hughes BR, Cunliffe WJ, Bailey CC. Excess benign melanocytic naevi after chemotherapy for malignancy in childhood. BMJ 1989; 299:88–91.

Kincannon J, Bartzale C. The physiology of pigmented nevi. Pediatrics 1999; 10(4 Pt 2):1042–1045.

Luo S, Sepehr A, Tsao H. Spitz nevi and other Spitzoid lesions. Part I. Background and diagnoses. J Am Acad Dermatol 2011; 65:1073–1084.

Luo S, Sepehr A, Tsao H. Spitz nevi and other Spitzoid lesions. Part II. Natural history and management. J Am Acad Dermatol 2011; 65:1087–1092.

Luther H, Altmeyer P, Garber C, et al. Increase of melanocytic nevus counts in children during 5 years of follow-up and analysis of associated factors. Arch Dermatol 1996; 132:1473–1478.

Mehregan AH, Mehregan DA. Malignant melanoma in childhood. Cancer 1993; 71:4096–4103.

Mones JN, Ackerman AB. Melanomas in prepubescent children: review comprehensively, critique histologically, criteria diagnostically, and course biologically. Am J Dermatopathol 2003; 24:223–238.

Nicholls EM. Development and elimination of pigmented moles, and the anatomical distribution of primary malignant melanoma. Cancer 1973; 32:191–195.

Nino M, Bruncetti B, Delfino S, et al. Spitz nevus: follow-up study of 8 cases of childhood starburst type and proposal for management. Dermatology 2009; 218:48–51.

Novakovic B, Clark WH Jr, Fears TR, et al. Melanocytic nevi, dysplastic nevi, and malignant melanoma in children from melanoma-prone families. J Am Acad Dermatol 1995; 33:631–636.

Pappo AS. Melanoma in children and adolescents. Eur J Cancer 2003; 39:2651–2661.

Pfahberg A, Uter W, Kraers C, et al. Monitoring nevus density in children as a method to detect shifts in melanoma risk in the population. Prev Med 2004; 38:382–387.

Piccolo D, Ferrari A, Peris K. Sequential dermoscopic evolution of pigmented Spitz nevus in childhood. J Am Acad Dermatol 2003; 49:556–558.

Smith CH, McGregor JM, Barker JN, et al. Excess melanocytic nevi in children with renal allografts. J Am Acad Dermatol 1993; 28:51–55.

Soura E, Eliades PJ, Shannon K, et al. Hereditary melanoma: update on syndromes and management: genetics of familial atypical multiple mole melanoma syndrome. J Am Acad Dermatol 2016; 74(3):395–407.

Tlougan BE, Orlow SJ, Schaffer JV. Spitz nevi: beliefs, behaviors, and experiences of pediatric dermatologists. JAMA Dermatol 2013; 149(3):283–291.

Weedon D, Little JH. Spindle and epithelioid cell nevi in children and adults. A review of 211 cases of the Spitz nevus. Cancer 1977; 40:217–225.

Hypopigmented Macules

DiLerna V. Segmental nevus depigmentosus: analysis of 20 patients. Pediatr Dermatol 1999; 16:349–353.

Fitzpatrick TB, Szabo G, Hori Y, et al. White leaf-shaped macules. Arch Dermatol 1968; 98:1–6.

Hossler EW, Lountzis NI, Black DR. Hypopigmented macules. J Am Acad Dermatol 2010; 62(3):e13–e14.

Lee HS, Chun YS, Hann SK. Nevus depigmentosus: clinical features and histologic characteristics in 67 patients. J Am Acad Dermatol 1999; 40:21–26.

Lio PA. Little white spots: an approach to hypopigmented macules. Arch Dis Child Educ Pract Ed 2008; 93(3):98–102.

Norio R, Oksanen T, Rantanen J. Hypopigmented skin alterations resembling tuberous sclerosis in normal skin. J Med Genet 1996; 33:184–186.

Randle SC. Tuberous sclerosis complex: a review. Pediatr Ann 2017; 46(4):e166–e171.

Staley BA, Vail EA, Thiele EA. Tuberous sclerosis complex: diagnostic challenges, presenting symptoms, and commonly missed signs. Pediatrics 2011; 127(1):e117–e125.

Ullah F, Schwartz RA. Nevus depigmentosus: review of a mark of distinction. Int J Dermatol 2019; 58:1366–1370.

Vanderhooft SL, Francis JS, Pagon RA, et al. Prevalence of hypopigmented macules in a healthy population. J Pediatr 1996; 129:355–361.

Xu AE, Huang B, Li YW, et al. Clinical, histopathological and ultrastructural characteristics of naevus depigmentosus. Clin Exp Dermatol 2008; 33(4):400–405.

Nevus Anemicus

Fleisher TL, Zeligman I. Nevus anemicus. Arch Dermatol 1969; 100:750–755.

Nevoid Hypopigmentation (Incontinentia Pigmenti Achromians)

Delaporte E, Janin A, Blondel V, et al. Linear and whorled nevoid hypermelanosis versus incontinentia pigmenti: is pigment incontinence really a distinctive feature? Dermatology 1996; 192:70–72.

Happle R. Tentative assignment of hypomelanosis of Ito to 9q33-qter. Hum Genet 1987; 75:98–99.

Ishikawa T, Kanayama M, Sugiyama K, et al. Hypomelanosis of Ito associated with benign tumors and chromosomal abnormalities: a neurocutaneous syndrome. Brain Dev 1985; 7:45–49.

Kuster W, Kong A. Hypomelanosis of Ito: no entity, but a cutaneous sign of mosaicism. Am J Med Genet 1999; 85:346–350.

Nehal KS, PeBenito R, Orlow SJ. Analysis of 54 cases of hypopigmentation and hyperpigmentation along the lines of Blaschko. Arch Dermatol 1996; 132:1167–1170.

Sybert VP. Hypomelanosis of Ito: a description, not a diagnosis. J Invest Dermatol 1994; 103(Suppl 5):1415–1438.

Piebaldism

Janjua SA, Khachemoune A, Guldbakke KK. Piebaldism: a case report and a concise review of the literature. Cutis 2007; 80(5):411–414.

Oiso N, Fukai K, Kawada A, et al. Piebaldism. J Dermatol 2013; 40(5):330–335.

Vitiligo

Alikhan A, Felsten LM, Daly M, et al. Vitiligo: a comprehensive overview part I. Introduction, epidemiology, quality of life, diagnosis, differential diagnosis, associations, histopathology, etiology, and work-up. J Am Acad Dermatol 2011; 65(3):473–491.

Bacigalupi RM, Postolova A, Davis RS. Evidence-based, non-surgical treatments for vitiligo: a review. Am J Clin Dermatol 2012; 13(4):217–237.

Herane MI. Vitiligo and leukoderma in children. Clin Dermatol 2003; 21:283–295.

Ho N, Pope E, Weinstein M, et al. A double-blind, randomized, placebo-controlled trial of topical tacrolimus 0.1% vs. clobetasol propionate 0.05% in childhood vitiligo. Br J Dermatol 2011; 165(3):626–632.

Iannella G, Greco A, Didona D, et al. Vitiligo: pathogenesis, clinical variants and treatment approaches. Autoimmun Rev 2016; 15(4):335–343.

Kurtev A, Dourmishev AL. Thyroid function and autoimmunity in children and adolescents with vitiligo. J Eur Acad Dermatol Venereol 2004, 18:109–111.

Majumder PP, Nordlund JJ, Nath SK. Pattern of familial aggregation of vitiligo. Arch Dermatol 1993; 129:994–998.

Nisticò S, Chiricozzi A, Saraceno R, et al. Vitiligo treatment with monochromatic excimer light and tacrolimus: results of an open randomized controlled study. Photomed Laser Surg 2012; 30(1):26–30.

Nordlund JJ, Lerner AB. Editorial: vitiligo. It is important. Arch Dermatol 1982; 118:5–8.

Norris DA, Kissinger RM, Naughton GM, et al. Evidence for immunologic mechanisms in human vitiligo: patient's sera induce damage to human melanocytes in vitro. J Invest Dermatol 1988; 90:783–789.

Shullreuter KU, Lemke R, Brandt O, et al. Vitiligo and other diseases: coexistence or true association? Hamberg study of 321 patients. Dermatology 1994; 188:269–275.

Taieb A, Picardo M. Clinical practice. Vitiligo. N Engl J Med 2009; 360:160–169.

van Geel N, Wallaeys E, Goh BK, et al. Long-term results of non-cultured epidermal cellular grafting in vitiligo, halo naevi, piebaldism and naevus depigmentosus. Br J Dermatol 2010; 163(6):1186–1193.

Westerhof W, Nieuweboer-Krobotova L. Treatment of vitiligo with UV-B radiation vs topical psoralen plus UV-A. Arch Dermatol 1997; 13:1525–1528.

Albinism

Boissay RE, Nordlund JJ. Molecular basis of congenital hypopigmentary disorders in humans: a review. Pigment Cell Res 1997; 10:12–24.

Dessinioti C, Stratigos AJ, Rigopoulos D, et al. A review of genetic disorders of hypopigmentation: lessons learned from the biology of melanocytes. Exp Dermatol 2009; 18(9):741–749.

Grønskov K, Ek J, Brondum-Nielsen K. Oculocutaneous albinism. Orphanet J Rare Dis 2007; 2:43.

Hayashibe K, Mishima Y. Tyrosinase-positive melanocyte distribution and induction of pigmentation in human piebald skin. Arch Dermatol 1988; 124:381–386.

Huizzing M, Gahl WA. Disorders of vesicles of lysosomal lineage: the Hermansky-Pudlak syndrome. Curr Mol Med 2002; 2:451–467.

Oetting WS, Fryer JP, Shiram S, et al. Oculocutaneous albinism type 1: the last 100 years. Pigment Cell Res 2003; 16:307–311.

Orlow SJ. Albinism: an update. Semin Cut Med Surg 1997; 16:24–29.

Pingault V, Ente D, Dastot-Le Moal F, et al. Review and update of mutations causing Waardenburg syndrome. Hum Mutat 2010; 31(4):391–406.

Scheinfeld NS. Syndromic albinism: a review of genetics and phenotypes. Dermatology Online J 2003; 9:5.

Vachtenheim J, Borovanský J. 'Transcription physiology' of pigment formation in melanocytes: central role of MITF. Exp Dermatol 2010; 19(7):617–627.

Waardenburg PJ. A new syndrome combining developmental anomalies of the eyelids, eyebrows and nose root with pigmentary defects of the iris and head hair and with congenital deafness. Am J Hum Genet 1951; 3:195–253.

7

Reactive Erythema

George O. Denny and Bernard A. Cohen

INTRODUCTION

The term reactive erythema refers to a group of disorders characterized by erythematous patches, plaques, and nodules that vary in size, shape, and distribution. Unlike other specific and intrinsic dermatoses, these represent cutaneous reaction patterns triggered by a variety of either endogenous triggers or environmental agents. In children, the most common reactive erythemas include drug eruptions, urticaria, viral exanthems, erythema multiforme (EM), erythema nodosum (EN), vasculitis, photosensitive eruptions, and collagen vascular disorders. An algorithmic approach to diagnosis for reactive erythema is summarized at the end of the chapter (see Fig. 7.58).

DRUG ERUPTIONS

Of all patients admitted to hospital, approximately 27% experience an adverse drug reaction (ADR) and ~0.1–0.3% will experience a fatal ADR. Approximately half of ADRs will result in cutaneous findings. Drug-induced rashes are also a frequent diagnostic problem in the outpatient setting. Although the skin rash often occurs alone, it may be accompanied by fever, arthritis, and other systemic findings. The incidence of drug reactions increases with age and the number of medications used. Paradoxically, patients with hereditary or acquired immunodeficiency appear to be particularly prone to developing reactions from medications. For example, nearly 75% of human immunodeficiency virus–infected patients develop morbilliform eruptions from sulfonamides during their illness.

The overwhelming majority of medication-induced rashes are morbilliform. Depending upon the study population, 50–94% of patients with cutaneous ADR will present with this classic rash. The remainder of the rashes are urticarial in 25%, fixed drug reactions in 10%, and exfoliative erythroderma, Stevens–Johnson syndrome (SJS)/toxic epidermal necrolysis (TEN), vasculitic, lichenoid, and acneiform eruptions in less than 5% each. Early recognition of drug-related rashes and discontinuation of the inciting agent may prevent progressive, life-threatening complications and certainly reassure patients, parents, and practitioners.

Morbilliform Drug Eruptions (Including Drug Rash With Eosinophilia and Systemic Symptoms or Drug-Induced Hypersensitivity Syndrome)

Morbilliform (measles-like, maculopapular, exanthematous) rashes account for the majority of drug-induced rashes. Typically, after 1–2 weeks of drug therapy, red macules and papules erupt on the extremities and spread centrally to involve the trunk. Not infrequently, however, the trunk is the first area to be involved and the rash spreads centripetally (Fig. 7.1). Lesions may become confluent, but the perioral and perinasal areas are often spared. Conjunctival and oral mucosal erythema may be prominent. Although the rash can be asymptomatic, pruritus is common and may be severe. The skin may be the only organ system involved, but fever, arthralgias, and general malaise may follow. Occasionally, the rash resolves despite continuation of the medication, and rarely, eruptions evolve into SJS/TEN with widespread necrosis of the epidermis.

Almost any drug can trigger a morbilliform rash. Common categories include antibiotics, anticonvulsants, and antihypertensives. Prompt diagnosis and discontinuation of the drug usually result in improvement in 1–2 days and resolution within 1 week. Occasionally, the rash does not appear until several days after the drug course has been completed.

Patients with a simple morbilliform drug rash can often be treated with discontinuation of the offending medication, topical steroids as needed, and supportive care. It is advised that the patient avoid the offending medication in the future to prevent recurrence of the reaction.

Drug rash with eosinophilia and systemic symptoms (DRESS)/drug-induced hypersensitivity syndrome (DIHS) usually begins with a morbilliform eruption 2–6 weeks after initiation of the inciting medication. This timeline is important to keep in mind when evaluating a new patient with a cutaneous ADR, as DRESS/DIHS can have significantly higher morbidity and mortality compared with a simple morbilliform drug rash. Lesions first appear on the face, upper trunk, and proximal extremities, often with follicular accentuation, and disseminate quickly. Skin edema may be intense, resulting in the formation of vesicles, bullae, and pustules. Early clues to diagnosis are significant facial edema and widespread lymphadenopathy. High fever and multisystem involvement defines this disorder, and it should be suspected in any

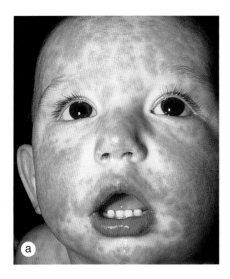
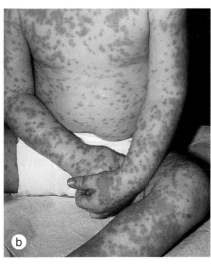

Fig. 7.1 A morbilliform reaction to phenobarbital developed in a toddler after 2 weeks of treatment for febrile seizures. Lesions were most prominent on **(a)** the face, and **(b)** the upper trunk and extremities. Note the perioral and perinasal sparing.

patient with morbilliform rash, fever, facial edema, and lymphadenopathy. Hepatitis (which may rarely be fulminant), generalized lymphadenopathy, myocarditis, pneumonitis, nephritis, thyroiditis (including a delayed thyroiditis months after a patient recovers from DRESS/DIHS), and meningoencephalitis may develop. Laboratory testing will often show atypical lymphocytes and eosinophilia, although these are not always present.

This condition is most often triggered by aromatic anticonvulsants (phenytoin, carbamazepine, and phenobarbital), lamotrigine, allopurinol, sulfonamides, dapsone, and other antibiotics. Although the pathogenesis of DRESS/DIHS is not fully understood, the reaction is thought to occur in genetically predisposed individuals who have a reduced capacity to metabolize medication metabolites. Toxic metabolites accumulate and activate T-lymphocytes, which drive the immunologic process, including eosinophilic infiltration of the skin and viscera. Interestingly, reactivation of viruses including human herpesvirus 6 (HHV6) and HHV7 in patients with DRESS/DIHS also supports an immunologic mechanism and perhaps a drug–viral interaction. Some centers have even begun to use serologic positivity for HHV6 and/or HHV7 as evidence for diagnosing a patient with DRESS/DIHS. Immediate discontinuation of the inciting medication is critical, and systemic steroids may be required to shut off the disorder, which may last for weeks to months (Fig. 7.2).

Unfortunately, morbilliform rashes often appear in febrile children who are placed on antibiotics for treatment of presumed bacterial infections such as sinusitis and otitis media. The differentiation of a viral infection with associated exanthem from a drug rash is usually impossible, and many of these children are labeled antibiotic allergic. In some patients, recognition of specific viral exanthems and serologic confirmation support an infectious etiology. Moreover, some drugs may interact with certain viruses to produce an exanthem such as the rash seen in up to 95% of children with mononucleosis who are treated with ampicillin (Fig. 7.3). The differential diagnosis also includes graft-vs-host disease and Kawasaki syndrome, but the medical history and associated findings help to exclude these disorders. Histologic findings in morbilliform drug reactions

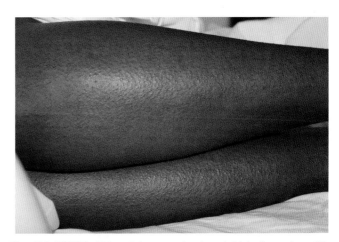

Fig. 7.2 DRESS. This adolescent developed high fever, hepatitis, generalized edema, and a progressive diffuse erythema with follicular prominence on her extremities after treatment of acne with oral trimethoprim-sulfamethoxazole tablets.

overlaps with viral exanthems and graft-vs-host disease, so skin biopsies usually do not help to distinguish these disorders.

Stevens–Johnson Syndrome/Toxic Epidermal Necrolysis

Although SJS and TEN were initially thought to represent severe variants of EM, further studies support the clinical separation of EM and SJS/TEN. Although SJS/TEN may be triggered by drugs and a number of other infectious and biological agents, EM has been most commonly associated with infectious agents, particularly herpes simplex virus and mycoplasma infections, in children and adults. SJS/TEN are defined by a severe mucositis of multiple mucous membranes and variable cutaneous involvement which may be life-threatening. SJS is distinguished by the amount of body surface area affected, with up to 10% in SJS, 10–30% in SJS/TEN overlap, and over 30% in TEN. It is important to contrast key clinical findings that distinguish SJS/TEN from EM, as the clinical prognosis for SJS/TEN is much worse (mortality for SJS/TEN can

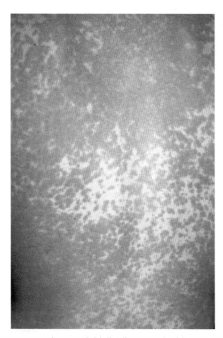

Fig. 7.3 A teenager who was initially diagnosed with streptococcal pharyngitis was started on ampicillin. After 4 days, a morbilliform rash erupted on the trunk and spread to the face and extremities. A monospot test was positive in the office, and the antibiotic was discontinued.

range from 5% to 95% based upon clinical features). In contrast to SJS/TEN, which commonly spares the palm and soles and consists of flat lesions, EM presents with characteristic raised targetoid lesions on the distal extremities. Additionally, although SJS/TEN and EM both can affect oral mucous membranes, the oral lesions in SJS/TEN are typically much more severe, more common, and persistent. Although SJS/TEN is rare, the clinician must recognize these clinical patterns early to avoid or effectively deal with potentially serious complications. Classic EM, SJS, and TEN are described in Chapter 4.

Fixed Drug Eruption

Fixed drug eruption is a distinctive reaction pattern characterized by the sudden onset of one or several EM-like annular, erythematous, edematous plaques ranging in size from 1 cm to over 5 cm in diameter. Lesions will typically recur in the same location when a patient is challenged with the causative medication. Lesions occur after exposure to a number of medications (Fig. 7.4). Lesions typically take a few days to develop after first-time medication exposure, but on subsequent exposure can develop in as little as 30 min. Intense edema may result in bulla formation. When the drug is withdrawn, lesions flatten, erythema fades, and prominent post-inflammatory hyperpigmentation persists for weeks to months. On re-exposure to the

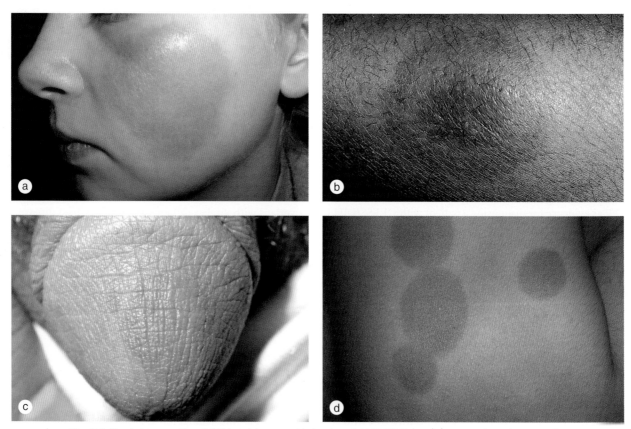

Fig. 7.4 Fixed drug eruption. **(a)** This adolescent girl developed a recurrent fixed drug reaction whenever she took a non-steroidal anti-inflammatory drug for menstrual cramps. **(b)** This 10-year-old, darkly pigmented boy developed a recurrent target lesion in the same spot on his arm after exposure to a cold remedy. Note the dusky center with marked hyperpigmentation. **(c)** Typical itchy violaceous plaques developed on the glans penis of this adolescent boy when he was started on doxycycline for treatment of acne. **(d)** Dramatic hyperpigmented macules persisted after a fixed drug eruption to an oral antibiotic resolved.

allergen, old lesions reappear and new plaques may develop and slowly progress. Widespread bullous eruptions rarely occur with recurrent exposure to the offending agent.

Although the rash may develop on any site, the face, lips, genitals, and buttocks are the most commonly involved. The most frequent triggering agents include trimethoprim-sulfamethoxazole, aspirin, tetracyclines, barbiturates, and non-steroidal anti-inflammatory drugs.

Although the mechanism is not known, T-lymphocytes that reside in the dermis and amplification by T-cells recruited from the circulation are thought to be responsible for the acute reaction, as well as the cutaneous memory function of the fixed drug eruption. Suppressor/cytotoxic T-lymphocytes recognize drug-haptens, which bind to proteins in basal keratinocytes and melanocytes to form a complete antigen, which stimulates the immunologically mediated process. Histologic findings are similar to those of EM, but pigment incontinence tends to be intense. This explains the impressive, discrete hyperpigmentation, which may be the only clinical finding between episodes. Once the diagnosis is considered, the allergen can be identified and avoided.

Urticaria

Urticaria, commonly known as hives, is characterized by the sudden appearance of transient, well-demarcated wheals that are usually intensely pruritic, especially when they arise as part of an acute, immunoglobulin (Ig)E-mediated hypersensitivity reaction (Fig. 7.5). Individual lesions usually last several minutes to several hours, but they may rarely persist for up to 24 h. Wheals may have a red center with an edematous white halo or the reverse: an edematous white center with a red halo. Size can vary from a few millimeters to giant lesions over 20 cm in diameter. Central clearing with peripheral extension may lead to the formation of annular, polycyclic, and arcuate plaques that simulate EM and erythema marginatum. The reaction may involve the mucous membranes and can spread to the subcutaneous tissue to produce woody edema known as angioedema (Fig. 7.6). Histopathology usually demonstrates a mild, lymphocytic, perivascular infiltrate with marked dermal edema.

Urticaria can be triggered by a variety of immunologic mechanisms, including IgE antibody response, complement activation, and abnormal response to vasoactive amines. Most cases of acute urticarial—defined as lasting less than 6 weeks—are caused by a hypersensitivity reaction to drugs, food, insect bites, contact antigens, inhaled substances, or acute infections. Physical agents, which include cold, heat, water, exercise, and mechanical pressure, may also trigger hives. Dermatographism or dermatographia (skin writing) refers to a variant of

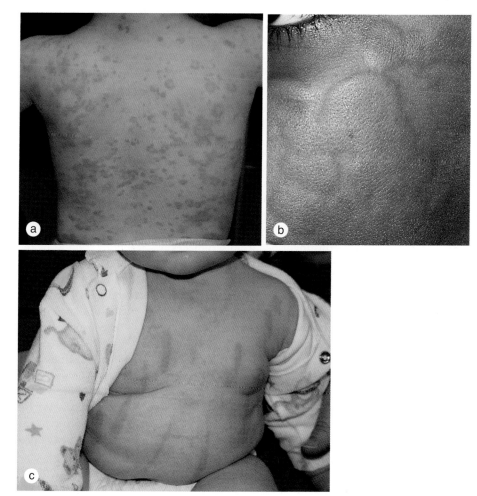

Fig. 7.5 Urticaria. **(a)** Pruritic papules and annular plaques recurred on the trunk and extremities of a toddler with chronic urticarial. **(b)** Wheals have become confluent on the face of this boy. **(c)** This infant developed recurrent urticaria and dermatographism, demonstrated here by vertical linear red plaques with surrounding pallor.

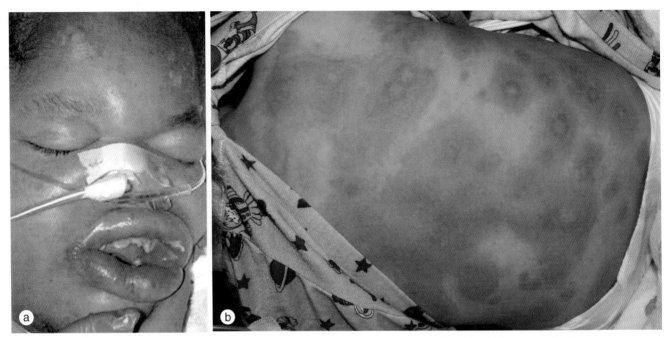

Fig. 7.6 (a) This 12-year-old boy developed diffuse angioedema with some airway involvement shortly after receiving intramuscular penicillin after a dental procedure. **(b)** Generalized migratory itchy papules and annular plaques with central purpura typical of urticarial multiforme developed on this 3-year-old girl with viral gastroenteritis.

physical urticaria, which occurs in 2–5% of the population and refers to hives triggered by rubbing or scratching the skin. Less than 5% of patients evolve into chronic urticaria, which lasts from 6 weeks to many years. Most commonly chronic urticaria is idiopathic in nature; however, its development has been associated with autoimmune disease and malignancy in adult patients.

Specific drugs and foods known to cause hives should be avoided because of the risk of inducing anaphylaxis on subsequent exposure. Exhaustive laboratory studies in an otherwise healthy child with acute urticaria are unlikely to be rewarding. Laboratory evaluation is guided by findings on history and physical examination. Patients with chronic disease require intermittent re-examination, particularly if other problems such as arthritis, diarrhea, or fever develop.

Extensive urticaria associated with pruritus may respond readily to both sedating H1 antihistamines (e.g., diphenhydramine, hydroxyzine, or chlorpheniramine) and non-sedating H1 antihistamines (e.g., cetirizine, loratadine, desloratadine, and fexofenadine). Dosages should be increased to twice the recommended level or until unacceptable adverse reactions are noted. Most children accommodate quickly to sedation associated with first-generation antihistamines, but many children respond to the non-sedating antihistamines and only require sedating antihistamines for night-time breakthrough symptoms. In resistant cases, the addition of an H2 antihistamine, such as cimetidine or ranitidine, and/or β-adrenergic agonists, such as ephedrine and terbutaline, may be helpful. Adrenaline (epinephrine) may be lifesaving in urticaria and angioedema that involve the airway. Systemic corticosteroids are reserved for patients with life-threatening disease.

Urticarial eruptions may appear early in the course of serum sickness reactions triggered by infectious agents or drugs. Asymptomatic or painful, red papules and expanding annular plaques with hemorrhagic borders are associated with fever, arthralgias, periarticular swelling, and occasionally arthritis. Skin lesions differ from classic urticaria by the lack of pruritus and persistence beyond 24 h. Serum sickness reactions have been reported with cefaclor, but may also occur with a number of other antibiotics (Fig. 7.7a). Skin biopsies usually demonstrate a lymphohistiocytic, dermal, inflammatory infiltrate, but occasionally vasculitis may be present.

Urticaria may also occur during the prodrome of Henoch–Schönlein purpura, which is characterized by leukocytoclastic vasculitis with palpable purpura. Urticarial-like eruptions triggered by viral infections referred to as urticaria multiforme can be distinguished from serum sickness reactions and EM by the presence of pruritus and a transient, rapidly evolving course. Unlike classic urticaria, individual expanding plaques in urticaria multiforme typically persist for several weeks and often develop a dusky center (Fig. 7.7b).

Erythema marginatum, one of the major criteria for rheumatic fever and which occurs in 20% of patients, may be confused with hives. This eruption is characterized by transient, asymptomatic, red papules that enlarge over several hours to form annular, scalloped, and serpiginous expanding plaques with narrow borders and central clearing (Fig. 7.8). Successive crops appear on the trunk and extremities as old plaques fade. New lesions typically flare with evening fever spikes, and involvement is restricted predominantly to the trunk and proximal extremities. The absence of pruritus helps distinguish erythema marginatum from hives, and skin biopsies show predominantly a perivascular neutrophilic

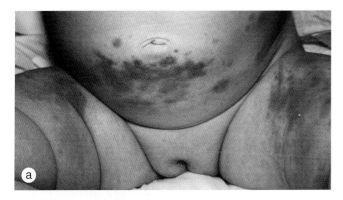

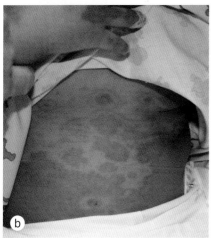

Fig. 7.7 (a) A 10-month-old girl developed urticaria on the lower trunk and thighs while being treated with cefaclor for an ear infection. Although the drug was stopped, the annular plaques progressed and became purpuric centrally. The rash was accompanied by arthralgias, joint swelling, and fever consistent with a serum sickness picture. **(b)** Generalized migratory itchy papules and plaques (urticaria multiforme) developed in this 4-year-old girl with a viral gastroenteritis.

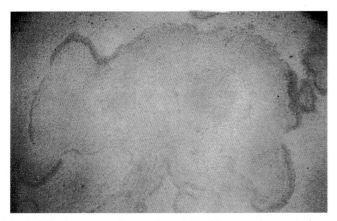

Fig. 7.8 Erythema marginatum in a child with acute rheumatic fever. Note the scalloped margins and distribution on the trunk.

infiltrate. The diagnosis of rheumatic fever is dependent on the recognition of other well-defined criteria.

Urticaria must also be distinguished from the figurate erythemas and other reactive erythemas, discussed later in this chapter.

Exfoliative, Lichenoid, and Acneiform Drug Reactions

Drugs can also trigger reactions that mimic other cutaneous conditions. In an exfoliative erythroderma, widespread inflammation in the skin is associated with generalized erythema and scale. The entire body surface can be involved, including the scalp, palms, and soles. Although this reaction pattern usually evolves from a primary cutaneous disorder, such as atopic dermatitis, seborrheic dermatitis, psoriasis, or T-cell lymphoma, a number of medications (including allopurinol, barbiturates, captopril, carbamazepine, cimetidine, diltiazem, griseofulvin, gold, thiazide diuretics, isoniazid, hydantoins, D-penicillamine, quinidine, and sulfonamides) have been implicated in some patients. A history of drug exposure, preceding rashes, and associated findings provide clues to the cause of the erythroderma. Histopathology usually reveals a chronic dermatitis. However, the presence of eosinophils may suggest a medication hypersensitivity reaction, while other distinct findings indicate an underlying skin disorder.

In lichenoid drug reactions, clinical findings are usually indistinguishable from those of lichen planus. However, the dermal infiltrate may contain eosinophils, which is unusual for classic lichen planus. Withdrawal of medications may result in improvement of the eruption over weeks to many months. Drugs that have been reported to cause lichenoid reactions include thiazide diuretics, streptomycin, isoniazid, gold, methyldopa, beta-blockers, naproxen, and captopril. Lichenoid drug reactions have also been seen in reaction to anti–tumor necrosis factor (TNF) therapy, as well as tyrosine kinase inhibitors. Lichenoid drug reactions may be difficult to distinguish from graft-vs-host disease in transplant patients.

Acneiform drug reactions may be differentiated from typical acne vulgaris by the presence of uniform, inflammatory papules and pustules (rather than mixed comedones and inflammatory lesions in acne vulgaris); involvement of the usual acne areas (face, shoulders, upper trunk), as well as the lower trunk, arms, and legs; acute onset with introduction of the inciting drug; and resistance to standard therapy. Medications may also exacerbate pre-existing acne. Commonly identified drugs include corticosteroids, corticotropin, isoniazid, lithium, iodides, cyclosporine, and anticonvulsants. Although the eruption may improve with systemic and topical acne preparations, severe or recalcitrant cases may require a decrease or discontinuation of the medication if possible.

Acute generalized exanthematous eruptive pustulosis (AGEP) may also mimic an acute flare of acne. Disseminated pustules appear within 1–3 days of initiation of the inciting medication and may involve the palms and soles. The lesions have a preference for flexural and intertriginous locations. Mild systemic complaints including fever, elevated liver enzymes, and rarely transient renal dysfunction have been reported. Lesions usually clear within 7–14 days of discontinuing the drug. The eruption has been associated with exposure to antibiotics (β-lactams, macrolides, cephalosporins), calcium channel blockers, carbamazepine, paracetamol, and a number of viral organisms (Fig. 7.9).

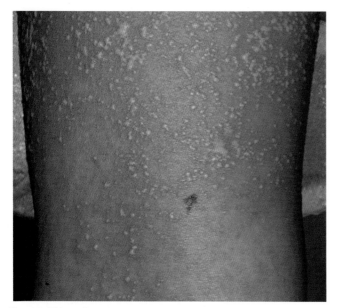

Fig. 7.9 This patient developed a generalized red papular eruption with central pustules while on an antibiotic for pharyngitis.

Chemotherapy-Induced Erythema

Many cytotoxic agents have been identified as causing a multitude of cutaneous adverse reactions. Although a complete discussion is beyond the scope of this book, two of the more common reactions present as reactive erythema of the hands and feet. Neutrophilic eccrine hidradenitis is classically associated with cytarabine exposure and presents as asymptomatic to painful edematous plaques on the hands and feet. Histology is diagnostic with neutrophilic infiltrate surrounding eccrine glands. These lesions may develop an acneiform appearance and may spread to seborrheic areas of the trunk and face (Fig. 7.10). Hand-foot syndrome (also known as palmoplantar dysesthesia syndrome) is most commonly associated with cytarabine, fluorouracil, and multi-kinase inhibitors. This condition typically presents as highly painful edematous plaques on the hands and feet, with a predilection for fat pads. The lesions can progress to bullae and peeling acral skin.

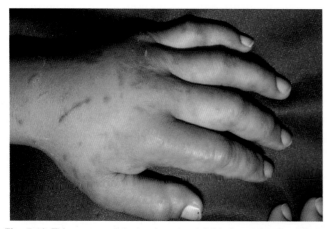

Fig. 7.10 This young adult developed painful indurated red confluent plaques on the palms and soles after infusion of bleomycin.

VIRAL EXANTHEMS

A number of viral infections have cutaneous manifestations that provide a clue to the diagnosis. In some, the skin rash is the major finding. Early recognition of distinct exanthems also helps differentiate viral infections from drug reactions, bacterial and rickettsial rashes, and other reactive erythemas.

In the early twentieth century, clinicians commonly referred to childhood exanthems by number. Scarlet fever and measles were known as "first" and "second" disease, but the two rashes were frequently confused. Rubella was established as an entity distinct from measles and known as "third" disease. In 1900, Duke described "fourth" disease, which probably does not represent a distinct condition, but a combination of rubella and scarlet fever. "Fifth" disease is recognized today as erythema infectiosum, and roseola finishes off the numbered exanthems as "sixth" disease. Many other viruses produce distinct reaction patterns in the skin. Infections from herpes- and poxviruses are readily diagnosed by their characteristic vesiculobullous eruptions, while infections from picornaviruses (which include the enteroviruses) are well recognized for their morbilliform exanthems.

Viruses trigger exanthems by a number of mechanisms. Direct infection of the skin occurs in varicella, enteroviruses, and herpetic infections. Other rashes, such as measles and rubella, probably result from a combination of viral spread to the skin and host immunologic response. Some host–viral interactions are activated by exposure to certain drugs, exemplified by the generalized exanthem that occurs in over 95% of individuals with Epstein–Barr virus infection who receive ampicillin.

Measles and Rubella

In the pre-vaccine era, measles and rubella were common, and their exanthems became a paradigm for other "morbilliform" rashes. Although the usual late-winter to early-spring epidemics have been interrupted by widespread vaccination in industrialized nations, starting in the early 2000s failure to immunize significant numbers of children has resulted in intermittent and increasing outbreaks in the United States.

Measles

Measles (rubeola, red measles, 10-day measles) is a highly contagious, potentially severe illness with a prodrome characterized by fever, malaise, dry cough, coryza, conjunctivitis, and severe photophobia (Fig. 7.11a). Several days into the course, diagnostic Koplik spots appear on the buccal and labial mucosae (Fig. 7.11b). These lesions consist of 1–3 mm diameter and bluish-white papules surrounded by red halos, which increase in number and fade over 2–3 days. Unfortunately, this characteristic enanthem is often transient and goes unnoticed.

On the third or fourth day of illness, the exanthem first appears on the face as an eruption of blanching, red macules and papules, which spreads cephalocaudally over 3 days and ultimately involves the palms and soles (Fig. 7.12). Once generalized, lesions become confluent on the face, trunk, and extremities in succession. Older lesions commonly develop a rusty hue from capillary leak and hemosiderin deposition. The rash begins to fade after 3 days and clearance is complete 3 days later, for a total

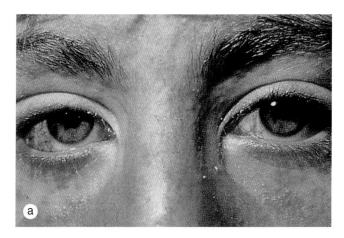

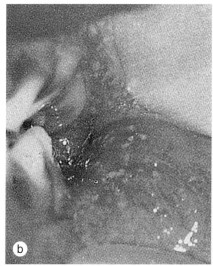

Fig. 7.11 Rubeola/measles. **(a)** During and after the prodromal period, the conjunctivae are injected and produce a clear discharge. This is associated with marked photophobia. **(b)** Koplik spots, bluish-white dots surrounded by red halos, appear on the buccal and labial mucosae a day or two before the exanthem and begin to fade with the onset of the rash.

duration of 10 days for the illness. Widespread desquamation may appear 1–2 weeks after resolution of the rash.

Patients are contagious 4 days before the exanthem until 4 days after it appears. During the illness, fever may be persistent and severe. Generalized adenopathy is common. Morbidity and mortality are highest in patients compromised by hereditary or acquired immunodeficiency, and in developing countries in which malnutrition is rampant (supplementation with vitamins, particularly vitamin A, may reduce the risk of death and complications). Potential complications that result from primary viral infection or secondary bacterial infection include conjunctivitis, otitis media, pneumonitis, meningitis, acute encephalitis, and obstructive laryngotracheitis.

Atypical measles is an unusual syndrome that occurs in individuals who received a killed measles vaccine, when it was available between 1963 and 1967, and are subsequently exposed to the measles virus. Unlike typical measles, the exanthem begins and remains primarily on the extremities and often develops a petechial component. Koplik spots are absent, fevers are high, and pneumonitis is usually severe. This disorder probably represents a hypersensitivity reaction to the virus and is most frequently confused with Rocky Mountain spotted fever and collagen vascular disease.

Rubella

Rubella (German measles) is known as 3-day measles because the pink exanthem, which mimics a mild case of measles, usually evolves over 1–3 days. In fact, nearly 25% of patients may have only mild upper respiratory symptoms with little or no rash.

Rubella is typically associated with several days of low-grade fever, adenopathy, headache, sore throat, and coryza. In young children, fever may last for less than 24 h. Forchheimer spots consist of transient, small, red papules on the soft palate and are seen in some patients at the beginning of the rash. This enanthem helps differentiate this otherwise non-specific eruption from other viral exanthems.

As with measles, peak incidence occurs in the late winter and early spring. Serologic testing may be useful to make a specific diagnosis, particularly if the patient is pregnant. Although complications

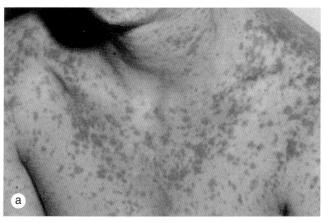

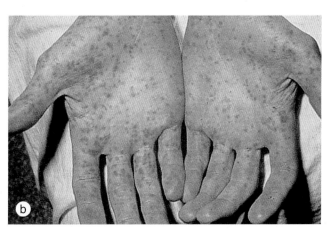

Fig. 7.12 The measles exanthem. **(a)** A blotchy, erythematous, blanching eruption appears at the hairline and spreads cephalocaudally over 3 days. **(b)** Ultimately, the exanthem involves the palms and soles. With evolution, lesions become confluent on the face, neck, and upper trunk.

are rare in children, the fetus is particularly vulnerable to intrauterine infection, with complications that include spontaneous abortion, diffuse cataracts, microphthalmia, glaucoma, and congenital heart disease. Up to 25% of infected newborns develop severe, disseminated disease with jaundice, pneumonitis, meningoencephalitis, bony abnormalities, thrombocytopenia, blueberry muffin lesions (extramedullary erythropoiesis), and a morbilliform exanthem. Babies with congenital infection may shed virus in urine, stools, and respiratory secretions for up to 1 year, and should be isolated from other infants and pregnant women.

Erythema Infectiosum (Fifth Disease)

In 1983, erythema infectiosum (or fifth disease) was linked to human parvovirus B19. Since then, investigators have defined the clinical features and epidemiology of infection in normal and compromised patients.

In its most commonly recognized clinical presentation, viral infection presents in children of school age with an asymptomatic "slapped cheek" erythema on the face and a lacy or reticulated, blanching erythema on the trunk and extremities (Fig. 7.13a–d). Although the exanthem usually fades over 2–3 weeks, lesions may recur for up to 3 months, especially when cutaneous blood flow is increased and after fever or vigorous physical activity.

The prevalence of B19 antibody is about 5–10% in children under 5 years of age and rises to over 50% in adults. Human volunteer studies suggest that the virus is spread in respiratory secretions. After an incubation period of 5–7 days, infectivity peaks during the viremia, which lasts 5–7 days. The end of viremia is

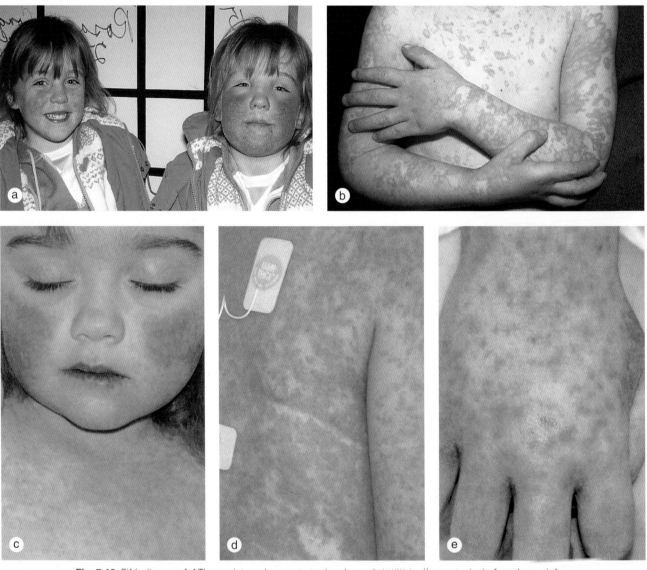

Fig. 7.13 Fifth disease. **(a)** These sisters demonstrate the slapped cheek erythema typical of erythema infectiosum. Despite the edema in one girl, both were completely asymptomatic. **(b)** A diffuse, lacy, and confluent annular eruption appeared on this otherwise healthy 9-year-old boy during a recent fifth disease epidemic. The reticulated erythema on his arms flared intermittently for 6 weeks. **(c)** Slapped cheek erythema and **(d)** a diffuse, reticulated, morbilliform eruption developed in this 4-year-old girl with high fever, arthralgias, and myalgias. **(e)** Four days into her illness she developed discrete and eventually confluent purpuric macules and papules on her hands and feet. Serology for parvovirus B19 was positive for acute infection.

marked by a rise in IgM and then IgG antibody and followed 2–5 days later by the appearance of the rash. Consequently, the risk of infection is low when the exanthem is diagnosed, and children can remain in school.

Associated symptoms, which include fever and arthralgias, are usually mild or absent in young children. However, arthralgias or frank arthritis may be severe in adolescents and adults. At least a quarter of patients with serologic evidence of disease do not develop the exanthem, and the arthropathy may develop before, after, or without the rash.

Early in the infection most patients experience a transient reticulocytopenia for 7–10 days and a clinically insignificant drop in hemoglobin level. This phenomenon, however, may trigger an aplastic crisis in patients with severe hemoglobinopathies. The virus has also been implicated as a cause of hydrops fetalis in pregnant women with no other evidence of clinical disease. However, recent reports suggest that parvovirus can rarely cause fetal malformations. In hereditary or acquired immunodeficiency syndromes, B19 may produce persistent infection and chronic, life-threatening anemia.

Human parvovirus B19 has also been isolated from children and adults with papular-purpuric gloves and socks syndrome (Fig. 7.13e). Although this painful, itchy erythema, edema, and purpura of the palms and soles occurs most commonly in the spring at the peak of the human parvovirus B19 season, it has also been associated with other viruses including Coxsackie virus B6 and HHV6. Red papules reminiscent of Koplik spots and erosions may also develop on the tongue, palate, and buccal mucosa, and fever and arthropathy are variable. Treatment is symptomatic, and the syndrome usually resolves in 1–2 weeks.

The reticulated exanthem of erythema infectiosum may be easily confused with livedo reticularis, thus some distinctions between these entities are required. Livedo reticularis is a persistent, lacy, blanching, violaceous erythema that occurs in primary and secondary forms (Fig. 7.14). In the idiopathic variant of livedo reticularis, lesions are symmetric and widespread with poorly defined borders. Unlike cutis marmorata in neonates (another benign reticulate erythema), the pattern does not resolve with warming. Livedo reticularis occurs most commonly in young women who are otherwise healthy. The secondary variant is more common in men and has been reported in association with polyarteritis nodosa, hepatitis, syphilis, and a number of other infections, connective tissue diseases, and malignancy.

Exanthema Subitum (Roseola)

Roseola, or exanthema subitum (the "surprise" rash), has been recognized by pediatricians for over a century. The classic clinical course occurs in children between 6 months and 3 years old. After a 3–5-day illness marked by high-spiking fevers, which occasionally trigger febrile seizures, a sudden end to the fever is followed by the appearance of a widely disseminated, pink, papular rash (Fig. 7.15). As in fifth disease, the end of viremia is marked by the development of the rash and a rise in antibody to the causative agent: HHV6. Consequently, the risk of infection is greatest during the febrile period and minimal after the appearance of the rash.

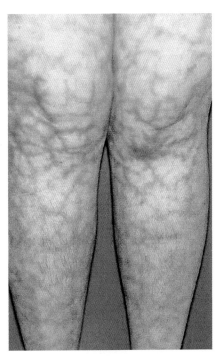

Fig. 7.14 Widespread livedo reticularis became particularly prominent on the extremities of this adolescent shortly after she started a neuroleptic medication for attention-deficit/hyperactivity disorder.

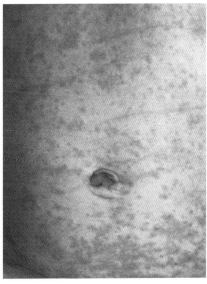

Fig. 7.15 Roseola/exanthema subitum. A generalized, pink, maculopapular rash suddenly appeared on this infant after 3 days of high fever.

Serologic studies show an almost universal exposure of the population to HHV6. Although only one-third of infants develop clinical disease, prevalence of antibody increases from less than 10% in children under 6 months of age to 75–90% in adults. Consequently, a large number of children develop asymptomatic infection. Conversely, seroprevalence studies of febrile infants demonstrate that viral infection may commonly produce a febrile illness without a rash. A similar febrile disorder has been associated with HHV7 in some children. HHV6 has also been linked to a mononucleosis-like illness in young adults.

Papular Acrodermatitis (Gianotti–Crosti Syndrome)

In 1955, Gianotti, while working in the Milan department of dermatology directed by Crosti, described a distinctive exanthem associated with anicteric hepatitis, lymphadenopathy, and hepatitis B surface antigenemia, subtype *ayw*. The skin rash consists of flat-topped, 3–10 mm diameter, skin-colored to red edematous papules that involve the arms, legs, buttocks, and face (Fig. 7.16). Lesions on the calves and extensor surfaces of

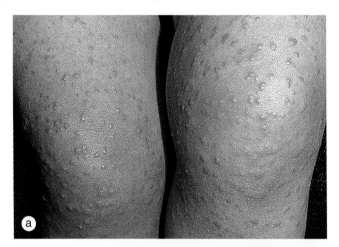
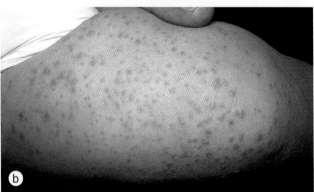
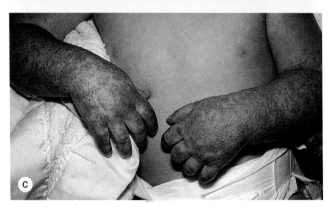

Fig. 7.16 Papular acrodermatitis. A symmetric, acrally distributed, red papular rash developed in this toddler with low-grade fever and loose stools. Note the discrete, edematous papules on the **(a)** knees and **(b)** thighs. **(c)** In some areas on his hands and forearms the lesions were confluent.

the arms may become so edematous as to appear vesicular, and occasionally frank vesicles are present.

During the past 15 years, it has become apparent that most cases in the United States are caused by various viruses, including enteroviruses, respiratory viruses, and Epstein–Barr virus. As most children are asymptomatic, no treatment is necessary. However, given its clinical appearance and protracted course, parents need to be counseled that the eruption may persist for up to several months.

Papular acrodermatitis can be differentiated from lichen planus, as the lesions in papular acrodermatitis are typically asymptomatic versus the severe pruritus seen in lichen planus. A negative history of recent drug exposure excludes a lichenoid drug eruption. Other viral eruptions may also be confused with papular acrodermatitis. Unfortunately, the histopathology is not specific and shows focal spongiosis and exocytosis in the epidermis overlying a perivascular, lymphocytic, dermal infiltrate.

Other Viral Exanthems

Exanthems associated with the enteroviruses are quite variable and usually follow a shorter incubation period than the classic viral exanthems. Although they occur all year round, the incidence peaks in the late summer and early fall. Morbilliform, vesicular, petechial, and urticarial eruptions are variably present, usually in association with fever (Fig. 7.17). Other symptoms may include meningitis, conjunctivitis, cough, coryza, pharyngitis, and pneumonia. Hand-foot-and-mouth disease is a distinctive entity associated with papulovesicular lesions on the palms, soles, palate, and (not infrequently) trunk, particularly the buttocks. The typical incubation period for development of this syndrome is 3–5 days, and it is important to note that the enanthem can occur without the exanthema and vice versa. Coxsackie viruses A1-6, A8, A10, A16, and A22 and enterovirus 71 have been identified in patients with this syndrome. With the recent introduction in the United States of a new Coxsackie A6 virus from Asia, there has been a shift in the exanthem to a papulovesicular-crusted eruption with prominence of lesions on the arms and legs, and around the mouth and diaper area, with relative sparing of mucous membranes. The rash also tends to koebnerize with increased aggregation of skin lesions in areas of pre-existing trauma, such as in patches of eczema, burns, and cuts and scrapes.

Unilateral laterothoracic exanthem (asymmetric periflexural exanthem of childhood) (Fig. 7.17c) is another distinct clinical pattern that may be triggered by a number of organisms, including the enteroviruses. The asymptomatic or minimally pruritic morbilliform or scarlatiniform eruption usually begins near one axilla and, although it often remains predominant on the initial side, spreads over the trunk in infants and preschool children. The mean age of onset is 2 years, and girls are affected twice as often as boys. Lesions usually heal without scarring over 5 weeks. Although there is no diagnostic test, a unique eccrine lymphocytic infiltrate is identified in skin biopsies.

Papulovesicular rashes may be differentiated from varicella zoster and herpes simplex infections by obtaining a polymerase chain reaction (PCR) swab of a lesion for both HVS (herpes simplex virus) 1/2 and VZV (varicella zoster virus) testing.

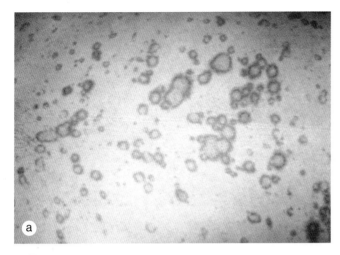

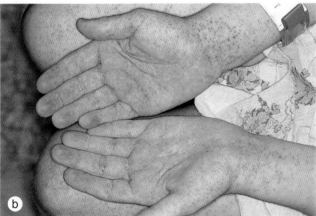

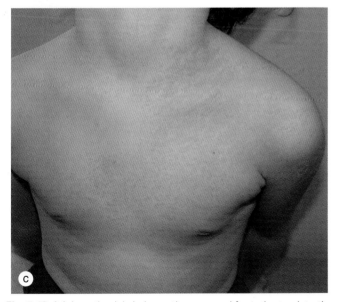

Fig. 7.17 (a) An urticarial viral exanthem spread from the trunk to the face and extremities in this infant. Lesions faded over several days. **(b)** A 6-year-old boy developed 1–2 mm red macules and petechiae on the distal extremities with involvement of the palms and soles. **(c)** This healthy 4-year-old boy developed a unilateral discrete and confluent papular eruption on his left chest, which generalized over several days.

Additionally, Tzanck smear, cultures, and serologic studies help to make a specific diagnosis. Although meningococcal infections tend to peak during the winter and spring, occasionally cases occur during the summer and fall enteroviral season. Consequently, the child with a petechial exanthem and presumed enteroviral meningitis must be evaluated carefully to exclude a bacterial infection.

Infection with cytomegalovirus, Epstein–Barr virus, and respiratory viruses may be associated with macular, morbilliform, or urticarial exanthems, which are difficult to differentiate from drug rashes. Children who require medications and develop intercurrent viral infections and resulting morbilliform exanthems may remain on their medications while under close observation. These minor viral exanthems usually fade in several days, while drug reactions tend to persist or intensify. However, drugs must be discontinued in any patients who develop urticaria, angioedema, SJS/TEN, or other signs of progressive allergic reactions.

SCARLATINIFORM RASHES

The rash of scarlet fever provides a model for a number of important disorders that must be differentiated by other signs and symptoms. Bacterial toxins, viral infections, drugs, and Kawasaki syndrome have all been associated with scarlatiniform eruptions.

Scarlet Fever

Scarlet fever is characterized by a fine, red, papular, sandpaper-like rash that begins on the face and neck and generalizes to the trunk and extremities within 1–2 days (Fig. 7.18). The skin is warm and flushed, and some patients complain of mild pruritus. Circumoral pallor is typical but not diagnostic. The rash ranges from a subtle pink to fiery red color and usually follows the onset of streptococcal pharyngitis by 24–48 h. Pastia lines are the accentuation of the rash from linear petechiae, which occurs in the flexural creases of the arms, legs, and trunk (Fig. 7.18b). Other associated symptoms include nausea, vomiting, fever, headache, general malaise, and abdominal pain. The palms, soles, and conjunctivae are usually spared. In classic cases, the pharynx is beefy red with palatal petechiae, purulent tonsillitis, and tender, cervical adenopathy. Early in the course the lingual papillae poke through a white membrane (white strawberry tongue; Fig. 7.19a). Shedding of the membrane by days 4–5 results in a bright red, strawberry tongue (Fig. 7.19b). In many patients, the throat infection is mild or completely asymptomatic. Scarlet fever may also be associated with streptococcal impetigo.

The rash is triggered by one of three antigenically distinct erythrotoxins, which are produced by most strains of Group A β-hemolytic streptococci. Development of antibodies against the streptococcal organism and erythrotoxin is protective and results in resolution of the symptoms and rash within 4–5 days. This is followed 1–2 weeks later by generalized desquamation, which is particularly marked on the fingertips and toes (Fig. 7.18c). Although both oral and cutaneous infections with nephritogenic streptococci can trigger glomerulonephritis, only pharyngeal infections have been associated with subsequent development of rheumatic fever. Treatment of patients with amoxicillin or penicillin (erythromycin or other macrolides in

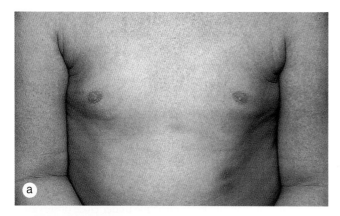

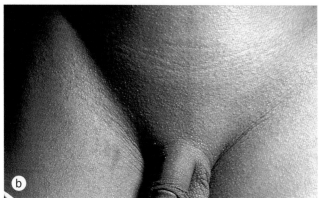

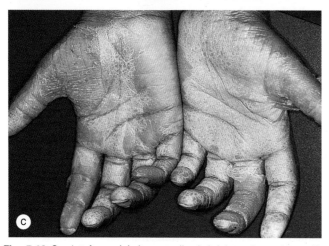

Fig. 7.18 Scarlet fever. **(a)** A generalized, bright red, sandpaper-like papular rash developed in a 7-year-old boy with a streptococcal pharyngitis. Note the accentuation of the rash at the neck and axillary and antecubital creases. **(b)** A 5-year-old boy demonstrated a similar eruption with Pastia lines in the groin creases. **(c)** Widespread desquamation appeared in this 8-year-old girl 10 days after the onset of symptoms and rash and was most prominent on the hands and feet.

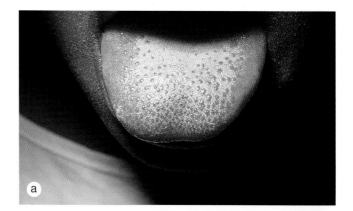

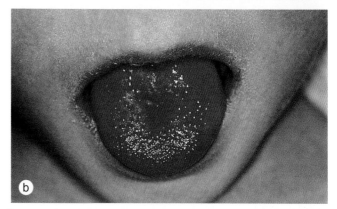

Fig. 7.19 Scarlet fever. **(a)** A white strawberry tongue is usually followed by **(b)** a red strawberry tongue as the erythrotoxin-mediated enanthema evolves.

penicillin-allergic patients) may shorten the course of fever and other symptoms. If antibiotics are initiated within 10 days of the onset of pharyngitis, the risk of rheumatic fever may be reduced from 3% to less than 1%. Unfortunately, early treatment of nephritogenic strains has not been shown to decrease the incidence of poststreptococcal renal disease. Moreover, asymptomatic pharyngeal infection may escape detection until after the development of late complications.

Several other toxin-mediated syndromes may be confused with scarlet fever. Children with staphylococcal scarlet fever develop a rash, which may be indistinguishable from streptococcal disease. Nikolsky sign may be present, but pharyngeal signs are usually absent. Cultures from the typical purulent conjunctivitis or the oral or nasal pharynx invariably demonstrate *Staphylococcus aureus*. Unlike streptococcal scarlet fever, desquamation begins early in the course (by day 2) and is complete within a week. The clinical signs and course probably vary with the source of the infection, amount of staphylococcal exotoxin present, and host response. A similar eruption may accompany toxic shock syndrome. However, the eruption is usually accompanied by hyperemia of the conjunctivae, oral and vaginal mucosa, a strawberry tongue, and severe multisystem disease. The early findings in both staphylococcal scalded-skin syndrome and TEN may mimic scarlet fever. However, the presence of Nikolsky sign and progression to widespread sloughing of skin quickly differentiate these disorders. Scarlatiniform viral exanthems may occur with a number of different organisms. The course may be similar to that of scarlet fever and can only be differentiated by serologic studies and the absence of streptococci in throat or skin cultures.

Kawasaki Syndrome

Although the exact etiology of Kawasaki syndrome is unknown, the epidemiology, clinical findings, and course suggest an as yet unidentified infectious agent. Cases occur all year round, with slight peaks in the late spring and late fall. Epidemics have also been reported. Although all races may be affected, the increased incidence among Japanese and intermediate risk of Japanese Americans supports a genetic predisposition.

Kawasaki syndrome is defined clinically by the presence of five out of six major criteria, which are fever (usually unresponsive to antipyretics for at least 5 days), conjunctivitis, pharyngitis, erythema and edema of the hands and feet, rash, and adenopathy (Fig. 7.20). The acute phase, which lasts 10–14 days, begins with an abrupt onset of high fever and extreme irritability. A rash usually appears shortly after the fever and may take

the form of a scarlatiniform, morbilliform, or urticarial exanthema, or a combination of them. It is commonly accentuated in intertriginous areas, where maceration and scaling may be prominent, particularly on the perineum and inguinal creases (Fig. 7.20f). Facial swelling and pallor are commonly present. Other findings during the acute phase include non-purulent, conjunctival injection, erythema, edema, and cracking of the lips, palatal erythema and a strawberry tongue, painful erythema and edema of the hands and feet, and painful, unilateral cervical adenopathy. Arthritis, diarrhea, abdominal pain, aseptic meningitis, hepatitis, urethritis, otitis, and hydrops of the

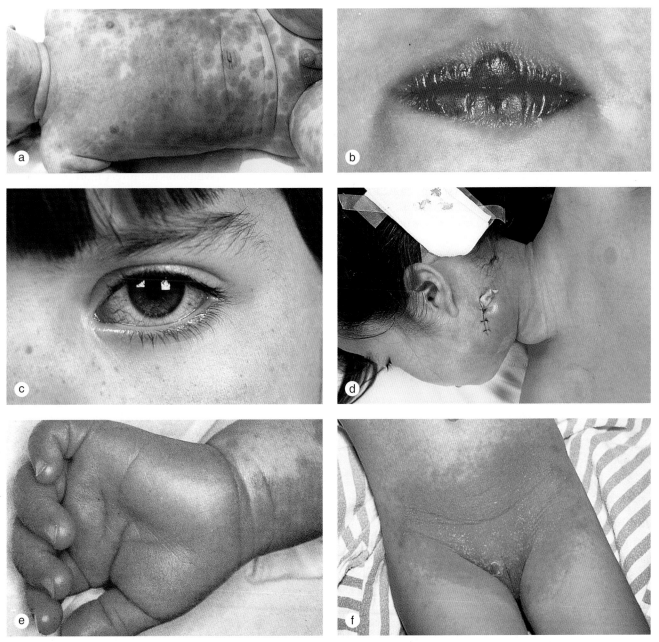

Fig. 7.20 Kawasaki syndrome. Characteristic clinical findings demonstrated include **(a)** a generalized, morbilliform, erythema multiforme-like rash, **(b)** erythema and fissuring of the lips, **(c)** conjunctival injection, **(d)** lymphadenopathy, **(e)** palmar and plantar erythema with edema of the hands and feet, and **(f)** erythema and scaling in the groin creases.

gallbladder may also be present. The improvement in acute-phase mucocutaneous and systemic symptoms is often so dramatic that many practitioners look to this response to confirm their clinical diagnosis.

The subacute phase begins 10–14 days after the onset of symptoms, as the fever and rash improve. It is during this period that carditis associated with coronary angiitis becomes apparent, particularly in untreated patients. By 3 weeks, most patients experience a thrombocytosis of over 1 million platelets/cm^3, which may further increase coronary morbidity. Widespread desquamation occurs 1–2 weeks after resolution of the rash, particularly over the fingers and toes, where the skin is shed in large sheets. Although no specific laboratory tests are available for Kawasaki syndrome, leukocytosis is common and acute-phase reactants, which include C-reactive protein and erythrocyte sedimentation rate, are markedly elevated.

The convalescent phase begins in the fourth or fifth week and ends when the sedimentation rate returns to normal. Children require cardiac re-evaluation at least through this stage and for a year or more if aneurysms are detected.

The differential diagnosis includes viral exanthems, toxin-mediated bacterial disorders, connective tissue disease, and a number of other reactive erythemas. Acral erythema and edema, one of the classic findings during the acute phase of Kawasaki syndrome, is also typical of papular acrodermatitis and other viral exanthems, Rocky Mountain spotted fever, erythromelalgia, pernio, and acrodynia (pink disease). Papular acrodermatitis is easily differentiated from Kawasaki syndrome by the lack of fever and other systemic symptoms. The specific criteria and course of Kawasaki syndrome usually help to differentiate it from other viral infections that produce urticarial lesions and edema of the extremities. The findings in rickettsial diseases are also distinctive.

Early recognition is important to minimize the risk of coronary artery abnormalities. Intervention with intravenous gamma globulin, 2 g/kg given over 10–12 h as a single infusion, can reduce the incidence of coronary artery aneurysm formation from 20% to less than 4%. Over 75% of patients are under 4 years old and 50% less than 2 years of age. High-dose aspirin is typically added to this treatment regimen, given as 30–100 mg/kg total daily until fevers have been absent for 48 h. However, meta-analysis has shown that the addition of aspirin does not affect the development of coronary artery aneurysms.

ACRAL ERYTHEMA

Erythromelalgia

Erythromelalgia is an unusual entity characterized by paroxysms of painful erythema of the hands and feet, which last for minutes to hours (Fig. 7.21). Patients often complain of warmth of the distal extremities followed by marked erythema and pain, which is initially improved by elevation, and then only by increasing periods of immersion in cold water. Although the primary variant is usually familial and inherited in an autosomal dominant pattern, secondary erythromelalgia may be triggered by polycythemia vera, lymphoproliferative disorders, hypertension, and disorders associated with hyperviscosity. When the underlying

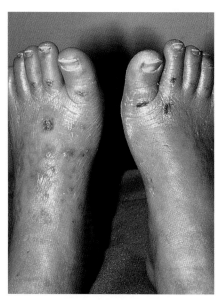

Fig. 7.21 Erythromelalgia. Necrotic blisters and ulcerations recurred chronically in this 11-year-old girl, who received relief from throbbing, debilitating foot pain by dunking her feet in near-freezing water for up to 12 h a day. Her brother also had erythromelalgia, but his symptoms were mild and usually resolved with leg elevation alone.

condition is treated, symptoms improve. Unfortunately, primary disease is often recalcitrant and cold-water exposure results in an "immersion foot" with progressive vascular injury, recurrent ulcerations, and secondary bacterial infection. The inherited form of erythromelalgia has been linked to mutations in voltage-gated sodium channel Nav1.7, which is expressed in peripheral nociceptors.

Erythromelalgia and the following acral erythemas can usually be distinguished from chemotherapy-induced hand-foot syndrome based on history and symptoms.

Pernio

Pernio, also known as chilblains, results from cold exposure, usually just above freezing, and recurrent trauma. It is commonly reported in temperate climates, where women and children are most commonly affected. Typical lesions consist of painful nodules and plaques that overlie bony prominences on the hands and feet (Fig. 7.22). Histopathology demonstrates intense edema of the papillary dermis and endothelial swelling associated with a mononuclear, perivascular infiltrate. Inflammation may extend to vessels in the deep dermis and fat. Thin girls and young women with a history of cold hands and feet, equestrians, scuba divers, and individuals who participate in fall and winter sports are particularly prone to developing lesions. The risk of recurrences can be reduced by keeping the distal extremities warm and protected from trauma. Patients should be instructed to avoid cold and damp exposures to the hands and to wear dry gloves or mittens in any cold environment. Chilblains should be distinguished from child abuse (in which cold exposure is not the primary trigger) and chilblain lupus. One should suspect child abuse when clinical findings seem inconsistent with environmental exposure, such as geographic lesions or highly asymmetric distributions (e.g., only one foot

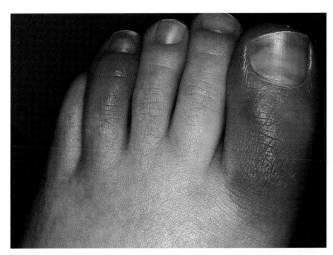

Fig. 7.22 Pernio. Painful, purple nodules developed on the sides of the feet and toes in this 13-year-old boy after walking with wet boots in a cold stream.

being involved). Chilblain lupus may represent an overlap of pernio and lupus, but in time, many patients with chilblain lupus develop features both clinically and histologically of discoid lupus in addition to their pernio lesions.

Acrodynia

Acrodynia, or pink disease, occurs in infants and toddlers as a result of chronic exposure to mercury. Painful, persistent erythema and swelling of the hands and feet are accompanied by other signs of sympathetic stimulation, which include tachycardia, hyperhidrosis, restlessness, and irritability. Treatment is directed toward removing the source of mercury exposure and chelation therapy.

PURPURAS AND VASCULITIDES

Bleeding into the skin may be an innocent finding in minor trauma or the first sign of a life-threatening disease. Early diagnosis and treatment, when necessary, requires that the practitioner recognizes and carefully evaluates any patient with purpura.

Cutaneous hemorrhage can be differentiated from hyperemia that results from increased blood flow through dilated vessels by failure of the hemorrhagic area to blanch when pressure is applied across the surface (diascopy). Diascopy can be demonstrated by pressing the skin apart between the thumb and index finger or by applying a glass or plastic slide. Pinpoint areas of hemorrhage are called petechiae; large, confluent patches are referred to as ecchymoses. Purpura results from extravascular, intravascular, and vascular phenomena.

Extravascular Purpura

Trauma is the most common cause of extravascular purpura in children. Non-blanching, purple patches caused by accidental trauma vary from a few millimeters to many centimeters in diameter and are usually located over bony prominences, such as the knees, elbows, the extensor surfaces of the lower legs,

forehead, nose, and chin. Petechiae are only occasionally present in otherwise healthy children, although they may occur on the face and chest after vigorous coughing or vomiting.

The presence of purpura on protected or non-exposed sites, such as the buttocks, spine, genitals, upper thighs, and upper arms, suggests the possibility of non-accidental trauma. In some cases, the shape of the bruise gives a clue as to the weapon used to inflict the injury.

Scars, sun damage, nutritional deficiency, inherited disorders of collagen and elastic tissue, and other factors that decrease the tensile strength of the skin may increase the risk of bruising caused by extravascular phenomena, even after minor trauma (Fig. 7.23).

Intravascular Purpura

Intravascular purpura results from any disorder that interferes with normal coagulation. Petechiae and ecchymoses are present on the skin, mucosal bleeding may be seen, and in severe cases bleeding may occur in the kidneys, gastrointestinal tract, and central nervous system. Among the causes are immune thrombocytopenic purpura (ITP), acute leukemia, aplastic anemia, sepsis, nutritional deficiencies, and clotting factor deficiencies.

Immune Thrombocytopenic Purpura

In children, ITP is the most common cause of intravascular purpura. Patients typically present in the late winter and early spring, a few weeks to several months after a viral illness, with purpura of all sizes and no history of trauma. When injuries occur, ecchymoses may be impressive. Bleeding of the gums occurs regularly with brushing, and occult blood may be detected in the urine and stool. Fortunately, severe bleeding is unusual and most cases are self-limited, with improvement in platelet counts from less than 10 000/mm³ to over 100 000/mm³ within 1–2 months. The presence of ITP is associated with the development of an IgG that binds to platelets and results in increased destruction by the reticuloendothelial system. Antiplatelet antibodies have also been reported in patients with lupus erythematosus, leukemia, lymphoma, and drug reactions. Moderate-to-severe cases usually respond to treatment with intravenous Ig. Resistant patients may require systemic corticosteroids and/or splenectomy.

Patients with ITP may be clinically indistinguishable from those with leukemia and aplastic anemia (Fig. 7.24). Associated symptoms, which include fatigue, general malaise, fever, weight loss, and bone pain, suggest the diagnosis of leukemia. In leukemia, blasts may be discovered in the peripheral smear, as well as the bone marrow. In ITP, the bone marrow demonstrates increased numbers of megakaryocytes, whereas they are usually decreased in leukemia. In aplastic anemia, purpura may be the first sign of marrow failure. When aplastic anemia develops, blood elements are decreased in the peripheral blood, as well as in the bone marrow, and severe bacterial infection is a common complication. In contrast to ITP, children with inherited clotting-factor disorders bruise easily and may develop hemarthroses and bleeding into viscera, but petechiae are not usually seen in these patients.

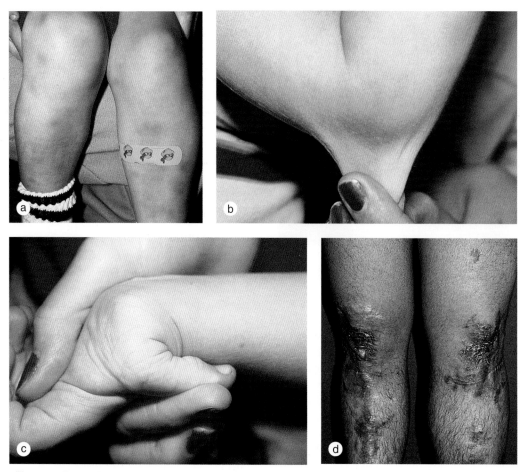

Fig. 7.23 Ehlers–Danlos syndrome. This child demonstrates a number of classic features of the disorder, which include **(a)** increased bruisability, **(b)** hyperelastic skin, and **(c)** hyperextensible joints. His father **(d)** had multiple, wide, atrophic purple scars over the shins, which accumulated over the years from trauma.

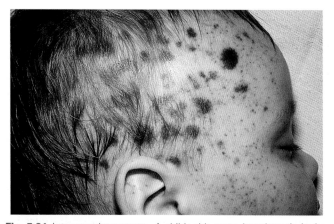

Fig. 7.24 Intravascular purpura. A child with acute lymphocytic leukemia shows bruises of various sizes, which are typically found in individuals with low platelet counts.

Disseminated Intravascular Coagulation

Bacterial sepsis, disseminated viral infection, malignancy, and medications may rarely trigger disseminated intravascular coagulation (DIC), with widespread bleeding into the skin and viscera. Rare benign infiltrative vascular tumors such as Kaposiform hemangioendotheliomas and tufted angiomas may also be associated with DIC known as the Kasabach-Merritt phenomenon.

This process is driven by a consumptive coagulopathy and fibrinolysis where platelets and clotting factors are consumed in the formation of clots in the microcirculation. Ecchymoses may progress rapidly to cover large areas of the body surface in minutes to hours (Fig. 7.25). Unfortunately, necrosis may develop in the center of some areas of purpura. In survivors, healing occurs with scarring and occasionally loss of digits or limbs.

Patients are usually critically ill, and death may ensue quickly unless supportive measures, including urgent volume expansion, vasopressors, and parenteral antibiotic therapy, are begun immediately. Some intensivists recommend treatment with heparin, fresh frozen plasma, platelet transfusion, and systemic steroids. However, the main goal in therapy should be directed at the underlying cause of the DIC. Laboratory studies demonstrate thrombocytopenia, decreased fibrinogen, prolonged bleeding time, and elevations in fibrin split products. In healthy children, meningococcemia, Rocky Mountain spotted fever, and streptococcal infections are the most common cause. In immunosuppressed patients, opportunistic organisms should also be considered.

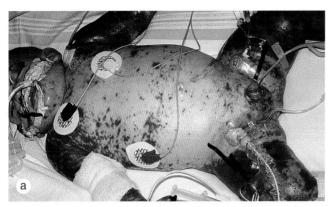
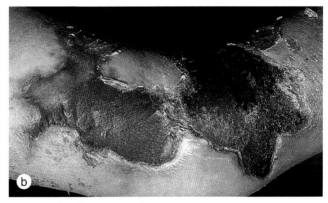

Fig. 7.25 Disseminated intravascular coagulation. **(a)** Purpura fulminans developed in this infant with meningococcemia. Widespread bleeding into the skin was noted, particularly on the extremities. **(b)** A toddler with staphylococcal sepsis and DIC developed widespread cutaneous necrosis on the legs.

Vascular Purpura

Vascular purpura develops when an inflammatory process involves the vessel wall (vasculitis). In leukocytoclastic vasculitis, the inflammation is predominantly neutrophilic. In lymphocytic vasculitis and late stages of leukocytoclastic vasculitis, vascular damage is caused by infiltrating mononuclear cells. Sweet syndrome shows primarily leukocytoclastic changes, whereas pyoderma gangrenosum shares features of leukocytoclastic and lymphocytic vasculitis. Granulomatous vasculitis is uncommon in children and usually presents in the setting of granulomatosis with polyangiitis (formerly called Wegener's) or eosinophilic granulomatosis with polyangiitis (formerly called Churg–Strauss).

Leukocytoclastic vasculitis results from immune complex deposition in dermal blood vessels and subsequent complement-activated leukocyte infiltration. Infections, medications, autoimmune disorders, and malignancy can all trigger vasculitis. Regardless the underlying cause, the clinical picture is typically palpable petechiae and purpura, which is more prominent on dependent areas such as the lower legs.

Leukocytoclastic vasculitis involves small, dermal blood vessels, usually postcapillary venules. Classic histologic findings include endothelial swelling, fibrin deposition within and around the vessels, neutrophilic infiltrate within the vessel walls, and nuclear dust (scattered nuclear fragments from neutrophils). Vascular destruction with hemorrhage may be prominent. Fresh biopsies demonstrate IgA and C3 deposition around the dermal blood vessels.

Henoch–Schönlein purpura. Henoch–Schönlein purpura (HSP) is the most common form of leukocytoclastic vasculitis to occur in children, with peak incidence between 4 and 8 years old. However, HSP can occur in infants and adults.

Although the rash is characterized by palpable purpura, the typical 2–10 mm diameter, purpuric papules may be preceded by several days of urticaria, hence HSP sometimes being referred to as anaphylactoid purpura or allergic vasculitis. Lesions most commonly pepper the buttocks and the extensor surfaces of the arms and legs. However, any site may be involved, including the face, ears, and trunk (Fig. 7.26). Crops erupt episodically for 2–4 weeks, and individual lesions usually fade over 3–5 days.

Confluent ecchymoses occasionally evolve from confluent small lesions, and rarely necrosis and hemorrhagic bullae develop. Scalp edema and periarticular swelling (Schönlein purpura) and paroxysmal abdominal colic with melena or frankly bloody stools (Henoch purpura) may occur before, during, or after the rash. Vasculitis may also involve vessels in the kidneys, lungs, and central nervous system.

Recurrences occur in about half of patients for up to several months, but these episodes are usually mild. In most cases, the visceral disease is self-limiting. However, acute renal failure develops rarely, and intussusception may complicate vasculitis in the bowel. More subtle renal disease may persist or develop over years and requires long-term monitoring.

Although most children with HSP may be observed at home, patients with progressive renal disease or severe abdominal pain require hospitalization. A normal blood count, platelet count, and coagulation studies help to differentiate HSP from intravascular forms of purpura. Identification of typical clinical findings and course, histopathology (leukocytoclastic vasculitis usually IgA positive), and other screening studies (e.g., antinuclear antibodies [ANA], rheumatoid factor, precipitin antibodies) exclude lupus erythematosus and other connective tissue disorders.

Acute hemorrhagic edema of infancy probably represents a variant of HSP occurring in children from 2 to 24 months old. However, skin lesions tend to be larger than those seen in HSP and characterized by discrete and confluent urticarial edematous plaques most commonly on the face and extremities, particularly the extensor surfaces of the arms. Edema of the hands and feet is common, and skin biopsies demonstrate a leukocytoclastic vasculitis similar to that seen in classic HSP but usually IgA negative. Fortunately, the course is usually shorter than HSP, recurrences are rare, and viscera are not usually involved.

Polyarteritis nodosa. Polyarteritis nodosa (PAN) is a leukocytoclastic vasculitis that involves small- and medium-sized arteries. A systemic form, which occurs extremely rarely in children, presents acutely with fever, weakness, abdominal pain, and cardiac failure. Despite treatment with high-dose corticosteroids and immunosuppressive agents, death may ensue

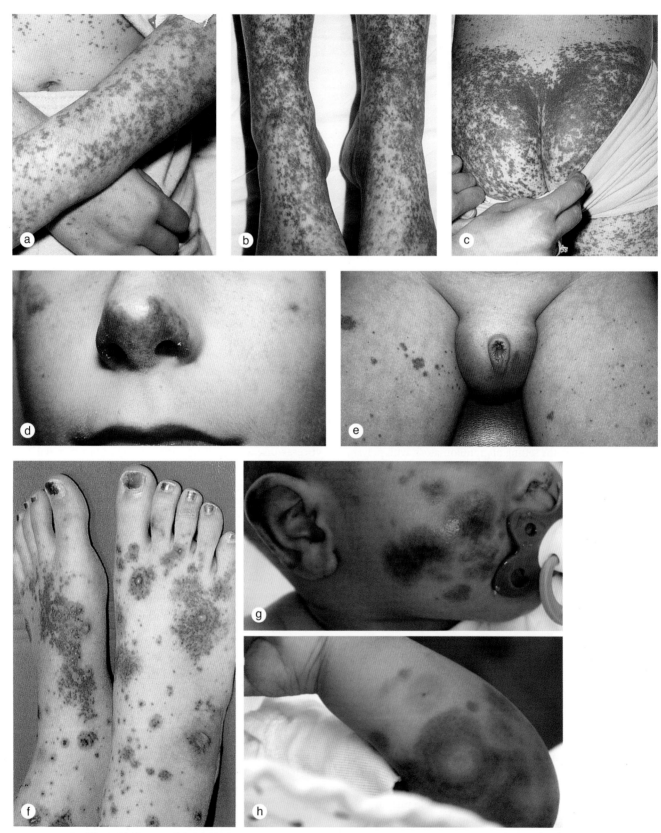

Fig. 7.26 Henoch–Schönlein purpura and acute hemorrhagic edema of infancy. Vasculitic lesions developed on the extensor surfaces of the **(a)** arms, **(b)** legs, and buttocks of this school age child. Any area including the **(d)** face and **(e)** genitals may be involved. Non-pitting edema of the face, chest, and genitals may be prominent, as in the child shown in **(e)**. **(f)** Necrosis of the skin overlying the vasculitic papules may result in vesicles and bullae, particularly on the feet. **(g,h)** This healthy 8-month-old boy had a brief febrile illness, followed by the development of large expanding annular red plaques with central purpura typical of acute hemorrhagic edema of infancy. He was asymptomatic and the rash resolved without recurrence 10 days later.

quickly from renal failure, gastrointestinal bleeding, and bowel perforation. Cutaneous lesions, which include livedo reticularis, erythema, and purpura on the lower extremities, are not diagnostic.

Cutaneous PAN is more likely to come to the attention of the dermatologist. In this distinct variant, cutaneous findings predominate and the viscera are usually spared. Crops of painful nodules and annular plaques blossom on the arms and legs, particularly the hands and feet, and less commonly on the trunk, head, and neck (Fig. 7.27). Urticaria, livedo, and cutaneous ulcerations may also develop. Episodes last for several weeks and tend to recur for years. Although severe systemic disease does not usually occur in the cutaneous form of PAN, fever and arthralgias frequently accompany flares in disease activity.

The diagnosis of cutaneous PAN is made by establishing the clinical pattern and histopathology, which demonstrates a leukocytoclastic vasculitis of medium-sized arteries. Patients usually respond quickly to prednisone, but resistant cases require methotrexate, azathioprine, intravenous immunoglobulin (IVIg), or cyclophosphamide. Nodules localized to the palms and soles melt away with intralesional corticosteroids. Long-term monitoring is required to detect those children who develop severe systemic involvement.

The painful nodules of cutaneous PAN may be difficult to differentiate from EN, cold panniculitis, and lupus panniculitis, particularly early in the course. Associated clinical findings and histopathology, however, are distinctive in these disorders.

Infectious Vasculitis

Although overwhelming infection with a number of bacterial organisms may trigger rapidly fatal DIC with widespread bleeding into the skin, mucous membranes, and viscera, many patients develop discrete vasculitic lesions. In fact, the presence of 0.5–2 cm diameter, angulated, pink-to-red hemorrhagic macules, papules, pustules, and plaques is associated with a relatively good prognosis (Fig. 7.28). Over several hours, lesions become hemorrhagic and central necrosis with bulla formation

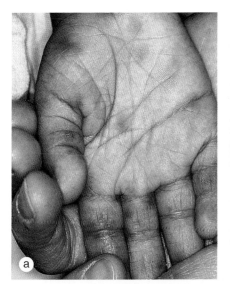
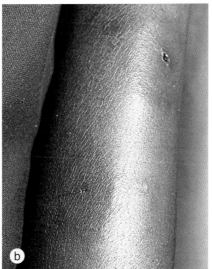
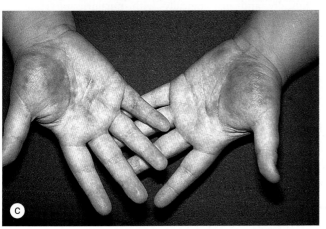
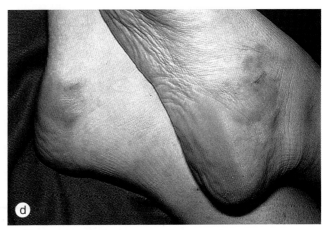

Fig. 7.27 Polyarteritis nodosa. Over several days a 3-year-old girl developed painful nodules on the trunk, face, and extremities. **(a)** Lesions on the hands were associated with arthritis. **(b)** Some of the nodules on the legs developed central necrotic vesicles. A 13-year-old girl with chronic cutaneous polyarteritis nodosa complained of recurrent, painful, violaceous nodules on her **(c)** hands and **(d)** feet.

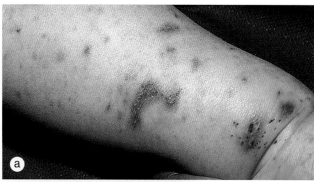

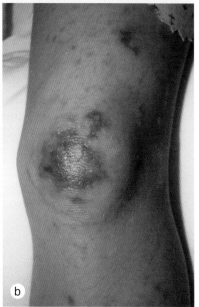

Fig. 7.28 Infectious vasculitis. **(a)** Sharply angulated, purpuric, and necrotic papules developed on the extremities of a toddler with meningococcemia. He presented with meningitis and responded quickly to parenteral antibiotics. **(b)** A similar rash appeared on the extremities of a 10-year-old boy with Rocky Mountain spotted fever. In both children, vasculitic papules and plaques spread to the palms and soles, and to a lesser extent, the trunk.

or ulceration may develop. Prompt recognition of this condition and the initiation of antibiotics and supportive care may be life-saving.

Although the rash may be caused by hematogenous dissemination of the organism to the skin, many lesions result from immune complex deposition in dermal vessels. For example, Osler nodes (tender nodules on the finger or toe pads) and Janeway lesions (small, painless nodules on the palms and soles) probably represent an immune-mediated vasculitic phenomenon (Fig. 7.29). *Neisseria meningitidis, Neisseria gonorrhoeae, Haemophilus influenzae* type B, *Streptococcus pneumoniae*, other *Streptococcus* spp., and *Staphylococcus aureus* have been cultured from blood and skin in normal hosts with infectious vasculitis (Fig. 7.29d). Rocky Mountain spotted fever may produce a similar clinical picture, but the inflammation tends to be primarily lymphocytic. In immunosuppressed individuals, these organisms, as well as opportunistic bacteria and fungi, must also be considered. Ecthyma gangrenosum, characterized

by a punched-out ulceration with a central opalescent eschar and a hemorrhagic border, is a prototypic infectious vasculitis. It typically results from *Pseudomonas* septicemia (Fig. 7.30). Lesions typically appear on the lower abdominal wall, thighs, and groin in patients with leukemia, burn patients, and other debilitated individuals who have been on antibiotics. Although most patients are severely ill with multiple lesions, in some cases only one or several indolent ulcers are present. Other Gram-negative organisms, as well as fungi such as *Candida* and *Aspergillus* spp., may produce the same type of skin lesions.

The diagnosis of ecthyma gangrenosum can be made by searching for organisms in Gram-stains obtained from pustules and necrotic ulcers. Identification of specific organisms from blood and tissue cultures is required to select the appropriate antibiotics. Skin biopsies show a necrotizing vasculitis with neutrophils and a variable number of bacteria within vessels. Aplastic patients may show minimal inflammation with large numbers of organisms.

Lymphocytic Vasculitis

Rather than being a distinct entity, lymphocytic vasculitis represents a reaction pattern in the skin found in a number of disorders in which lymphocytic inflammation predominates. Lymphocytic vasculitis has been described in cutaneous drug reactions as vasculitic lesions of Sjögren syndrome, and as a late phase of leukocytoclastic vasculitis. Pigmented purpuric dermatosis (PPD) is the prototypic lymphocytic vasculitis.

The development of asymptomatic localized patches of petechiae and larger patches of purpura, particularly on the lower extremities, characterizes PPD (Fig. 7.31a). Hemosiderin deposition and postinflammatory hyperpigmentation lead to shades of brown, gold, and bronze as lesions evolve. Confluent patches may form a reticulated pattern. Although lesions are usually flat and asymptomatic, fine scale and lichenoid papules may be associated with mild pruritus. In the lichen aureus variant, rusty brown patches on the trunk, particularly the lower back, have been misdiagnosed as child abuse (Fig. 7.31b). Occasionally, disseminated lesions erupt over a few days to a few weeks and resolve over 2–3 months. This variant of PPD may overlap clinically and histologically with purpuric pityriasis rosea (Fig. 7.31c).

Skin biopsies from active areas demonstrate lymphocytes around and within the walls of superficial dermal capillaries. Mild hemorrhage and hemosiderin deposition are also present.

Clinically and histologically, it may be impossible to differentiate PPD from a drug reaction, and occasionally practitioners have reported children with large patches over the lower back or buttocks for suspected abuse. Unfortunately, no treatment has proved satisfactory, and lesions may persist for years. Systemic and topical corticosteroids and pulsed-dye laser therapy may arrest progression temporarily.

Sweet Syndrome

Sweet syndrome—also referred to as acute febrile neutrophilic dermatosis—is not a true vasculitis, but it can be confused clinically for early vasculitic lesions and display some leukocytoclasia on histology. It is characterized by violaceous, 0.5–3 cm

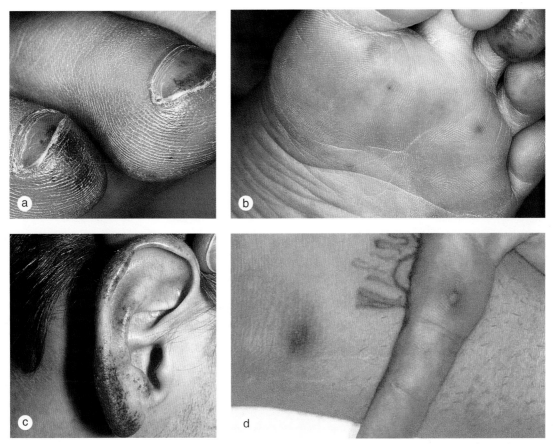

Fig. 7.29 Infectious vasculitis. **(a)** Osler nodes, splinter hemorrhages, and **(b)** Janeway lesions appeared on the hands and feet of this 10-year-old boy with acute bacterial endocarditis caused by *Staphylococcus aureus*. **(c)** Another child with subacute bacterial endocarditis developed vasculitis papules on his ears. **(d)** These exquisitely tender pustules on the right index finger and left ankle were the only cutaneous findings in a 16-year-old girl with gonococcal arthritis dermatitis syndrome. Blood cultures were negative, but cultures from the cervix grew *Neisseria gonorrhoeae*.

diameter nodules and plaques that erupt abruptly on the face and extremities (Fig. 7.32). Recurrent crops of nodules that appear over 1–8 months are heralded by high fever, arthralgias, and occasionally periarticular swelling and arthritis. Necrotic vesicles and bullae may also form. Although Sweet syndrome is self-limiting, symptoms may be debilitating. Skin lesions, arthralgias, and fever usually melt away with systemic corticosteroids; however, recurrences are common when the medication is tapered.

Although initially described in middle-aged women, a number of cases have been reported in infants and children. About 10% of adult cases are associated with myeloproliferative disorders, especially acute myelocytic or myelomonocytic leukemia. Children with this syndrome require a thorough physical examination and laboratory evaluation, including a blood count, peripheral smear, and bone marrow biopsy, to exclude any underlying disorder.

Sweet syndrome may be confused with EM, EN, viral exanthems, HSP, infectious vasculitis, and PAN. Although Sweet syndrome may be suspected because of the cutaneous lesions and clinical course, skin biopsy of a fresh lesion demonstrates diagnostic findings, which include a dense, perivascular, neutrophilic infiltrate and intense edema in the upper dermis; some leukocytoclasia without true vasculitis; and, in some cases, subepidermal bullae formation.

Pyoderma Gangrenosum

Pyoderma gangrenosum, similar to Sweet syndrome, can often be mistaken for a vasculitic process. It is characterized by painful pustules or nodules that develop central necrosis and an enlarging ulcer with a hemorrhagic, purple, undermined advancing border (Fig. 7.33). Ulcers range in size from about 1 cm in diameter when they first appear to over 10 cm as they evolve. One or several lesions may occur, and any area, including the face, trunk, and extremities, may be involved. Lesions rarely develop in the upper airway and trachea. Pathergy, or the development of new lesions at sites of trauma (e.g., venipunctures or biopsy) is a reliable diagnostic clue. An underlying systemic disease, such as inflammatory bowel disease, myelogenous leukemia, or rheumatoid arthritis, is associated with cutaneous lesions in half of the cases.

Skin biopsies show typical (but non-diagnostic) findings, which include a lymphocytic vasculitis at the advancing border and necrosis with abscess formation and reactive

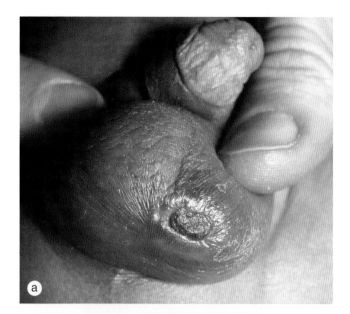

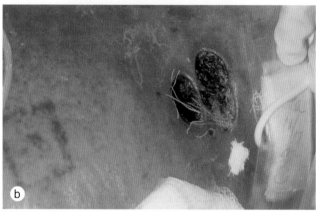

Fig. 7.30 Ecthyma gangrenosum. **(a)** An infant with an inherited immunodeficiency experienced recurrent episodes of Gram-negative septicemia. *Pseudomonas* grew from cultures obtained from blood and the necrotic, crusted ulcer on the scrotum. **(b)** This 6-year-old liver transplant recipient developed a high fever and black necrotic bullae, which ulcerated on his lower abdominal wall. A skin biopsy of the ulcer and blood cultures grew Gram-negative *Citrobacter*.

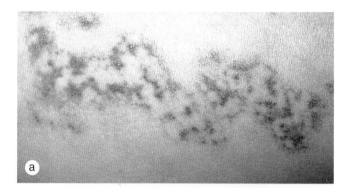

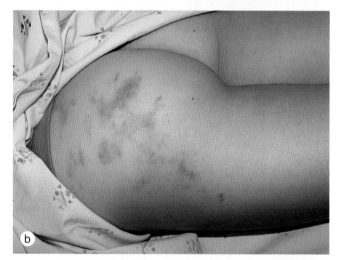

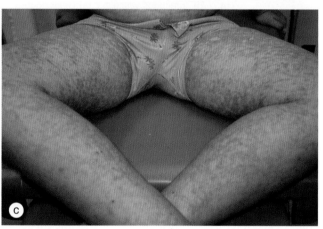

Fig. 7.31 Progressive pigmented purpuric dermatosis. **(a)** Reticulated hyperpigmented patches had slowly advanced across the leg of a 15-year-old girl for years. **(b)** A golden-brown eruption on this preschooler's left buttock was thought originally to represent physical abuse. **(c)** A diffuse asymptomatic eruption on this 9-year-old boy resolved without treatment 8 weeks after it appeared. Histologic findings were typical of pigmented purpura.

polymorphous inflammation that extends into the subcutaneous tissue.

Pyoderma gangrenosum usually responds to treatment of the underlying condition. Idiopathic cases can be treated with antibiotics, systemic corticosteroids, dapsone, or tumor necrosis factor inhibitors. Resistant cases may require immunosuppressive agents such as azathioprine, methotrexate, or cyclosporine.

Granulomatous Vasculitis

Granulomatous vasculitis is a term used to describe necrotizing granulomatous inflammation restricted to blood vessels. However, in granulomatosis with polyangiitis (formerly called Wegener's) or eosinophilic granulomatosis with polyangiitis (formerly called Churg–Strauss), which occasionally occur in children, granuloma formation typically occurs in extravascular sites.

In granulomatosis with polyangiitis, necrotizing vasculitis and granulomas involve the upper and lower respiratory tracts and are accompanied by a focal necrotizing glomerulonephritis. Arteries and veins in multiple organs can be involved, including the skin. Cutaneous lesions (Fig. 7.34) including painful papules, nodules, necrotic vesicles, and large ulcers resembling pyoderma gangrenosum may disseminate over the extensor

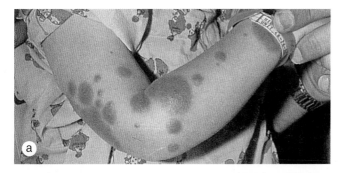

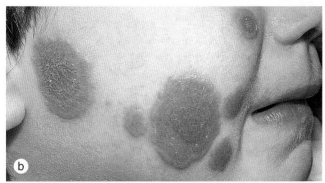

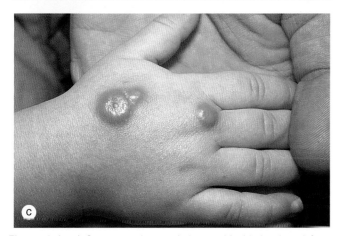

Fig. 7.32 (a–c) Sweet syndrome. A 2-year-old girl developed fever, arthritis, leukocytosis, and widely disseminated, red-to-violaceous plaques and nodules, which demonstrated intense neutrophilic inflammation on skin biopsy. An extensive evaluation failed to reveal any underlying disease. Although she responded quickly to systemic corticosteroids, it took nearly a year to wean her because of frequent recurrences.

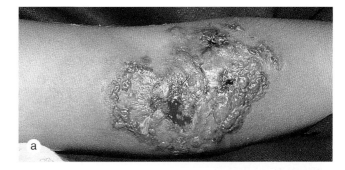

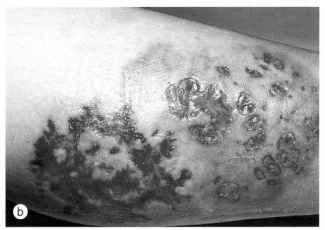

Fig. 7.33 Pyoderma gangrenosum. **(a)** A 9-year-old boy developed a painful, expanding, crusted, necrotic plaque with an undermined border on his arm. An exhaustive medical evaluation was unrevealing until bone marrow biopsy demonstrated chronic myelogenous leukemia. **(b)** A similar plaque in a teenager with Crohn disease shows cribriform scarring as inflammation abates. Lesions in both children healed after aggressive treatment of the underlying disorders.

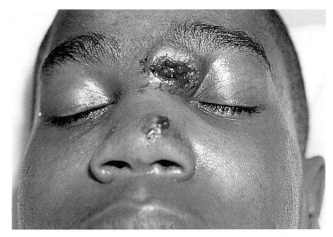

Fig. 7.34 Granulomatosis with polyangiitis (formerly called Wegener's granulomatosis). This 17-year-old boy developed ulcerated nodules on his nose in association with renal and pulmonary disease. All lesions cleared with systemic steroids and cyclophosphamide.

FIGURATE ERYTHEMA

A number of disorders are characterized by the development of annular plaques with a well-defined, advancing, red border and central clearing. Typical, but non-diagnostic, histologic findings include a tight, perivascular, mononuclear cell infiltrate in the

surfaces of the extremities and buttocks. Although not diagnostic, 80% of patients demonstrate antineutrophil cytoplasmic antibodies, usually of the cytoplasmic type (c-ANCA).

The cutaneous features of eosinophilic granulomatosis with polyangiitis overlap with those of granulomatosis with polyangiitis. However, this disorder is distinguished by the presence of systemic vasculitis associated with hypereosinophilia in the setting of pre-existing asthma and allergic rhinitis. Tender nodules may arise on the scalp or more widely on the extremities and less commonly the trunk. Distinctive histologic findings include a necrotizing vasculitis, tissue infiltration by eosinophils, and extravascular granulomas.

superficial dermis, with occasional extension to the mid- and deep-dermis. The overlying epidermis is normal or shows mild spongiosis. Erythema annulare centrifugum (EAC) and erythema chronicum migrans, now usually referred to as erythema migrans, are the most commonly recognized figurate erythemas in children.

Erythema Annulare Centrifugum

In EAC, one or multiple asymptomatic, expanding, annular or serpiginous red plaques with well-defined raised borders and trailing scales on the inner aspect of the border occur (Fig. 7.35). As lesions progress from <1 cm to over 20 cm in diameter over several weeks, new plaques may arise within the borders to produce concentric rings. The eruption typically spreads from the central trunk to the proximal extremities (centrifugal), and lesions continue to evolve for months to years.

Although EAC probably represents a hypersensitivity reaction to the same sort of phenomena that trigger urticaria and other reactive erythemas, a number of reports suggest a common association with chronic dermatophyte infection (e.g., tinea pedis, tinea cruris). Cases of EAC may erupt throughout childhood, but it occurs most commonly in adults. Annular erythema of infancy is undoubtedly a clinical variant of this disorder (Fig. 7.35c).

The persistence of individual lesions and lack of pruritus differentiate EAC from urticaria. The chronic course and absence of viral symptoms help to exclude an urticarial viral exanthem. Granuloma annulare may be excluded by the finding of epidermal changes (erythema and scale) in EAC. Although there are no specific laboratory tests for EAC, skin biopsy typically shows a tight, lymphocytic, perivascular infiltrate (coat-sleeve pattern) in the mid-dermis and deep dermis. Dermatitic changes may also be present in the epidermis.

When a fungal infection is identified, oral antifungal medications may result in clearing of the rash. Otherwise, no specific treatment is indicated.

Erythema Migrans

In erythema migrans, which marks the onset of Lyme disease, a single papule begins 3–30 days after a tick bite and expands quickly to form an enlarging, annular red plaque with central clearing (Fig. 7.36). New lesions resulting from hematogenous spread of the organism may continue to evolve successively or in crops over several months. Plaques over 4 cm in diameter are typical, and some may exceed 30 cm. Mild, influenza-like symptoms, which include headache, sore throat, arthralgias, and malaise, are commonly associated with the skin rash. If untreated, resolution of skin lesions is followed several months later by a pauciarticular arthritis that involves the knees, elbows, and/or wrists in 50% of patients. In 15% of cases, neurologic abnormalities, including meningoencephalitis, neuropathy, or facial palsy, occur 2 weeks to 8 months after the tick bite. Cardiac symptoms, which appear in 5% of patients, may mimic rheumatic fever.

Lyme disease is caused by the spirochete *Borrelia burgdorferi*, which can be carried by *Ixodes scapularis* and related ticks (Fig. 7.36e). These ticks are widely distributed

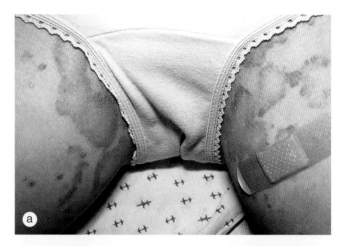

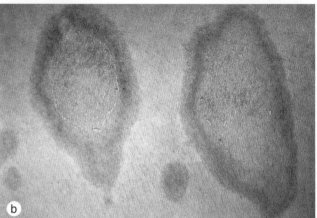

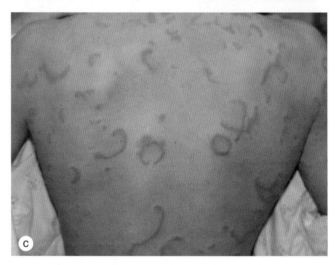

Fig. 7.35 Erythema annulare centrifugum. **(a)** Symmetric, annular, red plaques slowly expanded on the anterior thighs of a 10-year-old girl. **(b)** Another child with large lesions on the trunk demonstrates the bright red border with fine trailing scale and central clearing. **(c)** Like his father, this adolescent boy has had a generalized evolving annular eruption since early infancy.

throughout the United States and Europe, and in many places such as coastal New England, the Great Lakes states, and the mid-Atlantic coast, the infection has become endemic. The ticks can be the size of a pinhead, and up to 50% of patients do not recall the bite.

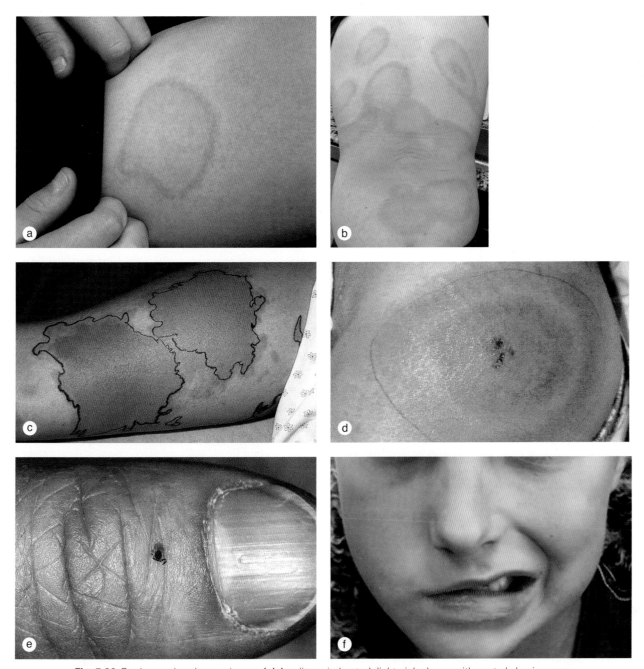

Fig. 7.36 Erythema chronicum migrans. **(a)** A solitary, indurated, light-pink plaque with central clearing grew over several weeks from a small, red papule at the site of a tick bite. The lesion, as well as associated arthralgias and intermittent low-grade fever, resolved within 48 h of starting oral amoxicillin. **(b)** A few days after removing a tick from his back this adolescent developed a single expanding annular red plaque on his back. Two days later he developed a fever and multiple lesions appeared on his face, trunk, and extremities. Within 24 h of starting oral doxycycline he defervesced and most of the plaques disappeared. **(c)** In this 12-year-old girl, two solid, dark-red patches were initially diagnosed and treated as cellulitis. **(d)** This adolescent boy developed several concentric expanding rings around the central tick bite. **(e)** The spirochete is transmitted from animals to humans by the tiny *Ixodes dammini* and related tick vectors. **(f)** This 11-year-old boy developed a low-grade fever, a headache, and a single expanding annular red plaque on the side of his scalp. He also improved quickly with oral doxycycline.

The incidence of Lyme disease is highest in children, particularly boys, in whom multiple lesions are common, but all ages are affected. Although the diagnosis is usually made clinically, more reliable serologic tests may aid in differentiation of the annular plaques of erythema migrans from urticaria, viral exanthems, erythema marginatum, and EAC. Skin biopsy specimens obtained from the expanding border or the center of lesions may demonstrate spirochetes with the use of special silver stains in up to 50% of cases. When available, PCR studies and immunoperoxidase staining of monoclonal antibodies to the axial filaments of *Borrelia* are highly sensitive and specific. It is important to note that in early Lyme disease (<2 weeks), serologic testing can be negative. Otherwise, the histopathologic findings are not diagnostic and show changes typical of insect-bite reactions.

Any individual in an endemic area who develops an annular eruption, especially if it is associated with viral symptoms and a tick bite, should be treated to reduce the risk of arthritis and other late complications. Although treatment recommendations vary, a 14–21-day course of doxycycline 100 mg twice a day is the choice for older children and adults, and amoxicillin at a dose of 25–50 mg/kg per day, with a maximum of 2 g daily given in three divided doses, is recommended for children younger than 8 years old. Children allergic to penicillin may be treated with cefuroxime, 30 mg/kg per day in two divided doses (maximum 1000 mg/day or 1.0 g/day for 14–21 days).

Avoiding tick-infested areas or wearing protective clothing reduces the risk of exposure. Tick repellents containing diethyltoluamide (DEET) are also effective. However, excessive use of diethyltoluamide, particularly in infants and young children, has been associated with neurotoxic reactions. Low-concentration lotions (Skedaddle 7.25% and OFF 10–30%) are as effective as traditional repellents with concentrations over 50% and have a much better safety profile; however, their effects may not last as long and require more frequent application. The American Academy of Pediatrics currently recommends the use of products containing 10–30% DEET. Alternative repellents containing picaridin may also be effective. Tick inspections after hikes and camping trips and removal of ticks within 24–48 h of attachment also reduce transmission of the spirochete. Prophylactic treatment of tick bites before the development of erythema migrans has not been shown to be effective.

PANNICULITIS

Panniculitis refers to a group of disorders in which an inflammatory process involves the fat lobules, intervening fat septae, or both. Clinically, patients present with deep-seated, poorly defined, tender, erythematous to violaceous nodules. The overlying epidermis is usually intact, although it may be taut and shiny. Because of the inflammation occurring in deeper tissue, epidermal scaling is not typically seen. If necrosis develops, ulcerations may occur.

Erythema Nodosum

EN is the most common panniculitis to appear in children, usually in adolescents. Typically, painful, red subcutaneous nodules and plaques, 1–5 cm in diameter, erupt on the shins, but lesions may also involve the arms and thighs, and rarely the trunk and face (Fig. 7.37). Nodules usually fade over several weeks, but recurrences are frequent. In some cases, crops can recur for months.

Over 100 years ago, the development of EN with tuberculosis was recognized. More recently, EN has been associated with a number of infections, including viral pharyngitis, streptococcal pharyngitis, histoplasmosis, coccidioidomycosis, and other deep fungi and atypical mycobacteria. Non-infectious inflammatory conditions, such as sarcoidosis, inflammatory bowel disease, lupus erythematosus, and medications (namely, oral contraceptives and non-steroidal anti-inflammatory drugs [NSAIDs]) may trigger the reaction.

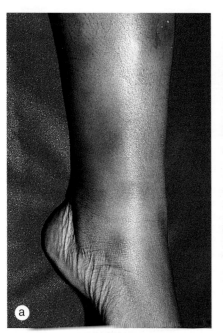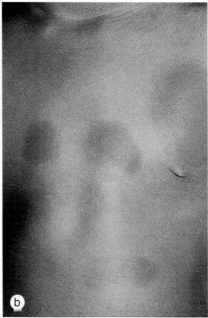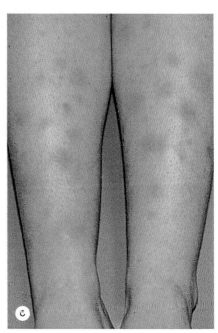

Fig. 7.37 Erythema nodosum. **(a)** Tender, deep-seated nodules appeared on the shins of a 16-year-old girl 2 weeks after starting birth-control pills. The lesions resolved when the medication was discontinued. **(b)** An 18-month-old boy developed (biopsy proved) erythema nodosum on the chest and abdomen after a cold. The nodules resolved without therapy over several weeks. **(c)** This 15-year-old girl developed recurrent biopsy-proven erythema nodosum on her shins with flares of her systemic lupus erythematosus.

On histology, the finding of a septal panniculitis without fat necrosis is characteristic of EN. Early in the course, neutrophilic inflammation is common. Later, lymphocytes, histiocytes, and giant cells predominate. Vessels show endothelial cell swelling, inflammation in the vascular walls, and hemorrhage.

In most children, EN is self-limiting and treatment, when necessary, is tailored to the underlying disorder. Leg elevation and NSAIDs may help to reduce the pain.

Cold Panniculitis

In infants and young children, cold injury can result in intracellular crystallization and rupture of fat cells with subsequent inflammation. Persistent, indurated red nodules and plaques appear most commonly on the cheeks, but the trunk and extremities may also be involved (Fig. 7.38). Ulceration and atrophy do not usually develop, and nodules resolve without treatment in several weeks to several months.

Although the cause is not known, the increased saturation of fatty acids in the subcutaneous fat of infants compared with adults makes their fat more prone to solidification at low temperatures. Morphologically, cold panniculitis may be confused with bacterial cellulitis (Fig. 7.39). However, in cel-

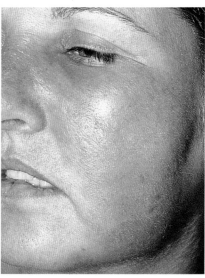

Fig. 7.39 Facial cellulitis/erysipelas. A painful, indurated red plaque spread within several hours across the cheek of this 17-year-old girl. She also had a fever and tender cervical adenopathy, which resolved on parenteral penicillin.

lulitis the indurated plaques are warm, tender, and progressive, and the patients are febrile and of toxic appearance. Other nodular erythemas, such as PAN and EN, are usually differentiated by the clinical course and skin biopsy findings when necessary.

Subcutaneous Fat Necrosis of the Newborn

Subcutaneous fat necrosis of the newborn is a variant of cold panniculitis that occurs within the first month of life. Several circumscribed lesions appear on the trunk and proximal extremities in an otherwise healthy infant. Nodules heal without scarring, but transient depression of the skin surface occurs frequently and ulceration on occasion. Even after the skin lesions have resolved, affected infants should be monitored for up to 6 months of age for hypercalcemia with resultant renal calcinosis and failure to thrive.

Sclerema Neonatorum

In contrast to infants with cold panniculitis, infants who develop sclerema neonatorum are severely ill. In this process, widespread, woody induration of the skin develops. This process probably results as a complication of multisystem failure and associated cooling of the skin and fat from decreased cutaneous perfusion. In skin biopsies from these infants, edema of the fibrous septae is found with no necrosis of fat cells. In contrast, subcutaneous fat necrosis of the newborn and cold panniculitis are associated with necrosis of fat cells and granulomatous inflammation.

Lupus Panniculitis

In lupus panniculitis, persistent, purple, painless nodules, 1–5 cm in diameter, develop on the face, extremities, and buttocks (Fig. 7.40). Although these lesions may occur in a child with other signs of systemic lupus erythematosus (SLE), they

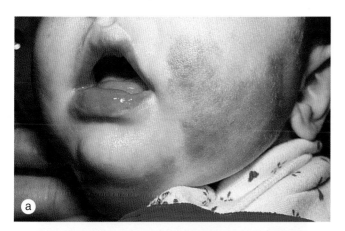

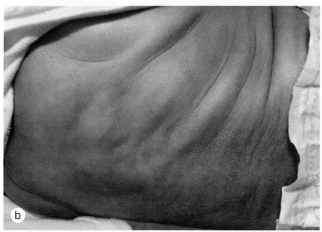

Fig. 7.38 (a) Cold panniculitis appeared on the cheeks and chin of this 6-month-old infant 1 day after he was given an ice-filled teething ring. (b) This healthy newborn had tender subcutaneous confluent nodules on her back at birth. All lesions resolved by 2 months of age, and calcium studies were normal.

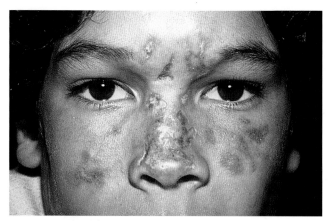

Fig. 7.40 Lupus panniculitis. A 13-year-old boy presented with chronic, recurring, deep-seated nodules and plaques, which healed with punched-out scars.

may be the first or only manifestation of the disease. Individual lesions may persist for months to years, and ulceration, scarring, and/or atrophy occur frequently. Unfortunately, lupus panniculitis is often resistant to treatment with antimalarial drugs, and the use of systemic corticosteroids and immunosuppressive agents should probably be guided by systemic symptoms.

Histopathology is non-specific and shows lymphohistiocytic inflammation within the fat lobules and hyalinization of fat cells. Inflammation and vasculitis may also occur in the fat septae.

PHOTOSENSITIVITY

Photosensitivity is a term used to describe a group of conditions marked by abnormal reactions to light. Sunburn is a phototoxic reaction that results from exposure to naturally occurring, short-wavelength ultraviolet (UV)B light. Longer wavelength (UVA) light is only weakly phototoxic; however, all individuals deliberately or accidentally exposed to high-enough doses of topical or oral UVA-photosensitizing agents may also develop burns. In photoallergic reactions, susceptible patients, who are exposed to certain photosensitizing chemicals or drugs, develop an immunologically mediated rash that is activated by light. A number of genetic and metabolic disorders are associated with photosensitivity, and the recognition of cutaneous findings may be a clue to diagnosis. Photodermatoses include several specific conditions that have unusual reactions to light. In some of these dermatoses, the action spectrum, or the wavelengths that trigger the skin findings, have been described. Finally, other diseases may be exacerbated by light. The recognition of this phenomenon may be important in managing these conditions.

Phototoxic and Photoallergic Reactions

Exposure of the skin to sunlight results in a number of biologic reactions. Small amounts of UVB activate the conversion of 7-dehydrocholesterol into vitamin D3. Large amounts of UV light produce erythema and swelling, known as sunburn (Fig. 7.41). Intense reactions may result in the development of blistering burns on sun-exposed surfaces. Healing is marked by desquamation, thickening, and hyperpigmentation of the skin.

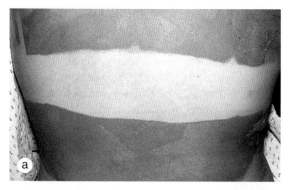

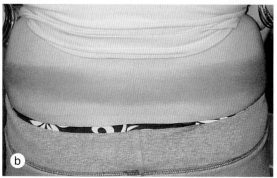

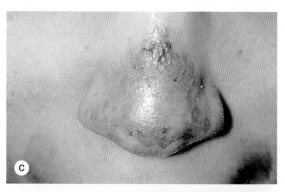

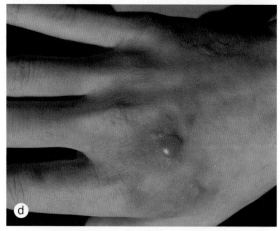

Fig. 7.41 Phototoxic reaction. **(a)** A severe sunburn developed in sun-exposed areas after this teenager applied a topical photosensitizing cream to her skin and spent the day outdoors. Note the areas of sparing under her bathing suit. **(b)** This adolescent lacrosse player was burned in a narrow, unprotected band above her waist. **(c)** A 16-year-old boy returned from a winter ski trip where he forgot to protect his nose with sunscreen. **(d)** This adolescent girl developed a phytophotodermatitis (phototoxic reaction) after she spilled lime juice on her hands at the beach and forgot to clean them and protect them from sun exposure.

Although UVB is 100 times more erythemogenic than UVA, the large quantity of UVA ($1000\times$ UVB) that reaches the ground contributes substantially to sunburn (10–15%). On overcast days, when 15–20% of UVB is absorbed and scattered by the cloud cover, the role of UVA is even greater. The minimum dose of light required to produce a discrete area of cutaneous erythema is referred to as the minimal erythema dose (MED). The MED tends to increase with increasing skin types. Individuals with skin type 1 always burn and never tan. These people have blonde or red hair and blue eyes, and often demonstrate freckling in sun-exposed sites. Skin type 2 denotes individuals who always burn at first but sometimes tan after repeated sun exposure. Type 3 people occasionally burn but tan readily. Olive-complected individuals who always tan fall into type 4. Types 5 and 6 include members of darkly pigmented races.

Factors that potentiate the development of sunburn include increasing elevation above sea level, wind, low humidity, and applications that result in thinning of the epidermis, such as peeling agents (topical retinoids, salicylic acid, lactic acid). Damage to DNA is the initiating event in the development of the erythema response. The subsequent production of inflammatory mediators (e.g., prostaglandins, histamine) triggers the clinical response. Factors that interfere with normal DNA repair mechanisms (hereditary defects in DNA repair enzymes or antimetabolites, such as methotrexate) result in an exaggerated, recurrent, or prolonged erythema response.

Wrinkling, elastosis, lentigines, and other "age"-related changes in the skin result from long-term exposure to sunlight; the majority of most individuals' lifetime exposure occurs during childhood and young adult life. It has been estimated that the incidence of non-melanoma skin cancers (basal cell carcinoma and squamous cell carcinoma) could be reduced by 75–80% if people used sun-protective clothing, sunscreens (chemicals that absorb UV light), and sunblocks (agents that reflect sunlight) from early childhood. Although most sunscreens (e.g., para-aminobenzoic acid, its esters, and cinnamates) provide good coverage against UVB, the number of UVA-protective agents is limited (see Chapter 1). The sun-protective factor (SPF) of a product is determined by calculating the ratio of the MED of unprotected skin to the MED of sunscreen-protected skin. In infants, who should not be left in the sun, sunscreens are only rarely necessary. Parents of ambulatory children, particularly individuals with light pigmentation, should be given aggressive counseling about sun protection. People with skin types 1 and 2 must use sunscreens/sunblocks with an SPF of at least 30 (preferably 50 or greater), whereas darker-pigmented individuals may be safe with lower SPFs, particularly after gradually increasing sun exposure has produced protective darkening of the skin. The U.S. Food and Drug Administration (FDA) is currently evaluating the ingredients in sunscreens, and its forthcoming rulings will likely result in dramatic changes to the compositions available.

Unlike phototoxicity, which can occur in any individual given enough UV radiation, photoallergic reactions involve an immunologic response in a small number of individuals who are sensitized to certain chemicals or drugs in the presence of sunlight. In many cases, a type 4 delayed hypersensitivity reaction results in the development of an eczematous dermatitis in a sun-exposed distribution, rather than a sunburn. A number of medications have been implicated in the production of both phototoxic and photoallergic reactions. Some of the most common photosensitizers are furocoumarins, nalidixic acid, dyes, salicylanilides, fragrances, para-aminobenzoic acid, phenothiazines, sulfonamides, tetracyclines, thiazides and related sulfonamide diuretics, and NSAIDs. Pseudoporphyria, cutaneous photosensitivity resulting in symptoms and skin findings mimicking porphyria in individuals without evidence of a defect in porphyrin metabolism, has been reported with exposure to a number of medications (most commonly NSAIDs). Patients on these drugs must be warned to protect themselves against the risk of photosensitivity.

Rarely, photoactivated, eczematous reactions persist for months or years. A persistent light reaction usually evolves from a previous photocontact allergic dermatitis, but oral medications have been implicated as well. In actinic reticuloid (also known as chronic actinic dermatitis), the chronic dermatitis often spreads to involve covered sites, the lesions become lichenified and nodular, and skin biopsies may show lymphoma-like infiltrates in addition to a chronic dermatitis. In these patients, the dermatitis may be reproduced on normal patches of skin by exposure to UVA, UVB, and sometimes visible light, and MEDs at various wavelengths of UV light are markedly decreased. Some patients with atopic dermatitis note a flare of disease activity in sun-exposed sites. These individuals may be differentiated from patients with photoactivated eczematous reactions by the absence of exposure to photosensitizing drugs and topical agents, negative photopatch tests, and an abnormal MED to UVB only.

Polymorphous Light Eruption

Several photo-induced dermatoses may be identified by distinctive clinical and histologic findings. Polymorphous light eruption (PMLE) is the most common childhood photodermatosis, accounting for over 75% of photo-induced rashes. In PMLE, crops of red macules, papules, vesicles, or plaques typically erupt on exposed areas several hours to several days after intensive sun exposure in the early spring (Fig. 7.42). The morphology of lesions varies from patient to patient. However, the rash tends to be monomorphous in a given individual. PMLE appears most commonly in girls and women under 30 years old and may recur each spring for years. Although the rash usually progresses for several weeks, complete regression occurs within 3–4 weeks, despite continued light exposure. It is thought that with continued exposure a "hardening" of the skin occurs, such that the previous light exposure that would elicit a reaction can no longer do so. In fact, phototherapy (psoralen-UVA, narrow band UVB, and UVA-1) has been used to trigger the reaction deliberately and treat or "harden" the skin in a controlled setting to avoid inconvenient expression of the rash. PMLE is most common in temperate or northern climates, where the hardening of the skin tends to wane during the winter months. In the sunbelt states and tropics, where sun exposure occurs all year round, the rash is less common and often spares the face and "V" of the neck, which are most prominently exposed and hardened all year round.

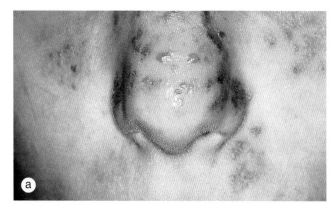

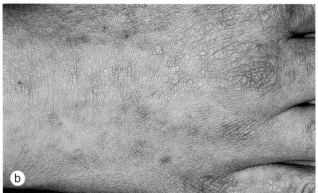

Fig. 7.42 Polymorphous light eruption. **(a)** Red papules and vesicles erupted on the face of a 14-year-old girl after a trip to the beach in the spring. She had experienced this phenomenon every spring for the previous 5 years. **(b)** An 8-year-old girl developed a mildly pruritic, papular rash on the tops of her hands and face after a spring picnic. In both girls the rashes peaked within several weeks and healed despite continuing sun exposure.

The histopathology of PMLE typically shows an intense, lymphocytic, perivascular infiltrate in the upper and mid-dermis. Dermal edema may also be prominent. Differential diagnosis from lupus erythematosus may be difficult clinically and histologically. The histology of lupus usually demonstrates inflammation at the dermal–epidermal junction and the dermal infiltrate often surrounds both adnexal structures and vessels. Laboratory evaluation with ANA and extractable nuclear antigens (ENA) can help distinguish these entities, as they should be negative in pure PMLE. However, early in the course of lupus, the histology may be non-specific, clinical findings may be confined to the skin, and serologic studies may be negative.

Solar Urticaria

Although urticaria after sun exposure may be caused by medications or associated with systemic illness, such as lupus or porphyria, a rare group of otherwise healthy individuals develops hives within minutes of sun exposure. Although the lesions may become quite itchy and extensive, symptoms usually abate with continued light exposure, similar to the hardening response seen in PMLE. Various wavelengths of light, including UV and visible radiation, have been associated with hives.

In many cases, solar urticaria is caused by a type 1 IgE-mediated reaction, and lesions result from the release of histamine and other vasoactive substances. In time, inflammatory mediators are depleted and lesions subside. Unfortunately, antihistamines only partially suppress solar urticaria. However, persistent light exposure can be maintained with phototherapy to keep the reaction under control.

Genetic Disorders

A number of inherited and metabolic disorders are associated with photosensitivity. In xeroderma pigmentosum (see Fig. 6.3), Bloom syndrome, Cockayne syndrome, and Rothmund–Thomson syndrome, light alone triggers an abnormal reaction in the skin and subsequent acute and chronic changes. These conditions all exhibit abnormal DNA repair or synthases, and their photosensitivity derive from an inability of keratinocytes to fix the UV-induced damage derived from regular levels of UV exposure. Disorders that result in pigment dilution, such as albinism, phenylketonuria, and other aminoacidopathies, markedly increase sensitivity to phototoxic reactions because of their lack of natural photoprotection. In congenital porphyrias, porphyria cutanea tarda, and Hartnup disease, endogenous metabolites function as potent photosensitizers (Fig. 7.43). In

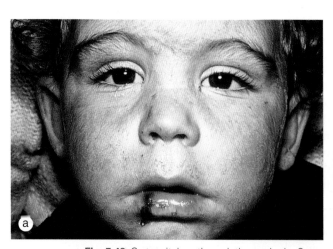

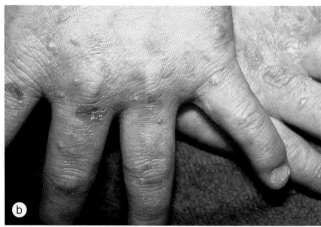

Fig. 7.43 Congenital erythropoietic porphyria. Severe photosensitivity from accumulation of cutaneous porphyrins results in recurrent blistering and scarring in sun-exposed areas. **(a)** Note scarring, erosions, and hirsutism on his face and **(b)** scarring with milia formation on his hands.

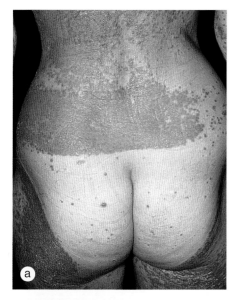
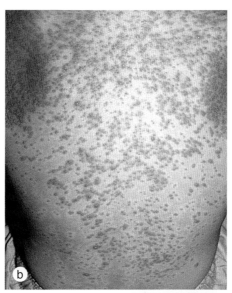
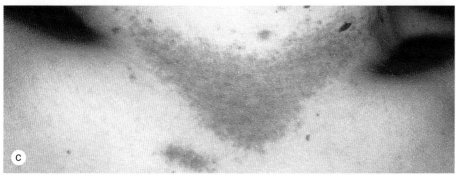

Fig. 7.44 Photoexacerbated conditions. **(a)** This 18-year-old girl with psoriasis developed recurrent skin lesions in sun-exposed areas after a sunburn (Koebner phenomenon). **(b)** Photoexacerbation was evident in this child with varicella. The bathing trunk area was relatively spared. **(c)** For this girl, vasculitic plaques of Henoch–Schönlein purpura erupted in sun-exposed sites.

many genetic disorders with photosensitivity, the clinical findings provide the key to diagnosis.

Other Photo-Exacerbated Disorders

Many disorders are triggered or aggravated by sunlight. For instance, although careful exposure to sun may result in improvement of psoriasis and repigmentation in vitiligo, sunburn often produces Koebner phenomenon and results in exacerbation of both disorders (Fig. 7.44). Sun exposure, particularly sunburn, is also known to exacerbate acne vulgaris, acne rosacea, EM, viral exanthems, autoimmune bullous disorders, lichen planus, lupus erythematosus, pityriasis alba, and herpes labialis.

COLLAGEN VASCULAR DISEASE

Collagen vascular disorders present with myriad confusing and overlapping cutaneous findings. Although the clinical picture and laboratory markers help to define a specific entity, often the practitioner is unable to make a definitive diagnosis. A number of autoantibody systems have been identified in these diseases. Antibodies target vascular endothelium and epithelial basement membrane zone structures, which results in cutaneous and visceral inflammation. In the skin, inflammation produces distinctive reaction patterns.

Lupus Erythematosus

Lupus is a chronic multisystem disorder that can affect any organ system. Although SLE was considered to be progressive, often with a fatal outcome as recent as 25 years ago, the aggressive use of systemic corticosteroids and immunosuppressive agents has greatly improved the prognosis. Early intervention requires immediate recognition of variable and sometimes subtle signs and symptoms. Cutaneous findings may suggest the diagnosis.

The most common variant of lupus in childhood is SLE. Although the incidence is only 1:200 000 in childhood, nearly 25% of all cases begin before the age of 20 years. In young children, boys are affected almost as often as girls. However, in adolescence, when the incidence begins to rise, girls account for 80–90% of cases. Other forms of lupus, which are uncommon in childhood, include discoid lupus (chronic cutaneous lupus), lupus panniculitis, subacute cutaneous lupus, and neonatal lupus (see Fig. 2.93).

Discoid lupus lesions are the most common skin rash found in childhood SLE. This eruption is characterized by red, coin-shaped plaques 0.5–5 cm in diameter, with central atrophy and hypopigmentation and peripheral hyperpigmentation (Fig. 7.45). Adherent scale, follicular plugging, and telangiectasias, especially in areas of atrophy, may be prominent. Although these plaques may develop on any area, sun-exposed sites, which include the face (in a malar distribution), scalp, ears,

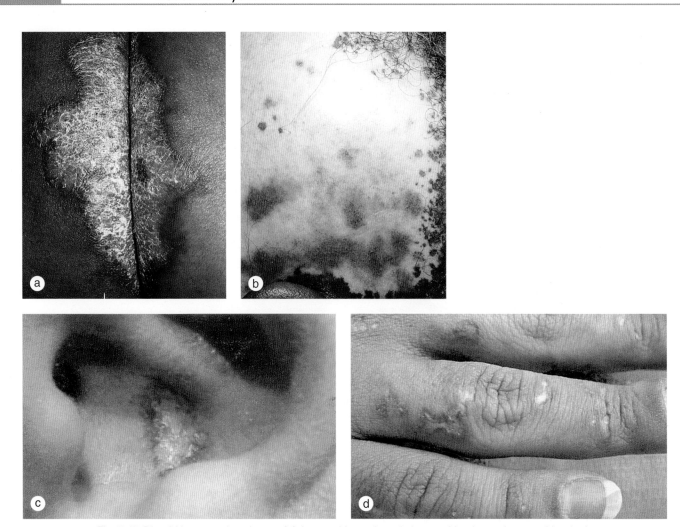

Fig. 7.45 Discoid lupus erythematosus. **(a)** An atrophic, scaly, red plaque with a hyperpigmented border in the gluteal cleft showed histologic changes typical of lupus. **(b)** Atrophy, depigmentation, scarring alopecia, and telangiectasias persisted in an old lesion. **(c)** Follicular plugging, scale, atrophy, and pigmentary changes were prominent on this adolescent's ears. **(d)** She also had lesions on the tops of her fingers.

neck, upper trunk, and extensor surfaces of the arms, are most commonly involved. Discoid lesions may be the sole cutaneous finding in SLE. However, when discoid lesions occur without systemic disease, the disorder is referred to as benign cutaneous lupus, discoid lupus erythematosus (DLE), or chronic cutaneous lupus erythematosus (CCLE). About 15–20% of patients with DLE eventually go on to develop SLE. These patients must be counseled and followed accordingly. Discoid plaques may progress and heal with extensive scarring and disfigurement. Topical corticosteroids, systemic corticosteroids, and antimalarial drugs are the mainstay of therapy, depending on the severity of the systemic disease. Topical retinoids have been used to remodel scars and treat hyperpigmentation when lesions go into remission.

Other cutaneous findings in SLE include the classic red and edematous malar rash, diffuse and annular psoriasis-like plaques in sun-exposed areas (subacute cutaneous lupus erythematosus), scarring and non-scarring scalp hair loss, rheumatoid nodules, nail fold telangiectasias, livedo reticularis, and palpable purpura that results from small vessel vasculitis (Fig. 7.46). Severe Raynaud phenomenon with digital infarcts

may also develop. Mucous membranes can be involved, with nasal and oral ulcerations and painful erosions on the lip.

In addition to cutaneous features, the most common presenting complaints in SLE are fevers and arthralgias. Other common findings include pulmonary disease (pleuritis, pneumonitis: 66% of patients), cardiac manifestations (pericarditis, myocarditis, endocarditis: 50% of patients), lupus nephritis (60% of patients), and central nervous system disease (50% of patients).

Serologic findings may be very useful in establishing the diagnosis (Table 7.1). Almost 100% of patients with SLE have a positive ANA. The rate of positivity varies, however, with the substrate used for the test. In the past, a subset of SLE patients were identified as ANA negative. Many of these patients have subsequently tested positive using HEp-2 cells, which are derived from a human tumor line, as a substrate. Although there is no direct correlation between ANA titers and disease activity, patients with high-titer ANA tend to have more active SLE. A number of other antibodies are also found in lupus patients and may correlate with certain aspects of disease activity. One of these antibody systems, Ro (SSA) and La (SSB), which is

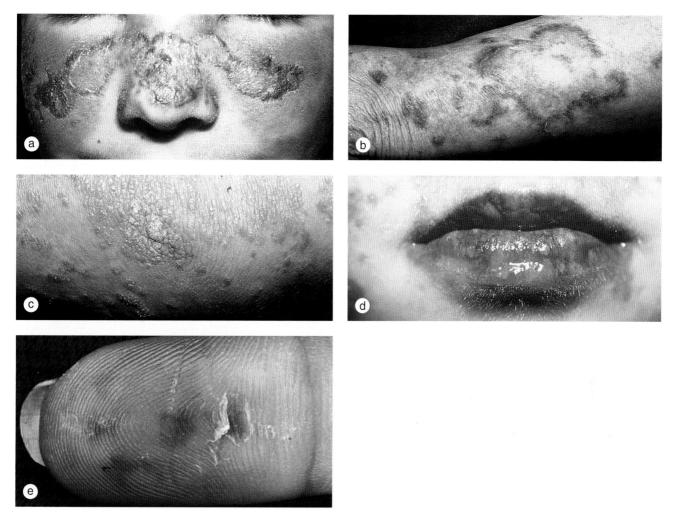

Fig. 7.46 Lupus erythematosus. **(a)** A 13-year-old girl with systemic lupus erythematosus developed malar erythema, edema, and erosions associated with a flare of nephritis after spending a day in the sun at the beach. Other lesions typical of lupus include **(b)** annular, scaly patches and plaques, **(c)** psoriasis-like plaques, **(d)** erosions on the oral mucosa and vermilion border, and **(e)** Raynaud phenomenon with digital infarcts.

directed against a small cytoplasmic ribonuclear protein, is associated with photosensitivity, neonatal lupus, and subacute cutaneous lupus erythematosus. Ro and La are also found in Sjögren syndrome in the absence of SLE. Patients with photosensitivity should be counseled about sunscreens, protective clothing, and judicious sun exposure. Occasionally, systemic disease can be triggered by excessive sun exposure.

The symptoms of juvenile rheumatoid arthritis (JRA) can easily be confused with lupus (Fig. 7.47). However, the rash of JRA is urticarial and evanescent, peaking with fever spikes. Unlike the destructive arthritis of JRA, the arthritis in lupus is often transient and does not impair function. Many of the other reactive erythemas may share features with lupus. However, the diagnosis of lupus is dependent on clearly defined criteria. The 1997 American College of Rheumatology (ACR) criteria and the 2012 Systemic Lupus International Collaborating Clinics (SLICC) criteria are both commonly used to make the diagnosis of lupus. Although both the ACR and the SLICC criteria can be easily used to make the diagnosis of lupus, the SLICC criteria is more sensitive.

Dermatomyositis

Dermatomyositis (DM) accounts for only 5% of pediatric collagen vascular disease. However, cutaneous lesions are distinctive and mark the onset of non-suppurative inflammation in the muscle. Unlike the adult variant, DM in childhood is self-limiting and not associated with underlying malignancy. Unfortunately, calcinosis cutis, which follows the disease and is more common in the pediatric form of DM, can be debilitating.

Most cases of childhood DM occur between 4 and 12 years of age. As in lupus, there is a 2:1 female predominance. There is no known inheritance pattern or racial predisposition.

Cutaneous findings may precede myositis for over a year, and the onset of signs and symptoms is usually insidious. Conversely, progressive, symmetric proximal muscle weakness may precede the rash by months. Patients often complain of easy fatigability with routine tasks such as brushing teeth, combing hair, and climbing steps. Muscle tenderness may be accompanied by anorexia, malaise, and fever. Dysphagia, dysphonia, and dyspnea occur in 10% of patients and signal palatal, esophageal, and thoracic involvement.

TABLE 7.1 Autoantibodies in Collagen Vascular Disorders

	Designation	Subtype	Antigen	Frequently Associated Disease States
Antinuclear antibodies	dsDNA		Double-stranded DNA	Lupus erythematosus, nephritis (high specificity for SLE)
	ssDNA		Single-stranded DNA	Lupus erythematosus, other non-rheumatic diseases
	ENA		Extractable nuclear antigen	Based on specific ENA subtype
		Sm	RNAase-resistant glycoprotein (U1, U2, U4, U5, and U6 small ribonucleoprotein)	Lupus erythematosus, nephritis (high specificity for SLE)
		RNP	RNAase-sensitive ribonucleoprotein (U1 small ribonucleoprotein)	Lupus erythematosus, discoid lupus erythematosus; mixed connective tissue disease, Raynaud phenomenon
		Leukocyte-specific		Rheumatoid arthritis, Felty syndrome
	SSC (RAP)		Trypsin-sensitive protein	Rheumatoid arthritis
	RANA			Rheumatoid arthritis
	NANA		Nucleolar ANA	Systemic sclerosis
	PM-1 (Mi)		Trypsin-sensitive protein	Polydermatomyositis
	DNP		DNA-histone	Drug-induced lupus erythematosus; rheumatoid arthritis; lupus erythematosus
	Centromere		Kinetochore	CREST syndrome
	Centriole		Centriole	Sclerosis–Raynaud phenomenon
	Scl-70		Non-histone nuclear protein	Systemic sclerosis, CREST syndrome
Anticytoplasmic antibodies	ssRNA		Single-stranded RNA	Systemic sclerosis
	Ro (SSA)		Acidic glycoprotein	Lupus erythematosus, photosensitivity, Sjögren syndrome, neonatal lupus
	Ribosomal		Ribosome	Lupus erythematosus
	La (SSB)		RNA-protein	Lupus erythematosus, neonatal lupus
Antineutrophilic cytoplasmic antibodies	c-ANCA			Wegener granulomatosis
Anticardiolipin, antiphospholipid antibodies			Platelet membrane phospholipid	Lupus anticoagulant syndrome

DNA, Deoxyribonucleic acid; *SLE*, systemic lupus erythematosus; *ENA*, extractable nuclear antigen; *RNA*, ribonucleic acid; *RNP*, ribonucleoprotein; *RANA*, rheumatoid arthritis nuclear antigen; *NANA*, nucleolar antinuclear antibodies; *ANA*, antinuclear antibodies; *DNP*, dinitrophenol; *CREST*, calcinosis cutis, Raynaud phenomenon, esophageal dysfunction, sclerodactyly, telangiectasia; *ANCA*, antineutrophil cytoplasmic antibodies.

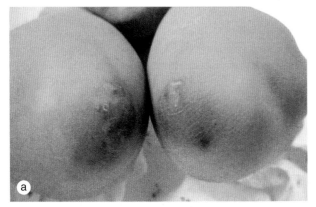
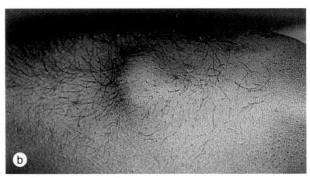

Fig. 7.47 Rheumatoid nodule. This adolescent girl developed rheumatoid-factor-positive rheumatoid arthritis and systemic lupus erythematosus. The painless nodules appeared on her forearms. **(b)** Another adolescent girl with systemic lupus developed similar nodules on her forearms.

Nearly 75% of children with DM develop a diagnostic rash. Periorbital findings include a periorbital dermatitis, with or without edema, which gives a violaceous hue and is known as heliotrope (Fig. 7.48). A psoriasis-like rash can develop that involves the extensor surfaces of the elbows, knees, and knuckles (Fig. 7.49). When over the distal interphalangeal joints, these changes are referred to as Gottron papules and are pathognomonic for the diagnosis of DM. A malar rash reminiscent of lupus is variably present. Periungual and facial telangiectasias may become prominent. Diffuse erythema and scaling with

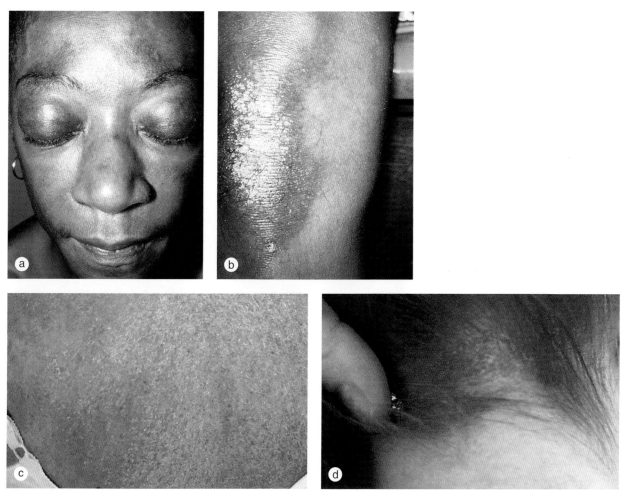

Fig. 7.48 Dermatomyositis. **(a)** Heliotrope. A young woman with dermatomyositis presented with violaceous erythema and edema of the upper eyelids. **(b)** A 10-year-old boy with a psoriasis-like dermatitis on the elbows and knees for 6 months developed rapidly progressive proximal muscle weakness. Erythema and scaling were prominent over the trunk **(c)** and scalp **(d)** of this 16-year-old girl, who also developed diffuse alopecia.

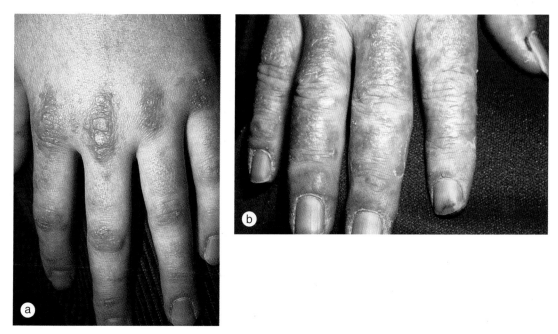

Fig. 7.49 Gottron papules **(a)** in a child with dermatomyositis are contrasted with **(b)** a psoriasis-like dermatitis on the hands of a patient with systemic lupus erythematosus. Note the sparing of the knuckles in lupus.

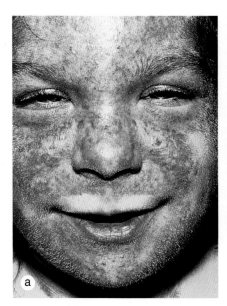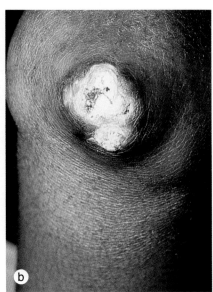

Fig 7.50 Dermatomyositis. **(a)** Despite resolution of cutaneous inflammation and myositis with systemic corticosteroids, telangiectasias progressed on the face of this 6-year-old girl. **(b)** Extensive cutis calcinosis, particularly over bony prominences, resulted in chronic, painful, draining ulcers and cellulitis in this 12-year-old boy with burned-out dermatomyositis. Note the white, chalk-like calcium deposits at the base of an ulcer on his knee.

alopecia may be prominent (Fig. 7.48d). Atrophy, fibrosis, hypopigmentation, and hyperpigmentation progress gradually, which results in telangiectasias (Fig. 7.50a) and poikiloderma with salt-and-pepper-like mottling.

Up to 50% of children with DM develop dystrophic calcification in skin and muscle, probably secondary to necrosis and scarring of the involved tissues (Fig. 7.50b). In some patients, painful, chronic ulceration of calcified nodules, recurrent cellulitis, and progressive contractures continue to limit recovery, even after active inflammation resolves. Complications may also occasionally result from gastrointestinal, cardiac, and pulmonary involvement. Treatment consists of aggressive use of systemic corticosteroids and physical therapy to preserve muscle function. In severe cases, methotrexate or other immunosuppressives may be required. Persistent, widespread telangiectasias and calcinosis cutis are typically resistant to therapy.

Clinical diagnosis is usually confirmed by detecting elevated muscle enzymes, typical electromyographic (EMG) findings, and muscle biopsy. In many centers, magnetic resonance imaging (MRI) has replaced muscle biopsy and EMG studies for diagnostic evaluation. In DM, as in lupus, the inflammatory process targets blood vessels in the involved tissues. Skin biopsies from the heliotrope rash, Gottron papules, and the psoriasiform dermatitis demonstrate perivascular and dermal–epidermal junction changes indistinguishable from those of lupus.

Sclerosing Collagen Vascular Disease

Sclerosing conditions of the skin represent a broad spectrum of disease, from the benign to the life-threatening. Scleroderma (systemic sclerosis) represents the more malignant end of the spectrum, and conditions such as morphea the more benign. Systemic sclerosis is uncommon, accounting for only 5% of collagen vascular disease in childhood. Morphea, previously called localized scleroderma, is a closely related localized process that can be very subtle and is probably underdiagnosed.

Morphea can present in a plaque (the most common pattern), linear, guttate, or generalized pattern (Fig. 7.51). Sclerotic plaques with an ivory-white center and an advancing lilac-colored border characterize active morphea. During the course, hyperpigmentation may also be marked. In the most common form, one or several lesions from 1 to 10 cm in diameter appear on the trunk. In generalized morphea (not to be confused with systemic sclerosis), similar widespread lesions develop on the trunk and extremities. Occasionally, multiple small, oval lesions reminiscent of lichen sclerosis et atrophicus erupt on the upper trunk in the guttate variant. Morphea can also progress in a linear pattern, particularly on the scalp, face, and extremities. En coup de sabre describes a subset of linear morphea cases in which a furrow extends vertically from the scalp across the forehead and down the face. Involvement of the underlying soft tissue and bone may result in severe disfigurement. Central nervous system involvement in association with lesion on the face and scalp is also probably more common than previously suspected. Intracranial lesions can result in significant morbidity and should be evaluated with brain MRI. Progressive facial hemiatrophy (Perry–Romberg syndrome) probably represents a variant of en coup de sabre with minimal fibrosis but prominent atrophy and high risk of ocular, oral, and central system involvement. Over months to years, the lesions of morphea heal with softening of the involved areas and atrophy. In children, cutaneous disease with no systemic symptoms is not associated with progression to systemic sclerosis.

Laboratory findings in morphea are not specific or prognostic. Occasionally, eosinophilia is present on a complete blood count, and rheumatoid factor may be elevated. In 10–15% of cases, ANA are present. Skin biopsies from new lesions or from the advancing borders of established lesions show lymphocytic inflammation between collagen bundles and around blood vessels in the deep dermis, which extends into the subcutis. Some areas of fat may be replaced by newly formed collagen. In late sclerotic plaques, thick, homogeneous collagen extends from the dermal–epidermal junction into the subcutaneous tissue. Adnexal structures appear to be enveloped in collagen, and little if any inflammatory infiltrate remains.

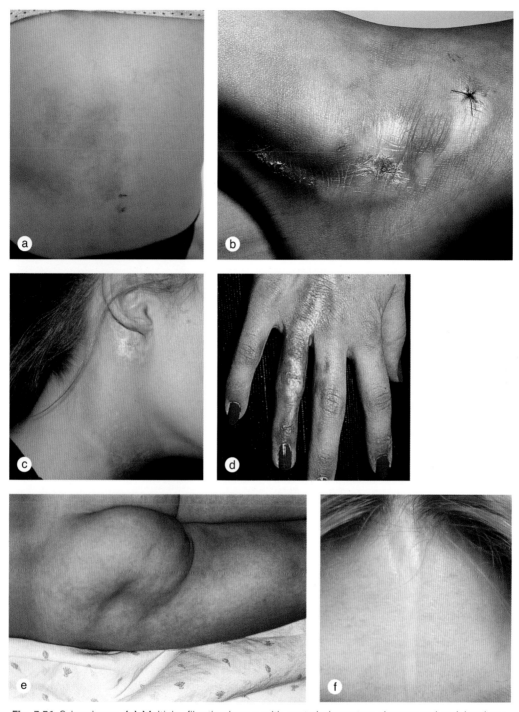

Fig. 7.51 Scleroderma. **(a)** Multiple, fibrotic plaques with central pigmentary changes and peripheral erythema slowly enlarged on the back of an adolescent girl. **(b)** An atrophic, fibrotic, hypopigmented plaque extended around the ankle of a 10-year-old girl for 2 years. Fortunately, she did not experience functional impairment. **(c)** A girl developed a similar plaque by her ear. **(d)** Linear morphea produced fibrosis and atrophy of the soft tissue of this young woman's right fourth finger, while **(e)** this adolescent developed lipoatrophy of the left hip and posterior thigh. **(f)** An unusual variant of morphea that affects the scalp, coup de sabre (stroke of the saber), extends from the mid-frontal scalp down the forehead to the nasal bridge.

Unfortunately, therapy can be disappointing. For single localized lesions, topical or intralesional corticosteroids are often first-line therapy. Topical calcineurin inhibitors can also be used, but are often not potent enough to elicit a proper response. The use of penicillamine, even in severe localized disease, has never been proven to be beneficial. Systemic antimalarials, vitamin D

derivatives, and antimetabolites have been tried, with variable response. Short courses of high-dose corticosteroids (1–2 mg/kg per day) may help to shut off rapidly progressive linear morphea when it endangers important structures. When central system lesions are present, tapering courses of oral corticosteroids over 2–3 months, followed by 12–18 months of methotrexate, has been advocated by some investigators. Recently, therapy with PUVA (psoralen and ultraviolet A) and UVA-1 phototherapy has been used with some success for cutaneous lesions. Narrow band UVB (NBUVB) phototherapy is not helpful, as the light does not penetrate deeply enough into the dermis. Physical therapy may be necessary when lesions extend across joints.

Nephrogenic systemic fibrosis, previously known as nephrogenic fibrosing dermopathy, a recently described disorder associated with renal failure and renal dialysis, may clinically overlap with morphea and other disorders characterized by localized cutaneous fibrosis. Patients typically develop progressive thickening of the skin of the extremities, flank, and/or back, with sparing of the face and neck. Lesions are skin-colored or slightly red and painful, and often develop irregular ameboid borders. Contractures may be severe and incapacitating. Systemic involvement with fibrosis of eyes, lungs, bones, dura, and other organ systems has been described. Exposure to gadolinium-based contrast agents has been reported in many patients and should be avoided in individuals with renal failure. Histologic findings include a marked increase in fibroblast-like spindle cells and increased collagen and mucin deposition similar to scleromyxedema (a rare sclerosing condition associated with monoclonal gammopathy). Although lesions are usually restricted to the skin, rare cases with pulmonary involvement have been reported.

Systemic Sclerosis

Systemic sclerosis (SS), or scleroderma, is rare in childhood, and clinically the course is similar to that of adult cases. Raynaud phenomenon is present in 90% of patients and may precede the onset of systemic disease by years. Classic findings in the skin include tightening of the skin associated with woody induration, edema, and pigmentary changes. Life-threatening disease in the gastrointestinal tract, musculoskeletal system, heart, lungs, and kidneys may result from SS. Most patients with SS develop ANA, and nearly 50% have antinucleolar antibodies. A number of other antibody systems are also present in some cases of SS and may have special prognostic value.

Lichen Sclerosus et Atrophicus

Lichen sclerosus (LS, lichen sclerosus et atrophicus, or LS&A) occurs most commonly in postmenopausal women. However, about 10% of cases appear in children under 7 years old. Although it has been reported more commonly in girls than in boys, 14% of boys requiring circumcision for medical reasons had evidence of lichen sclerosus either clinically or histologically.

The anogenital area is the most common site of involvement. Typically, small, white, flat-topped papules arise on the cutaneous and mucous membrane surfaces of the labia, perineum, and perianal area. Confluent, white, atrophic patches may extend symmetrically in a figure-of-eight pattern around the vagina and rectum (Fig. 7.52). Scaling, vesiculation, and hemorrhage may be prominent, particularly after accidental trauma or rubbing and scratching from pruritus. A mild, watery discharge may be present. In some patients, extragenital patches on the trunk and extremities predominate (Fig. 7.53). In these lesions, follicular dimpling caused by hyperkeratosis with follicular plugging is characteristic. Truncal patches also share clinical and histologic

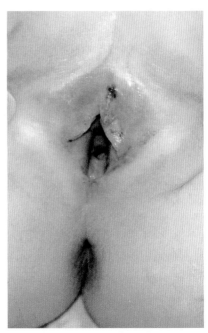

Fig. 7.52 Lichen sclerosus et atrophicus. A pruritic, atrophic, eroded, hypopigmented patch involved the genital skin and mucous membranes in this 5-year-old girl. Note the bruising from scratching on the labia minora.

features with morphea, and lesions typical of both entities have been described simultaneously in the same patients.

Girls with anogenital lesions typically complain of chronic pruritus, burning, erythema, scale, and erosions. However, the diagnosis should be considered in boys with recurrent erythema, balanitis, and tightening of the foreskin, which can lead to phimosis. It was generally believed that lichen sclerosus resolves spontaneously at puberty, but recent series do not support this. Symptoms may abate, but atrophy and fibrosis tend to persist, and early intervention with high-potency topical steroid applied daily and then tapered over several months may induce remission. Many patients will require maintenance with either topical steroids or topical calcineurin inhibitors. Although the cause is unknown, the association with morphea suggests an immunologic basis.

Histopathologic findings are often diagnostic. In addition to scale and follicular plugging, thinning of the mid-epidermis, hydropic degeneration of the basal layer, edema and homogenization of the upper dermis, and a band-like lymphohistiocytic infiltrate beneath the zone of homogenization are observed.

Clinically, LS must not be confused with child abuse, candidiasis, or streptococcal perianal or vaginal dermatitis. Cultures may be obtained to exclude bacterial and herpetic infections. The symmetric pattern and characteristic morphology of LS also help to eliminate child abuse as a serious consideration. In vitiligo, which may also present in a symmetric pattern in the anogenital area, the skin is completely normal except for depigmentation (Fig. 7.54). Inflammatory bowel disease may present with vaginal and perianal nodules, sinus tracts, and ulcers (Fig. 7.55). Other symptoms of gastrointestinal disease may be absent. Skin biopsies in these cases demonstrate granulomas typical of Crohn disease. Primary bullous dermatoses may also present a diagnostic dilemma. If the clinical presentation is not

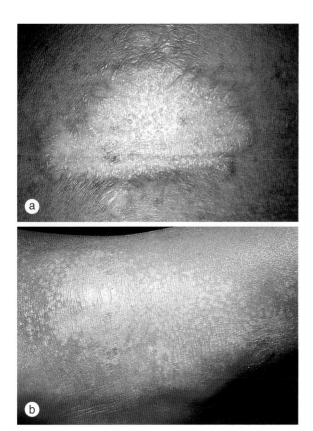

Fig. 7.53 Lichen sclerosis et atrophicus. Atrophic, hypopigmented, scaly papules coalesced into confluent patches on **(a)** the trunk and **(b)** the extremities of a 10-year-old girl.

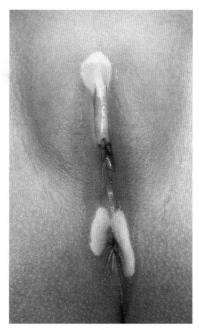

Fig. 7.54 Vitiligo developed around the vagina and anus of a 2-year-old girl, mimicking the pattern of lichen sclerosis et atrophicus.

distinctive, a skin biopsy with direct immunofluorescence may be necessary to make the diagnosis.

Necrobiosis Lipoidica

In necrobiosis lipoidica, reddish-yellow, indurated plaques typically appear on the shins (Fig. 7.56). Although this disease has a strong correlation with diabetes, not all patients who develop this condition will have diabetes, and not all diabetics will develop it. As the lesions expand from less than 1 to 4 cm in diameter or larger over months, the center of the plaque becomes shiny and atrophic. Telangiectasias extend from the center. Although lesions may remain stable and occasionally heal without treatment, most persist or slowly progress, and minor trauma may result in chronic, painful ulcerations. Some patients improve with topical or intralesional corticosteroids injected into the expanding red border.

About 75% of patients with necrobiosis lipoidica are female and over half have diabetes mellitus (hence the previous name of this condition, necrobiosis lipoidica diabeticorum). In some

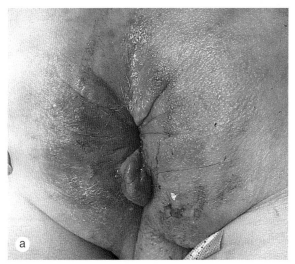

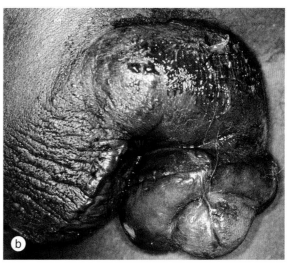

Fig. 7.55 Inflammatory bowel disease. **(a)** A 2-year-old girl was treated for chronic diaper dermatitis and candidiasis for months before the diagnosis of Crohn disease was considered. A biopsy of the perianal skin showed granulomas. **(b)** This 10-year-old boy had non-tender swelling of the penis for almost a year before the diagnosis of Crohn disease was made. Granulomas were noted on biopsy of his penis and colon.

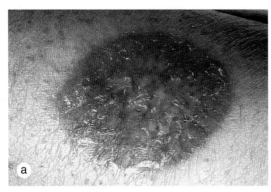

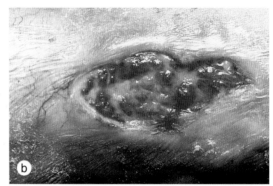

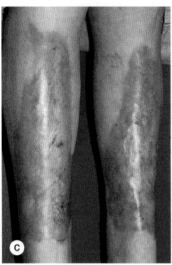

Fig. 7.56 Necrobiosis lipoidica. **(a)** A plaque on the shin of a 17-year-old diabetic demonstrates the typical red border and yellow, shiny, atrophic center with telangiectasias. **(b)** This patient developed a chronic, painful ulcer after repeated trauma. The ulcer healed after several months of treatment with occlusive dressings. **(c)** A healthy 20-year-old woman developed shiny atrophic fibrotic yellowish-pink plaques on her shins when she was 12 years old. She had no personal or family history of diabetes and all glucose metabolism studies were normal.

cases, necrobiosis lipoidica precedes the onset of clinical diabetes by years. Although the cause is unknown, investigators have suggested that some sort of vascular insult triggered by diabetes initiates the necrobiotic changes in collagen. Histologically, granulomatous inflammation is observed around altered and degenerating collagen, which extends in large bands into the deep reticular dermis. The overlying epidermis is atrophic, and ulceration may be present. Thickening of vascular walls, endothelial cell proliferation, and occasionally, vascular occlusion are seen throughout the dermis. The yellow color is imparted by deposition of lipid around necrobiotic collagen.

Necrobiosis lipoidica is usually differentiated from granuloma annulare, which does not develop epidermal changes. In some patients, fibrotic or atrophic plaques in scleroderma or LS&A mimic necrobiosis. The clinical course and skin biopsy findings, however, are distinctive. One-third of juvenile diabetics develop diffuse, non-pitting, waxy edema of the hands during the first 2 decades of life (Fig. 7.57). Although this process may be associated with progressive joint contractures, distinctive cutaneous lesions, atrophy, and pigmentary changes do not occur. Histology demonstrates increased dermal collagen, which is thought to be caused by increased glycosylation of the proteins in the collagen matrix and by dermal fibroblast proliferation (see the algorithm in Fig. 7.58).

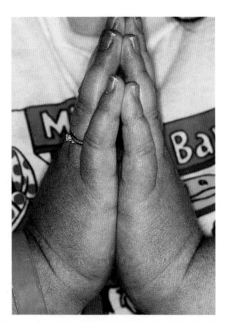

Fig. 7.57 Prayer sign. This 16-year-old type I diabetic developed progressive, waxy, non-pitting edema of her hands, associated with joint contractures.

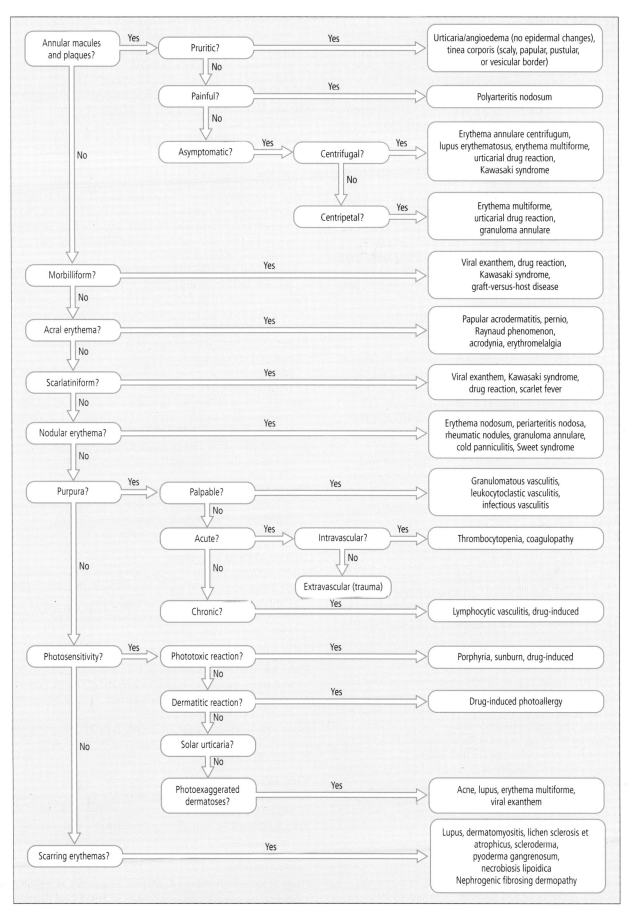

Fig. 7.58 Algorithm for evaluation of reactive erythema.

FURTHER READING

Drug Eruptions

Brahimi N, Routier E, Raison-Peyron N, et al. A three-year-analysis of fixed drug eruptions in hospital settings in France. Eur J Dermatol 2010; 20(4):461–464.

Carroll MC, Yueng-Yue KA, Esterly NB, et al. Drug-induced hypersensitivity syndrome in pediatric patients. Pediatrics 2001; 108:485–492.

Chen YC, Chiu HC, Chu CY. Drug reaction with eosinophilia and systemic symptoms: a retrospective study of 60 cases. Arch Dermatol 2010; 146(12):1373–1379.

Crowson AN, Brown TJ, Magro CM. Progress in the understanding of the pathology and pathogenesis of cutaneous drug eruptions: implications for management. Am J Clin Dermatol 2003; 4:407–428.

Friedmann PS, Lee MS, Friedmann AC, et al. Mechanisms in cutaneous drug hypersensitivity reactions. Clin Exp Allergy 2003; 33:861–872.

Hogan DJ. Morbilliform drug eruptions. J Am Acad Dermatol 2009; 61(1):152.

Hunziker T, Kunzi UP, Braunschweig S, et al. Comprehensive hospital drug monitoring (CHDM): adverse skin reactions, a 20 year survey. Allergy 1997; 52:388–393.

Ibia EO, Schwartz RH, Wiedemann BL. Antibiotic rashes in children: a survey in a private practice setting. Arch Dermatol 2000; 83:347–352.

Kano Y, Hiraharas K, Sakuma K, et al. Several herpesviruses can reactivate in a severe drug-induced multiorgan reaction in the same sequential order as in graft-versus-host disease. Br J Dermatol 2006; 155(2):301–306.

Kardaun SH, Sekula P, Valeyrie-Allanore L, et al. RegiSCAR study group. Drug reaction with eosinophilia and systemic symptoms (DRESS): an original multisystem adverse drug reaction. Results from the prospective RegiSCAR study. Br J Dermatol 2013; 169(5):1071–1080.

Khuo BP, Giam YC. Drug eruptions in children: a review of 111 cases seen in a tertiary skin referral centre. Singapore Med J 2000; 41:525–529.

Lazarou J, Pomeranz BH, Corey PN. Incidence of adverse drug reactions in hospitalized patients: a meta-analysis of prospective studies. JAMA 1998; 279(15):1200–1205.

Milikan LE, Feldman M. Pediatric drug allergy. Clin Dermatol 2002; 20:29–35.

Newell BD, Horii KA. Cutaneous drug reactions in children. Pediatr Ann 2010; 39(10):618–625.

Piñana E, Lei SH, Merino R, et al. DRESS-syndrome on sulfasalazine and naproxen treatment for juvenile idiopathic arthritis and reactivation of human herpesvirus 6 in an 11-year-old Caucasian boy. J Clin Pharm Ther 2010; 35(3):365–370.

Segal AR, Doherty KM, Leggott J, et al. Cutaneous reactions to drugs in children. Pediatrics 2007; 120(4):e1082–e1096.

Shin HT, Chang MW. Drug eruptions in children. Curr Prob Pediatr 2001; 31:207–234.

Shiohara T. Fixed drug eruption: pathogenesis and diagnostic tests. Curr Opin Allergy Clin Immunol 2009; 9(4):316–321.

Urticaria

Bailey E, Shaker M. An update on childhood urticaria and angioedema. Curr Opin Pediatr 2008; 20(4):425–430.

Champion RH, Roberts SO, Carpenter RG, et al. Urticaria and angioedema. A review of 554 cases. Br J Dermatol 1969; 81:588–597.

Charlesworth EN. Urticaria and angioedema: a clinical spectrum. Ann Allergy Asthma Immunol 1996; 76:484–499.

Confino-Cohen R, Chodick G, Shalev V, et al. Chronic urticaria and autoimmunity: associations found in a large population study. J Allergy Clin Immunol 2012; 129(5):1307–1313.

Greaves M. Management of urticaria. Hosp Med 2000; 61:63–69.

Greaves MW. Chronic urticaria in childhood. Allergy 2000; 55:309–320.

Kauppinen K, Juntunen K, Lanki H. Urticaria in children. Retrospective evaluation and follow-up. Allergy 1984; 39:469–472.

Kröpfl L, Maurer M, Zuberbier T. Treatment strategies in urticaria. Expert Opin Pharmacother 2010; 11(9):1445–1450.

Leech S, Grattan C, Lloyd K, et al.; Science and Research Department, Royal College of Paediatrics and Child Health. The RCPCH care pathway for children with urticaria, angio-oedema or mastocytosis: an evidence and consensus based national approach. Arch Dis Child 2011; 96(Suppl 2):i34–i37.

Legrain V, Taieb A, Sage T, et al. Urticaria in infants: a study of forty patients. Pediatr Dermatol 1990; 7:101–107.

Pomerantz RG, Mirvish ED, Geskin LJ. Cutaneous reactions to epidermal growth factor receptor inhibitors. J Drugs Dermatol 2010; 9(10):1229–1234.

Riten K, Shahina Q, Jeannette J, et al. A severe case of acute generalized exanthematous pustulosis (AGEP) in a child after the administration of amoxicillin-clavulanic acid: brief report. Pediatr Dermatol 2009; 26(5):623–625.

Shah KN, Honig PJ, Yan AC. 'Urticaria multiforme': a case series and review of acute annular urticarial hypersensitivity syndromes in children. Pediatrics 2007; 119(5):e1177–e1183.

Somekh E, Mizrahi A, Hanukoglu A. Chronic urticaria in children: expanding the 'autoimmune kaleidoscope.' Pediatrics 2000; 106:1139–1141.

Thakur BK, Kaplan AP. Recurrent 'unexplained' scalp swelling in an 18-month-old: an atypical presentation of angioedema causing confusion with child abuse. J Pediatr 1996; 129:163–165.

Weston WL, Badgett JT. Urticaria. Pediatr Rev 1998; 19:240–244.

Lichenoid Drug Eruptions

Asarch A, Gottlieb AB, Lee J, et al. Lichen planus-like eruptions: an emerging side effect of tumor necrosis factor-alpha antagonists. J Am Acad Dermatol 2009; 61(1):104–111.

Halevy S, Shai A. Lichenoid drug eruptions. J Am Acad Dermatol 1993; 29(2 Pt 1):249–255.

Chemotherapy-Induced Erythema

Miller KK, Gorcey L, McLellan BN. Chemotherapy-induced hand-foot syndrome and nail changes: a review of clinical presentation, etiology, pathogenesis, and management. J Am Acad Dermatol 2014; 71(4):787–794.

Susser WS, Whitaker-Worth DL, Grant-Kels JM. Mucocutaneous reactions to chemotherapy. J Am Acad Dermatol 1999; 40(3):367–398.

Viral Exanthems

Asano Y, Yoshikawa T. Human herpesvirus 6 and parvovirus B19 infections in children. Curr Opin Pediatr 1993; 5:14–20.

Bello S, Meremikwu MM, Ejemot-Nwadiaro RI, et al. Routine vitamin A supplementation for the prevention of blindness due to measles infection in children. Cochrane Database Syst Rev 2011; (4):CD007719.

Drago F, Rampini E, Rebora A. Atypical exanthems: morphology and laboratory investigation may lead to an aetiological diagnosis in about 70% of cases. Br J Dermatol 2002; 147:255–260.

Fölster-Holst R, Kreth HW. Viral exanthems in childhood–infectious (direct) exanthems. Part 1: classic exanthems. J Dtsch Dermatol Ges 2009; 7(4):309–316.

Fölster-Holst R, Kreth HW. Viral exanthems in childhood–infectious (direct) exanthems. Part 2: other viral exanthems. [Article in English, German] J Dtsch Dermatol Ges 2009; 7(5):414–419.

Fölster-Holst R, Kreth HW. Viral exanthems in childhood. Part 3: Parainfectious exanthems and those associated with virus-drug interactions. J Dtsch Dermatol Ges 2009; 7(6):506–510.

Hampton T. Outbreaks spur measles vaccine studies. JAMA 2011; 306(22):2440–2442.

McCuaig CC, Rudo P, Powell J, et al. Unilateral laterothoracic exanthem. A clinicopathologic study of 48 patients. J Am Acad Dermatol 1996; 34:979–984.

Okada K, Ueda K, Kusuhara K, et al. Exanthem subitum and human herpesvirus 6 infection: clinical observations in 57 cases. Pediatr Infect Dis J 1993; 12:204–208.

Sata T, Urishibata O, Kurata T. The rash of measles is caused by a viral infection in the cells of the skin: a case report. J Dermatol 1994; 21:741–745.

Scott LA, Stone MS. Viral exanthems. Dermatol Online J 2003; 9:4.

Smith PJ, Lindley MC, Rodewald LE. Vaccination coverage among US children aged 19–35 months entitled by the Vaccines for Children program. Public Health Pub 2009; 126(Suppl 2):109–123.

Kawasaki Syndrome

Alves NR, Magalhães CM, Almeida Rde F, et al. Prospective study of Kawasaki disease complications: review of 115 cases. [Article in English, Portuguese] Rev Assoc Med Bras 2011; 57(3):295–300.

Durongpisitkul K, Gururaj VJ, Park JM, et al. The prevention of coronary artery aneurysm in Kawasaki disease: a meta-analysis on the efficacy of aspirin and immunoglobulin treatment. Pediatrics 1995; 96(6):1057–1061.

Gerding R. Kawasaki disease: a review. J Pediatr Health Care 2011; 25(6):379–387.

Kawasaki T, Kosaki F, Okawa S, et al. A new infantile acute febrile mucocutaneous lymph node syndrome (MLNS) prevailing in Japan. Pediatrics 1974; 54:271–276.

Meissner HC, Leung DY. Kawasaki syndrome: where are the answers? Pediatrics 2003; 112(3 Pt 1):672–676.

Acral Erythema

Davis MD, O'Fallon WM, Rogers RS 3rd, et al. Natural history of erythromelalgia: presentation and outcome in 108 patients. Arch Dermatol 2000; 136:330–336.

Davis MD, Sandroni P, Rooke TW, et al. Erythromelalgia vasculopathy, neuropathy, or both? A prospective study of vascular and neurophysiologic studies in erythromelalgia. Arch Dermatol 2003; 139:137–143.

Drenth JP, te Morsche RH, Guillet G, et al. SCN9A mutations define primary erythermalgia as a neuropathic disorder of voltage gated sodium channels. J Invest Dermatol 2005; 124(6):1333–1338.

Farr KP, Safwat A. Palmar-plantar erythrodysesthesia associated with chemotherapy and its treatment. Case Rep Oncol 2011; 4(1):229–235.

Gardinal-Galera I, Pajot C, Paul C, et al. Childhood chilblains is an uncommon and invalidant disease. Arch Dis Child 2010; 95(7):567–568.

Hedrich CM, Fiebig B, Hauck FH, et al. Chilblain lupus erythematosus—a review of literature. Clin Rheumatol 2008; 27(8):949–954.

Lampert A, Dib-Hajj SD, Eastman EM, et al. Erythromelalgia mutation L823R shifts activation and inactivation of threshold sodium channel Nav1.7 to hyperpolarized potentials. Biochem Biophys Res Commun 2009; 390(2):319–324.

Lokich JL, Moore C. Chemotherapy-associated palmar-plantar erythrodysesthesia syndrome. Ann Intern Med 1984; 101:798–800.

McLellan B, Kerr H. Cutaneous toxicities of the multikinase inhibitors Sorafenib and Sunitinib. Dermatol Ther 2011; 24(4):396–400.

Millot F, Auriol F, Brecheteau P, et al. Acral erythema in children receiving high-dose methotrexate. Pediatr Dermatol 1999; 16:398–400.

Sano S, Itami S, Yoshikawa K. Treatment of erythromelalgia with ciclosporin. N Engl J Med 2003; 249:816–817.

Vargas-Diez E, Abajo P, Fraga J, et al. Chemotherapy-induced acral erythema. Acta Derm Venereol 1999; 79:173–175.

Purpura Fulminans

Auletta MJ, Headington JT. Purpura fulminans. A cutaneous manifestation of severe protein C deficiency. Arch Dermatol 1988; 124:1387–1391.

Bergmann F, Hoyer PF, D'Angelo SV, et al. Severe autoimmune protein S deficiency in a boy with idiopathic purpura fulminans. Br J Haematol 1995; 89:610–614.

Chalmers E, Cooper P, Forman K, et al. Purpura fulminans: recognition, diagnosis and management. Arch Dis Child 2011; 96(11):1066–1071.

Chuansumrit A, Hotrakitya S, Kruavit A. Severe acquired neonatal purpura fulminans. Clin Pediatr (Phila) 1996; 35:373–376.

Darmstadt GL. Acute infectious purpura fulminans: pathogenesis and medical management. Pediatr Dermatol 1998; 15:169–183.

Januário G, Ramroop S, Shingadia DV, et al. Postinfectious purpura fulminans secondary to varicella-induced protein S deficiency. Pediatr Infect Dis J 2010; 29(10):981–983.

Pathan N, Faust SN, Levin M. Pathophysiology of meningococcal meningitis and septicaemia. Arch Dis Child 2003; 87:601–607.

Pipe SW, Schmaier AH, Nichols WC, et al. Neonatal purpura fulminans in association with factor VR506Q mutation. J Pediatr 1996; 128:706–709.

Robby SI, Mihm MC, Colman RC, et al. The skin in disseminated intravascular coagulation. Br J Dermatol 1973; 88:221–229.

Warren PM, Kagan RJ, Yakaboff KP, et al. Current management of purpura fulminans: a multicenter study. J Burn Care Rehabil 2003; 24:119–126.

Leukocytoclastic Vasculitis

Ballinger S. Henoch-Schönlein purpura. Curr Opin Rheumatol 2003; 15:591–594.

Batu ED, Ozen S. Pediatric vasculitis. Curr Rheumatol Rep 2012; 14(2):121–129.

Fiore E, Rizzi M, Simonetti GD, et al. Acute hemorrhagic edema of young children: a concise narrative review. Eur J Pediatr 2011; 170(12):1507–1511.

Jennette JC, Falk RJ. Small-vessel vasculitis. N Engl J Med 1997; 337:1512–1522.

Ozen S. The spectrum of vasculitis in children. Best Pract Res Clin Rheumatol 2002; 16:411–425.

Watson L, Richardson AR, Holt RC, et al. Henoch Schönlein purpura—a 5-year review and proposed pathway. PLoS One 2012; 7(1):e29512.

Yalcindag A, Sundel R. Vasculitis in childhood. Curr Opin Rheumatol 2001; 13:422–427.

Granulomatous Vasculitis

Belostotsky VM, Shah V, Dillon MJ. Clinical factors in 17 paediatric patients with Wegener granulomatosis. Pediatr Nephrol 2002; 17:754–761.

Bosco L, Peroni A, Schena D, et al. Cutaneous manifestations of Churg–Strauss syndrome: report of two cases and review of the literature. Clin Rheumatol 2011; 30(4):573–580.

Polyarteritis Nodosa

Akikusa JD, Schneider R, Harvey EA, et al. Clinical features and outcome of pediatric Wegener's granulomatosis. Arthritis Rheum 2007; 57(5):837–844.

Bansal NK, Houghton KM. Cutaneous polyarteritis nodosa in childhood: a case report and review of the literature. Arthritis 2010; 2010:687547.

Bauzo A, Espana A, Idoate M. Cutaneous polyarteritis nodosa. Br J Dermatol 2002; 146:694–699.

Jones SK, Lane AT, Golitz LE, et al. Cutaneous periarteritis nodosa in a child. Am J Dis Child 1985; 139:920–922.

Kumar L, Thapa BR, Sarkar B, et al. Benign cutaneous polyarteritis nodosa in children below 10 years of age—a clinical experience. Ann Rheum Dis 1995; 54:134–136.

Ozen S, Besbas N, Saatci U, et al. Diagnostic criteria for polyarteritis nodosa in childhood. J Pediatr 1992; 120:307–314.

Siberry GK, Cohen BA, Johnson B. Cutaneous polyarteritis nodosa. Report of cases in children and review of the literature. Arch Dermatol 1994; 130:884–889.

Ecthyma Gangrenosum

Doriff GI, Geimer NF, Rosenthal DR, et al. Pseudomonas septicemia. Illustrated evolution of its skin lesion. Arch Intern Med 1971; 128:591–595.

Levy I, Stein J, Ashkenazi S, et al. Ecthyma gangrenosum caused by disseminated Exserohilum in a child with leukemia: a case report and review of the literature. Pediatr Dermatol 2003; 20(6):495–497.

Pouryousefi A, Foland J, Miche C, et al. Ecthyma gangrenosum as a very early herald of acute lymphoblastic leukaemia. J Paediatr Child Health 1999; 35:505–506.

Secord E, Mills C, Shah B, et al. Picture of the month. Ecthyma gangrenosum. Am J Dis Child 1993; 147:795–796.

Zamorrodi A, Wald ER. Ecthyma gangrenosum: consideration in a previously healthy child. Pediatr Infect Dis J 2002; 21:161–164.

Progressive Pigmented Purpuric Dermatosis

Gelmett C, Cerri D, Grihalt R. Lichen aureus in childhood. Pediatr Dermatol 1991; 8:280–283.

Kano Y, Hirayama K, Orihara M, et al. Successful treatment of Schamberg disease with pentoxifylline. J Am Acad Dermatol 1997; 36:827–830.

Newton RC, Raimer SS. Pigmented purpuric eruptions. Dermatol Clin 1985; 3:165–169.

Price ML, Jones EW, Calnan CD, et al. Lichen aureus: a localized persistent form of pigmented purpuric dermatitis. Br J Dermatol 1985; 112:307–314.

Torrelo A, Requena C, Mediero IG, et al. Schamberg's purpura in children: a review of 13 cases. J Am Acad Dermatol 2003; 48(1):31–33.

Tristani-Firouzi P, Meadous KR, Vanderhooft S. Pigmented purpuric eruption of childhood. Pediatr Dermatol 2001; 18:299–304.

Sweet Syndrome

Boatman BW, Taylor RC, Klein LE, et al. Sweet erythema in children. South Med J 1994; 87:193–196.

Brady RC, Morris J, Connelly BL, et al. Sweet's syndrome as an initial manifestation of pediatric human immunodeficiency virus infection. Pediatrics 1999; 104(5 Pt 1):1142–1144.

Hazen PG, Kark EC, Davis BR, et al. Acute febrile neutrophilic dermatosis in children: report of two cases in male infants. Arch Dermatol 1983; 119:998–1002.

Itami S, Nishioka K. Sweet syndrome in infancy. Br J Dermatol 1980; 103:449–451.

Levin DL, Esterly NB, Herman JJ, et al. The Sweet syndrome in children. J Pediatr 1981; 99:73–78.

Seidel D, Huguet P, Lebbe C, et al. Sweet syndrome as the presenting manifestation of chronic granulomatous disease in an infant. Pediatr Dermatol 1994; 11:237–240.

Pyoderma Gangrenosum

Crowson AN, Mihm MC Jr, Mayro C. Pyoderma gangrenosum: a review. J Cutan Pathol 2003; 30:97–107.

Gilman AL, Cohen BA, Wrbach AH, et al. Pyoderma gangrenosum a manifestation of leukemia in children. Pediatrics 1988; 81:846–848.

Graham JA, Hansen KK, Rabinowitz LG, et al. Pyoderma gangrenosum in children. Pediatr Dermatol 1994; 11:7–10.

Hayani A, Steuber CP, Mahoney DH, et al. Pyoderma gangrenosum in childhood leukemia. Pediatr Dermatol 1990; 7:296–298.

Leon JT, Atherton MT, Byrne JP. Neutrophilic dermatoses: pyoderma gangrenosum and Sweet syndrome. Postgrad Med J 1997; 73:65–68.

Mika RB, Riahi J, Fenniche S, et al. Pyoderma gangrenosum: a report of 21 cases. Int J Dermatol 2002; 41:65–68.

Figurate Erythema

Bhate C, Schwartz RA. Lyme disease: part I. Advances and perspectives. J Am Acad Dermatol 2011; 64(4):619–638.

Bhate C, Schwartz RA. Lyme disease: part II. Management and prevention. J Am Acad Dermatol 2011; 64(4):639–654.

Bressler GS, Jones RE. Erythema annulare centrifugum. J Am Acad Dermatol 1981; 4:597–602.

Eppes SC. Diagnosis, treatment, and prevention of Lyme disease in children. Pediatr Drugs 2003; 5:363–372.

Feder HM Jr. Lyme disease in children. Infect Dis Clin North Am 2008; 22(2):315–326.

Gerber MA, Shapiro ED, Burke GS, et al. Lyme disease in southeastern Connecticut. Pediatric Lyme disease study group. N Engl J Med 1996; 335:1270–1274.

Hogan P. Annular skin lesions with a smooth surface. Aust Fam Physician 1998; 27:133–134.

Huppertz HI. Lyme disease in children. Curr Opin Rheumatol 2001; 13:434–440.

Kim KJ, Chang SE, Choi JH, et al. Clinicopathologic analysis of 66 cases of erythema annulare centrifugum. J Dermatol 2002; 29:61–67.

Lee JL, Naguwa SM, Cheema GS, et al. Acute rheumatic fever and its consequences: a persistent threat to developing nations in the 21st century. Autoimmun Rev 2009; 9(2):117–123.

Murray TS, Shapiro ED. Lyme disease. Clin Lab Med 2010; 30(1):311–328.

Ravisha MS, Tullu MS, Damat JR. Rheumatic fever and rheumatic heart disease: clinical profile of 550 cases in India. Arch Med Res 2003; 34:382–387.

Ziemer M, Eisendle K, Zelger B. New concepts on erythema annulare centrifugum: a clinical reaction pattern that does not represent a specific clinicopathological entity. Br J Dermatol 2009; 160(1):119–126.

Panniculitis

Crowson AN, Magro CM. Idiopathic perniosis and its mimics: a clinical and histologic study of 38 cases. Hum Pathol 1997; 28:478–484.

Garty BZ, Poznanski O. Erythema nodosum in Israeli children. Isr Med Assoc J 2000; 2:145–146.

Koransky JS, Esterly NB. Lupus panniculitis (profundus). J Pediatr 1981; 98:241–244.

Labbe L, Maleville J, Taieb A. Erythema nodosum in children: a study of 27 patients. Pediatr Dermatol 1996; 13:447–450.

Polcari IC, Stein SL. Panniculitis in childhood. Dermatol Ther 2010; 23(4):356–367.

Rotman H. Cold panniculitis in children. Arch Dermatol 1966; 94:720–724.

Shuval SJ, Frances A, Valderramo E, et al. Panniculitis and fever in children. J Pediatr 1993; 122:372–378.

Ter Poorten JC, Herbert AA, Ilkiw R. Cold panniculitis in a neonate. J Am Acad Dermatol 1995; 33:383–385.

Weingartner JS, Zedek DC, Burkhart CN, et al. Lupus erythematosus panniculitis in children: report of three cases and review of previously reported cases. Pediatr Dermatol 2012; 29(2):169–176.

Wimmershoff MB, Hohenleutner U, Landthaler M. Discoid lupus erythematosus and lupus profundus in childhood: a report of 2 cases. Pediatr Dermatol 2003; 20:140–145.

Photosensitivity

Allen JE. Drug induced photosensitivity. Clin Pharmacol 1993; 12:580–587.

Beattie PE, Dawe RS, Ibbotson SH, et al. Characteristics and prognosis of idiopathic solar urticaria: a cohort of 87 cases. Arch Dermatol 2009; 139:1149–1154.

Ferguson J. Diagnosis and treatment of the common idiopathic photodermatoses. Australas J Dermatol 2003; 44:90–96.

Fotiades J, Soter NA, Lim HW. Results of evaluation of 203 patients for photosensitivity in a 7.3 year period. J Am Acad Dermatol 1995; 33:597–602.

Fourtanier A, Moyal D, Seité S. Sunscreens containing the broad-spectrum UVA absorber, Mexoryl SX, prevent the cutaneous detrimental effects of UV exposure: a review of clinical study results. Photodermatol Photoimmunol Photomed 2008; 24:164–174.

Frick MA, Soler-Palacín P, Martín Nalda A, et al. Photosensitivity in immunocompromised patients receiving long-term therapy with oral voriconazole. Pediatr Infect Dis J 2010; 29(5):480–481.

Gonzalez E, Gonzalez S. Drug photosensitivity, idiopathic photodermatoses, and sunscreens. J Am Acad Dermatol 1996; 35:871–885.

Harris A, Burge SM, George SA. Solar urticaria in an infant. Br J Dermatol 1997; 136:105–107.

Hönigsmann H. Polymorphous light eruption. Photodermatol Photoimmunol Photomed 2008; 24(3):155–161.

Kerr HA, Lim HW. Photodermatoses in African Americans: a retrospective analysis of 135 patients over a 7-year period. J Am Acad Dermatol 2007; 57(4):638–643.

Kotrulja L, Ozanic-Bulic S, Sjerobabski-Masnec I, et al. Photosensitivity skin disorders in childhood. Coll Antropol 2010; 34(Suppl 2):263–266.

Schauder S, Ippen H. Contact and photocontact sensitivity to sunscreen: review of a 15-year experience and of the literature. Contact Dermatitis 1997; 37:221–232.

Stern RS, Weinstein MC, Baker SG. Risk reduction for nonmelanoma skin cancer with childhood sunscreen use. Arch Dermatol 1986; 122:537–545.

Taylor CR, Sober AS. Sun exposure and skin disease. Ann Rev Med 1996; 47:181–191.

Connective Tissue Disease

Batthish M, Feldman BM. Juvenile dermatomyositis. Curr Rheumatol Rep 2011; 13(3):216–224.

Buckley D, Barnes L. Childhood subacute cutaneous lupus erythematosus associated with a homozygous complement 2 deficiency. Pediatr Dermatol 1995; 12:327–330.

Campos LM, Kiss MH, D'Amico EA, et al. Antiphospholipid antibodies and antiphospholipid syndrome in 57 children and adolescents with systemic lupus erythematosus. Lupus 2003; 12:820–826.

Chang C. Neonatal autoimmune diseases: a critical review. J Autoimmun 2012; 38(2–3):J223–J238.

Chiu YE, Co DO. Juvenile dermatomyositis: immunopathogenesis, role of myositis-specific autoantibodies, and review of rituximab use. Pediatr Dermatol 2011; 28(4):357–367.

Christianson HB, Dorsey CS, O'Leary PA, et al. Localized scleroderma: a clinical study of 235 cases. Arch Dermatol 1956; 74:629–639.

Fett N, Werth VP. Update on morphea: part I. Epidemiology, clinical presentation, and pathogenesis. J Am Acad Dermatol 2011; 64(2):217–228.

Fett N, Werth VP. Update on morphea: part II. Outcome measures and treatment. J Am Acad Dermatol 2011; 64(2):231–242.

George PM, Tunnessen WW Jr. Childhood discoid lupus erythematosus. Arch Dermatol 1993; 124:613–617.

Lee LA. Neonatal lupus erythematosus: clinical findings and pathogenesis. J Int Dermatol Symp Proc 2004; 9:52–56.

Lee LA. Cutaneous lupus in infancy and childhood. Lupus 2010; 19(9):1112–1117.

Lee LA, Weston WL. Cutaneous lupus erythematosus during neonatal and childhood periods. Lupus 1997; 6:132–138.

Lehman TJ. Systemic and localized scleroderma in children. Curr Opin Rheumatol 1996; 8:576–579.

Lythgoe H, Morgan T, Heaf E, et al. UK JSLE Study Group. Evaluation of the ACR and SLICC classification criteria in juvenile-onset systemic lupus erythematosus: a longitudinal analysis. Lupus 2017; 26(12):1285–1290.

Martin V, Lee LA, Askanase AD, et al. Long-term followup of children with neonatal lupus and their unaffected siblings. Arthritis Rheum 2002; 46:2377–2383.

McCammack E, Haggstrom AN. Cutaneous manifestations of connective tissue disease. Adolesc Med State Art Rev 2011; 22(1):35–53.

Nelson AM. Localized forms of scleroderma, including morphea, linear scleroderma, and eosinophilic fasciitis. Curr Opin Rheumatol 1996; 8:473–476.

Robinson AB, Reed AM. Clinical features, pathogenesis and treatment of juvenile and adult dermatomyositis. Nat Rev Rheumatol 2011; 7(11):664–675.

Rockerbie NR, Woo TY, Callen JP, et al. Cutaneous changes of dermatomyositis precede muscle weakness. J Am Acad Dermatol 1989; 20:629–632.

Santimyire-Rosenberger B, Dugan EM. Skin involvement in dermatomyositis. Curr Opin Rheumatol 2003; 15:714–722.

Sonntag M, Lehmann P, Megahed M, et al. Lupus erythematosus tumidus in childhood. Report of 3 patients. Dermatology 2003; 207:188–192.

Yokota J. Mixed connective tissue disease in childhood. Acta Paediatr Jpn 1993; 35:472–479.

Nephrogenic Fibrosing Dermopathy

Jan F, Segal JM, Dyer J, et al. Nephrogenic fibrosing dermopathy: 2 pediatric cases. J Pediatr 2003; 143:678–681.

Mackag-Wiggin JM, Cohen DJ, Ardí YA, et al. Nephrogenic sclerosing dermopathy (scleromyxedema-like illness of renal disease). J Am Acad Dermatol 2003; 48:55–60.

Zou Z, Zhang HL, Roditi GH, et al. Nephrogenic systemic fibrosis: review of 370 biopsy-confirmed cases. JACC Cardiovasc Imaging 2011; 4(11):1206–1216.

Lichen Sclerosis et Atrophicus

Becker K. Lichen sclerosus in boys. Dtsch Arztebl Int 2011; 108(4):53–58.

Bohm M, Frieling U, Luger TA, et al. Successful treatment of anogenital lichen sclerosus with topical tacrolimus. Arch Dermatol 2003; 139:922–924.

Chi CC, Kirtschig G, Baldo M, et al. Topical interventions for genital lichen sclerosus. Cochrane Database Syst Rev 2011; (12):CD008240.

Murphy R. Lichen sclerosus. Dermatol Clin 2010; 28(4):707–715.

Loening-Baucke V. Lichen sclerosis et atrophicus in children. Am J Dis Child 1991; 145:1058–1061.

McLelland J. Lichen sclerosus in children. J Obstet Gynaecol 2004; 24(7):733–735.

Poindexter G, Morrell DS. Anogenital pruritus: lichen sclerosus in children. Pediatr Ann 2007; 36(12):785–791.

Sahn EE, Bluestein EL, Oliva S. Familial lichen sclerosis et atrophicus in childhood. Pediatr Dermatol 1994; 11:160–163.

Tasker GL, Wojnarowska R. Lichen sclerosus. Clin Exp Dermatol 2003; 28:128–133.

Necrobiosis Lipoidica

Kavanagh GM, Novelli M, Hartog M, et al. Necrobiosis lipoidica—involvement of atypical sites. Clin Exp Dermatol 1993; 18:543–544.

Kelly WF, Nicholas J, Adams J, et al. Necrobiosis lipoidica diabeticorum: association with background retinopathy, smoking, and proteinuria. A case controlled study. Diabet Med 1993; 10:725–728.

O'Toole EA, Kennedy U, Nolan JS, et al. Necrobiosis lipoidica: only a minority of patients have diabetes mellitus. Br J Dermatol 1999; 140:283–286.

Ullman S, Dahl MV. Necrobiosis lipoidica. Arch Dermatol 1977; 113:1671–1673.

Verotti A, Chiarelli F, Amerio P, et al. Necrobiosis lipoidica diabeticorum in children and adolescents: a clue for underlying renal and retinal disease. Pediatr Dermatol 1995; 12:220–223.

8

Disorders of the Hair and Nails

Saleh Rachidi, Anna M. Bender, and Bernard A. Cohen

INTRODUCTION

Diseases of the hair and nails are an important part of pediatric dermatology. Both hair and nails are composed of keratin, produced by the hair follicle and nail matrix. Some diseases are specific to these structures, while others affect the skin and other organ systems. In many cases, important diagnostic clues to skin and systemic disease can be found in related abnormalities of the hair and nails. Algorithmic approaches to diagnosis for disorders of the hair and nails are summarized at the end of the chapter (Figs. 8.69 and 8.70).

HAIR DISORDERS

Embryology and Anatomy

Hair follicles begin to form around 9–12 weeks of gestation on the face. They develop as a down-budding of the epidermis in association with proliferating mesenchyme, which eventually becomes the dermal papilla. The development of hair follicles continues cephalocaudally on the remainder of the body around 16–20 weeks of gestation. No new hair follicles develop after birth.

In the premature infant, the scalp, forehead, and trunk are covered by variable amounts of fine, soft, long, lightly pigmented lanugo hair (Fig. 8.1). Lanugo is usually shed *in utero* at 7–8 months of gestation. The second covering of subtle lanugo is shed shortly after birth and replaced by short, fine, non-pigmented vellus hair. Terminal hair is thicker and more darkly pigmented and usually grows on the scalp, eyebrows, and eyelashes before puberty and the sites of sexual hair after puberty.

At term, most infants have full scalp coverage with normal terminal hair. However, shortly before or up to 4 months after birth, infants undergo a period of brisk physiologic hair shedding when actively growing hairs convert to the resting phase and are then synchronously shed (Fig. 8.2). In blonds and redheads, the process is often complete before birth, and the hair is sparse at delivery. Shedding may be delayed in dark-haired individuals and may occur rapidly during early infancy. Parents should be reassured that this is a normal physiologic process.

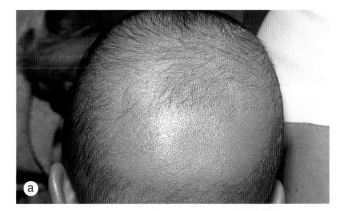

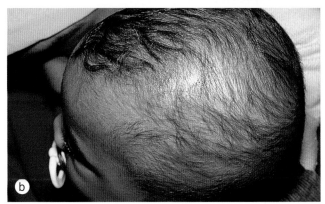

Fig. 8.2 Physiologic hair shedding. **(a,b)** These infants demonstrate the physiologic hair shedding that occurs in dark-haired babies at 3–5 months of age. **(a)** Note the band of exaggerated alopecia, probably brought on by trauma that girdles the occiput.

Fig. 8.1 Lanugo hair. A 31-week premature infant had extensive lanugo hair that covered most of the back. At term, this hair is usually shed before delivery.

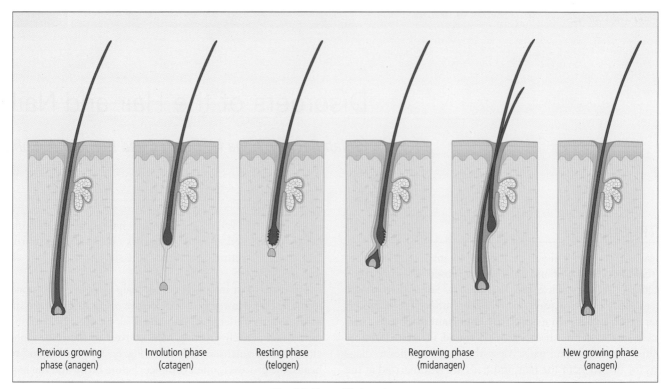

Previous growing   Involution phase   Resting phase   Regrowing phase   New growing phase
phase (anagen)   (catagen)   (telogen)   (midanagen)   (anagen)

Fig. 8.3 Normal hair cycle.

Throughout life, each hair follicle undergoes normal hair cycling, consisting of three phases (Fig. 8.3): anagen (growth phase), catagen (regression phase), and telogen (resting phase). The growth phase, anagen, typically lasts approximately 2–6 years. The length of anagen is genetically determined, varies by anatomic location, and dictates the final length of hair. After anagen, catagen (regression phase) occurs and typically lasts 2–3 weeks. During this phase, the lower two-thirds of the hair follicle involutes. Finally, the resting phase, telogen, occurs and typically lasts 3 months. During the telogen phase, the proximal end of the hair shaft forms a characteristic club shape as is seen in telogen effluvium (Fig. 8.4). After the telogen phase, the hair shaft is shed and anagen occurs again. It is normal for a typical adult to shed approximately 100 scalp hairs per day.

In the newborn, hair growth is synchronous, with all scalp hairs existing in the same phase of the hair cycle described earlier. Conversely, in adults, hair growth is asynchronous, with individual scalp hairs existing in different phases of the hair cycle. At any given time, approximately 85–90% of adult scalp hairs exist in anagen, 10–15% in telogen, and less than 1% in catagen. The adult pattern of asynchronous hair growth generally becomes established anywhere between 4 months and 2 years of life. The normal ratio of hairs existing in anagen and telogen may be altered in certain hair disorders. For example, patients on chemotherapy may lose their hair in a process called anagen effluvium, where dividing cells in the anagen hair bulb arrest and hair is shed within 1–2 weeks. Such patients may show a greatly increased ratio of telogen hairs on their scalp. An increased ratio of telogen hairs on the scalp also occurs in alopecia areata and telogen effluvium.

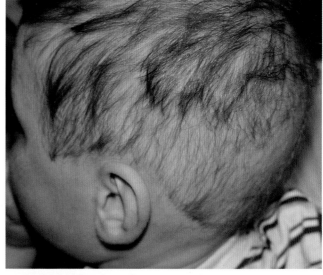

Fig. 8.4 Telogen effluvium. This 3-year-old boy developed rapid diffuse thinning of scalp hair 3 months after an acute febrile illness. This telogen hair loss was associated with a dramatic but transient increase in shedding of club hairs.

Congenital and Hereditary Disorders

The normal pattern of hair growth and shaft morphology may be disturbed in a number of hereditary disorders and congenital syndromes (Table 8.1).

Localized patches of alopecia may be associated with epidermal and connective tissue nevi, pigmented nevi, vascular tumors, and hamartomas, interrupting normal hair

TABLE 8.1 Selected Hair Anomalies

Alopecia (Localized)
Non-scarring
    Hamartomatous nevi (e.g. epidermal, sebaceous)
    Pigmented nevi
    Hemangiomas
    Triangular alopecia
Scarring
    Incontinentia pigmenti
    Halo scalp ring
    Aplasia cutis

Hirsutism (Localized)
Congenital pigmented nevus
Congenital smooth muscle and pilar hamartoma
Repeated trauma

Alopecia (Generalized)
Hypohidrotic ectodermal dysplasia
Congenital hemidysplasia with ichthyosiform erythroderma and limb defects (CHILD) syndrome
Clouston syndrome
Cockayne syndrome
Dyskeratosis congenita
Hallermann–Streiff syndrome
Hay–Wells syndrome
Homocystinuria
Menkes syndrome
Progeria
Trichorhinophalangeal syndrome
Trichothiodystrophy
Cartilage–hair hypoplasia
Papillon–Lefèvre syndrome
Acrodermatitis enteropathica

Hirsutism (Generalized)
Berardinelli lipodystrophy syndrome
Cerebro-oculo-facio-skeletal syndrome
Coffin–Siris syndrome
Fetal hydantoin syndrome
Frontometaphyseal dysplasia
Mucopolysaccharidoses
Leprechaunism
Marshall–Smith syndrome
Trisomy 18
Schinzel–Giedion syndrome
Fetal alcohol syndrome

Hair Shaft Anomalies
Monilethrix (beaded hair)
Pili torti (twisted hair)
    Menkes kinky hair syndrome
    Wooly hair syndrome
    Wooly hair nevus
    Bazex syndrome
    Crandall syndrome
    Björnstad syndrome
    Scurvy
Pili trianguli et canaliculi
    Uncombable hair syndrome
    Ectodermal dysplasia
Trichorrhexis invaginata
    Netherton syndrome
Ribbon-like hair
    Trichothiodystrophy

growth (Fig. 8.5a–e). Perinatal events such as vascular compromise produced by trauma to the scalp during passage through the birth canal can lead to halo scalp ring, an annular patch of non-scarring alopecia, with hair regrowth in the following 6 months. Scarring has been reported but is uncommon.

Triangular alopecia is a distinctive, non-scarring, congenital hair anomaly that may not become evident until later in childhood (Fig. 8.5f). This condition presents with a stable patch of triangular, round, or rectangular hair loss with the base of the lesion characteristically at the junctions of the frontal and temporal scalp. Lesions are usually unilateral but occasionally bilateral. They could be completely devoid of hair or contain vellus hairs and diminished terminal hairs.

Aplasia cutis congenita presents on the scalp or elsewhere on the skin with an ulcer or depressed scar. Peripheral hypertrichosis surrounding the lesion (hair collar sign) could signify underlying neural tube defect (Fig. 8.6). Incontinentia pigmenti is an X-linked disease of females (embryonic lethal in males) with four stages: vesicular, verrucous, hyperpigmentation, and hypopigmentation/atrophy. The fourth stage can manifest as atrophic Blaschkoid plaques with alopecia.

Generalized sparse or abnormal hair growth suggests an inherited hair shaft anomaly or genodermatosis (Figs. 8.7 and 8.8). Monilethrix is a relatively common developmental hair defect that presents in infancy and sometimes after puberty. Affected individuals are born with normal hair, which is then replaced by the abnormal beaded hair in the neonatal period. It is characterized by brittle, beaded hair with nodes separated at relatively uniform intervals (Fig. 8.9). The condition is inherited in autosomal-dominant or recessive patterns. It is mainly seen in the occipital scalp but can affect the entire scalp and other body areas. The condition persists throughout life but may improve in adolescence or adulthood.

Pili torti is another structural defect in which the hair shaft is twisted on its axis (Fig. 8.10). Pili torti may be localized or generalized, and classic presentation is brittle hair in the first year of life in a blond-haired child, although a rarer variant presents around puberty in individuals with black hair. It can occur as an isolated hair defect or in association with a multisystem disorder such as Menkes kinky hair syndrome (an inherited disease of copper metabolism that also affects the central nervous, cardiovascular, and skeletal systems).

Trichorrhexis invaginata (bamboo hair) manifests as brittle, sparse hair in early infancy, which may improve with age. The

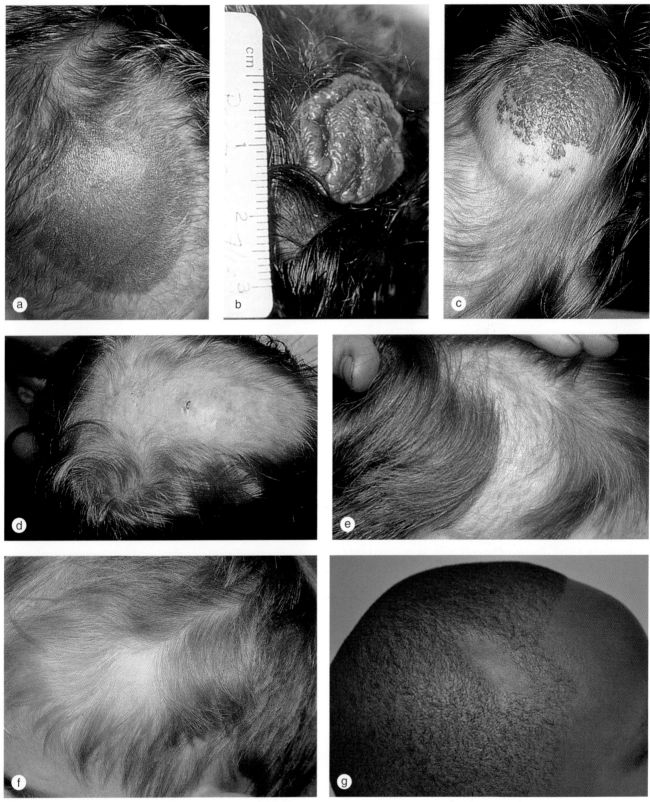

Fig. 8.5 Congenital localized alopecia. **(a)** Marked hair thinning was present in a congenital pigmented nevus on the scalp. At 12 months of age, the hair overlying the nevus was sparse, dark, long, and coarse. **(b)** An area of complete alopecia was noted at birth in a cerebriform nevus sebaceous. **(c)** A 1-year-old infant had sparse hair overlying an involuting hemangioma on the scalp. **(d)** A patch of permanent, scarring alopecia extended across the mid-scalp of a child with amniotic band syndrome. **(e)** An arcuate patch of sparse hair above the ear marked the site of an epidermal nevus in an adolescent boy. **(f)** A healthy 8-year-old boy had a patch of "triangular" alopecia with fine vellus hairs on the right temple for at least 5 years. **(g)** This 10-year-old boy had this triangular patch of alopecia at birth. Vellus hairs were noted on dermoscopy typical of temporal triangular alopecia.

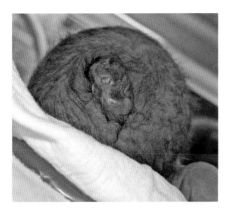

Fig. 8.6 Aplasia cutis congenita with hair collar sign. This premature newborn was noted to have two contiguous round atrophic violaceous plaques on her scalp with surrounding dense hair.

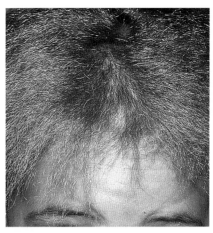

Fig. 8.8 Uncombable hair syndrome is characterized by light blond, frizzy, unruly hair that does not lie flat on the scalp, which makes combing almost impossible. Diagnosis may be made by identifying the triangular-shaped hairs with longitudinal grooves along the hair shaft using light microscopy. Although some cases appear to be autosomal dominant, most are sporadic.

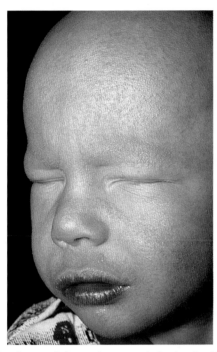

Fig. 8.7 Ulerythema of the eyebrows and cheeks. In this variant of keratosis pilaris, inflammation of the pilosebaceous structures is associated with progressive alopecia and atrophy of the involved hair follicles. This may occur as an isolated disorder of keratinization or in association with other anomalies.

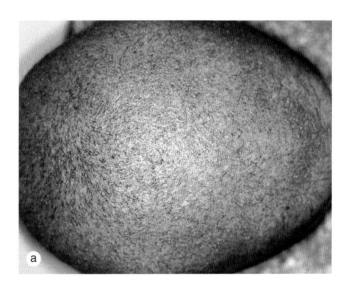

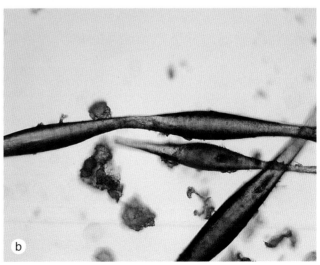

Fig. 8.9 Monilethrix. (a) Short, broken hairs give the appearance of diffuse alopecia. (b) Microscopically, periodic narrowing of the hair shafts is seen. Hairs are brittle and break off at constricted points near the scalp.

hair shaft demonstrates a ball-in-socket morphology where the distal end intussuscepts in the proximal portion. It is seen in Netherton syndrome, an autosomal-recessive dermatosis consisting of severe atopic dermatitis, ichthyosis linearis circumflexa (serpiginous erythematous annular plaques with double-edge scale), and trichorrhexis invaginata (Fig. 8.11).

In the ectodermal dysplasia syndromes, a heterogeneous group of genodermatoses, sparse hair is associated with dysmorphic facies and abnormalities of other structures, which include nails, sweat glands, and teeth (Fig. 8.12). In the hypohidrotic variants, early diagnosis may be life-saving by preventing fatal hyperthermia, which may develop during otherwise self-limited childhood infections.

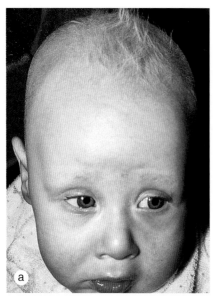

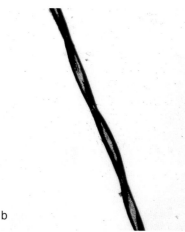

Fig. 8.10 Menkes syndrome. **(a)** This child presented with lightly pigmented skin, blue eyes, sparse hair that demonstrated pili torti, seizures, and loss of developmental landmarks. Copper and ceruloplasmin levels in the serum were low. **(b)** Twisting along the longitudinal axis is noted.

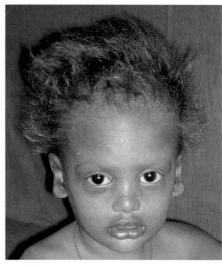

Fig. 8.12 Hypohidrotic ectodermal dysplasia. This child demonstrates the typical findings of sparse hair, absent eyebrows and lashes, frontal bossing, supraorbital ridges, periorbital hyperpigmentation, and thick, everted lips.

Trichothiodystrophy is a hair shaft defect of autosomal-recessive inheritance characterized by deficiency in sulfur-containing amino acids, which manifests in increased hair fragility, splitting of the hair, and alternating light and dark transverse bands on polarizing microscopy (Fig. 8.13). Clinically, the hair is sparse, dull, and brittle. It presents either with isolated hair findings or with a constellation of findings summarized in the acronym PIBIDS: photosensitivity, intellectual impairment, brittle hair, ichthyosis, decreased fertility, and short stature.

Children with congenital hair disorders require a careful medical and neurodevelopmental evaluation. Family history aids in establishing a pattern of inheritance. Hairs are examined microscopically to detect specific anomalies.

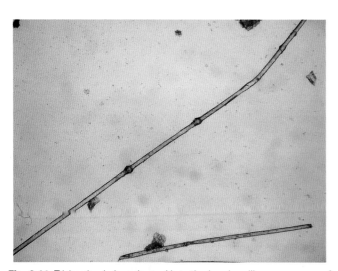

Fig. 8.11 Trichorrhexis invaginata. Note the bamboo-like appearance of the hair shaft from a toddler with Netherton syndrome.

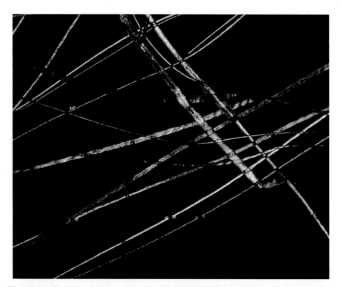

Fig. 8.13 Polarized light microscopy demonstrates hairs with alternating dark and light bands referred to as tiger tails.

Acquired Alopecia

Acquired alopecias may be differentiated by the presence or absence of clinical scarring. In non-scarring processes, inflammation may be clinically evident, subtle, or absent. Non-scarring disorders may be further subdivided by the presence of localized or diffuse involvement. Importantly, chronic non-scarring alopecia can ultimately result in scarring.

Scarring (Cicatricial) Alopecia

Cicatricial alopecia is a broad umbrella encompassing different diseases. It presents with scarring patches of hair loss with absence of follicular ostia. A number of inflammatory disorders may involve the hair follicle primarily or by spread from contiguous skin. In this section we discuss the most common etiologies of scarring alopecia.

Discoid lupus erythematosus (DLE) presents with scaly erythematous plaques in the early phases, then progresses to atrophic, hypopigmented scarred plaques, often with peripheral hyperpigmentation and complete loss of follicular ostia. It most commonly presents as an isolated skin disease but can also be associated with systemic lupus erythematosus. DLE mainly presents on the head and neck and can involve oral mucosa, especially the hard palate, with characteristic shallow erythematous ulcers and white borders. In hair-bearing areas, inflammation around the hair follicle is seen early in the disease and later results in irreversible scarring (Fig. 8.14). Treatment involves topical steroids, topical calcineurin inhibitors, intralesional steroids, and systemic immunomodulators (e.g. hydroxychloroquine, methotrexate, mycophenolate mofetil).

Lichen planopilaris presents with perifollicular erythema and scale, cuffing the hair shaft at its exit from the scalp. Interfollicular erythema can also be observed. This later results in destruction of the hair follicle and scarred patches (Fig. 8.14), which are often described as footprints in the snow. Treatment is largely similar to DLE.

Acne keloidalis is a scarring folliculitis that presents with inflamed papules and pustules at the nape of the neck and occipital scalp in post-pubescent African American men (Fig. 8.15). These later heal with scarring, often resulting in hypertrophic scars and keloids. Treatment includes topical steroids and topical or systemic antibiotics.

Folliculitis decalvans is a severe variant of non-infectious folliculitis that produces slowly but relentlessly enlarging areas of cicatricial alopecia (Fig. 8.16), often affecting the crown. Pili multigemini, multiple hairs arising from a single follicular opening, is often observed (hair tufting or doll's hair). Some treatments include topical or intralesional steroids, vitamin D derivatives, antibiotics, isotretinoin, and biologics including tumor necrosis factor (TNF)-α inhibitors.

Dissecting cellulitis of the scalp may present with boggy, suppurative nodules; abscesses; and sinus tracts with patches of alopecia (Fig. 8.17). It heals with disfiguring scars and/or keloids, most often involving the crown. It mainly affects young men of African ancestry but can affect children, too. Long-standing disease poses increased risk of squamous cell carcinoma. Treatment options include systemic antibiotics, isotretinoin, intralesional steroids, and biologics.

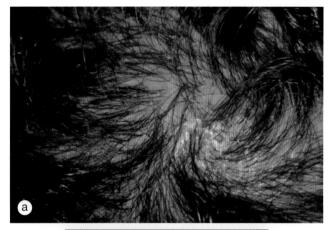
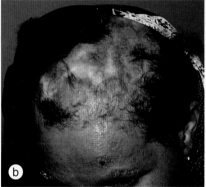

Fig. 8.14 (a) Lichen planopilaris. Lichen planopilaris presents with follicular papules with collarets of scale leading to progressive scarring alopecia. **(b)** Discoid lupus. This woman had an 11-year history of slowly progressive pink scaly plaques on the sun-exposed areas of the face and scalp along with scarring alopecia. The well-demarcated pink scarring plaques presented with classical depigmentation centrally along with a peripheral rim of hyperpigmentation.

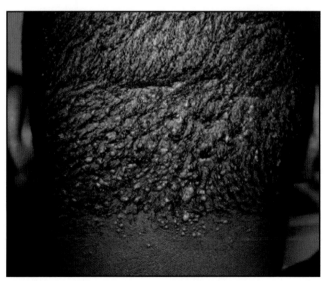

Fig. 8.15 Acne keloidalis nuchae. This healthy teenage boy developed follicular pustules on the back of his scalp, which healed with itchy fibrotic papules.

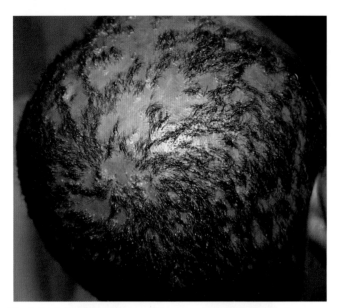

Fig. 8.16 Folliculitis decalvans. This young man complained of recurrent pustules on the scalp leading to progressive patchy hair loss. His follicular papules and pustules improved with oral antibiotics and topical steroids; however the irregular bald patches remained. Note the areas of tufted folliculitis seen as multiple tufts of hair emanating from dilated follicular openings within the scarred patches.

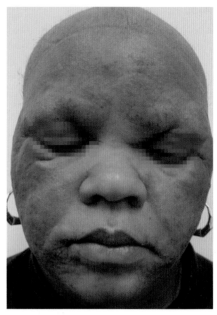

Fig. 8.18 Follicular mucinosis. This young woman developed slowly progressive, asymptomatic violaceous hyperpigmented follicular papules and infiltrative plaques for 2 years. Lesions started on her scalp and face and spread to her neck and trunk. Skin biopsy showed changes typical of follicular mucinosis.

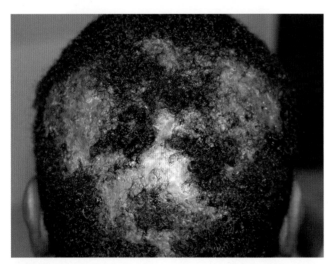

Fig. 8.17 Dissecting folliculitis. This man had a 10-year history of recurrent scarring hair loss associated with boggy fluctuant hairless plaques, suppuration, and a periphery of studded crusts and pustules.

Physical agents including allergens, irritants (acids and alkalis), thermal burns, and blunt trauma may cause necrosis of the skin and non-specific scarring. Examples include alkali burns from hair-grooming products, surgical scars, and radiation-induced injuries. Scarring alopecia may also result from severe infection of the scalp. In addition, scarring alopecia may be associated with infiltrative disorders such as granulomatous infiltration in sarcoidosis or mucin infiltration in alopecia mucinosa (Fig. 8.18).

Patients with scarring alopecia deserve a careful examination of the skin, nails, and mucous membranes to identify clues for diagnosis. When the cause is not readily apparent, a skin biopsy is considered. A delay in diagnosis and treatment may result in widespread patches of disfiguring, scarring alopecia.

Non-Scarring Alopecia

Most hair loss in children occurs without scarring. Clinically, hair loss can be localized or diffuse and may or may not be associated with scaling or inflammation (erythema, pustules, etc.).

Tinea Capitis

Tinea capitis is the most common cause of hair loss in children between ages 2 and 10 years (Fig. 8.19). It is mainly caused by *Trichophyton* and *Microsporum* species and is most common among African American children, but it can also be seen in adults and children of other races.

Tinea capitis has two major patterns: ectothrix, which has dermatophyte infection of the outside and inside of the hair shaft, and endothrix, which involves only the inside. A variety of clinical presentations of tinea capitis occur. Some present with mild redness and scaling in areas of partial alopecia. Others display widespread hair breakage caused by invasion of the hair shaft by the fungus, creating the appearance of black dots on the scalp with short, broken-off hairs poking up on the surface of the scalp. Occasionally, scalp lesions are annular, like patches of tinea corporis. In some children, there is associated edema and pustule formation. As the pustules rupture and the area weeps, thick, matted, yellow crusts form, which simulates impetigo. Less commonly, intense inflammation causes the formation of raised, tender, boggy plaques studded with pustules, known as kerions. Large, occasionally painful, occipital, postauricular, and preauricular adenopathy occurs with inflammatory tinea.

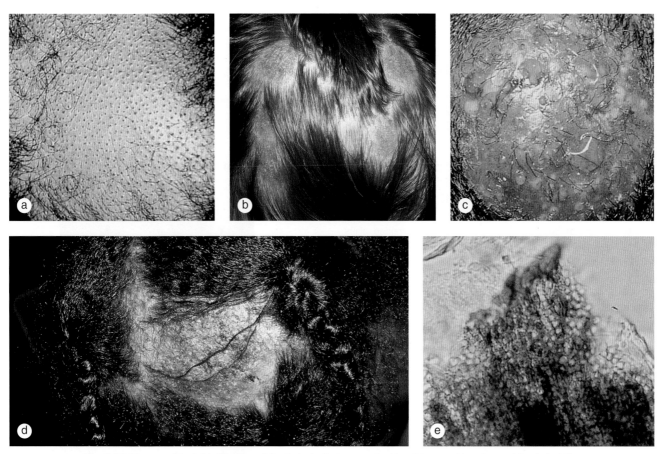

Fig. 8.19 Tinea capitis. **(a)** Infiltration of the hair shafts has resulted in widespread breakage of the hair at the scalp to produce a "salt-and-pepper" appearance known as black dot ringworm. **(b)** Multiple, crusted patches developed in this child with tinea caused by *Microsporum canis*. **(c)** A boggy mass has formed as a result of an intense, inflammatory response known as a kerion. **(d)** A 10-year-old girl developed scarring alopecia after successful treatment of a large kerion with a 2-week course of prednisone and 4 months of griseofulvin. **(e)** Microscopic appearance of hair shafts infected with fungi. Note the tight packing of fungal arthrospores that cause hair shaft fragility and breakage (KOH mount for endothrix).

Unless treated promptly and aggressively with oral antifungal agents and, in severe cases, oral corticosteroids, kerions may heal with scarring and permanent hair loss. Incision and drainage are not indicated.

Fungal infection of the scalp is readily confirmed by a potassium hydroxide (KOH) preparation of infected hairs. The best hairs for examination are those that are broken off at the surface. A good specimen may be obtained by scraping hairs and scale onto a glass slide with a #15 blade. A toothbrush may be used to brush hairs and scale from large areas of the scalp directly onto fungal medium for culture. Before 1970, most cases of tinea capitis in the United States were caused by *Microsporum* species, which fluoresce bright blue-green under Wood light. This screening tool is of little value today because the endothrix infection produced by *Trichophyton tonsurans* does not fluoresce. Favus is an uncommon, severe form of tinea capitis presenting with yellowish crust adherent to the hair shafts and in a honeycomb pattern. It is mainly caused by *Trichophyton schoenleinii*.

Tinea capitis is treated with systemic antifungals as a result of dermatophyte infection of the hair follicle, which cannot be targeted by topical therapies. Terbinafine has the highest efficacy

against *T. tonsurans*, the most frequent pathogen, and is given for 4–8 weeks. It is also effective against *Microsporum canis* and other dermatophyte species. Griseofulvin, given for at least 8 weeks, has slightly better efficacy than terbinafine against *M. canis*; however, given the established safety, efficacy, and shorter treatment duration of terbinafine, the latter remains first-line therapy for *M. canis* as well. Fluconazole and itraconazole are possible alternatives, while systemic ketoconazole should be avoided given its risk of hepatotoxicity. Only fluconazole is available in a liquid formulation.

Although this usually eradicates infection, the risk of reinfection is high. Recurrent infection prompts a careful examination and possible culture of other family members to identify untreated cases. Concurrent use of antifungal shampoos such as selenium sulfide or ketoconazole may help minimize the risk of recurrence and spread.

Although most children who present with scalp pustules have tinea capitis, bacterial folliculitis should also be considered, particularly if pustules are small, are superficial, are not associated with hair loss, and appear at the base of hairs under tension, providing a breach for which bacteria invades. This disorder, termed impetigo of Bockhart, is easily treated by regular

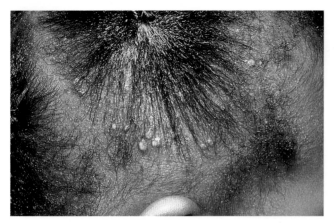

Fig. 8.20 Impetigo of Bockhart. A toddler with tightly braided plaits developed follicular pustules in the area of greatest traction.

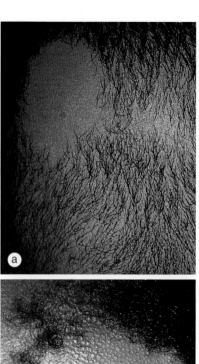

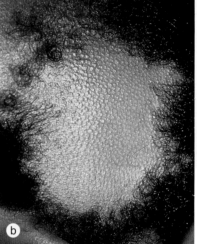

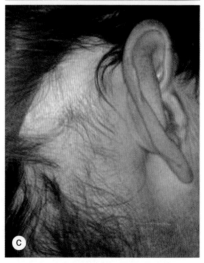

shampooing and loosening of the hair (Fig. 8.20). Occasionally, an oral antibiotic is required. Seborrhea may be difficult to differentiate from tinea. However, seborrhea presents with diffuse patches of fine, flaky, or greasy scale. A child with patches of scalp "seborrhea" warrants a KOH preparation and fungal culture to exclude tinea.

Alopecia Areata

Alopecia areata presents with patches of complete hair loss on the scalp, eyebrows, lashes, extremities, and/or trunk (Fig. 8.21). Occasionally, hair loss progresses to involve the entire scalp (alopecia areata totalis) or the whole body (alopecia areata universalis) (Fig. 8.22). The insult that triggers alopecia areata is unknown. Although clinical signs of inflammation are absent, skin biopsies from sites of active disease show perifollicular, lymphocytic inflammation, as well as deposition of antibody and immune complexes.

Clues to diagnosis include the absence of erythema and scaling in involved areas of the scalp and sometimes the presence of short (3–6 mm), easily epilated hairs at the margins of the patch. Under magnification, these hair stubs resemble exclamation points, as the hair shaft is narrower as they exit the scalp than at the distal end. Yellow dots, which represent enlarged sebaceous glands, are often seen in post-pubertal patients. Another finding in many patients with alopecia areata is Scotch-plaid pitting of the nails, which consists of rows of pits that cross in a transverse and longitudinal pattern. Alopecia areata is also a common cause of trachyonychia in children, which is nail dystrophy with sandpaper texture of the nail plates.

The course of alopecia areata is unpredictable. In adolescents and young adults, hair loss usually resolves without permanent alopecia over months to years. In infants and young children, particularly when alopecia is diffuse, the prognosis is more guarded. Atopic dermatitis is associated with earlier onset and worse prognosis of alopecia areata.

Treatment includes safe measures that do not carry the risk of systemic toxicity. Topical and intralesional corticosteroids, local irritants (e.g. tar preparations, dithranol), topical minoxidil, topical sensitizers (e.g. squaric acid dibutyl ester), calcipotriene, and ultraviolet light therapy have been used with

Fig. 8.21 Alopecia areata. **(a)** Multiple, round patches of alopecia continued to progress despite treatment with griseofulvin for presumed tinea capitis. Cultures for fungus were negative, and the lesions of alopecia areata waxed and waned for years before resolving. **(b)** A round patch of alopecia, with no scale or inflammation, appeared on the scalp of this 10-year-old boy. The shiny, complete alopecia is typical of alopecia areata. **(c)** This woman developed patches of smooth non-scarring alopecia in a headband-like pattern extending from behind the ears around to her occipital scalp. The lack of inflammation or other changes in the skin was typical of alopecia areata.

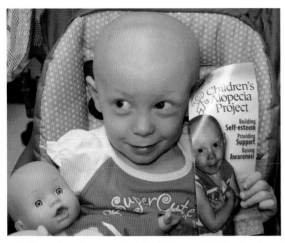

Fig. 8.22 Alopecia universalis. This healthy preschooler developed total body hair loss.

some success. Although oral corticosteroids may induce hair regrowth, these medications do not change prognosis. Consequently, their use should be restricted to short courses in selected patients with widespread, rapidly progressive disease. Studies until 2020 have demonstrated promising results with JAK inhibitors (ruxolitinib and tofacitinib), but controlled clinical trials are still lacking.

Traumatic Hair Loss

A common form of benign hair loss in infants is observed on the occipital scalp because of rubbing in infants who commonly sleep on their back. Parents should be reassured that this is a benign process and hair will grow back.

Traction alopecia is a form of traumatic alopecia common in young girls and women whose hairstyles, such as ponytails, plait, and braids, maintain a tight pull on the hair shafts (Fig. 8.23). This traction causes shaft fractures, as well as follicular damage. If prolonged, permanent scarring can result. When this affects the frontal or temporal scalp, an important clue is the fringe sign, where shorter hairs along the frontotemporal hairline are preserved as they are not included and pulled with the rest of the hair.

Trichotillomania, or hair pulling, is a common disorder seen in toddlers, children of school age, and adolescents resulting from repetitive pulling and/or twisting of hair (Fig. 8.24). It often presents with oddly shaped patches of hair loss, often in broad, linear bands on the vertex or sides of the scalp, where the hair is easily twisted and pulled out. Rarely, the entire scalp, eyebrows, and eyelashes are involved. Hair pulling is most often confused with alopecia areata and can be distinguished based on the bizarre pattern of alopecia and presence of short, broken-off hairs of various lengths. Skin biopsy of the scalp from an area of recent hair pulling may demonstrate large numbers of catagen hairs, perifollicular hemorrhage, and trichomalacia. Shaving the hair in a given area results in normal hair regrowth as the hairs cannot be grabbed and pulled, thus supporting the diagnosis.

Although hair pulling may occur in children with severe obsessive-compulsive disorder or other psychiatric diseases, many cases, particularly in preschool children, are associated with habitual behavior or situational stress (Fig. 8.25). In young, habitual hair twirlers, positive reinforcement or replacement of hair twirling with other socially acceptable behaviors usually succeeds in extinguishing hair pulling. Adolescents and their parents often deny adamantly that hair loss could be caused by the child; thus, the diagnosis rests on a high index of suspicion and recognition of the clinical findings.

Traumatic alopecia may also be caused by breakage of the hair shaft resulting from acquired structural defects of the hair occurring by traumatic hair care practices. The most common defect is acquired trichorrhexis nodosa, which can develop at any age as brittle, short hairs that are easily broken. Microscopically, the distal ends of the hairs are frayed, resembling a broomstick (Fig. 8.26). Other hairs may have nodules that resemble two broomsticks stuck together on microscopy. Acquired trichorrhexis nodosa most commonly occurs in black patients arising from trauma of combing tightly curled hairs or from excessive use of hot combs, hairdryers, hair straighteners, or other chemicals. This disorder is self-limited and normal hairs regrow when the source of damage is eliminated.

Other forms of deliberate and accidental physical, thermal, and chemical injury to the hair shaft and scalp can also cause

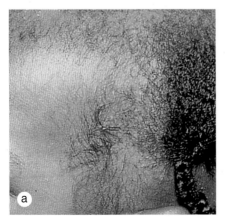
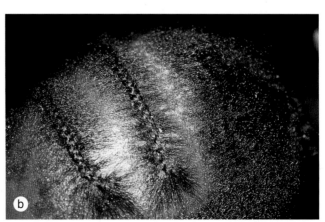

Fig. 8.23 Traction alopecia. Alopecia is most prominent at **(a)** the periphery of the scalp and **(b)** along the parts in the hair. These areas are under the most traction.

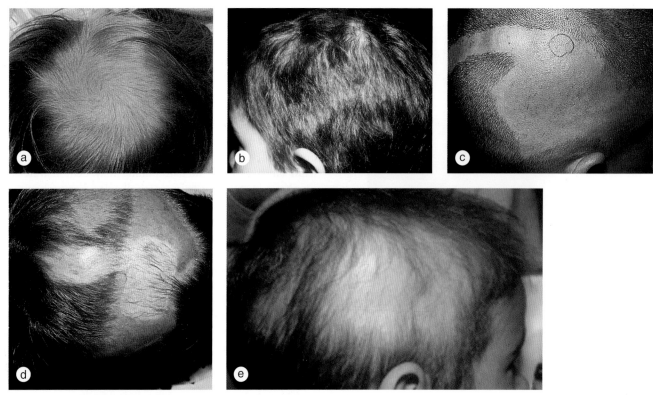

Fig. 8.24 Hair pulling. **(a)** Alopecia from hair pulling is found most commonly on the occiput. **(b)** Hairs broken off and regrowing at various lengths may produce a moth-eaten appearance. **(c,d)** Bizarre patterns that defy anatomic landmarks are typical. **(c)** A short haircut failed to camouflage the alopecia. **(d)** Note the rectangular area of regrowth in the mid scalp, which followed 1 month of covering with an occlusive dressing. **(e)** This healthy 4-year-old girl was observed twirling her hair at naptime and bedtime, resulting in well-demarcated patches of hair thinning. She also had dry, lusterless hairs of varying lengths giving a moth-eaten appearance. The hair loss disappeared a year later when she entered kindergarten.

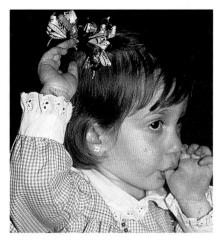

Fig. 8.25 Hair pulling occurs frequently as a habitual behavior. At bedtime and naptime, this happy, healthy toddler pulls and twirls her hair and sucks her thumb.

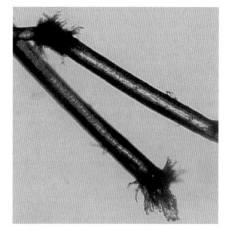

Fig. 8.26 Trichorrhexis nodosa ("split ends") is a brittle hair shaft defect, usually caused by overmanipulation of the hair or chemical use. The frayed broom appearance is typical.

alopecia. Examples include child abuse and pressure necrosis of the skin (Fig. 8.27).

Telogen Effluvium

Telogen effluvium is the most common form of non-inflammatory, non-scarring, diffuse hair loss in children (Fig. 8.4). It displays diffuse hair loss involving the entire scalp, resulting in varying amounts of hair loss, which can be up to half of the scalp's hair. In normal conditions, 10–15% of scalp hairs are in telogen phase at any given time. Duration of the telogen phase is 2–3 months, at the end of which hairs are shed. In telogen effluvium, a stressor results in a significant amount of hairs

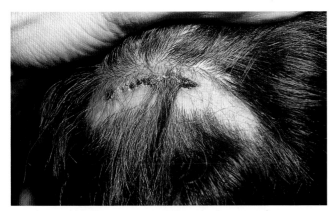

Fig. 8.27 An 11-year-old boy developed pressure necrosis of the skin on the occiput and a linear patch of alopecia several days after liver transplant surgery. The area of injury conformed to the shape of a rubber doughnut, on which his head had been placed at the beginning of surgery.

entering the telogen phase, followed by diffuse shedding of those telogen hairs a few months later. Systemic insults include infections, autoimmune diseases, medications, hormonal changes, nutrient deficiencies, surgery, or other physiological and psychological stressors. Although quite distressing, telogen effluvium is temporary (lasts 6–12 months if the insult is withdrawn) and rarely produces more than 50% hair loss. Chronic diseases such as systemic lupus erythematosus can lead to chronic telogen effluvium lasting for years. In some children, telogen loss occurs repeatedly after recurrent ear infections and upper respiratory infections. Even in these cases, the prognosis for full recovery is excellent. Neither treatment nor laboratory studies are usually required if the insult can be identified by history. Otherwise, laboratory studies including iron, zinc, vitamin D, and thyroid function may be done if such etiologies are suspected. Patients describe hair loss from the roots instead of hair shaft breakage. Diagnosis may be confirmed by examination of hairs pulled from the scalp, which demonstrates an increased percentage of telogen hairs (white hair bulb at the root). Parents are also reminded that hair grows only about 1 cm per month, so the return to pre-telogen effluvium hair length takes many months.

Anagen Effluvium

In anagen effluvium, sudden loss of growing hairs is caused by abnormal cessation of the anagen phase from medications, radiation, or infections. This occurs most commonly in cancer patients who are treated with radiation or systemic chemotherapy, especially cytotoxic agents. In this process, diffuse loss of up to all of scalp hairs occurs over several days to weeks. Eyebrows, lashes, and body hair are affected as well. The extent of hair loss is determined by the toxicity of the agent, dose, and length of exposure. In anagen effluvium, the hair shaft tapers proximally like a pencil point and subsequently loses adhesion to the follicle. Scalp hypothermia is used to decrease this side effect in patients receiving chemotherapy, and randomized clinical trials have demonstrated its efficacy. Hair regrowth usually occurs when the toxic agent is discontinued and is observed as early as 2 months after insult cessation. Anagen effluvium has also been reported with toxic levels of boric acid, thallium, arsenic, bismuth, warfarin, and lead, as well as colchicine.

Loose Anagen Syndrome

Loose anagen syndrome is an autosomal-dominant disorder characterized by actively growing hairs that are loosely anchored to the follicle and easily and painlessly pulled from the scalp (Fig. 8.28). Although the typical patients described are blonde girls between 2 and 5 years old, children of both sexes and children with dark hair color may be affected. These children demonstrate short, variably sparse scalp hair and rarely require haircuts. A hair pull shows dystrophic anagen hairs with ruffled cuticles and darkly pigmented, misshapen hair bulbs with a "baggy stocking" appearance. There is no known therapy, but many patients improve during adolescence.

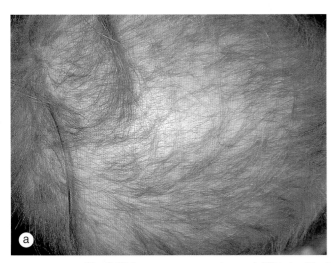

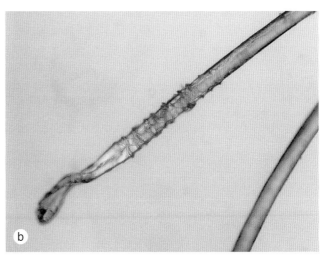

Fig. 8.28 Loose anagen syndrome. **(a)** This healthy toddler had diffusely sparse hair, which was readily epilated. **(b)** The anagen hair bulb is misshapen, and the inner and outer root sheaths are missing. Note the wrinkling of the cuticle giving a "baggy stocking" appearance.

Androgenetic Alopecia

Androgenetic alopecia (AGA) may occur in both males and females and may be seen as early as late childhood or adolescence. Patients usually complain of thinning of scalp hair instead of shedding. In females, the frontal hairline is usually intact, but there is decreased density and miniaturized hairs in the frontal scalp and crown. This can begin as a widened central part (Fig. 8.29). Male pattern androgenetic alopecia consists of bilateral recession of the frontotemporal hairline and thinning of the vertex scalp hair (Fig. 8.30). Dermoscopy reveals miniaturized hairs or hair loss with preserved follicular ostia. Treatment includes topical minoxidil 5% twice daily or oral finasteride, which is only approved for males over 18 years old. Spironolactone orally and oral contraceptive pills have been shown to be useful in adult female patients with androgenetic alopecia

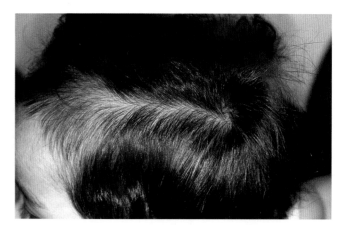

Fig. 8.31 Flag sign. A light pigmented band of hair appeared on the scalp of this 6-year-old girl with cystic fibrosis after several months of inadequate pancreatic enzyme replacement. When her medication was adjusted, the hair pigment returned to normal, and the light band of hair continued to grow outward.

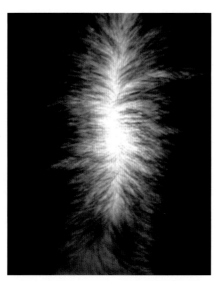

Fig. 8.29 Androgenetic alopecia. This woman presented with widening of the central part on the top of her scalp in a Christmas-tree-like pattern. The density of scalp hair on her occipital scalp remained normal.

(female pattern hair loss [FPHL]). Topical minoxidil 5% once daily can be used in females as well. Females could experience undesired facial hair growth. Use of lower concentration (2%) or cessation of minoxidil would be necessary in that case, with subsequent spontaneous resolution of undesired hair. Female patients should be counseled against applying minoxidil close to bedtime as the medication can rub on the pillow and reach their face.

Generalized changes in the color and/or texture of the hair may also accompany a number of medical disorders (e.g. hypothyroidism, hyperthyroidism), the use of certain medications (e.g. antimalarials), and nutritional deficiencies (e.g. zinc, copper, iron, protein; Fig. 8.31). These disorders fall under the umbrella of telogen effluvium.

Hypertrichosis and Hirsutism

Hypertrichosis refers to localized patches of increased hair growth, whereas hirsutism refers to excessive hair growth, usually in children and women, in an adult male pattern. Generalized increase in hair at birth may occur as a normal physiologic variant. However, unusual patterns or persistence beyond early infancy should prompt a careful evaluation for potentially serious hereditary aberrations (e.g. hypertrichosis lanuginosa, Cornelia de Lange syndrome) (Fig. 8.32). Localized hypertrichosis occurs frequently in Becker nevi, congenital melanocytic nevi, plexiform neurofibromas, and congenital smooth muscle hamartomas. The application of topical corticosteroids or androgens may also stimulate localized hair growth. Post-cast hypertrichosis is also frequently observed after application of a cast for a prolonged period, especially in adolescents and young adults. Widespread hypertrichosis may appear in hypothyroidism, porphyria, and following the use of certain medications, such as phenytoin, cyclosporine, and minoxidil.

Hirsutism presents with excess hair growth in a male sexual distribution such as the upper lip, cheeks, chin, chest, upper back, abdomen, and thighs (Fig. 8.33). Hirsutism may appear as a physiologic variant in an otherwise healthy child. However, an endogenous or exogenous source of androgens must be

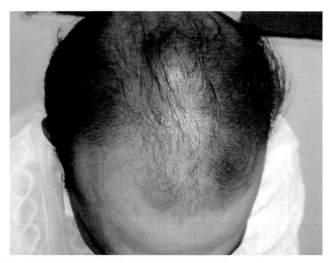

Fig. 8.30 Androgenetic alopecia. This 30-year-old man developed gradual thinning of hair on the frontoparietal scalp and bitemporal recession over the last several years. His father had a similar pattern of hair loss.

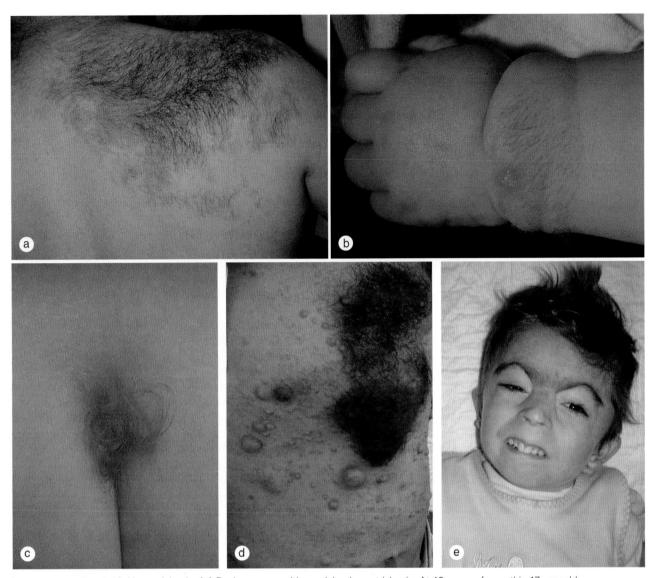

Fig. 8.32 Hypertrichosis. **(a)** Becker nevus with overlying hypertrichosis. At 12 years of age, this 17-year-old boy developed an irregularly shaped uniformly tan patch on the upper back and shoulder. Several years later, dark coarse hair began to appear over the patch. These changes are typical of a Becker nevus also known as a hairy epidermal nevus. **(b)** Congenital smooth muscle hamartoma. This healthy newborn had an asymptomatic flesh-colored plaque on his left wrist at birth associated with subtle coarse dark hair. Rubbing of the plaque led to "pseudo-Darier's sign" mimicking urtication resulting from transient piloerection. A skin biopsy showed changes typical of a smooth muscle hamartoma. **(c)** Faun tail nevus. This 7-year-old girl had an abnormal tuft of hair present in the lumbosacral area since birth. Imaging studies of the underlying spine were normal. **(d)** Plexiform neurofibroma. This man presented with a pigmented plaque with terminal hairs with a "bag of worms" consistency on palpation. He also had multiple neurofibromas and café-au-lait macules. **(e)** Cornelia de Lange syndrome. This 4-year-old boy had microcephaly; mental retardation; bushy eyebrows that met in the midline (synophrys); small, upturned nose; and prominent eyelashes.

excluded, especially if other signs of hyperandrogenism are present or if a patient has signs of premature puberty. Cushing syndrome, acromegaly, and congenital adrenal hyperplasia, along with ovarian, adrenal, or pituitary neoplasms, may be associated with hirsutism. The most common cause of medically significant hirsutism is polycystic ovarian syndrome (PCOS). In PCOS, patients present with evidence of hyperandrogenism, insulin resistance, oligomenorrhea, and/or cystic ovaries. Endocrinologic evaluation is guided by careful history and physical examination. Once terminal hairs develop, correction of the underlying medical condition does not reverse hirsutism, which in turn could be treated with laser, electrolysis, topical eflornithine, or other depilatory agents.

Acne

Acne Vulgaris

This is a disorder of the pilosebaceous apparatus and is the most common skin problem of adolescence (Fig. 8.34). Lesions may appear on the face as early as 8 years of age but usually begin to develop with the onset of puberty. Areas with

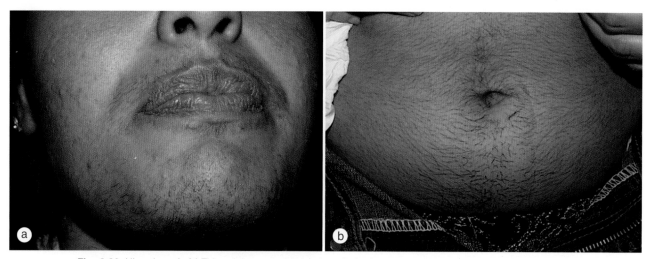

Fig. 8.33 Hirsutism. **(a,b)** This adolescent girl developed slowly progressive generalized hirsutism when she was 14 years old. She showed coarse, dark hairs in the male distribution of the upper lip, lower cheeks, and chin.

prominent sebaceous hair follicles, such as the face, upper chest, and back, are involved.

The exact pathogenesis of acne is unknown. However, abnormalities in follicular keratinization are thought to produce the acne lesion that develops earliest, the microcomedone. In time, microcomedones may grow into clinically apparent, open comedones (blackheads; Fig. 8.34a) and closed comedones (whiteheads; Fig. 8.34b). The entire process is fueled by androgens, which stimulate sebaceous-gland growth, and the production of sebum. The proliferation of *Propionibacterium acnes* in non-inflammatory comedones, and the leak of comedone contents into the surrounding dermis, triggers inflammatory papules, pustules, and cysts (Fig. 8.34c–e). Cystic acne is characterized by nodules and cysts scattered over the face, chest, and back. This variant frequently leads to disfiguring scarring.

Although therapy must be individualized, patients with mild-to-moderate comedonal and/or inflammatory acne are treated with a combination of topical retinoids (e.g. tretinoin, adapalene, tazarotene), benzoyl peroxide, antibiotics, dapsone, and azelaic acid. Moderate-to-severe inflammatory acne warrants oral antibiotics in combination with topical retinoids. Oral 13-cis-retinoic acid (isotretinoin) should be used in patients with moderate to severe acne not responding to the mentioned regimens, and low threshold for its use should be used if scarring is observed. In adolescent and adult females with a hormonal distribution of acne (along the jawline and chin), which often flares before menses, spironolactone and/or estrogen-progesterone OCPs (oral contraceptive pills) can be very effective. Fortunately, acne is usually self-limited and winds down by early adult life. However, some middle-aged adults, especially females, continue to experience breakouts well into adulthood.

Evaluation of a patient with acne includes a careful medical and family history and physical examination. Although no special laboratory studies are usually necessary, signs and symptoms of precocious puberty, hyperandrogenism, or ovarian dysfunction warrant further investigation.

Acne conglobata is a severe form of nodulocystic acne, presenting with interconnecting comedones, cysts, abscesses, and sinus tracts in a typical acne distribution. Treatment includes oral isotretinoin and systemic steroids in the first month to avoid further flare upon isotretinoin initiation.

Acne fulminans is a form of severe cystic acne that occurs abruptly, usually in young males, with fever, myalgia, arthralgia, leukocytosis, and osteolytic bone lesions (Fig. 8.35). Treatment should begin with systemic corticosteroids, then low-dose isotretinoin can be initiated and systemic steroids tapered once the inflammatory phase and systemic symptoms subside. Note that treatment of severe nodulocystic acne with oral isotretinoin can be an inciting factor for acne fulminans, and systemic steroids should be used in that case. Acne conglobata and acne fulminans can be manifestations of genetic syndromes such as SAPHO (synovitis, acne, pustulosis, hyperostosis, and osteitis), PAPA (pyogenic arthritis, pyoderma gangrenosum, and acne), PASH (pyoderma gangrenosum, acne, and suppurative hidradenitis), and PAPASH (pyogenic arthritis, pyoderma gangrenosum, acne, and suppurative hidradenitis).

Acne may occur commonly in the first 2 months of life and is referred to as neonatal acne or neonatal cephalic pustulosis. This usually manifests as small papules and pustules on the face and usually resolves without treatment by 3–6 months of age (Fig. 8.36). Neonatal acne is thought to be related to exposure to maternal androgens and *Pityrosporum* species. Topical ketoconazole can be effective but is unnecessary as this acne is self-resolving. Infantile acne occurs between 3 and 24 months of age. It presents with comedones, erythematous papules, and pustules and sometimes deeper nodules that may be more persistent and difficult to treat (Figs. 8.37 and 8.34d). This is thought to be secondary to adrenal dehydroepiandrosterone (DHEA), and other signs of hyperandrogenism are absent. Treatment includes topical retinoids, benzoyl peroxide, topical or oral antibiotics, and low-dose isotretinoin in severe cases, especially for scarring disease. Acne vulgaris in children 2–7 years of age can be physiologic but warrants investigation

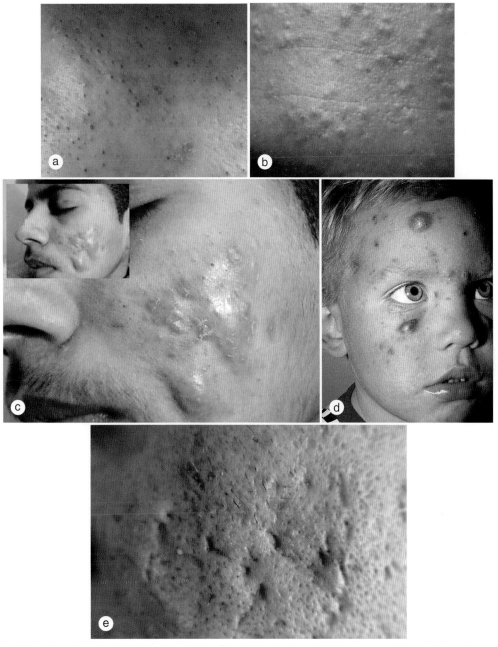

Fig. 8.34 Acne. **(a)** Open comedones (blackheads) dot the forehead of this 16-year-old boy. **(b)** Closed comedones (whiteheads) cover the forehead of this 14-year-old girl. **(c)** Nodulocystic acne. This 18-year-old boy had a 3-year history of severe cystic acne consisting of deep tender nodules, violaceous cysts, pustules, and comedones. He improved dramatically with a 20-week course of oral 13-cis-retinoic acid (isotretinoin). **(d)** Papules, pustules, and cysts spread over the face, neck, and scalp of this toddler. He also responded well to 13-cis-retinoic acid. Both his parents had scars from previous cystic acne. **(e)** Pitted acne scarring. Multiple pitted scars remained after this patient's active acne was treated.

of secondary hormonal causes such as congenital adrenal hyperplasia or neoplasms.

Acneiform reactions differ from classic acne vulgaris by the presence of lesions in a widespread distribution, which may extend to involve the arms, legs, and lower trunk (Fig. 8.38). Endogenous corticosteroids (e.g. Cushing syndrome), prednisone, anabolic steroids, isoniazid, anticonvulsants, lithium, epidermal growth factor receptor (EGFR) inhibitors, and other medications may trigger acneiform eruptions. When the medication cannot

be decreased or discontinued, traditional management with topical and oral acne preparations may help.

Folliculitis

Acne vulgaris may be confused with folliculitis (Fig. 8.39); however, the latter lacks comedones and distribution varies depending on the etiology. Folliculitis can be bacterial, fungal, or sterile or a result of other infectious etiologies (e.g. viral, mycobacterial, *Demodex*). Most commonly, folliculitis is sterile or grows

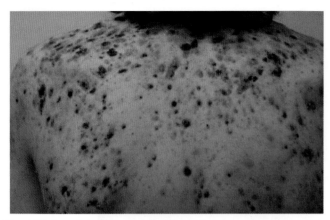

Fig. 8.35 Acne fulminans. This healthy adolescent with severe nodulo-cystic acne developed widespread ulcerations and crusts shortly after starting oral 13-cis-retinoic acid. Oral corticosteroids were added to his regimen and slowly tapered over 2 months.

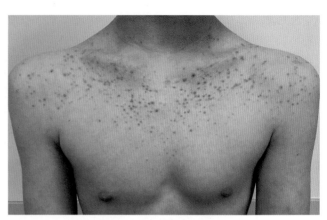

Fig. 8.38 Acneiform eruption. Uniform pustules on an inflamed base appeared on the upper chest and shoulders of this 14-year-old boy who was placed on high dose oral corticosteroids to treat his inflammatory bowel disease. The eruption cleared when he was tapered off the steroids.

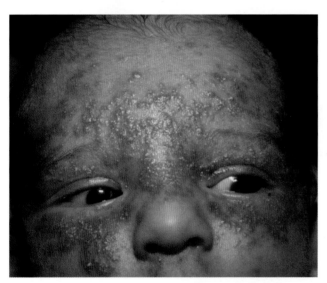

Fig. 8.36 Neonatal acne. This healthy newborn developed numerous closed comedones and pustules on the face. The eruption resolved without therapy 1 month later.

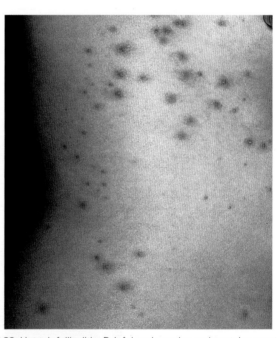

Fig. 8.39 Hot-tub folliculitis. Painful, red papules and pustules erupted (in a bathing suit distribution) on this teenage girl 24 h after lounging in a neighbor's hot tub. *Pseudomonas* grew from pus obtained from one of the lesions. Fortunately, she remained well, and the folliculitis resolved over 3 days without treatment.

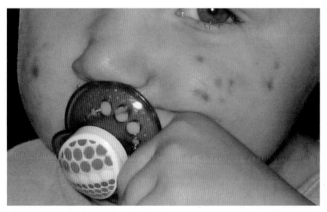

Fig. 8.37 Infantile acne. This healthy infant presented with several atrophic pink papules in various stages of healing on the bilateral cheeks.

various staphylococcal species, many of which are normal skin flora, and is seen on the trunk and proximal extremities. Treatment involves topical antiseptics, topical or oral antibiotics, and topical antibiotics in the nares and perianally in case of *Staphylococcus aureus* carriers.

Pityrosporum folliculitis is an intensely pruritic papular and pustular eruption on the upper trunk and face. Risk factors include systemic corticosteroids and antibiotics, heat, humidity, and occlusive garments. Treatment includes oral fluconazole or itraconazole, topical ketoconazole, or ciclopirox in milder disease.

Pseudomonas folliculitis (hot-tub folliculitis) is due to exposure of pseudomonas in hot tubs or swimming pools, especially with inadequate chlorine levels. The eruption develops on the trunk and buttocks within a few days from exposure and presents as pruritic or tender follicular-based papules and pustules. It is self-resolving but can be treated with oral or topical antipseudomonal antibiotics.

Gram stains, KOH preparations, and cultures help to differentiate folliculitis from acne. Occasionally, an acne patient on long-standing antibiotics develops an acute worsening of acne in association with a gram-negative folliculitis. This probably results from selection of a resistant gram-negative organism. Pustules usually resolve with an alternative antibiotic or isotretinoin.

Acne rosacea is differentiated from acne vulgaris by the presence of red papules, pustules, cysts, and often telangiectasias but the absence of comedones (Figs. 8.40 and 8.41). Acne rosacea first occurs mostly in young and middle-aged patients.

Hidradenitis Suppurativa

Hidradenitis suppurativa (HS), also known as "acne inversa," is part of the follicular occlusion tetrad: HS, acne conglobata, pilonidal cysts, dissecting cellulitis of the scalp. It may develop in association with any of these or as a separate entity (Fig. 8.42). Hidradenitis is a non-infectious inflammatory process that involves the axillae, groin, suprapubic, perianal, and inframammary areas. As with acne, hyperkeratosis of the follicular epithelium leading to follicular occlusion is probably the initiating event. In the acute form, tender pustules and deep-seated nodules become fluctuant and discharge pus. Over time, many patients develop chronic draining abscesses, sinus tracts, and severe scarring. HS is associated with obesity and insulin resistance and worsened by smoking and high-glycemic diet. Treatment consists of topical antibiotics and antiseptics and oral antibiotics for mild–moderate disease, and biologics such as TNF-α and Th17 inhibitors for moderate-to-severe disease. Smoking cessation in smokers and weight loss in obese patients should be encouraged. For patients with localized

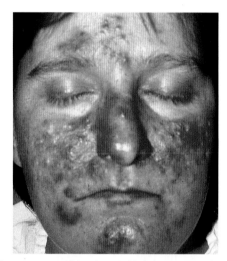

Fig. 8.40 Acne rosacea. This 19-year-old demonstrates the classic rash with red papules, pustules, cysts, and telangiectasias.

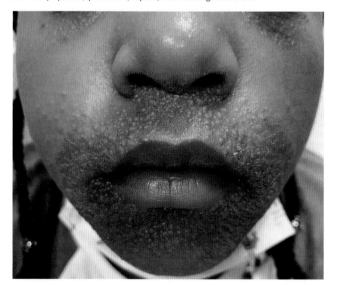

Fig. 8.41 Perioral dermatitis. This 10-year-old girl developed asymptomatic red, discrete, and confluent papules around her mouth, eyes, and nose typical of perioral dermatitis. This is considered a variant of rosacea that can be associated with the use of topical or oral steroids, but her parents denied exposure to steroids. A 6-week course of oral erythromycin resulted in complete and long-term clearing of the eruption.

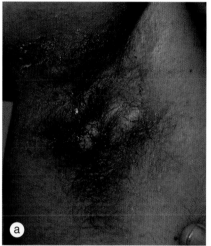

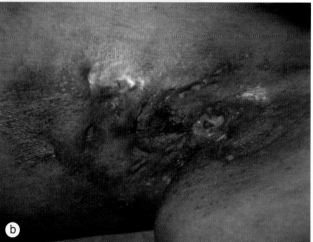

Fig. 8.42 Hidradenitis suppurativa. **(a)** This young man had recurrent inflammatory papules and nodulocystic lesions in the axillae and groin for 5 years. Although lesions initially improved with oral antibiotics, he subsequently developed draining sinus tracts. **(b)** This young woman had multiple indurated sinus tracts, nodules, and ulcers with purulent and necrotic drainage in her axillae.

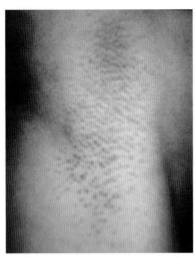

Fig. 8.43 Fox–Fordyce disease (apocrine miliaria). This young woman complained of persistent itchy skin-colored papules in her bilateral axillae that developed during adolescence.

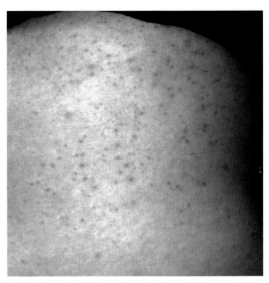

Fig. 8.44 Miliaria rubra. This patient developed itchy non-follicular pink papules while in a hot and humid environment. The rash was more pronounced in areas of skin occluded by clothing.

disease, excision of the active foci can be curative. Intralesional steroids are an effective modality for localized symptomatic nodules as well. Incision and drainage of abscesses is not indicated, as these are sterile, but can be performed for relief of pressure and patient comfort.

Fox–Fordyce disease, also known as apocrine miliaria, presents as pruritic dome-shaped skin-colored papules in areas of apocrine-bearing skin such as the axillae, areolae, pubic, and perineal areas (Fig. 8.43). It is thought to result from retention of keratin in follicular infundibula and is most commonly seen in post-pubescent females. Treatment is with topical steroids and retinoids.

Miliaria

Miliaria are a common presentation of eccrine duct obstruction and include multiple subtypes depending on the level of obstruction in the skin. Miliaria crystallina is caused by eccrine duct obstruction superficially within or just beneath the stratum corneum, resulting in clear, easily ruptured, asymptomatic vesicles that appear in crops. It more commonly occurs in the first few weeks of life as a result of eccrine duct immaturity. Miliaria rubra, also known as prickly heat, is due to deeper obstruction of the eccrine duct within the epidermis. It occurs as "heat rash," consisting of non-follicular, pruritic, erythematous papules in areas of occlusion (Fig. 8.44). It can be seen with excess sweating such as in children who are over-swaddled or bed-ridden or in older children and adults with fever or in hot climates, particularly in occluded areas of the skin. When pustules form within miliaria rubra, they are termed miliaria pustulosa. Treatment is avoidance of excessive heat and topical steroids if needed to alleviate symptoms.

NAIL DISORDERS

As with hair disorders, abnormalities of the nails may provide clues to the diagnosis of multisystem hereditary or acquired diseases. Patients may also seek the advice of practitioners for nail problems because of pain or cosmetic concerns.

Embryology and Anatomy

Nails are first delineated as a fold in the skin of the developing fetus at 10–11 weeks. By the 15th week, the nail plate has already begun to keratinize, well before other epidermal structures. At birth, the nail is fully formed.

The major part of the nail includes the hard nail plate, which arises from the matrix beneath the proximal nail fold (Fig. 8.45). The pink color of the nail bed is derived from the extensive plexus of vessels that lies beneath the normally transparent nail plate. A white, crescent-shaped lunula, which extends from under the proximal nail fold, represents the distal portion of the nail matrix. As the nail plate emerges from the matrix, its lateral borders are enveloped by the lateral nail folds. The skin that underlies the free end of the nail is referred to as the hyponychium, which connects the nail bed with the adjacent skin on the tips of the digits. Abnormalities in any part of the nail anatomy may result in characteristic clinical findings.

Congenital and Hereditary Disorders

Absence, hypoplasia, or dysplasia of the nails may occur as an isolated phenomenon or as part of an ectodermal dysplasia or another genodermatosis (Table 8.2).

Isolated Malformations

Clubbing and spooning (koilonychia) of the nails may occur as autosomal-dominant abnormalities with no other anomalies (Fig. 8.46). Congenital ingrown toenails may result from congenital malalignment of the great toenails and resolve only with surgical realignment, but most cases are self-limiting and not related to an anatomic nail defect (Fig. 8.47). In the spontaneously regressing type, the ingrown nail may result from transient hypoplasia of the toenails, particularly the great toenails, which

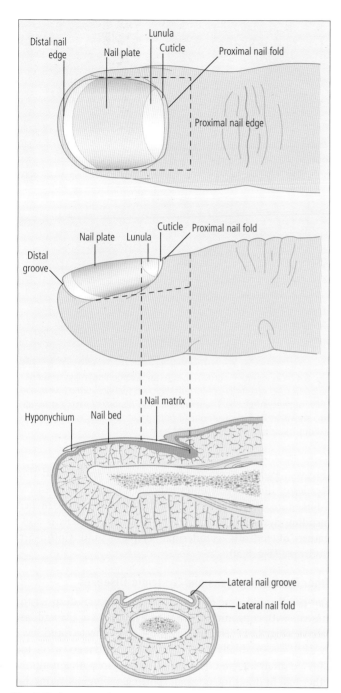

Fig. 8.45 Anatomy of the nail.

TABLE 8.2	Selected Nail Anomalies

Anonychia
Deafness, onycho-osteodystrophy, mental retardation (DOOR) syndrome
Nail–patella syndrome
Hallermann–Streiff syndrome
Coffin–Siris syndrome
Klein syndrome

Hereditary Ectodermal Dysplasias
(Variable findings in which alopecia, dental defects, nail defects, or anhidro-
sis occur in combination with one sign affecting other structures of epidermal origin)

Chromosomal Anomalies
Monosomies 4p, 9p
Trisomies 3q partial, 7q, 8, 8p, 9p, 13, 18, 21
Turner syndrome
Noonan syndrome
Group G-ring chromosome

Hyperplastic Nails
palmoplantar keratoderma
Ichthyosis
Pachonychia congenita
Group G-ring chromosome

Koilonychia (Spoon Nails)
Mal de Meleda keratoderma
Monilethrix
Nail–patella syndrome
Incontinentia pigmenti
Trichothiodystrophy

Drug-Induced Malformations
Phenytoin, trimethadione, paramethadione
    Hyperpigmentation
    Hypoplasia
Warfarin
    Hypoplasia
Fetal alcohol syndrome
Hypoplasia

Miscellaneous Disorders With Nail Dystrophy
Epidermolysis bullosa
Acanthosis nigricans
Acrodermatitis enteropathica
Diabetes
Gingival fibromatosis
Hyper-IgE syndrome
Hyperuricemia
Lesch–Nyhan syndrome
Tuberous sclerosis

usually resolves within 12–18 months. Nail changes may be exacerbated by external trauma and recurrent/chronic paronychia.

Ectodermal Dysplasias

Many of the ectodermal dysplasias are associated with nail
abnormalities; some may be characteristic and diagnostic. In
pachonychia congenita, an autosomal-dominant disorder with
variable penetrance, hyperkeratosis of the nail bed, which develops in the first few months of life, is followed by vertical
thickening and elevation of the nail plate with yellow-brown
discoloration (Fig. 8.48). Minor trauma may induce painful

separation of the nail plate from the nail bed and bleeding.
Hyperhidrosis of the palms and soles, as well as callosities and
blistering are common. Other findings include leukokeratosis
of the oral mucosa (not associated with malignant degeneration), thickening of the tympanic membranes (which results in
deafness), leukokeratosis of the cornea, and cataracts. Hyperkeratotic papules on the extensor surfaces of the extremities,
dermoid cysts, and steatocystoma multiplex are other findings.

Pachonychia congenita Jadassohn–Lewandowsky type, which
is not associated with eye findings, is caused by a mutation in the

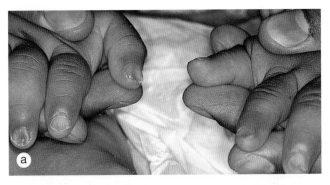

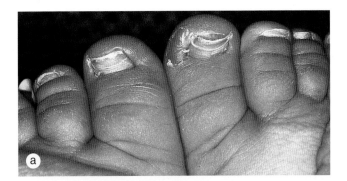

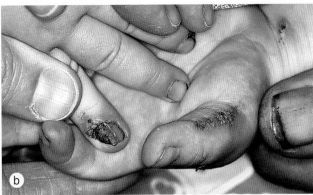

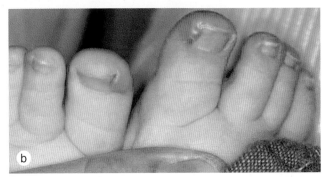

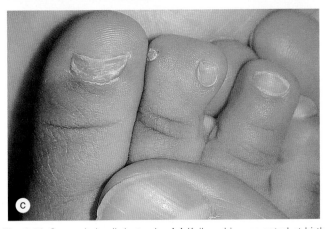

Fig. 8.47 Congenital ingrown nails. **(a)** Congenital malalignment of the great toes resulted in recurrent ingrown toenails, which were eventually repaired surgically. There was a family history of similar problems. **(b)** This infant had involvement of both great toenails, which improved without treatment by 12 months of age.

Fig. 8.46 Congenital nail dystrophy. **(a)** Koilonychia was noted at birth in this infant whose mother had similar nails. **(b)** An extensive congenital epidermal nevus involved this infant's left thumb and right fifth fingernail. **(c)** Isolated congenital bifid nails were present in this infant and several other members of his father's family.

keratin 16 (*KRT16*) or keratin 6A (*KRT6A*) genes. Defects in keratin 17 (*KRT17*) or keratin 6B (*KRT6B*) genes are associated with the Jackson–Lawler type where corneal dystrophy is found without oral leukoplakia.

Dyskeratosis congenita may be confused with pachonychia congenita. However, in dyskeratosis congenita, which may be X linked, autosomal dominant, or autosomal recessive, the nail plate is thinned with longitudinal ridging and pterygium formation (Fig. 8.49). In dyskeratosis congenita, poikiloderma with reticulated pigmentation, telangiectasias, and atrophy is most prominent on the neck and trunk. Leukoplakia of the oral mucosae may develop into squamous cell carcinoma. Other malignancies of the gastrointestinal tract are also

observed. Pancytopenia is common in the second and third decades of life and resembles Fanconi anemia. Most cases are X-linked recessive because of mutations in the Xq28 gene encoding dyskerin (*DKC1*). Hypoplasia of the nails is also a feature of hidrotic ectodermal dysplasia and Coffin–Siris syndrome (Fig. 8.50).

Other Genodermatoses and Systemic Diseases

Nail-patella syndrome is an autosomal-dominant disorder that presents with congenital absence or hypoplasia of the nails and patellae (Fig. 8.51). Thumbs are most often affected, and severity decreases gradually from the first to fifth fingers, while toenails are rarely affected. Triangular lunulae are pathognomonic. Other nail findings include nail splitting, pterygia, koilonychia, and brittle nails. Besides the patella, bone dysplasia is observed in the pelvis and elbows. Glomerulonephritis occurs in a small percentage of cases and is rarely fatal. Heterochromia iris, keratoconus, and cataracts have also been reported.

Periungual fibromas (Koenen tumors) arise adjacent to the proximal nail fold and are major criteria of tuberous sclerosis (TS). Although the fibromas do not appear until later childhood or adult life, they may provide the first clue to diagnosis in individuals who are otherwise mildly affected (Fig. 8.52). They can also develop after trauma in unaffected individuals, but their presence should raise suspicion for TS. Other nail findings in TS include longitudinal grooves and erythronychia.

Congenital hypoplasia of the nails in infants with intrauterine exposure to anticonvulsants, alcohol, warfarin, or other

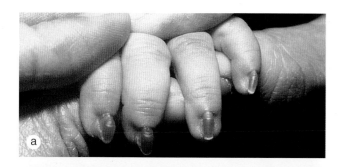

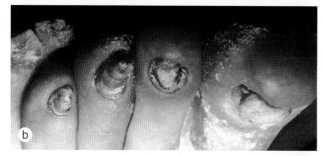

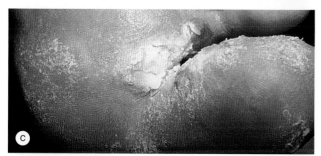

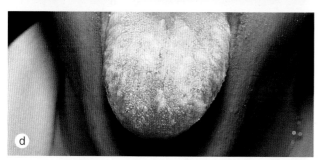

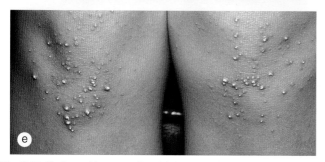

Fig. 8.48 Pachonychia congenita. **(a)** At 3 months of age, all 20 of this child's nails showed early changes of pachonychia with yellowing and pinched-up hyperplasia. **(b,c)** His father had marked involvement of all nails, as well as painful callosities on the dorsal and plantar aspects of the feet. **(d)** Leukokeratosis without a risk of malignant degeneration usually appears in infancy or early childhood and may involve the tongue, gingivae, and oral mucosae. **(e)** Hyperkeratotic papules on the extensor surfaces of the extremities are also common, particularly over the knees and elbows.

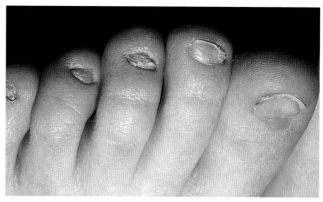

Fig. 8.49 Dyskeratosis congenita. Unlike pachonychia congenita, the nails are usually thin, fragile, and hypoplastic.

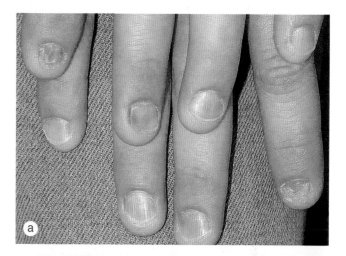

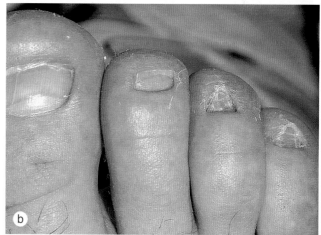

Fig. 8.50 Hypohidrotic ectodermal dysplasia. This child's **(a)** fingernails and **(b)** toenails were thin, somewhat hypoplastic, frequently dystrophic, and fractured by minor trauma.

teratogens should prompt a thorough evaluation for other drug-induced stigmata (Fig. 8.53).

Acquired Nail Disorders

Paronychia

Paronychia is a common childhood disorder. It presents as a red, tender swelling of the proximal or lateral nail fold.

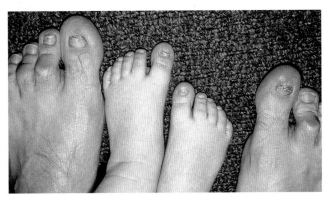

Fig. 8.51 Nail-patella syndrome. Both father and son had hypoplastic patellae and dystrophic, hypoplastic nails.

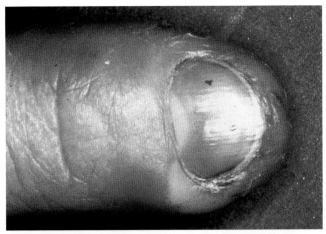

Fig. 8.54 Paronychia. An acute, staphylococcal paronychia developed after this child picked at a hangnail.

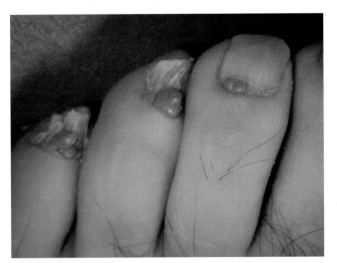

Fig. 8.52 Periungual fibromas, in the proximal nail groove. This is a common finding in patients with tuberous sclerosis.

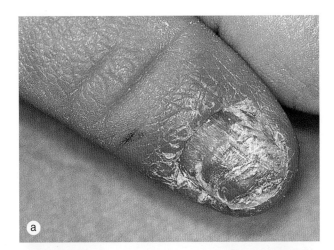

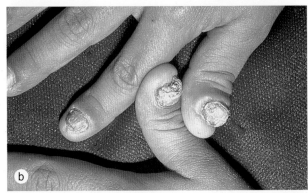

Fig. 8.55 Chronic paronychia. **(a)** A chronic, candidal paronychia recurred for over a year on the finger of an otherwise healthy toddler. Note the erythema at the base of the nail and loss of the cuticle. **(b)** All 20 nails were discolored and hyperplastic in this 8-year-old boy with chronic mucocutaneous candidiasis. The chronic paronychia and nail dystrophy resolved on long-term treatment with oral ketoconazole.

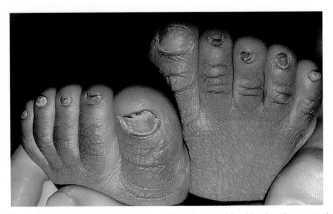

Fig. 8.53 Fetal alcohol syndrome. This 3-year-old with developmental delay, dysmorphic facies, and other stigmata of fetal alcohol syndrome had multiple congenital hypoplastic and dysplastic nails.

In the acute form, exquisite pain, sudden swelling, and sometimes abscess formation around one nail are caused by bacterial invasion after trauma to the cuticle (Fig. 8.54). Chronic paronychia may involve one or several nails. There is usually a history of frequent exposure to water (dishwasher's or thumb-sucker's paronychia). Tenderness is mild, and a small amount of pus may sometimes be expressed. In chronic cases, the nail may be discolored and dystrophic (Fig. 8.55). The causative organisms are *Candida* species, usually *C. albicans*.

Acute paronychia responds quickly to drainage of the abscess and warm tap-water soaks. Occasionally, oral anti-staphylococcal antibiotics are required. Chronic lesions resolve with topical antifungal agents and avoidance of water. Parents of toddlers must be reassured that recurrent candidal paronychia eventually heals without scarring when thumb-sucking ends. Intermittent, chronic use of antifungal creams in young children is effective and safe.

Nail Dystrophy

Nail dystrophy (distortion and discoloration of normal nail plate structure) may result from any traumatic or inflammatory process that involves the nail matrix, nail bed, or surrounding tissues. Although onychomycosis, the result of dermatophyte fungal infection, is the most common cause of nail dystrophy in adults, it is unusual in children before puberty (Fig. 8.56). Dystrophic nails occur frequently as a complication

of trauma (Fig. 8.57) or underlying dermatoses, such as psoriasis, atopic dermatitis, lichen planus, and alopecia areata (Figs. 8.58–8.61).

Trauma to the nail may cause a subungual hematoma, which results in a brown-black discoloration. This is particularly likely after crush injuries. Usually, the diagnosis is simple, unless trauma is subtle. Although most hematomas resolve without treatment, large, painful collections of blood may be drained by drilling a small hole in the nail plate using a sterile, large-bore needle. This relieves pain and reduces the risk of infection. Dark pigmentation at the base of the great toenail, caused by jamming the toe into the end of the shoe at a sudden stop, is called "turf toe" and also results from subungual hemorrhage (Fig. 8.62). This must be differentiated from melanoma and melanonychia (Fig. 8.63). Hemorrhage may be identified by the presence of purple-brown pigment in the distal nail and normal proximal outgrowth of the nail. In melanonychia, gray-brown streaks of pigment of varying width extend longitudinally from the proximal nail fold of one or several nails. Although this finding is common in darkly pigmented individuals, it may occur in individuals of any race at any age. Irregular or changing pigment streaks require a nail biopsy to confirm their innocent nature and exclude melanoma. Extension of a dark longitudinal streak to the proximal nail fold is called the Hutchinson sign and is very suggestive of melanoma.

Nail biting, grooming, and chronic manipulation of any sort may also result in nail dystrophy. Repeated trauma to the cuticle may produce leukonychia (transverse white lines) and constant picking of the nail plate leads to median nail dystrophy (central longitudinal ridging; Fig. 8.64).

Twenty-nail dystrophy (trachyonychia) is a disorder of otherwise healthy children of school age and is characterized by yellowing, pitting, increased friability, and other dystrophic changes that progress over several months to involve most or all of the nails, giving them a roughened texture (Fig. 8.65). Although the course is variable, in many cases the dystrophy

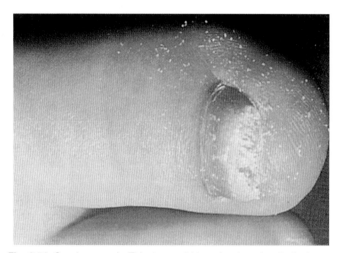

Fig. 8.56 Onychomycosis. This 4-year-old boy developed a single dystrophic toenail, which grew *Trichophyton rubrum* on fungal culture. His father had chronic athlete's foot.

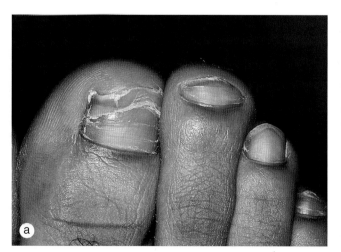
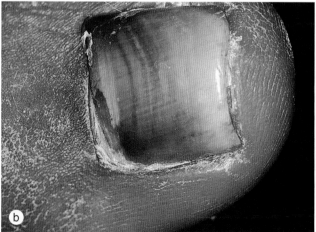

Fig. 8.57 Traumatic nail dystrophy. **(a)** Onychoschizia (transverse splitting of the nail at the distal free edge) occurred in both great toenails as a result of recurrent trauma from basketball in this high-school athlete. **(b)** Another adolescent athlete developed chronic *Pseudomonas* infection in a dystrophic great toenail.

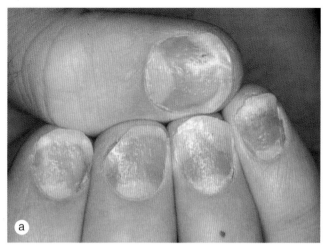
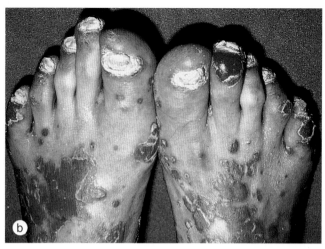

Fig. 8.58 Nail psoriasis. **(a)** This 26-year-old male presented with pits on the fingernail surface, onycholysis, and mild subungual hyperkeratosis, as well as generalized psoriatic plaques and **(b)** yellow, friable, flaking nails in another child with severe psoriatic arthritis.

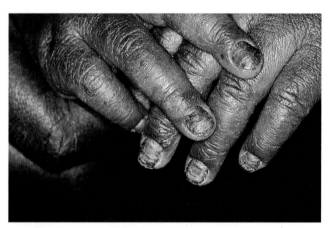

Fig. 8.59 Atopic nails. Multiple, transverse ridges and splitting of the nails developed in an atopic patient with generalized skin disease, which included severe hand involvement.

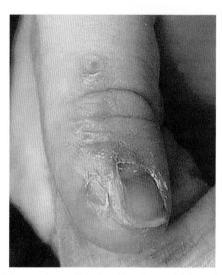

Fig. 8.61 Lichen striatus. This healthy 7-year-old boy developed an asymmetric nail dystrophy as a linear lichenoid eruption extended down his left arm to the lateral aspect of his thumb. A biopsy of the skin showed changes typical of lichen striatus.

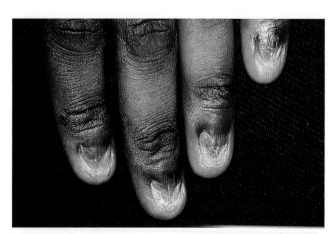

Fig. 8.60 Lichen planus. An adolescent girl demonstrates the characteristic nail changes in lichen planus, which include onychorrhexis (longitudinal splitting) and pterygium formation (forward growth of the skin at the proximal nail fold, which results from scarring).

resolves without scarring over a period of several years. This disorder probably includes a number of conditions that cannot be differentiated unless other cutaneous findings appear. Major causes of trachyonychia include lichen planus, alopecia areata, and psoriasis.

Nail dystrophy may accompany other skin disorders and help with their diagnosis. For example, alopecia areata is associated with characteristic Scotch-plaid pitting of the nails (Fig. 8.66). Psoriasis in the nail matrix results in scattered pits that are larger, deeper, and less numerous and more randomly arranged than those found in alopecia areata (Fig. 8.58a). Psoriasis of the nail bed, especially under the distal nail, causes separation of the nail plate from the underlying skin (onycholysis) and oil-drop discoloration with heaped-up scaling (Fig. 8.58b). Onycholysis alone, without

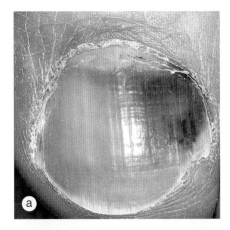

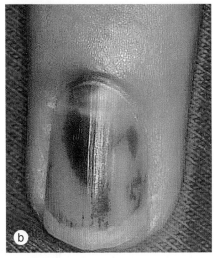

Fig. 8.62 Traumatic subungual hematoma. **(a)** Discoloration as a result of traumatic hemorrhage under the toenail is common in children and athletic adults. It is a result of repeated jamming of the toe into the end of the shoe while running or stopping suddenly (turf toe). **(b)** This 10-year-old boy slammed his finger in a car door a week ago.

pits or discoloration, may be caused by trauma, infection, nail-polish hardeners, or phototoxic reactions to drugs such as tetracyclines (Fig. 8.67).

Nail Changes and Extracutaneous Systemic Disease

Nail findings may provide a clue to the diagnosis of underlying medical disorders (Fig. 8.68). For example, clubbing may be associated with chronic pulmonary disease or congenital heart disease with a right-to-left shunt. Splinter hemorrhages in the nail bed are a physical sign of bacterial endocarditis. Cyanosis of the nail beds in Raynaud phenomenon and periungual telangiectasias may support a diagnosis of collagen vascular disease. Thickened, yellow, slow-growing nails (yellow nail syndrome) are associated with bronchiectasis and lymphedema. Koilonychia has been reported in hemochromatosis and iron deficiency. Color changes where the proximal nail appears white and the distal nail pink probably result from edema and changes in blood flow in the nail bed associated with kidney failure, heart failure, and cirrhosis. Leukonychia totalis may present at birth or develop in childhood. Although it may arise sporadically, it is most frequently inherited as an autosomal-dominant trait and may be associated with other features such as epithelial cysts and renal calculi. The white color results from retention of nuclei within the nail plate rather than a disorder of the nail bed. Uniform, transverse, white lines and/or grooves in the nail that move distally with nail growth (Beau lines) result from growth arrest during periods of stress including acute childhood infections, surgery, chemotherapy, and flares of systemic disorders (Fig. 8.68). Mees lines are transverse white lines of the nail plate and are seen with arsenic or thallium poisoning.

See Figs. 8.69 and 8.70 for diagnostic algorithms for disorders of the hair and nails.

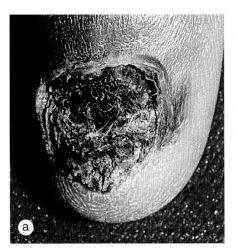

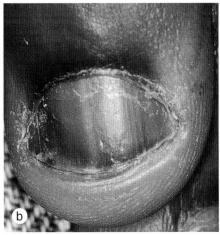

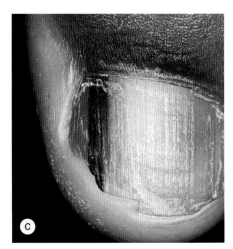

Fig. 8.63 (a) In this patient with an acral melanoma, which arose in the nail matrix or nail bed, the nail has become dystrophic and the nail bed is infiltrated with pigmented, malignant cells. **(b,c)** In melanonychia, neat, hyperpigmented streaks extend vertically across the nail from the proximal nail fold. This can appear in **(b)** a diffuse pattern or **(c)** in narrow bands.

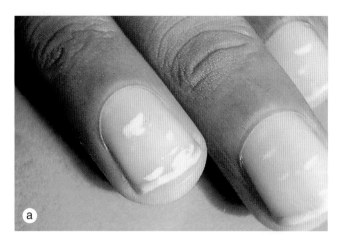

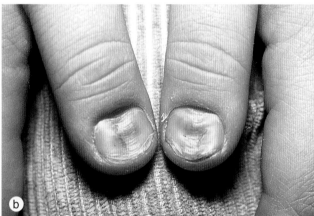

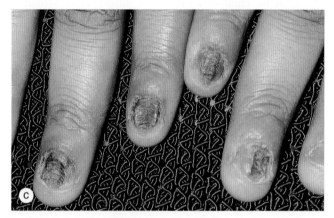

Fig. 8.64 Traumatic nail changes. **(a)** Leukonychia consists of punctate lesions or transverse white lines that grow out along the nail plate and frequently result from trauma to the nail at the cuticle. **(b)** Median nail dystrophy developed in this teenage boy, who admitted to chronically picking at his nails. **(c)** This adolescent was an obsessive nail picker. In addition to median nail dystrophy, he developed crusting and hemorrhage of fingers finger and toenails.

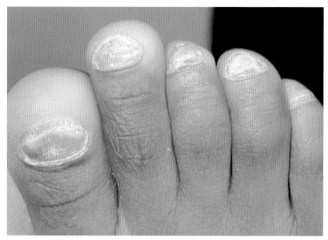

Fig. 8.65 Trachyonychia. This otherwise-healthy 9-year-old boy developed an asymptomatic nail dystrophy, which progressed to involve all 20 nails. Note the increased ridging, opalescence, and sandpaper-like roughness of all his nails. These nail changes can occur in association with lichen planus, psoriasis, atopic dermatitis, and alopecia areata.

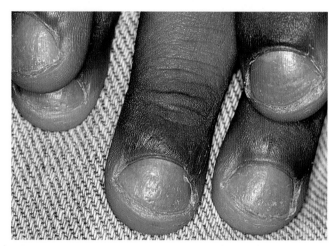

Fig. 8.66 Scotch-plaid pitting, transverse rows of regularly spaced pits, was associated with alopecia areata in this teenager.

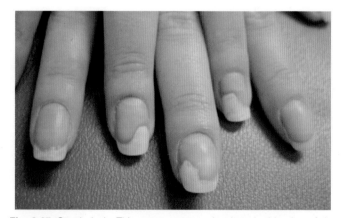

Fig. 8.67 Onycholysis. This young woman developed whitening of the distal nail plate with distal separation of the nail plate from the nail bed. It can be seen in inflammatory skin disorders such as psoriasis and secondary to chemical irritants, trauma, and medications. Onycholysis resulting from sunlight exposure is called photo-onycholysis and may occur in individuals taking oral doxycycline.

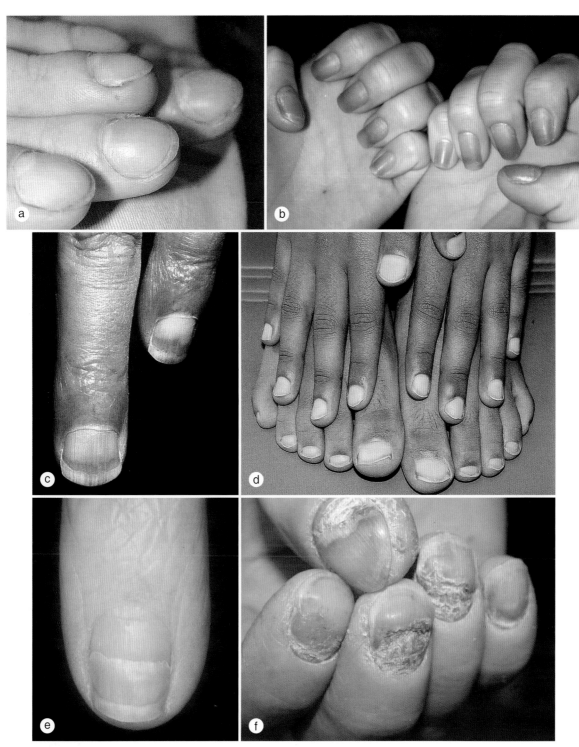

Fig. 8.68 Nail changes and systemic disease. **(a)** Clubbing may occur as an isolated, inherited defect or a complication of chronic lung or heart disease. **(b)** Yellow nail syndrome with chronic yellowing and slow growth of all nails was noted in this patient with Hodgkin disease. **(c)** Half-and-half nails (proximal nail bed white and distal nail bed red) were a marker for uremia in this 14-year-old girl with chronic renal failure. **(d)** White nails developed in this healthy 9-year-old boy. There was no family history of leukonychia, and a complete physical examination failed to reveal other significant cutaneous or systemic findings. **(e)** Beau line. This patient developed a transverse groove several months after a serious systemic infection from which she recovered 6 months earlier. These growth arrest lines affected all 20 nails and slowly grew toward the distal edge of the nail plate. **(f)** Onychomadesis. This man presented with crusting and scaling at the base of the nail associated with nail shedding. Onychomadesis has been reported in patients with bullous dermatoses, febrile illnesses, psoriasis, and cutaneous drug eruptions, particularly Stevens–Johnson syndrome and toxic epidermal necrolysis.

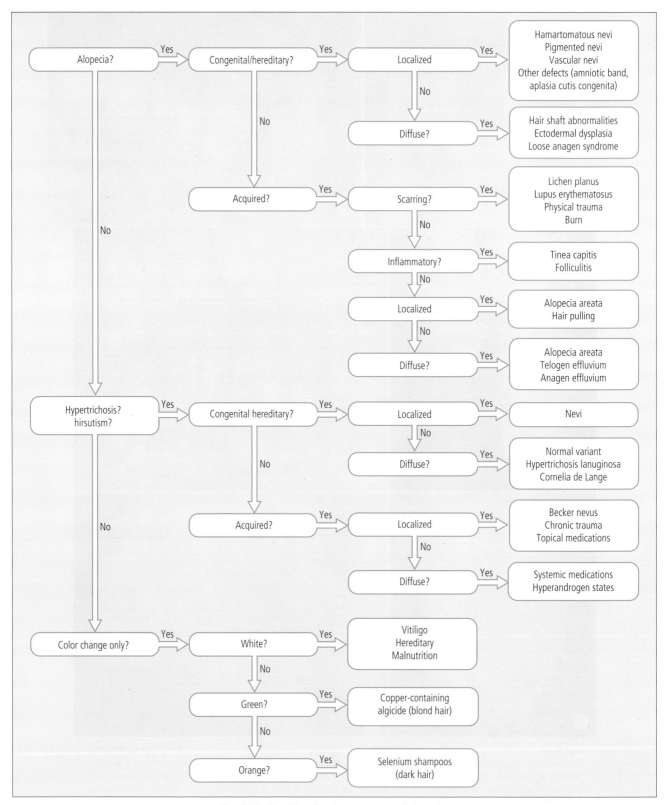

Fig. 8.69 Algorithm for the evaluation of the hair.

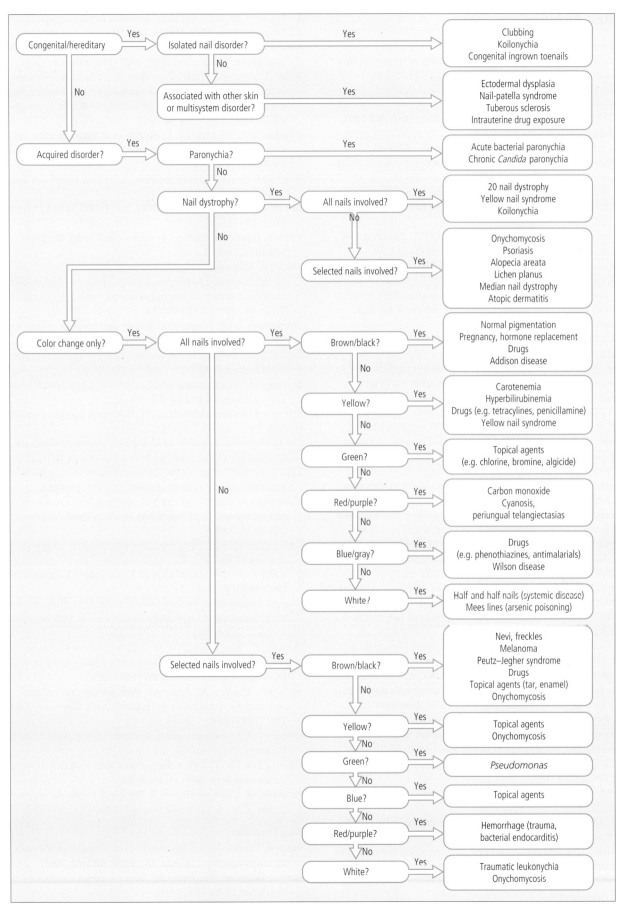

Fig. 8.70 Algorithm for evaluation of disorders of the nails.

FURTHER READING

Hair Disorders

Akoglu G, Emre S, Metin A, et al. High frequency of hypertrichosis after cast application. Dermatology 2012; 225(1):70–74.

Baden HP. Diseases of the hair and nails. Yearbook Medical Publishers, Chicago, 1987.

Barth JH. Normal hair growth in children. Pediatr Dermatol 1987; 4:173–184.

Bolognia J, Jorizzo JL, Rapini RP (eds). Hair, nails and mucous membranes. In: Dermatology, 2nd edn. Mosby/Elsevier, St Louis, 2008, pp. 965–1074.

Burk C, Hu S, Lee C, et al. Netherton syndrome and trichorrhexis invaginata—a novel diagnostic approach. Pediatr Dermatol 2008; 25(2):287–288.

Centers for Disease Control and Prevention (CDC). Pseudomonas dermatitis/folliculitis associated with pools and hot tubs—Colorado and Maine, 1999–2000. MMWR Morb Mortal Wkly Rep 2000; 49(48):1087–1091.

Chen X, Jiang X, Yang M, et al. Systemic antifungal therapy for tinea capitis in children: an abridged Cochrane Review. J Am Acad Dermatol 2017; 76(2):368–374.

Cheng AS, Bayliss SJ. The genetics of hair shaft disorders. J Am Acad Dermatol 2008; 59(1):1–26.

Elman SA, Joyce C, Nyberg F, et al. Development of classification criteria for discoid lupus erythematosus: results of a Delphi exercise. J Am Acad Dermatol 2017; 77(2):261–267.

Frieden IJ. Genetic hair disorders. In: Alper JC (ed). Genetic disorders of the skin. Mosby Year Book, St Louis, 1990, pp. 209–221.

Friedlander SF, Baldwin HE, Mancini AJ, et al. The acne continuum: an age-based approach to therapy. Semin Cutan Med Surg 2011; 30(3 Suppl):S6–S11.

Furdon SA, Clark DA. Scalp hair characteristics in the newborn infant. Adv Neonatal Care 2003; 3(6):286–296.

Guo L, Feng S, Sun B, et al. Benefit and risk profile of tofacitinib for the treatment of alopecia areata: a systemic review and meta-analysis. J Eur Acad Dermatol Venereol 2020; 34:192–201.

Hafsi W, Badri T. Acne conglobata. StatPearls. https://www.ncbi.nlm.nih.gov/pubmed/29083736. Accessed July 2020.

Harrison S, Sinclair R. Optimal management of hair loss (alopecia) in children. Am J Clin Dermatol 2003; 4:757–770.

Hordinsky MK, Sawaya ME, Scher RK (eds). Atlas of hair and nails. Churchill Livingstone, New York, 1999.

Ilkit M. Favus of the scalp: an overview and update. Mycopathologia 2010; 170(3):143–154.

Ingram JR, Collier F, Brown D, et al. British Association of Dermatologists guidelines for the management of hidradenitis suppurativa (acne inversa) 2018. Br J Dermatol 2019; 180:1009–1017.

Itin PH, Pittelkow MR. Trichothiodystrophy: review of sulfur-deficient brittle hair syndromes and association with the ectodermal dysplasias. J Am Acad Dermatol 1990; 22:705–717.

Jemec GB. Clinical practice. Hidradenitis suppurativa. N Engl J Med 2012; 366(2):158–164.

Kanwar AJ, Narang T. Anagen effluvium. Indian J Dermatol Venereol Leprol 2013; 79(5):604–612.

Levy ML. Disorders of the hair and scalp in children. Pediatr Clin North Am 1991; 38:905–919.

Liu CI, Hsu CH. Rapid diagnosis of monilethrix using dermoscopy. Br J Dermatol 2008; 159(3):741–743.

Malinali-Brenner F, Bergfeld WF. Hair loss: an overview. Dermatol Nurs 2001; 13:269–272, 277–278.

McMichaels AS. Hair and scalp disorders in ethnic populations. Dermatol Clin 2003; 21:629–644.

Mukherjee N, Burkhart CN, Morrell DS. Treatment of alopecia areata in children. Pediatr Ann 2009; 38(7):388–395.

Paller A, Mancini AJ (eds). Disorders of the hair and nails. In: Hurwitz's clinical pediatric dermatology: a textbook of skin disorders of childhood and adolescence, 4th edn. Saunders, Edinburgh, 2011, pp. 130–166.

Prindaville B, Belazarian L, Levin NA, et al. Pityrosporum folliculitis: a retrospective review of 110 cases. J Am Acad Dermatol 2018; 78(3):511–514.

Rogers M. Hair shaft abnormalities, part I. Australas J Dermatol 1995; 36:179–184.

Rogers M. Hair shaft abnormalities, part II. Australas J Dermatol 1996; 37:1–11.

Rook A, Dawber R. Diseases of the hair and scalp. Blackwell Scientific, Oxford, 1982.

Shah VV, Wikramanayake TC, DelCanto GM, et al. Scalp hypothermia as a preventative measure for chemotherapy-induced alopecia: a review of controlled clinical trials. J Eur Acad Dermatol Venereol 2018; 32(5):720–734.

Shimomura Y, Christiano AM. Biology and genetics of hair. Annu Rev Genomics Hum Genet 2010; 11:109–132.

Skelsey MA, Price VH. Noninfectious hair disorders in children. Curr Opin Pediatr 1996; 8:378–380.

Sperling LC. Hair anatomy for the clinician. J Am Acad Dermatol 1991; 25(Suppl 1, Pt 1):1–17.

Springer K, Brown M, Stulberg DL. Common hair loss disorders. Am Fam Physician 2003; 68(1):93–102.

Tan E, Martinka M, Ball N, et al. Primary cicatricial alopecias: clinicopathology of 112 cases. J Am Acad Dermatol 2004; 30:25–32.

Tay YK, Levy ML, Metry DW. Trichotillomania in childhood: case series and review. Pediatrics 2004; 113(5):e494–e498.

Thompson W, Shapiro J, Price VH. Alopecia areata: understanding and coping with hair loss. Johns Hopkins University Press, Baltimore, 2000.

Tosti A, Pazzaglia M. Drug reactions affecting hair: diagnosis. Dermatol Clin 2007; 25(2):223–231, vii.

Tosti A, Peluso AM, Miscali C, et al. Loose anagen hair. Arch Dermatol 1997; 133:1089–1093.

National Organization for Rare Disorders (NORD). Trichothiodystrophy. https://rarediseases.org/rare-diseases/ichthyosis-trichothiodystrophy/. Accessed Jan 04, 2018.

Tziotzios C, Brier T, Lee JYW, et al. Lichen planus and lichenoid dermatoses: conventional and emerging therapeutic strategies. J Am Acad Dermatol 2018; 79(5):807–818.

Vashi RA, Mancini AJ, Paller AS. Primary generalized and localized hypertrichosis in children. Arch Dermatol 2001; 137(7):877–884.

Whiting DA. Structural abnormalities of the hair shaft. J Am Acad Dermatol 1987; 16:1–25.

Whiting DA, Dy LC. Office diagnosis of hair shaft defects. Semin Cutan Med Surg 2006; 25(1):24–34.

Yamazaki M, Irisawa R, Tsuboi R. Temporal triangular alopecia and a review of 52 past cases. J Dermatol 2010; 37(4):360–362.

Nail Disorders

Baran R, Dawber RPR, DeBerker D, et al. Diseases of the nails and their management, 3rd edn. Blackwell, Oxford, 2001.

Barnett JM, Scher RK, Taylor SC. Nail cosmetics. Dermatol Clin North Am 1991; 38:921–940.

Bolognia JL, Jorizzo JL, Rapini RP (eds). Hair, nails and mucous membranes. In: Dermatology. Mosby, Philadelphia, 2003, pp. 10007–11113.

Cohen JL, Scher RK, Pappert AS. Congenital malalignment of the great toenails. Pediatr Dermatol 1991; 8:40–42.

Daniel CR, Scher RK. Nail changes secondary to systemic drugs and ingestants. J Am Acad Dermatol 1987; 17:1012–1016.

Deberker D. Childhood nail diseases. Dermatol Clin 2006; 24(3):355–363.

Fawcett RS, Linford S, Stulberg DL. Nail abnormalities: clues to systemic disease. Am Fam Physician 2004; 69(6):1417–1424.

Fistarol SK, Itin PH. Nail changes in genodermatoses. Eur J Dermatol 2002; 12:119–128.

Fleckman P, Omura EF. Histopathology of the nail. Adv Dermatol 2001; 17:385–406.

Léauté-Labrèze C, Bioulac-Sage P, Taïeb A. Longitudinal melanonychia in children. A study of 8 cases. Arch Dermatol 1996; 132:167–169.

Lembach L. Pediatric nail disorders. Clin Podiatr Med Surg 2004; 21(4):641–650.

Norton LA. Genetic nail disorders. In: Alper JC (ed). Genetic disorders of the skin. Mosby Year Book, St Louis, 1990, pp. 195–208.

Pappert AS, Scher RK, Cohen JL. Nail disorders in children. Pediatr Clin North Am 1991; 38:921–940.

Scher RK, Norton LA, Daniel CR. Disorders of the nails. J Am Acad Dermatol 1986; 15:523–528.

Schulz-Butulis BA, Welch MD, Norton SA. Nail-patella syndrome. J Am Acad Dermatol 2003; 49(6):1086–1087.

Stratigos AJ, Baden H. Unraveling the molecular mechanisms of hair and nail genodermatoses. Arch Dermatol 2001; 137:1465–1471.

Telfer NR. Congenital and hereditary nail disorders. Semin Dermatol 1991; 10:2–6.

9

Oral Cavity

Nikhil Shyam and Bernard A. Cohen

INTRODUCTION

A comprehensive skin examination should always include close inspection of the mucous membranes, particularly the mouth. Clinical findings in the oral mucosa may provide clues to the diagnosis of an underlying systemic disease (Fig. 9.1), and some cutaneous disorders are associated with specific oral findings (Fig. 9.2). Many lesions commonly identified in the skin occur in the mouth (Fig. 9.3a) or extend into the oral mucosa from perioral skin (Fig. 9.3b). Some lesions arise in the mouth before extending to or disseminating to the skin (Fig. 9.4).

Several lesions arise from structures in the mouth and are usually confined to the oral mucosa and contiguous structures. This chapter will focus on these disorders. An algorithmic approach to the evaluation of oral pathology is summarized at the end of the chapter (see Fig. 9.36).

ANATOMY OF THE ORAL CAVITY

The opening of the oral cavity (Fig. 9.5) is surrounded by the lips, two flexible muscular folds that extend from the corners of the mouth to the base of the nasal columella above and the mentolabial sulcus (fold above the chin) below (Fig. 9.5a). The lip is divided into three anatomic zones. The outer skin above and below the vermillion border is similar to skin at other sites and includes adnexal structures such as hair follicles, eccrine sweat glands, and sebaceous glands. The vermillion is a transitional zone with a thin stratum corneum and increased numbers of dermal blood vessels that impart a distinctive reddish-purple color. Although hair follicles and sweat glands are absent, ectopic sebaceous glands (Fordyce granules, see Fig. 9.26) may be present. The labial mucosa covers the inside of the lip and meets the alveolar mucosa. It contains large numbers of mucous-producing salivary glands.

The lips are anchored to the adjacent gingiva by the labial frenulum. The oral cavity is formed by the arch of the hard and soft palates above, the teeth and cheeks laterally, and the tongue on the floor of the mouth. The lips and teeth are separated by a shallow vestibule. The sides of the oral cavity are formed by the smooth pink to light-red buccal and labial mucosa. It merges with the alveolar mucosa, which is loosely attached to the underlying periosteum. The opening of the parotid gland (Stensen's duct) is a triangular papilla located on the buccal mucosa of the vestibule opposite the second molars. The linea alba or occlusal line is a pale-white to pink streak along the line of dental occlusion.

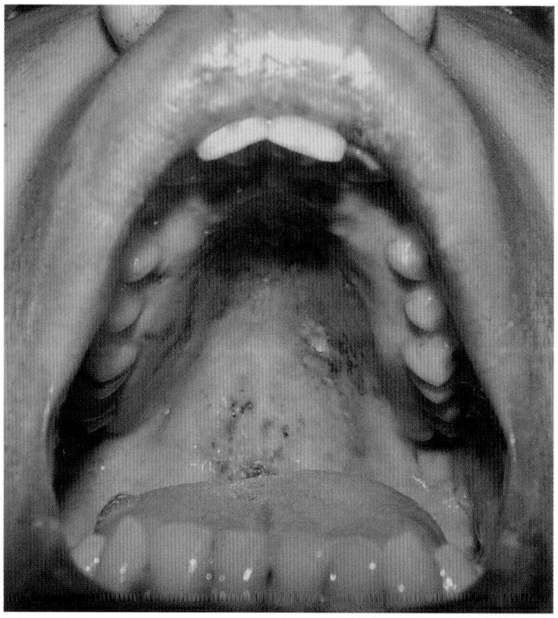

Fig. 9.1 Systemic lupus erythematosus. Erosions and scarring on the palate were early findings in this 16-year-old boy.

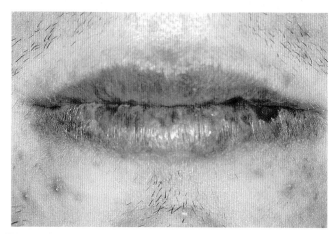

Fig. 9.2 Graft-vs-host disease. White lichenoid patches and ulcerations on the vermillion border extending into the mouth were associated with widespread cutaneous findings in this adolescent who had received a bone marrow transplant 3 weeks earlier.

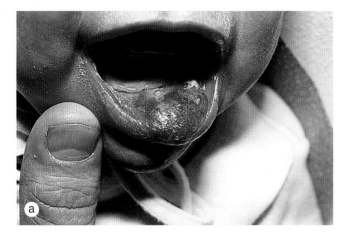

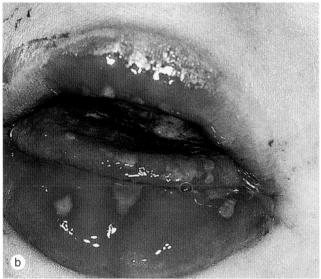

Fig. 9.3 (a) Hemangioma. Rapidly growing hemangioma on the inner aspect of the lower lip. **(b)** Herpetic gingivostomatitis. Vesicles and erosions on the lip and tongue.

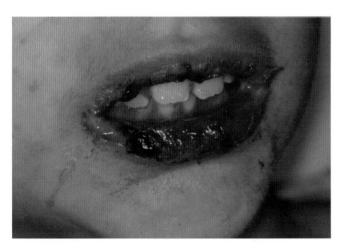

Fig. 9.4 Pemphigus vulgaris. Extensive lip and gingival ulcerations were the first manifestation of pemphigus in this 8-year-old boy.

The gingiva is divided into the fixed gingiva, which is fixed to the alveolar process, and the free gingiva, which is adjacent to the teeth and extends into the tissue that fills the space between the teeth and the interdental papillae. Although the free gingival is not usually pigmented, the attached gingiva appears stippled and other parts of the buccal mucosa may appear highly pigmented in dark-skinned individuals.

The anterior two-thirds of the palate is known as the hard palate, which is formed from the medial and two lateral palatine processes. The overlying mucosa is fixed to the underlying bone and has a rough appearance and a median raphe. The soft palate continues the roof of the mouth posteriorly as a fold of mucosa and muscle that ends centrally in the uvula and laterally in the folds merging with the tonsillar pillars and the tongue. The palatine tonsils sit between the anterior and posterior pillars. Additional lymphoid tissue lies at the base of the tongue.

The tongue is a mass of intersecting muscles divided into the inner and outer tongue muscles (Fig. 9.5b). The anterior two-thirds of the tongue, which is derived from the first pharyngeal arch, ends in a thin narrow tip or lingual apex, while the posterior third, which is derived from the third and fourth pharyngeal arches, is known as the lingual root. The junction of the root and the rest of the tongue forms a V-shaped groove known as the terminal sulcus that points toward the throat. The posterior end of the V marks the foramen caecum, the origin of the thyroid gland. The dorsum of the tongue represents the surface and extends from the tip to the epiglottis, while the ventral portion is known as the base, which merges with the loose mucosa on the floor of the mouth. The dorsum of the tongue, which is adapted for taste and mastication, is covered by specialized papillae. Filiform papillae appear as pointed spikes and are uniformly distributed over the surface, giving the tongue a rough texture. They are primarily responsible for mechanical movements such as licking. Fungiform papillae are red mushroom-shaped structures that are interspersed among the filiform papillae but more concentrated on the anterior surface. They distinguish between the sense of sweet and salty taste. The circumvallate papillae are the largest and most prominent papillae. They are located along the terminal sulcus and are responsible for sensing bitter taste. The vestigial foliate papillae are located on the posterior lateral portion of the tongue and are usually associated with the lingual tonsils.

The floor of the mouth is formed by the lingual aspect of the mandible and posteriorly by the base of the tongue. It is divided in the center by the lingual frenulum, which extends from the midline of the mandible to the ventral tip of the tongue. The plica sublingualis are symmetric mucosal folds with a fringed free edge on the ventral aspect of the tongue between the lingual frenulum and the lateral border of the tongue. Wharton's duct, the main excretory duct of the submandibular gland, exits at the sublingual caruncle adjacent to each side of the lingual frenulum.

Humans possess two sets of teeth: 20 primary teeth and 32 permanent teeth (Fig. 9.5c). Usually eruption of the primary teeth begins at 6 months of age and continues at a rate of one tooth a month until 2 or 2.5 years. The normal number of teeth for a given age can be estimated by subtracting six from the

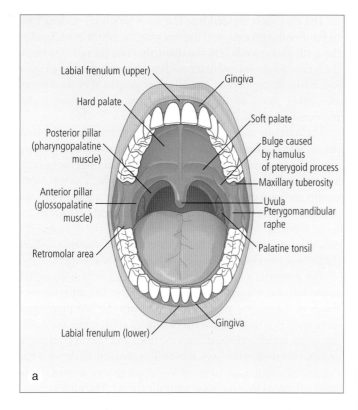

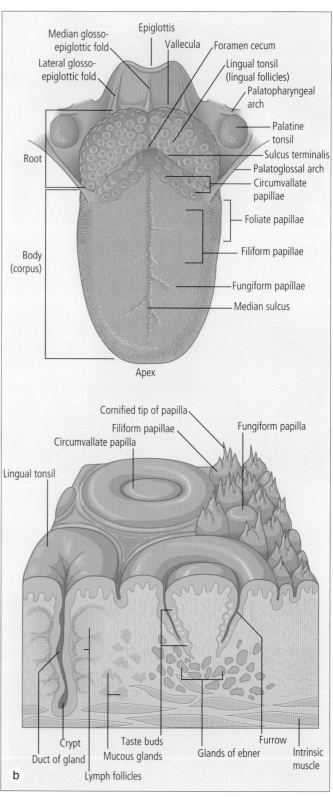

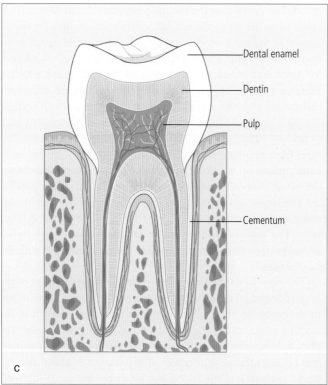

Fig. 9.5 (a) Oral cavity. **(b)** Tongue. **(c)** Tooth.

child's age in months up to 2 years of age. Eruption of the permanent teeth usually begins at age 6 years with appearance of the first molars. Calcification of the primary teeth begins at 3–4 months *in utero*, and calcification of the permanent teeth begins at birth and continues for 8–10 years. The structure of a tooth comprises the dental enamel (thin outer protective barrier), dentin (hard tissue that constitutes the bulk of teeth), cementum (cement like substance that anchors dentin to the periodontal ligament), and pulp (loose connective tissue containing blood vessels and nerves).

BUCCAL MUCOSA

White Sponge Nevus

White sponge nevus is a rare genodermatosis first described by Cannon in 1935 (Fig. 9.6). This autosomal-dominant disorder has a high degree of penetrance but variable expression, and results from mutations in genes coding for keratins 4 and 13, which are found in the spinous layer of the oral mucosa. Defects in these keratin filaments result in thickening of the oral mucosa and formation of mucosal folding, giving a spongy, white, leathery texture. The mucosa appears swollen, and there may be areas where the upper layers are pulled away, leaving fissures.

White sponge nevus may be present at birth, develop early in childhood, or be delayed until adolescence. Broad asymptomatic plaques usually involve the buccal mucosa bilaterally and may extend to the ventral surface of the tongue, labial mucosa, soft palate, alveolar mucosa, and the floor of the mouth. Rarely other mucosa, including the vagina, rectum, nose, and esophagus, may be involved.

Histologic findings include acanthosis and parakeratosis. The upper epithelial layers are vacuolated and contain pyknotic nuclei. Occasionally epidermolytic hyperkeratosis, characteristic of congenital ichthyosiform erythroderma, is seen.

These histologic and clinical features may overlap with the oral mucosal plaques found in patients with pachyonychia congenita and early dyskeratosis congenita. In type I pachyonychia congenita, the most common variant, white sponge nevus of the oral mucosa is associated with extensive nail plate thickening, follicular hyperkeratosis on the extensor surfaces of the arms and legs, palmoplantar keratoderma, and hyperkeratosis. Patients with the type II variant demonstrate no mucous membrane findings but may present with natal teeth.

Early oral mucous membrane plaques in patients with dyskeratosis congenita are indistinguishable from pachyonychia congenita, but oral leukoplakia in these patients does not usually appear until their early 20s. In early childhood, reticulated hyperpigmentation develops on the chest, neck, and arms, and generalized poikiloderma evolves by adolescence. Hypoplastic and dysplastic nail changes are a characteristic finding in dyskeratosis congenita in infancy or early childhood, and 50% of patients develop pancytopenia of the Fanconi type. Leukoplakia, which often involves multiple mucous membrane sites, is associated with a high risk of malignant degeneration, unlike in type I pachyonychia congenita.

Leukoedema may also be confused with white sponge nevus (Fig. 9.7). This asymptomatic process manifests as diffuse

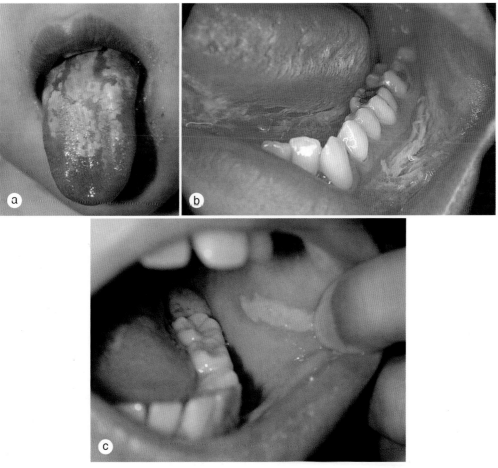

Fig. 9.6 White sponge nevus. **(a)** This 9-year-old girl with pachyonychia congenita had asymptomatic plaques on her tongue and buccal mucosa noted shortly after birth. **(b,c)** Congenital asymptomatic plaques confined to the oral cavity in a healthy adolescent and left buccal mucosa in a healthy 6-year-old girl.

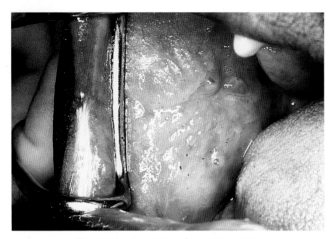

Fig. 9.7 Leukoedema of buccal mucosa.

whitening of the buccal mucosa and may extend to the labial mucosa and tongue, but fixed mucosa is not affected. Although there may be shallow folds, the mucosa is not usually thickened, and unlike white sponge nevus, the whitening decreases or disappears with stretching. Leukoedema is common particularly in dark-pigmented individuals, where it is often considered a normal variant.

White sponge nevus and leukoedema are asymptomatic, and treatment is not warranted.

Thrush (Pseudomembranous Candidiasis)

Thrush can be recognized by the characteristic white dots, patches, and plaques that develop most commonly on the buccal and labial mucosa, often extending to the ventral tongue and palate as well (Fig. 9.8). Rubbing of the white lesions leaves a red patch and occasionally superficial bleeding erosions. In immunosuppressed individuals, lesions may become widespread throughout the oral cavity. In both immunocompetent and immunocompromised hosts, candidiasis can present with angular cheilitis as well.

Of newborns, 10–15% present with thrush, acquired most frequently from maternal vaginal candidiasis. Nursing mothers can also transmit infection to their offspring when their breasts are involved. In infants, the buccal mucosa, tongue, and soft palate are most commonly involved, but lesions may appear on the posterior oral pharynx and lateral commissures of the mouth as well.

Persistent, widespread, or resistant candidiasis at any age should suggest the diagnosis of hereditary or acquired immunodeficiency. Thrush has also been reported in association with leukemia, lymphoma, inflammatory bowel disease, Addison disease, malnutrition, antibiotics, and oral corticosteroids.

The differential diagnosis includes leukoplakia, leukoedema, lichen planus, and white sponge nevus. These lesions can usually be distinguished by clinical findings, potassium hydroxide preparation of material from the white membrane, associated symptoms, and histologic evaluation if necessary.

Predisposing factors should be identified and treated if possible, and severe or persistent disease should prompt an evaluation for immunodeficiency. Although topical imidazoles in cream, solution, or troche formulation may be effective, resistant cases may require oral fluconazole or itraconazole. Fluconazole is available in convenient oral formulations of 10 mg/cc and 40 mg/cc for infants and young children.

TONGUE

Congenital Malformations

Ankyloglossia is often a minor developmental anomaly of the tongue resulting from a congenital short, thick lingual frenulum (Fig. 9.9). In the most severe variant, the tongue may be fused with the floor of the mouth. Mild ankyloglossia occurs in 2–4% of newborns, but is severe enough to require consultation in only 2–3/10 000 individuals.

Although limitation of movement of the tongue may be present, there is usually no interference with eating, swallowing, or speech development. However, there are rare reports of problems with breastfeeding.

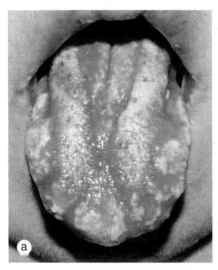
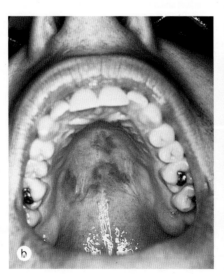
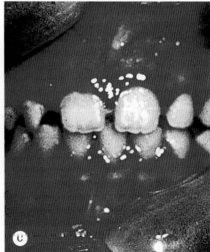

Fig. 9.8 (a) Oral candidiasis with white plaques on the tongue. **(b)** White plaques and erosions on the palate and **(c)** confluent beefy red plaques on the gingiva. Note the angular cheilitis in the child in Fig. 9.8a.

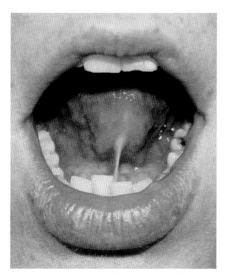

Fig. 9.9 Ankyloglossia. A 16-year-old girl was unable to fully extend her tongue.

The tongue normally tends to be short at birth and lengthens with increasing age. Consequently, most patients adapt to mild ankyloglossia, which likely improves or resolves spontaneously. However, if functional problems persist, frenulectomy is usually curative.

Rarely, accessory frenula may be found in association with ankyloglossia and should prompt investigation for other anomalies of the oral cavity, including cleft lip, cleft palate, and, specifically, orofaciodigital syndrome type I.

Congenital vascular malformations, ranula, thyroglossal duct cysts, dermoid cysts, and ectopic thyroid will be discussed later with tumors arising at the base of the tongue and macroglossia.

Geographic Tongue (*Stomatitis areata* Migrans, Erythema Migrans, Benign Migratory Glossitis)

Geographic tongue is a common tongue lesion that is often detected on routine oral examination (Fig. 9.10). It affects 1–2% of adolescents and young adults, girls more often than boys, and typically begins in childhood. Lesions are usually asymptomatic, but occasionally painful, especially when exposed to sour or spicy foods. Although the tongue is most often affected, other mucosal sites may be affected, including the buccal and labial mucosa and the soft palate.

Geographic tongue results from atrophy of the filiform papillae, while uninvolved fungiform papillae appear as red dots. The margin of lesions is slightly elevated, whitish, and thickened. Typically, a few 0.5–1cm patches begin on the edge or dorsum of the tongue and expand and increase in number over 3–5 days to form multiple serpiginous, annular, confluent patches, giving a map-like appearance. Lesions persist for 10–14 days and recur periodically for years, although the frequency of recurrences tends to decrease with increasing age.

Although patches most commonly occur as an isolated finding, geographic tongue may be associated with fissured tongue, psoriasis, and atopic dermatitis. Histologic features resemble psoriasis with acanthosis, hyperkeratosis, central atrophy, and a neutrophilic infiltrate in the lamina propria and epithelium. Geographic tongue may also be associated with balanitis circinata, a finding characteristic of Reiter syndrome.

Although no therapy is usually necessary, some patients experience mild stinging with acidic or spicy foods. Rarely, when symptoms are severe, temporary relief can be achieved with topical anesthetics.

Black Hairy Tongue (*Lingua Villosa Nigra*)

Hairy tongue, which can range in color from yellow to brownish-black, results from benign hyperkeratosis and elongation of the filiform papillae on the dorsal lateral surfaces of the tongue and probably represents exaggeration of the normal coating of the tongue (Fig. 9.11). Asymptomatic scaling usually begins just anterior to the terminal sulcus and spreads anteriorly and laterally, forming a triangular pattern.

Histopathology shows hyperkeratosis of the filiform papillae, overgrowth of bacteria and yeast, and non-specific inflammation.

Although the cause is unclear, hairy tongue may result from a microbial trigger that alters normal mouth flora. Oral and topical antibiotics, systemic and topical corticosteroids, methotrexate, antihypertensives, and tricyclic antidepressants have

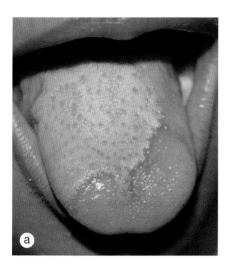

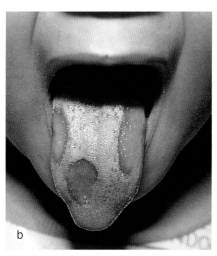

Fig. 9.10 Geographic tongue. Atrophic patches in (a) a 6-year-old girl and (b) a toddler.

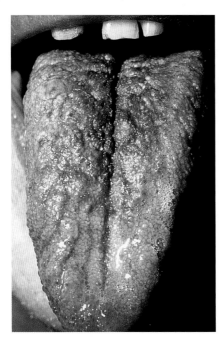

Fig. 9.11 Black hairy tongue followed a course of oral antibiotics.

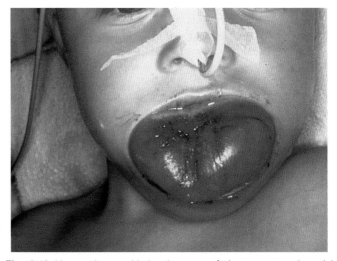

TABLE 9.1   Causes of Macroglossia
Congenital and Hereditary
Vascular malformations
Lymphangioma
Venous malformation
Combined lymphatic-venous malformation
Hemangioma
Hemihyperplasia
Congenital hypothyroidism (cretinism)
Beckwith–Wiedemann syndrome
Trisomy 21
Mucopolysaccharidoses
Neurofibromatosis
Acquired
Infiltrative processes
Amyloidosis
Myxedema
Granulomatous inflammation
Acromegaly
Angioedema
Tumors

Modified from Neville BW, Damm DD, Allen CM, et al. Oral and maxofacial pathology. WB Saunders, Philadelphia, 2002, p. 9.

been associated with the development of hairy tongue. Chronic use of oral topical antiseptics containing hydrogen peroxide, chlorhexidine, and similar agents may also trigger the reaction.

Darkening of hairy tongue probably results from chromogenic bacteria that colonize the scaly mass. The use of tobacco, certain food products, bismuth, and iron supplements may also contribute to the dark pigmentation.

Although hairy tongue may be resistant to treatment, elimination of triggers and routine brushing of the dorsum of the tongue with a toothbrush usually produces gradual improvement. Topical keratolytics such as urea and retinoic acid may also help.

Macroglossia

Enlargement of the tongue can be transient or persistent, unilateral or bilateral, and congenital or acquired (Table 9.1).

Transient swelling of the tongue results from anaphylaxis, C1-esterase deficiency (acquired or hereditary), insect-bite reactions, and systemic disorders associated with generalized edema such as renal, hepatic, and cardiac failure. Accidental injuries (e.g. burns, blunt trauma) and abscesses can produce asymmetric painful enlargement of the tongue.

Persistent macroglossia can be associated with tumors, metabolic disease, and endocrinologic disorders. Deep hemangiomas can lead to dramatic tongue enlargement that may interfere with eating and swallowing and cause partial or complete airway obstruction (Fig. 9.12). Surface changes from the superficial component of the hemangioma may provide a diagnostic clue. Early recognition and intervention may be life-saving with rapidly growing lesions.

Unlike hemangiomas, which slowly regress after 12 months of age, venous and lymphatic malformations persist indefinitely, and increasing ectasia may cause gradual progression of symptoms (Fig. 9.13).

Fig. 9.12 Hemangioma with involvement of the tongue and partial airway obstruction.

The mouth is a common site for lymphangiomas, which most commonly involve the tongue (Fig. 9.13b,c). Furthermore, vascular malformations are the most common cause of macroglossia in childhood. Lymphatic malformations can also involve the lips, buccal mucosa, and palate. Deep or feeder lymphatics arise at the angle of the mandible and produce persistent unilateral facial swelling. Most lesions are solitary, are poorly demarcated, and contain a deep component. Lymphangiomas less than 1 cm in diameter may occur in up to 4% of African American infants along the alveolar ridge. They occur twice as frequently in girls compared with boys and are often bilateral. These small lymphangiomas usually resolve without treatment within several months.

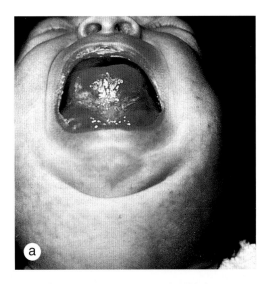

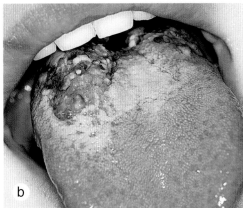

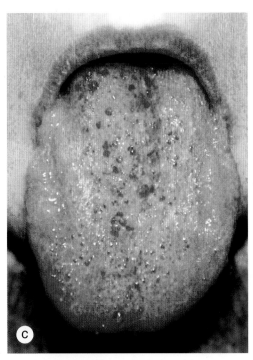

Fig. 9.13 Lymphangioma. **(a)** A massive lesion of the tongue was associated with a cystic hygroma in the neck of this infant. **(b)** This superficial lymphangioma of the posterior tongue was slowly enlarging in this 10-year-old boy. **(c)** This toddler demonstrates a subtle asymptomatic lymphangioma covering the dorsal surface of the tongue.

Vascular malformations tend to wax and wane in size, particularly after accidental trauma. Asymptomatic lesions can be followed clinically and with magnetic resonance imaging studies. Progressive lesions may improve with laser, excisional, and/or sclerotherapy. However, recurrences are common, particularly with lymphatic malformations, which may respond to low dose oral sirolimus.

Macroglossia can also occur with deposition disorders including scleredema, amyloidosis, lipoid proteinosis, and lysosomal storage disorders, which rarely present in children. Congenital malformation syndromes associated with macroglossia include trisomy 21, Winchester syndrome, anhidrotic ectodermal dysplasia, Zellweger syndrome, and Beckwith–Wiedemann syndrome. Tongue enlargement has also been noted in endocrinologic disorders such as acromegaly and hypothyroidism, as well as chronic inflammatory disorders such as cheilitis.

Median Rhomboid Glossitis (Central Papillary Atrophy)

Median rhomboid glossitis refers to a frequent asymptomatic finding in the middle of the tongue that is associated with a decrease or absence of papillae and appears as a smooth-topped red to violaceous plaque (Fig. 9.14). The area first becomes apparent during adolescence and is most frequently found by a dentist rather than the patient. The incidence in adults approaches 0.2%.

Although typically flat-topped, median rhomboid glossitis may be slightly elevated or markedly thickened and scaly. Lesions tend to form annular plaques in the middle-third of the tongue and take on the characteristic oval or rhomboid configuration as they progress posteriorly.

Although initially thought to represent a developmental defect of the midline of the tongue or a complication of candidiasis, it is now considered to result from loss of the filiform papillae in the area with or without *Candida*. Moreover, even when yeast is identified on cultures or biopsies, oral antifungal therapy may not result in clinical improvement.

When median rhomboid glossitis presents with a thick plaque or nodule, lesions must be distinguished from a lingual thyroid, thyroglossal duct cyst, and other tumors.

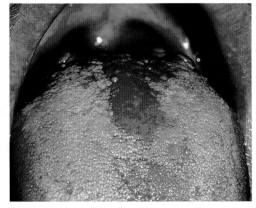

Fig. 9.14 Median rhomboid glossitis. An asymptomatic atrophic red patch on the posterior aspect of the dorsal tongue was noted on a routine dental examination.

Granular Cell Tumor

Granular cell tumor was initially described by Abrikossoff in 1926 as granular cell myoblastoma because the tumor cells were initially identified as immature muscle cells or myoblasts. Over the last decade electron microscopic and immunohistochemical findings suggest a Schwann cell or neuroendocrine origin.

Although most common on the dorsal surface of the tongue, these tumors may appear throughout the oropharynx, and 40% of tumors occur on the skin in the subcutaneous tissue (Fig. 9.15). There are also reports of lesions in the esophagus, stomach, appendix, larynx, bronchus, pituitary gland, uvea, and skeletal muscle. Most tumors are solitary, but up to 64 have been described in a single patient.

Granular cell tumors typically present as 0.5–3.0 cm well-circumscribed, raised, firm nodules. Lesions are occasionally tender or itchy and may have a warty white surface. The histopathology of the surface often reveals pseudoepitheliomatous hyperplasia, but within the lamina propria the characteristic sheets of polygonal cells with multiple cytoplasmic granules can be found. Consequently, when granular tumors are suspected, superficial biopsies are inadequate and may be misinterpreted as invasive carcinoma. Excision is usually curative, as recurrences are rare.

Traumatic Fibroma (Irritation Fibroma)

Traumatic fibroma is a benign nodule that commonly develops on the tongue, particularly on the tip of the tongue, buccal mucosa, and lips in areas prone to trauma (Fig. 9.16). This reactive process, which results from recurrent sucking, picking, and biting, usually presents as a solitary 0.05–1.0 cm nodule, although multiple lesions may be present.

Fibromas may be sessile or pedunculated, and occasionally the surface may be eroded. Histologic findings include hyperplasia with dense collagen deposition and an overlying fibropurulent membrane. Inflammation is usually minimal unless ulceration is present.

Irritation fibroma responds well to surgical excision and recurrences are rare.

Tumors at the Base of the Tongue
Lingual Thyroid

A lingual thyroid occurs when follicles of thyroid tissue are found in the substance of the tongue (Fig. 9.17). These lesions may arise from thyroid anlage that failed to migrate from the foramen cecum to the predestined site in the neck or from anlage remnants left behind in the tongue.

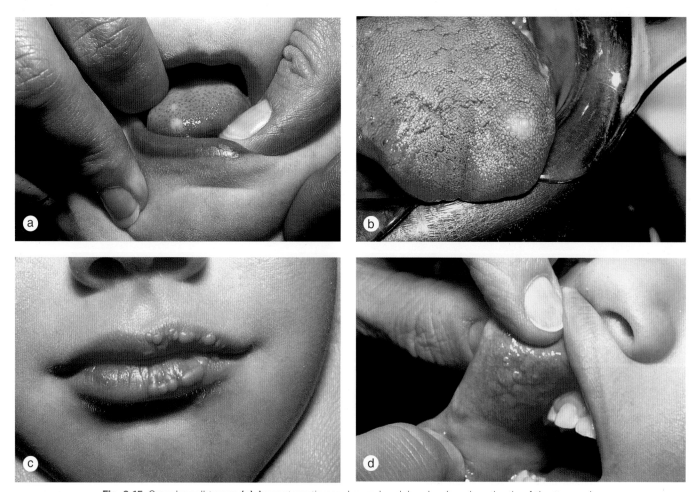

Fig. 9.15 Granular cell tumor. **(a)** Asymptomatic papules and nodules developed on the tip of the tongue in a toddler and **(b)** the dorsolateral surface of the tongue in an adolescent. **(c)** Lesions were noted at birth on the lips and **(d)** buccal mucosa of a 4-year-old boy.

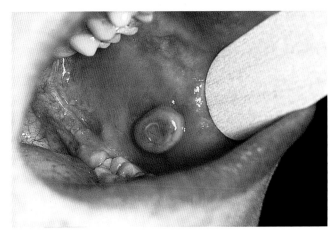

Fig. 9.16 Traumatic fibroma on the buccal mucosa.

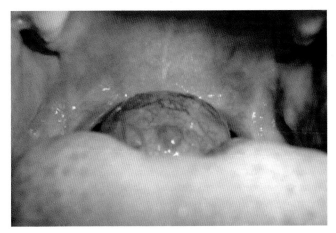

Fig 9.17 Lingual thyroid. This large tumor at the base of the tongue was associated with intermittent dysphagia.

Lingual thyroid usually presents as a 2–3 cm dark vascular tumor with overlying vessels at the base of the tongue and may be associated with dysphagia, dysphonia, hemorrhage with pain, and a feeling of fullness in the throat.

Lesions usually develop in or slightly lateral to the midline between the anterior two-thirds and posterior third of the tongue near the foramen cecum. However, ectopic thyroid can be found anywhere from the foramen cecum to the perilaryngeal and, rarely, substernal areas. There is a 6:1 female predominance, and most cases become apparent early in life.

Interestingly 10% of tongues demonstrate a lingual thyroid at autopsy. Of individuals who develop symptomatic lesions, 70% lack normal cervical thyroid glands altogether. Moreover, 1% of patients with lingual thyroids reported in the literature developed thyroid carcinoma.

Before symptomatic lingual thyroid tissue can be surgically excised, patients should have a careful assessment of thyroid function, and the presence of normal thyroid tissue must be established. When the ectopic gland is the only thyroid present, it can often be moved to a safer, more convenient site.

Thyroglossal Duct Cysts

As the thyroid anlage descends to the normal position below the thyroid cartilage by the seventh embryonic week, an epithelial tract or duct, which remains attached to the base of the tongue, is formed. Although the thyroglossal duct epithelium usually undergoes atrophy, occasionally remnants may persist and give rise to cysts along the tract, known as thyroglossal duct cysts (Fig. 9.18).

Thyroglossal duct cysts typically occur in the midline anywhere from the foramen cecum at the base of the tongue to the suprasternal notch. However, the majority develop below the hyoid bone. Cysts can appear at any age but most are detected within the first 2 decades. The majority of cysts are less than 3 cm in diameter and typically present as a painless, mobile, compressible mass unless they are infected. Lesions at the base of the tongue can lead to laryngeal obstruction. If they remain attached to the hyoid bone or tongue, they tend to move vertically with extension of the tongue and on swallowing.

Although there is at least a 10% risk of recurrence, cysts are most effectively treated with surgical excision. This risk can be reduced by removal of the midline section of the hyoid bone and muscular tissue along the entire thyroglossal duct tract.

Lingual Tonsils

Lingual tonsils are usually associated with the foliate papillae and are recognized as bilateral red, glistening papules and nodules on the posterolateral border of the tongue (Fig. 9.19). Although lymphoid tissue is part of the foliate papillae normally found in this area, papillae may become enlarged after

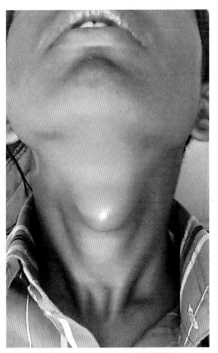

Fig. 9.18 Thyroglossal duct cyst. Although this cyst was first noted in early childhood, it did not become symptomatic until the third decade when it was surgically excised.

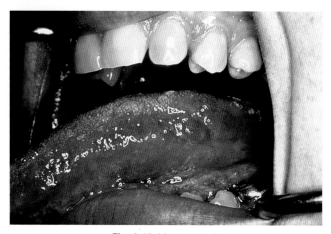

Fig. 9.19 Lingual tonsil.

trauma or with viral or bacterial pharyngitis. Hyperplasia of the foliate papillae may be mistaken for carcinoma.

Lymphoid tissue on the posterior third of the dorsum of the tongue, which is part of the oropharyngeal lymphoid tissue ring of Waldeyer, may also become intermittently or permanently enlarged with recurrent infections or chronic allergic sinusitis. Persistent hyperplasia is seen more commonly in atopic children and may be associated with dysphagia, dysphonia, a feeling of fullness in the throat, and obstructive sleep apnea. Symptomatic lesions can be ablated surgically.

FLOOR OF THE ORAL CAVITY

Ranula

Ranula is a clinical term for a mucocele or mucous retention cyst located on the floor of the mouth and arises from trauma to the sublingual or submandibular salivary glands (Fig. 9.20). These lesions can be acquired or congenital, and most are unilateral, although they can rarely be bilateral. Ranula usually present as a gray or bluish, glistening swelling that can reach a large size (over 5 cm in diameter).

There are two types of ranula; the most common or simple variant is usually confined to the oral cavity and the cervical ranula, which can extend from the sublingual space around or through the mylohyoid muscle to the submandibular space. Ranula are usually treated by marsupialization.

Ranula should be distinguished from lymphangiomas that arise in a similar location in the floor of the mouth. Lymphangiomas also tend to infiltrate between structures in the neck and are difficult to remove surgically. Cystic hygromas in the neck can be confused with cervical ranula. Other tumors such as lipomas and dermoid cysts rarely develop in the floor of the mouth and can only be excluded by biopsy.

Pigmentary Changes of the Oral Mucosa
Physiologic Pigmentation

Physiologic mucosal pigmentation, produced by mucosal melanocytes, is genetically acquired and tends to be more prominent in African Americans and Asians and with increasing age (Fig. 9.21). Pigment may appear diffusely or in discrete linear or spotted patterns. Although pigmentation is usually most prominent on the buccal mucosa along the bite line, any oral structure may be involved.

Postinflammatory Hyperpigmentation

Postinflammatory hyperpigmentation may develop after any injury to the oral mucosa. However, it is commonly seen in association with dermatologic disorders that produce full-thickness insults to the mucous membranes, such as lichen planus and lupus erythematosus. Pigmentary changes also tend to be more prominent in darker-pigmented individuals.

Systemic and Local Hyperpigmentation

Mucous membrane pigmentation may also provide a clue to underlying systemic disease. Irregular or patchy mucosal hyperpigmentation commonly appears in Addison disease and occasionally in acromegaly. Oral café-au-lait macules can develop in neurofibromatosis and McCune–Albright syndrome. Other

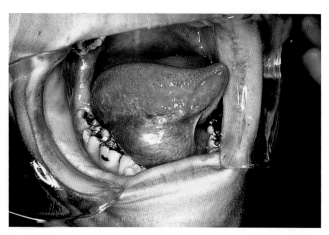

Fig. 9.20 Ranula. A purple mass at the base of the tongue gradually increased in size after it first became apparent in early adolescence.

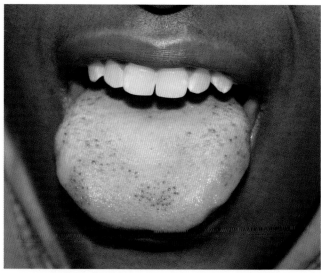

Fig. 9.21 Physiologic pigmentation of the tongue.

systemic triggers of pigmentation include heavy metal exposure, Wilson disease, hemochromatosis, Peutz–Jeghers syndrome (see Fig. 6.6), acquired immunodeficiency syndrome, and melanoma. Numerous medications including antimalarials, azidothymidine (AZT), oral contraceptives, phenolphthalein, chlorpromazine, and quinidine may also increase mucosal melanin. Bluish-green pigment from minocycline may occasionally be deposited in the gingiva with or without concomitant involvement of cutaneous lesions.

The use of tobacco products and topical agents containing heavy metals can result in focal or diffuse hyperpigmentation of the oral mucosa. Silver-containing solutions such as silver nitrate can leave black or gray mottled staining. Mercury may leave blue-gray pigmentation, and tin- and bronze-containing agents can produce brown to black pigmentation.

Melanotic Macules

Melanotic macules appear most commonly on the lower lip and usually measure less than 3 mm (Fig. 9.22a). However, the buccal mucosa, gingival, or palate may also be involved (Fig. 9.22b–d). These innocent macules usually represent a freckle, lentigo, or junctional nevus, and in adults they must be distinguished from malignant melanoma.

The presence of multiple labial macules should raise the suspicion of a variety of syndromes and prompt a careful

examination of the entire skin surface, as well as oral and genital mucosa (see Fig. 6.4) (Table 9.2).

Hypopigmentation/Depigmentation

Loss of pigmentation occurs most commonly from vitiligo, and the lips are most commonly involved (Fig. 9.23). Frequently vitiligo koebnerizes in a perioral distribution, spreading from the corners of the mouth to the inner aspect of the lips, and occasionally over the entire vermillion border. Depigmentation can be subtle in patients with light complexion but disfiguring in darker-pigmented individuals.

LIP

Congenital Malformations

A complete discussion of lip (and palate) anomalies is beyond the scope of this chapter. However, it is important to recognize the significance of these findings. Although congenital lip pits and fistulas of the lower lip are rare, they may be associated with clefting of the upper lip and palate and a number of underlying genetic disorders (e.g. Van der Woude syndrome, popliteal pterygium syndrome, orofaciodigital syndrome). Anomalies of the eyes, ears, nails, and feet and some forms of ichthyosis have also been reported. Lesions may be single or multiple and range from subtle dimples to fistulas up to 25 mm.

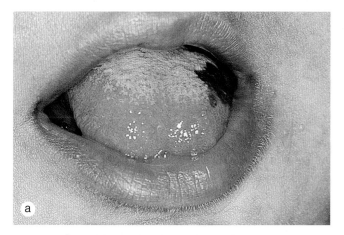
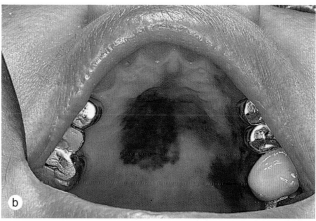
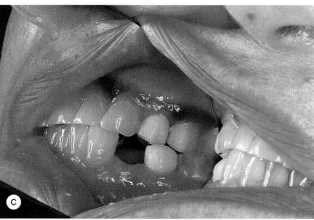
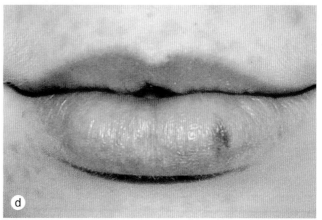

Fig. 9.22 Melanotic macules. **(a)** A small pigmented nevus was noted at birth on the left side of this infant's tongue. **(b)** Lentigines developed on the palate, **(c)** gingiva, and **(d)** lower lip.

TABLE 9.2 Disorders Associated With Pigmentary Changes in the Oral Mucosa

Disorder	Oral/Cutaneous Findings	Associated Findings
Laugier–Hunziker syndrome	Oral, genital pigmented macules; longitudinal melanonychia	None
Peutz–Jeghers syndrome (see Fig. 6.6)	Labial, oral, genital, distal extremity pigmented macules; melanonychia; striata	Hamartomatous polyps; colonic carcinoma; pancreatic carcinoma; ovarian, testicular tumors
Carney complex (NAME/LAMB syndrome) (**N**evi, **A**trial myxomas, **M**yxoid neurofibroma, **E**phelides/**L**entigines, **A**trial myxoma, **M**ucocutaneous myxomas, **B**lue nevi)	Oral, cutaneous freckles, nevi, lentigines	Pigmented nodular adrenocortical disease; mammary fibroadenomas; testicular, thyroid, pituitary tumors
LEOPARD syndrome (Fig. 6.4) (**L**entigines, **E**KG abnormalities, **O**cular hypertelorism, **P**ulmonary stenosis, **A**bnormalities of genitals, **R**etardation of growth, **D**eafness)	Oral lentigines	Mental retardation; hypertrophic obstructive cardiomyopathy
Lentiginosis profusa	Pigmented macules on skin, oral mucosa	None

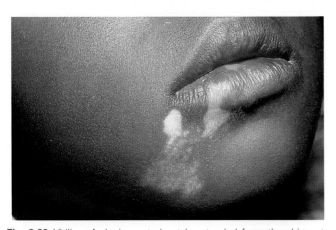

Fig. 9.23 Vitiligo. A depigmented patch extended from the chin onto the lower vermillion border.

Clefts of the lip, jaw, and/or palate occur more commonly with an incidence of 0.5–1.3 : 1000 births. In nearly one-third of patients, there is a family history of similar defects, and in 10% lesions are associated with specific syndromes (e.g. trisomy 13, orofaciodigital syndrome 1, fetal hydantoin syndrome, Stickler syndrome, Pierre Robin syndrome, ectrodactyly–ectodermal dysplasia, ankyloblepharon–ectodermal dysplasia clefting).

Cheilitis

Cheilitis results from a number of different disorders that produce inflammation of the lips and clinical findings that vary with the underlying trigger. The most common causes of cheilitis are irritant and allergic contact dermatitis, atopic dermatitis, and seborrheic dermatitis.

Cheilitis Simplex

Cheilitis simplex or chapped lips refers to one of the most common forms of cheilitis that presents clinically with cracking, fissuring, and scaling of both lips, but more commonly the lower lip. Chronic cases can progress to crusting, hemorrhage, and blister formation. Causes include acute and chronic sun exposure, atopic dermatitis, seborrheic dermatitis, and irritant and allergic contact dermatitis. However, repetitive biting, licking, and rubbing are the most common culprits.

Aggressive use of barrier lubricants such as petrolatum usually results in dramatic improvement. However, patients with obsessive-compulsive behavior may require psychiatric intervention, and in some patients, this may be the first manifestation of primary psychiatric disease.

Contact Dermatitis

Contact irritant and allergic dermatitis typically present with pruritic or burning, scaling, and fissuring of the lips with perioral extension. Occasionally angular cheilitis or perlèche is the only clinical sign.

Toothpaste and mouthwash, which spill over from the mouth where they only rarely cause symptoms, are the most common cause of contact irritant and allergic reactions on the lips. The components associated with contact reactions include clove oil, pimento oil, anise oil, menthol, and preservatives such as parabens and ethylenediamine. Allergic contact cheilitis from tartar control toothpastes usually results from exposure to pyrophosphates. Topical medications such as antivirals, antibiotics, sunscreens, and disinfectants, as well as food products such as apples and citrus fruits, have also been reported to cause reactions. In patients sensitized to rhus allergen, mango rinds can cross react with poison ivy and produce an intense allergic contact cheilitis.

Successful treatment requires some detective work to identify the irritant or allergen, but patch testing may be necessary in some patients. Other conservative measures such as cool compresses, emollients, topical steroids, and topical non-steroidal anti-inflammatory agents will help while the patient undergoes evaluation.

Lip-Licker's Dermatitis

Lip-licker's dermatitis is a variant of chronic irritant contact cheilitis that occurs more commonly in children than in adults (Fig. 9.24; see Fig. 3.36). Although the vermillion border may be involved exclusively, red papules, scaling, and occasionally fissures and crusting may form a well-demarcated circumferential ring around the lips. The lesions extend as far as the tongue can reach and invariably spare the angle of the mouth.

Lip-licker's dermatitis results from repetitive wetting and drying of the perioral skin and tends to flare during the cold, dry winter months. Aggressive application of bland emollients

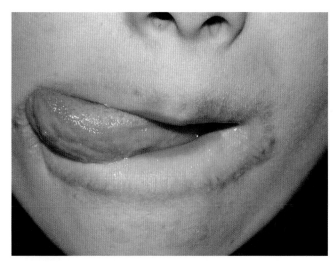

Fig. 9.24 Cheilitis. Dermatitis was restricted to the vermillion border and immediately contiguous skin in this chronic lip-licker.

can improve lesions, but healing is not complete until the lip-licking behavior is eliminated.

Angular Cheilitis

Cheilitis at the commissures of the mouth may present acutely or chronically with erythema, scale, crusts, fissures, and maceration (Fig. 9.8a). Lesions may spread to the adjacent skin and extend along the nasolabial folds. *Candida* and bacterial organisms, particularly *Staphylococcus aureus* and Group A β-hemolytic *Streptococcus*, may produce secondary infection.

Atopic dermatitis, seborrheic dermatitis, and contact irritant dermatitis from drooling may trigger angular cheilitis. In children, associated systemic disorders include diabetes mellitus, anemia, conditions that increase or decrease saliva production (e.g. medications), immunosuppression (e.g. acquired immunodeficiency syndrome, immunosuppressive medications), and nutritional deficiencies. Irritation from malocclusion of the mouth caused by abnormalities of the teeth, lips, or tongue and mechanical stretching of the corners of the mouth (e.g. dental procedures, intubation) can also predispose to the development of angular cheilitis.

Primary triggers should be identified and eliminated, and secondary infection should be treated. Prophylaxis with topical antibiotics, antifungals, and emollients may prevent recurrence of lesions in the setting of chronic systemic disease. Attention to good oral hygiene and dental care is also critical.

Cheilitis (Orofacial) Granulomatosa

Painless persistent swelling of the lip associated with fissured tongue and facial palsy should suggest the diagnosis of cheilitis granulomatosa or Melkersson–Rosenthal syndrome (Fig. 9.25).

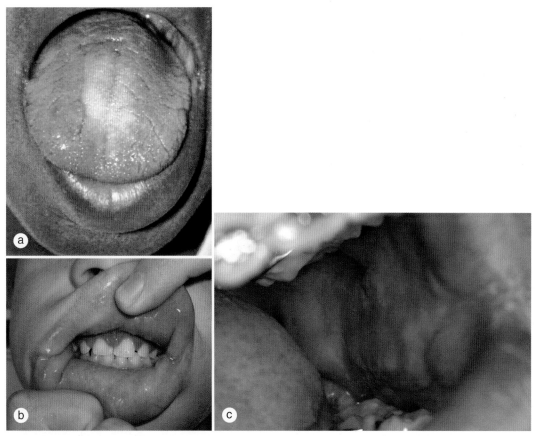

Fig. 9.25 Cheilitis granulomatosa. **(a)** This 12-year-old boy had a 1-year history of persistent woody induration of the lower lip and an enlarged fissured tongue. Another 12-year-old boy complained of **(b)** persistent lip swelling and gingival hypertrophy for over 6 months. **(c)** Note thickening of the buccal mucosa as well. Lip biopsy showed granulomatous inflammation and endoscopy showed ileitis consistent with Crohn disease.

(In 1928, Melkersson described a patient with facial palsy and chronic lip swelling. Years later, Rosenthal added fissured tongue to the clinical syndrome.)

Cheilitis granulomatosa represents a subset of patients with orofacial granulomatosa, which encompasses a number of clinical presentations that reveal granulomatous inflammation on biopsy. Although the lips and tongue are most commonly involved, orofacial granulomatosa may include the cheeks and other parts of the face, palate, gingiva, and buccal mucosa. Lesions restricted to the lips alone are referred to as cheilitis granulomatosa of Miescher.

Of patients with orofacial granulomatosa, 20–70% present with the full triad of lip swelling, fissured tongue, and facial palsy. The disorder peaks between ages 20 and 40 years and occurs equally in men and women. Although most patients present sporadically, familial cases have been described.

Lip swelling, particularly of the upper lip, is usually the first symptom. Painless attacks, which can start with the lower lip or both lips, may last for days to weeks and clear completely between episodes. Eventually, many patients complain of persistent swelling.

Facial palsy, typically unilateral, occurs in only 20–30% of patients, and rarely other cranial nerves can be involved. Fissured tongue, which occurs in 10–15% of normal individuals, is found in 50% of patients.

Histologic changes include non-caseating granulomatous inflammation with edema of the superficial lamina propria. Special stains for bacteria, fungi, and mycobacteria and a careful search for foreign material are negative. Chronic lesions demonstrate fibrosis.

Systemic granulomatous disorders including inflammatory bowel disease, sarcoidosis, and tuberculosis should be excluded by careful medical evaluation. Local causes of cheilitis such as oral infections, foreign body reactions, and contact dermatitis may also be discovered by careful history, review of systems, and other clues on physical examination.

Treatment is often challenging, although temporary relief of symptoms can be achieved with topical and intralesional steroids. Oral anti-inflammatory and immunosuppressive medications may help in chronic cases. Surgical reduction may be indicated in patients with persistent swelling associated with fibrosis.

Fordyce Granules

Fordyce granules, or ectopic sebaceous glands, are the most common structural anomaly found in the mouth, with a prevalence approaching 80% in adults. They were initially described by Kölliken in 1861 but were named after Fordyce, who described them in 1896.

Fordyce spots, which are most commonly present on the lips as tiny yellow papules, occasionally coalesce to form larger asymptomatic plaques (Fig. 9.26). The buccal mucosa is also commonly involved and occasionally the tongue, gingival, frenulum, and palate.

Lesions are likely present at birth but do not become clinically evident until, during, or after puberty. Fordyce granules are found in 20% of children, 30% of adolescents, and 70–80% of adults. They may become subtle or disappear altogether in the elderly.

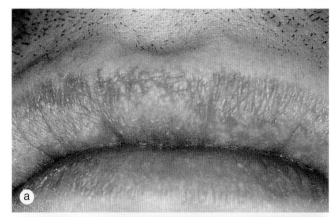

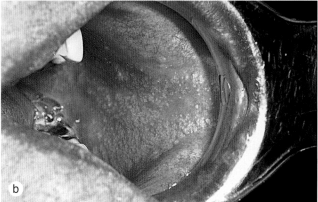

Fig. 9.26 Fordyce granules. Asymptomatic papules developed on **(a)** the vermillion and **(b)** the buccal mucosa.

Biopsies reveal normal sebaceous glands that are not associated with hair follicles. Although no treatment is necessary, superficial carbon dioxide laser can be used to ablate cosmetically disfiguring lesions.

Mucocele

Mucocele (mucous extravasation phenomenon) develops most commonly on the inner aspect of the lower lip and occasionally on the palate, upper lip, and buccal mucosa (Fig. 9.27). These

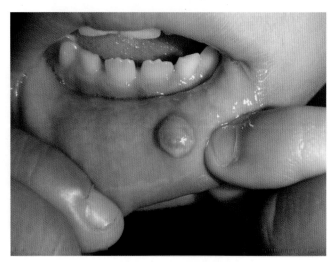

Fig. 9.27 Mucocele. This boy admitted to picking and biting at his lower lip. This lesion was shaved and cauterized.

mucous retention or extravasation cysts result from rupture of a salivary gland duct and release of mucin into the surrounding soft tissues. They are usually tense, small (<2 cm), non-tender, and fluid-filled, appearing most commonly in children and young adults. The presence of mucin in the superficial soft tissue often gives a bluish translucent hue. They may rupture after trauma from teeth and tend to recur after spontaneous rupture or surgical intervention including cryosurgery, carbon dioxide laser ablation, and surgical excision.

Mucocele, which lacks an epithelial lining, differs from the salivary duct cyst that arises from salivary gland tissue and consists of an epithelial-lined cavity with mucoid secretions in the lumen.

Aphthae

Aphthae, or canker sores, considered to be one of the most common oral lesions, present as painful mucosal erosions that start as red edematous papules that become necrotic and ulcerate (Fig. 9.28). They typically appear as small crateriform

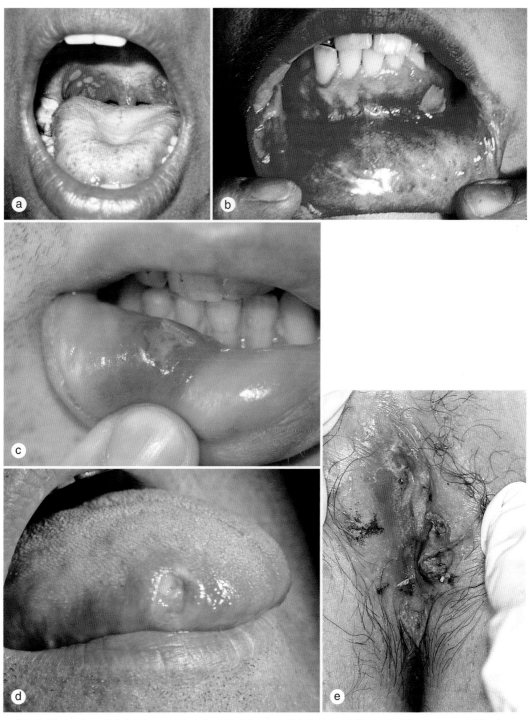

Fig. 9.28 Aphthae. Painful ulcers recurred on the **(a)** palate, **(b)** gingiva, **(c)**, lower lip, **(d)** tongue, and **(e)** vulva.

ulcers less than a centimeter in diameter, with an overlying white-to-yellow fibrin membrane and a red halo. Minor aphthae heal within 1–2 weeks, usually without scarring.

Recurrent aphthae occur in 10% of healthy individuals, often in a familial pattern, and more commonly in females than males. Although onset usually occurs between ages 10 and 30 years, they can occur at any time. Minor aphthae are characterized by the development of 1–5 lesions at a time between 2 and 5 mm in size. Although any site on the oral mucosa can be involved, aphthae favor movable anterior oral mucosal surfaces such as the labial mucosa, floor of the mouth, and lateral borders of the tongue. The frenulum and the uvula may also be involved. Rarely, the epiglottis, pharynx, and gastrointestinal tract are involved, but these locations should raise the possibility of underlying inflammatory bowel disease and Behçet disease. Fixed mucosal surfaces, particularly the keratinized epithelium of the hard palate and the vermillion, are usually spared.

Major aphthae are defined as lesions over a centimeter in diameter, more than five lesions at a time, involvement of the posterior oral mucosa, and persistence for weeks to months. Ulcers are deep and exquisitely painful and may be associated with genital lesions that typically involve the labia or scrotum (Fig. 9.28e). Major aphthae may be associated with Crohn disease and ulcerative colitis, as well as human immunodeficiency virus infection and acquired immunodeficiency syndrome. Although the oral lesions of Behçet disease may be indistinguishable from major aphthae, the following should allow for distinction from isolated major aphthae: arthritis, uveitis, cutaneous lesions, and central nervous system involvement. Recurrent, episodic aphthous stomatitis in association with fever should also raise the possibility of PFAPA syndrome (periodic fever, aphthous stomatitis, pharyngitis, and adenitis). This rare, self-limited periodic fever syndrome occurs most commonly in children under 5 years old.

Similar oral ulcers may be seen in gluten-sensitive enteropathy, malabsorption syndromes, drug reactions, trauma, herpangina, herpes gingivostomatitis, and herpes zoster (shingles).

Although the cause is unclear, some investigators have suggested a triggering role for trauma, psychosocial factors, food intolerance, and medications. Anti-epithelial antibodies have been detected in many patients with major aphthae. However, they are also present in 10% of normal individuals and may represent an epiphenomenon in patients with disease.

Aphthae can be managed with topical and oral analgesics, topical (e.g. fluocinonide gel 0.05%) and intralesional corticosteroids, and topical tacrolimus ointment. Recent studies describe a role for oral thalidomide as well.

PALATE

Palatal Cysts of the Newborn

Palatal cysts, including Epstein pearls and Bohn nodules, appear in 75% of newborns and resolve within several weeks without treatment (Fig. 9.29). Epstein pearls were originally described as 1–5 mm whitish-yellow nodules occurring most commonly on the mid palatal raphe at the junction of the hard and soft palates. These cysts are thought to arise from remnants

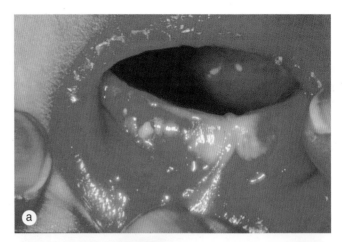

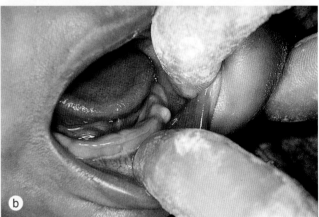

Fig. 9.29 Palatal and gingival cysts. **(a)** Cysts were present on the right maxillary alveolus and palate and **(b)** left mandibular alveolus in these healthy newborns.

of epithelium trapped between the palatal shelves and the nasal process. Bohn nodules appear as similar nodules scattered over the hard palate, often near the soft palate junction, and are thought to be derived from the minor salivary glands. These terms are frequently used interchangeably, and are also used to describe similar-appearing gingival cysts. The histology of palatal cysts shows a keratin-filled cyst identical to that of gingival cysts (Fig. 9.29).

GINGIVA

Gingival Cysts of the Newborn

Dental lamina cysts present as solitary or multiple 1–3 mm nodules on the alveolar processes in the newborn (Fig. 9.29). Similar to palatal cysts (Epstein pearls, Bohn nodules), these keratinized cysts also develop in 75% of newborns and resolve without treatment within several weeks to several months. They appear most commonly on the maxillary alveolus and are thought to arise from remnants of the dental lamina remaining after tooth formation.

Congenital Epulis

Epulis is a general term used to describe a number of reactive gingival lesions with vascular, fibroblastic, and granulation

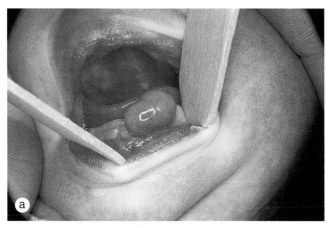

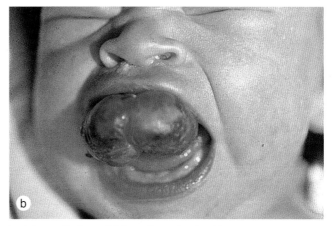

Fig. 9.30 Congenital epulis. Lesions may arise from the **(a)** mandibular and **(b)** maxillary alveolar ridges.

tissue proliferation. Congenital epulis or congenital gingival granular cell tumor refers to an exophytic congenital tumor that arises from the alveolar ridge and has histologic features identical to those of granular cell tumors (Fig. 9.30).

Congenital epulis typically presents as a 1–3 cm mucosal colored sessile or pedunculated tumor protruding from the alveolar ridges (maxillary or mandibular) of newborns. Rarely large tumors may interfere with feeding or obstruct the airway and require immediate surgical intervention. Some of these lesions have been diagnosed *in utero* by ultrasound and excised prenatally or shortly after delivery.

Although the histologic findings in congenital epulis resemble those of granular cell tumors, immunohistochemical analysis shows that, unlike granular cell tumor, the tumor cells in congenital epulis are negative for S100 protein. Although radical surgery of complicated lesions may cause injury to the alveolar ridge and result in abnormal dental development, conservative excision usually results in cure without sequelae.

Melanotic Neuroectodermal Tumor of Infancy

Melanotic neuroectodermal tumor of infancy is a rare, pigmented neoplasm that usually occurs during the first 2 years of life (Fig. 9.31). Although nearly 70% appear on the maxilla, tumors have been reported to arise at other sites. The most frequent extra-maxillary locations include the skull, mandible, brain, epididymis, and testis.

Although melanotic neuroectodermal tumors are benign, they may push on vital structures such as the airway and require early surgical intervention. Rare malignant variants may metastasize.

Histologic features include nests of round cells separated by fibrous connective tissue. Large melanin-producing cells sit at the periphery of these nests.

Clinical findings overlap with congenital epulis, and the diagnosis should be confirmed with a biopsy. Excision is recommended, but recurrences may exceed 15%.

Pyogenic Granuloma

Pyogenic granuloma is a benign neoplasm composed of granulation tissue that may represent a response to local

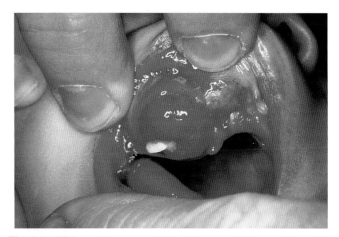

Fig. 9.31 Melanocytic neuroectodermal tumor of infancy. This rapidly expanding tumor developed on the anterior maxilla in this toddler.

irritation or trauma. Although most oral lesions arise on the gingiva, pyogenic granulomas may develop on the tongue, lips, and buccal mucosa (Figs. 9.4 and 9.32). Lesions are more common on the maxillary gingiva than the mandibular gingiva, and are more often located anterior than posterior. Although they may develop at any age, they are more common in children and young adults. Lesions are particularly common in pregnancy, when they are often referred to as granuloma gravidarum.

Although the cause is unclear, growth hormones such as estrogens and progesterone, which increase throughout pregnancy, may trigger the reaction. Growth hormone and other factors that promote growth and development in rapidly growing children may also play a role.

Granuloma gravidarum may regress spontaneously postpartum. However, irritated, bleeding, or symptomatic pyogenic granulomas can be treated with excision and cautery.

Gingival Hyperplasia

Gingival hyperplasia (Table 9.3) may result from local inflammation or gingivitis and infiltrative processes that provide a

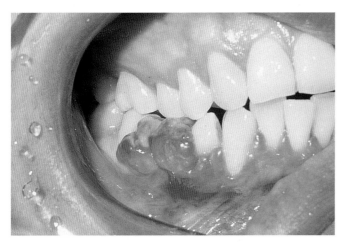

Fig. 9.32 Pyogenic granuloma. This friable reddish-purple nodule developed on the gingiva of a pregnant adolescent.

TABLE 9.3 Causes of Gingival Hyperplasia

Exogenous
Drugs (phenytoin, cyclosporine, oral contraceptives, nifedipine)
Hyperplastic gingivitis from mouth breathing
Nutritional deficiency (scurvy)
    Poor dental hygiene/bacterial infection

Endogenous
Granulomatous disorders
    Sarcoidosis
    Wegner granulomatosis
    Orofacial granulomatosis (Melkersson–Rosenthal syndrome)
    Inflammatory bowel disease
Other infiltrative processes
    Mucopolysaccharidoses
    Mucolipidoses
    Juvenile hyaline fibromatosis
    Hereditary gingival fibromatosis
    Amyloidosis
    Leukemia

clue to underlying systemic disease. In acute reactive gingival hyperplasia the gums are red, and boggy and bleed easily with minor trauma. In chronic fibrotic gingival hyperplasia, chronic fibrosis, which resembles scarring, eventually covers the teeth. These two processes overlap and may be triggered by similar disorders (Fig. 9.33).

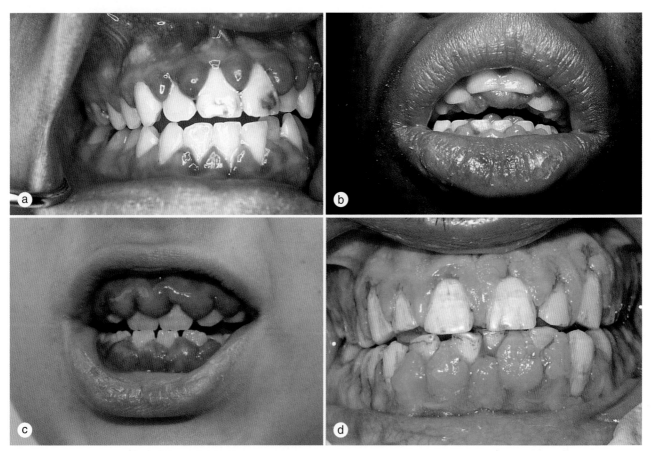

Fig. 9.33 Gingival hyperplasia. **(a)** Diffuse hypertrophy of the gingiva developed in this chronic mouth breather and **(b)** seizure patient on phenytoin therapy. **(c)** A 4-year-old girl with myelomonocytic leukemia and **(d)** an adolescent on chronic cyclosporine therapy after liver transplantation.

Acute gingivitis most commonly results from poor dental hygiene, which may be a problem in chronically ill or debilitated children (e.g. acquired immunodeficiency syndrome), poorly controlled diabetics, and pregnancy. Gingival hyperplasia can develop in scurvy and granulomatous disorders such as Crohn disease and Melkersson–Rosenthal syndrome. Although acute monocytic leukemia is most commonly associated with malignant infiltration of the gums, other leukemias can produce acute and chronic gingival hyperplasia. Drug-related gingival hyperplasia results from an increase in collagen, but acute and chronic inflammatory changes may also be present. Although investigators have established a strong association with cyclosporine, phenytoin, and nifedipine, numerous other medications (e.g. anticonvulsants such as carbamazepine, ethosuximide, felbamate, phenobarbital, and sodium valproate; calcium channel blockers verapamil, felodipine, and diltiazem; erythromycin; oral contraceptives) have been anecdotally reported to trigger gingival thickening. The prevalence peaks with phenytoin (50% of patients) and is notable with cyclosporine and nifedipine (25% of patients).

Gingival fibromatosis, which results in non-inflammatory fibrous change, may follow any inflammatory gingivitis or develop in the setting of hereditary congenital gingival fibromatosis. Similar findings occur in a wide variety of fibromatoses and other syndromes (e.g. tuberous sclerosis).

Gingival hyperplasia can be minimized by careful attention to dental hygiene, but repeated surgery may be necessary in severe cases.

DENTAL DEVELOPMENT AND ANOMALIES

Dental anomalies may represent a local phenomenon or provide clues to underlying multisystem disease. As the teeth are derived from both ectoderm and mesoderm, occult malformations of other structures derived from these embryonic tissues may be reflected in dental defects. By 6–8 weeks of intrauterine development, the dental buds, which arise from the oral epithelium, appear on the upper and lower jaws. Subsequently, the outer protective layer of enamel develops from the epithelium. The mesenchyme beneath the dental buds condenses to form the dental papillae. The mesenchyme in contact with the buds transforms into dentin, while the remaining mesenchyme forms the neurovascular core known as pulp.

The roots of the teeth are anchored to sockets in the mandible and maxilla by the periodontal membrane, through which the neurovascular supply passes to the root apex. The bony processes between the teeth are referred to as the interdental septae. After the teeth erupt, the visible portion is referred to as the crown, and the space between the crowns and the gingivae

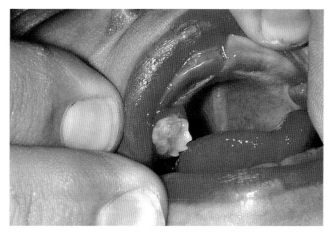

Fig. 9.34 Natal tooth. This loosely anchored natal tooth was extracted to eliminate the risk of aspiration.

is called the gingival crevice. The interdental papillae refer to the gingivae located between the teeth.

Although there may be some variation in the chronology of dental development, marked delay in eruption or loss of teeth may also indicate underlying systemic disease (e.g. hyperimmunoglobulin E syndrome). At approximately 6 months of age, the mandibular central incisors erupt, followed shortly by the maxillary central incisors, and the maxillary and mandibular lateral incisors. At 2 years, all of the primary teeth have erupted except the second primary molars that appear by age 3. Until 2 years of age, a rough estimate of the appropriate number of teeth for a given age can be calculated by subtracting six from the age in months. The eruption of permanent teeth begins with the first molars at age 6 and continues for approximately 6 years.

Occasionally, teeth are present in the newborn or erupt within the first month of life (Fig. 9.34). Although some investigators have suggested that these natal teeth represent predeciduous supernumerary teeth, most probably represent prematurely erupted deciduous teeth. If natal teeth are mobile and aspiration is a concern, removal is appropriate. However, stable teeth should be retained. Traumatic fibromas and ulceration of adjacent soft tissue known as Riga–Fede disease may occur during breastfeeding. However, protective measures may prevent local irritation.

Although environmental factors such as medications, syphilis, rubella, and irradiation may cause dental anomalies, most dental abnormalities are hereditary in nature. A number of genodermatoses (Fig. 9.35) may be associated with dental anomalies, and in some patients the dental findings may provide the first clues of a genodermatosis (Table 9.4).

See diagnostic algorithm in Fig. 9.36.

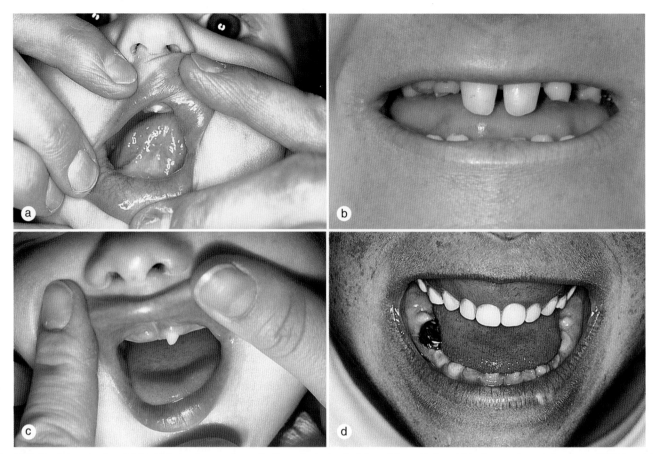

Fig. 9.35 Dental anomalies. **(a)** Multiple teeth were hypoplastic and missing in this toddler with hypohidrotic ectodermal dysplasia. **(b)** This adolescent with hidrotic ectodermal dysplasia had multiple missing and malformed teeth. **(c)** Hypodontia and pegged teeth were the primary complication of incontinentia pigmenti in this 3-year-old girl. **(d)** This adolescent with epidermolysis bullosa developed chronic gingivitis and severe dental caries requiring extensive dental restoration.

TABLE 9.4 Dental Anomalies

Disorder	Inheritance	Dental Anomalies	Associated Anomalies
Dentinogenesis imperfecta	Variable	Discolored, fragile teeth	Osteogenesis imperfecta
Ectodermal dysplasias			
Hypohidrotic	XLR	Absent or sparse abnormally formed teeth	Sparse hair; hypohidrosis; dysmorphic facies
Tooth and nail syndrome	AD	Hypodontia of permanent teeth	Sparse hair; small, brittle nails
Trichodentoosseous syndrome	AD	Hypoplasia of dental enamel; taurodontia	Kinky hair; thin, brittle nails
Rapp–Hodgkin syndrome	AD	Small, decreased number; conical teeth prone to caries	Coarse, wiry hair; short, thick nails; hypohidrosis; midfacial hypoplasia; cleft palate
Ankyloblepharon, ectodermal, dysplasia, cleft lip/palate		Hypodontia, small discolored conical teeth	Cleft lip/palate; scalp erosions; absent/dystrophic nails; hypohidrosis

XLR, X-linked recessive; *AD,* autosomal dominant.

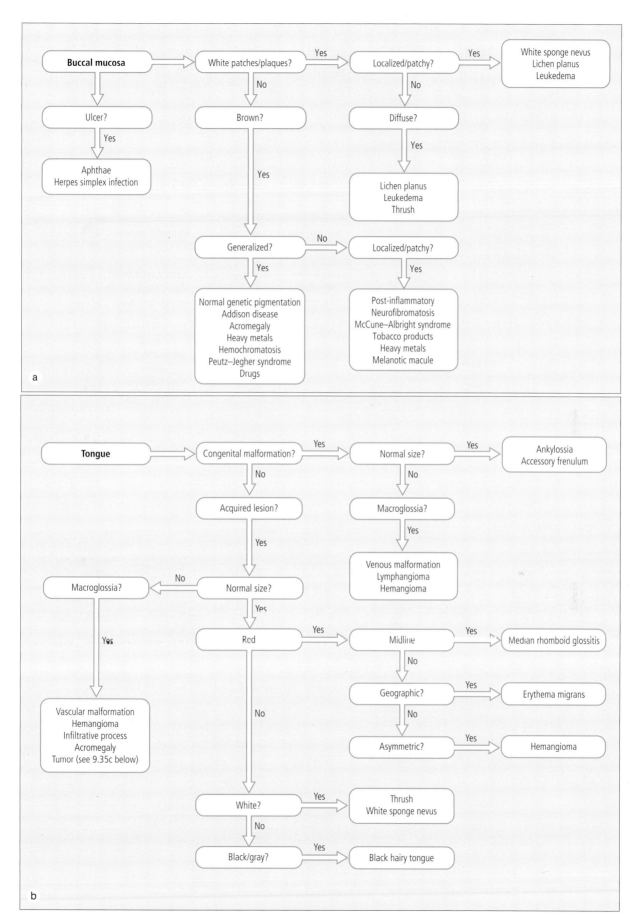

Fig. 9.36 Algorithm for the evaluation of oral pathology including lesions on the **(a)** Buccal Mucosa, **(b)** Tongue, **(c)** Floor of the mouth, **(d)** Lip, and **(e)** Roof of the mouth and gums.

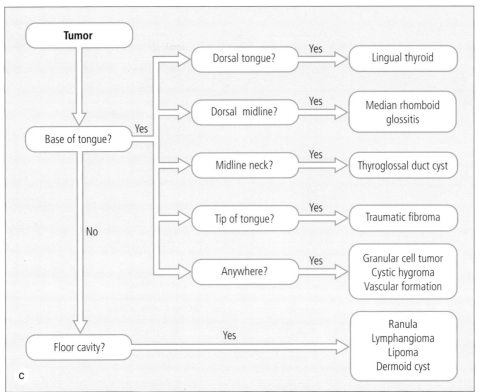

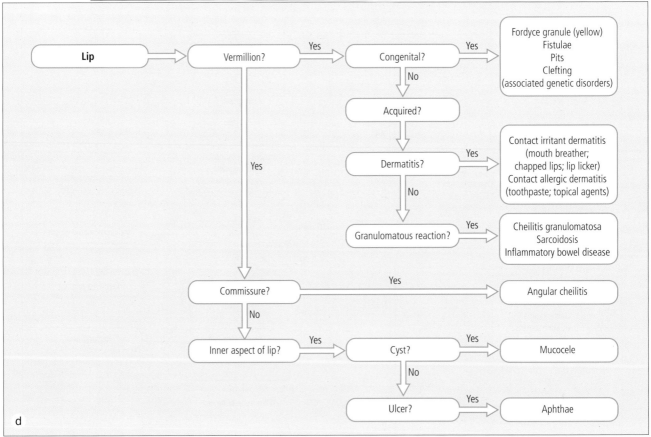

Fig. 9.36—cont'd.

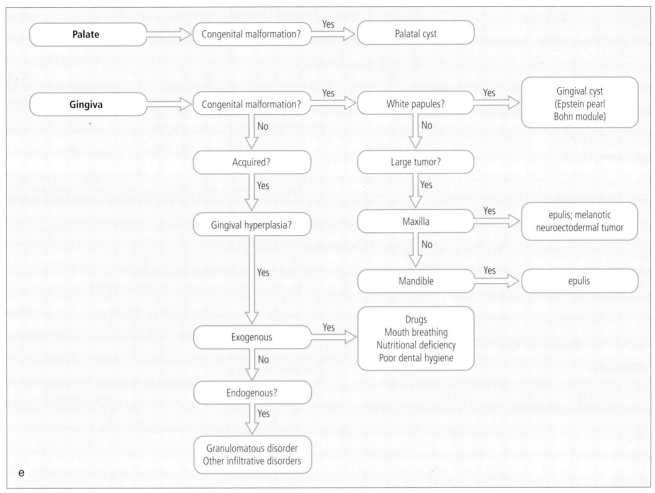

Fig. 9.36—cont'd.

FURTHER READING

White Sponge Nevus
Songu M, Adibelli H, Diniz G. White sponge nevus: clinical suspicion and diagnosis. Pediatr Dermatol 2012; 29(4):495–497.

Jones KB, Jordan R. White lesions in the oral cavity: clinical presentation, diagnosis, and treatment. Semin Cutan Med Surg 2015; 34(4):161–170.

Liu X, Li Q, Gao Y, Song S, Hua H. Mutational analysis in familial and sporadic patients with white sponge naevus. Br J Dermatol 2011; 165(2):448–451.

Satriano RA, Errichetti E, Baroni A. White sponge nevus treated with chlorhexidine. J Dermatol 2012; 39(8):742–743.

Rugg EL, Magee GJ, Wilson NJ, et al. Identification of 2 novel mutations in keratin 13 as the cause of white sponge naevus. Oral Dis 1999; 5:321–324.

Thrush (Pseudomembranous Candidiasis)
Fotos PG, Vincent SD, Hellstein JW. Oral candidiosis: clinical, historical, and therapeutic features of 100 cases. Oral Surg Oral Med Oral Pathol 1992; 74:41–49.

Hacimustafaoglu M, Celebi S. Candida infections in non-neutropenic children after the neonatal period. Expert Rev Anti Infect Ther 2011; 9(10):923–940.

Pienaar ED, Young T, Holmes H. Interventions for the prevention and management of oropharyngeal candidiasis associated with HIV infection in adults and children. Cochrane Database Syst Rev 2010; (11):CD003940.

Taudorf EH, Jemec GBE, Hay RJ, et al. Cutaneous candidiasis—an evidence-based review of topical and systemic treatments to inform clinical practice. J Eur Acad Dermatol Venereol 2019; 33(10):1863–1873.

Ankyloglossia
Block SL. Ankyloglossia: when frenectomy is the right choice. Pediatr Ann 2012; 41(1):14–16.

Walsh J, McKenna Benoit M. Ankyloglossia and other oral ties. Otolaryngol Clin North Am 2019; 52(5):795–811.

Walsh J, Tunkel D. Diagnosis and treatment of ankyloglossia in newborns and infants: a review. JAMA Otolaryngol Head Neck Surg 2017; 143(10):1032–1039.

Han SH, Kim MC, Choi YS, et al. A study on the genetic inheritance of ankyloglossia based on pedigree analysis. Arch Plast Surg 2012; 39(4):329–332.

Rowan-Legg A. Ankyloglossia and breastfeeding. Paediatr Child Health 2011; 16(4):222.

Erythema Migrans (Geographic Tongue)
Majorana A, Bardellini E, Flocchini P, et al. Oral mucosal lesions in children from 0 to 12 years old: ten years' experience. Oral Surg Oral Med Oral Pathol Oral Radiol Endod 2010; 110(1):e13–e18.

Gonzalez-Alvarez L, Garcia-Pola MJ, Garcia-Martin JM. Geographic tongue: predisposing factors, diagnosis and treatment. A systematic review. Rev Clin Esp 2018; 218(9):481–488.

Redman RS, Shapiro BL, Gorlin RJ. Hereditary component in the etiology of benign migratory glossitis. Am J Human Genet 1972; 24:124–133.

Shulman JD. Prevalence of oral mucosal lesions in children and youths in the USA. Int J Paediatr Dent 2005; 15(2):89–97.

Ugar-Cankal D, Denizci S, Hocaoglu T. Prevalence of tongue lesions among Turkish schoolchildren. Saudi Med J 2005; 26(12):1962–1967.

Zargari O. The prevalence and significance of fissured tongue and geographical tongue in psoriatic patients. Clin Exp Dermatol 2006; 31(2):192–195.

Black Hairy Tongue

Poulopoulos AK, Antoniades DZ, Epivatianos A, et al. Black hairy tongue in a 2-month-old infant. J Paediatr Child Health 2008; 44(6):377–379.

Schlager E, St Claire C, Asha K, et al. Black hairy tongue: predisposing factors, diagnosis, and treatment. Am J Clin Dermatol 2017; 18(4):563–569.

Thompson DF, Kessler TL. Drug-induced black hairy tongue. Pharmacotherapy 2010; 30(6):585–593.

Macroglossia

Perkins JA. Overview of macroglossia and its treatment. Curr Opin Otolaryngol Head Neck Surg 2009; 17(6):460–465.

Simmonds JC, Patel AK, Mildenhall NR, et al. Neonatal macroglossia: demographics, cost of care, and associated comorbidities. Cleft Palate Craniofac J 2018; 55(8):1122–1129.

Vogel JE, Muliken JB, Kaban LB. Macroglossia: a review of the condition and a new classification. Plast Reconstr Surg 1986; 78:715–723.

Wolford LM, Cottrell DA. Diagnosis of macroglossia and indications for reduction glossectomy. Am J Orthod Dentofac Orthop 1996; 110:170–177.

Median Rhomboid Glossitis (Central Papillary Atrophy)

Goregen M, Miloglu O, Buyukkurt MC, et al. Median rhomboid glossitis: a clinical and microbiological study. Eur J Dent 2011; 5(4):367–372.

Hellstein JW, Marek CL. Candidiasis: red and white manifestations in the oral cavity. Head Neck Pathol 2019; 13(1):25–32.

Goregen M, Miloglu O, Buyukkurt MC, et al. Median rhomboid glossitis: a clinical and microbiological study. Eur J Dent 2011; 5(4):367–372.

Granular Cell Tumor

Apisarnthanarax P. Granular cell tumor (review). J Am Acad Dermatol 1981; 5:171–181.

Freitas VS, dos Santos JN, Oliveira MC, et al. Intraoral granular cell tumors: clinicopathologic and immunohistochemical study. Quintessence Int 2012; 43(2):135–142.

López V, Santonja N, Jordá E. Granular cell tumor on the sole of a child: a case report. Pediatr Dermatol 2011; 28(4):473–474.

Schafer DR, Glass SH. A guide to yellow oral mucosal entities: etiology and pathology. Head Neck Pathol 2019; 13(1):33–46.

Nagaraj PB, Ongole R, Bhujanga-Rao BR. Granular cell tumor of the tongue in a 6-year-old girl—a case report. Med Oral Patol Oral Cir Bucal 2006; 11(2):E162–E164.

Stewart CM, Watson RE, Eversole LR, et al. Oral granular cell tumor: a clinical and immunohistochemical study. Oral Surg Oral Med Oral Pathol 1988; 65:427–435.

Lingual Thyroid Tumors

Aguirre A, de la Piedra M, Ruiz R, et al. Ectopic thyroid tissue in the submandibular region. Oral Surg Med Oral Pathol 1991; 71:73–76.

Batsakis JG, El-Naggar AK, Luna MA. Thyroid gland ectopias. Ann Otol Rhinol Laryngol 1996; 105:996–1000.

Toso A, Colombani F, Averono G, et al. Lingual thyroid causing dysphagia and dyspnoea. Case reports and review of the literature. Acta Otorhinolaryngol Ital 2009; 29(4):213–217.

Yoon JS, Won KC, Cho IH, et al. Clinical characteristics of ectopic thyroid in Korea. Thyroid 2007; 17(11):1117–1121.

Thyroglossal Duct Cysts

Li W, Ren YP, Shi YY, et al. Presentation, management, and outcome of lingual thyroglossal duct cyst in pediatric and adult populations. J Craniofac Surg 2019; 30(5):e442–446.

Josephson GD, Spencer WR, Josephson JS. Thyroglossal duct cyst: the New York Eye and Ear Infirmary experience and a literature review. Ear Nose Throat J 1998; 77:642–651.

LaRiviere CA, Waldhausen JH. Congenital cervical cysts, sinuses, and fistulae in pediatric surgery. Surg Clin North Am 2012; 92(3):583–597, viii.

Sameer KS, Mohanty S, Correa MM, et al. Lingual thyroglossal duct cysts—a review. Int J Pediatr Otorhinolaryngol 2012; 76(2):165–168.

Lingual Tonsils

Guimaraes CV, Kalra M, Donnelly LF, et al. The frequency of lingual tonsil enlargement in obese children. AJR Am J Roentgenol 2008; 190(4):973–975.

Kluszynski BA, Matt BH. Lingual tonsillectomy in a child with obstructive sleep apnea: a novel technique. Laryngoscope 2006; 116(4):668–669.

Knapp MJ. Oral tonsils: location, distribution, and histology. Oral Surg Oral Med Oral Pathol 1970; 29:155–161.

Ranula

Bonet-Coloma C, Minguez-Martinez I, Aloy-Prósper A, et al. Pediatric oral ranula: clinical follow-up study of 57 cases. Med Oral Patol Oral Cir Bucal 2011; 16(2):e158–e162.

Zhi K, Wen Y, Zhou H. Management of the pediatric plunging ranula: results of 15 years' clinical experience. Oral Surg Oral Med Oral Pathol Oral Radiol Endod 2009; 107(4):499–502.

Harrison JD. Modern management and pathophysiology of ranula: literature review. Head Neck 2010; 32(10):1310–1320.

Cheilitis (Orofacial) Granulomatosa

Critchlow WA, Chang D. Cheilitis granulomatosa: a review. Head Neck Pathol 2014; 8(2): 209–213.

Rose AE, Leger M, Chu J, et al. Cheilitis granulomatosa. Dermatol Online J 2011; 17(10):15.

Armstrong DKB, Burrows D. Orofacial granulomatosis. Int J Dermatol 1995; 34:830–834.

Khouri JM, Bohane TD, Day AS. Is orofacial granulomatosis in children a feature of Crohn's disease? Acta Paediatr 2005; 94(4):501–504.

Lynde CB, Bruce AJ, Orvidas LJ, et al. Cheilitis granulomatosa treated with intralesional corticosteroids and anti-inflammatory agents. J Am Acad Dermatol 2011; 65(3):e101–e102.

Fordyce Granules

Daley TD. Pathology of intraoral sebaceous glands. J Oral Pathol Med 1993; 22:241–245.

Elston DM, Meffert J. Photo quiz. What is your diagnosis? Fordyce spots. Cutis 2001; 68(1):24, 49.

Madani FM, Kuperstein AS. Normal variations of oral anatomy and common oral soft tissue lesions: evaluation and management. Med Clin North Am 2014; 98(6):1281–1298.

Mucocele

Bahadure RN, Fulzele P, Thosar N, et al. Conventional surgical treatment of oral mucocele: a series of 23 cases. Eur J Paediatr Dent 2012; 13(2):143–146.

Martins-Filho PR, Santos Tde S, da Silva HF, et al. A clinicopathologic review of 138 cases of mucoceles in a pediatric population. Quintessence Int 2011; 42(8):679–685.

Khandelwal S, Patil S. Oral mucoceles—review of the literature. Minerva Stomatol 2012; 61(3):91–99.

Moraes Pde C, Teixeira RG, Thomaz LA, et al. Liquid nitrogen cryosurgery for treatment of mucoceles in children. Pediatr Dent 2012; 34(2):159–161.

Shapira M, Akrish S. Mucoceles of the oral cavity in neonates and infants—report of a case and literature review. Pediatr Dermatol 2014; 31(2):e55–58.

Aphthae

Chiang CP, Yu-Fong Chang J, et al. Recurrent aphthous stomatitis—etiology, serum autoantibodies, anemia, hematinic deficiencies, and management. J Formos Med Assoc 2019; 118(9):1279–1289.

Rogers RS. Recurrent aphthous stomatitis: clinical characteristics and associated systemic disorders. Semin Cutan Med Surg 1997; 16:278–283.

Vigo G, Zulian F. Periodic fevers with aphthous stomatitis, pharyngitis, and adenitis (PFAPA). Autoimmun Rev 2012; 12(1):52–55.

Palatal and Gingival Cysts of the Newborn

Binnie WH. Periodontal cysts and epulides. Periodontol 2000 1999; 21:16–32.

Fromm A. Epstein's pearls, Bohn's nodules, and inclusion-cysts of the oral cavity. J Dent Child 1967; 34:275–287.

Gilhar A, Winterstein G, Godfried E. Gingival cysts of the newborn. J Dermatol 1988; 27:261–262.

Hayes PA. Hamartomas, eruption cyst, natal tooth, and Epstein pearls in a newborn. ASDC J Dent Child 2000, 67:365–368.

Mueller DT, Callanan VP. Congenital malformations of the oral cavity. Otolaryngol Clin North Am 2007; 40(1):141–160, vii.

Congenital Epulis

Kovacs L, Volpe C, Laberge JM, et al. Gingival mass in a newborn infant diagnosed in utero. J Pediatr 2002; 141:837.

Kokubun K, Matsuzaka K, Akashi Y, et al. Congenital epulis: a case and review of the literature. Bull Tokyo Dent Coll 2018; 59(2):127–132.

Kumar P, Kim HH, Zahtz GD, et al. Obstructive congenital epulis: prenatal diagnosis and perinatal management. Laryngoscope 2002; 112:1935–1939.

Merglová V, Mukensnabl P, Andrle P. Congenital epulis. BMJ Case Rep 2012; ii.

Neuroectodermal Tumor of Infancy

Gonçalves CF, Costa Ndo L, Oliveira-Neto HH, et al. Melanotic neuroectodermal tumor of infancy: report of 2 cases. J Oral Maxillofac Surg 2010; 68(9):2341–2346.

Kruse-Lösler B, Gaertner C, Bürger H, et al. Melanotic neuroectodermal tumor of infancy: systematic review of the literature and presentation of a case. Oral Surg Oral Med Oral Pathol Oral Radiol Endod 2006; 102(2):204–216.

Pyogenic Granuloma

Kamal R, Dahiya P, Puri A. Oral pyogenic granuloma: Various concepts of etiopathogenesis. J Oral Maxillofac Pathol 2012; 16(1):79–82.

Saravana GH. Oral pyogenic granuloma: a review of 137 cases. Br J Oral Maxillofac Surg 2009; 47(4):318–319.

Lee J, Sinno H, Tahiri Y, et al. Treatment options for cutaneous pyogenic granulomas: a review. J Plast Reconstr Aesthet Surg 2011; 64(9):1216–1220.

Zain RB, Khoo SP, Yeo JF. Oral pyogenic granuloma (excluding pregnancy tumor): a clinical analysis of 304 cases. Singapore Dent J 1995; 20:8–10.

Gingival Hyperplasia

Livada R, Shiloah J. Calcium channel blocker-induced gingival enlargement. J Hum Hypertens 2014; 28(1):10–14.

Agrawal AA. Gingival enlargements: differential diagnosis and review of literature. World J Clin Cases 2015; 3(9):779–788.

Bakaeen G, Scully C. Hereditary gingival fibromatosis in a family with Zimmerman-Laband syndrome. J Oral Pathol Med 1991; 20:457–459.

Ramnarayan BK, Sowmya K, Rema J. Management of idiopathic gingival fibromatosis: report of a case and literature review. Pediatr Dent 2011; 33(5):431–436.

Coletta RD, Graner E. Hereditary gingival fibromatosis: a systematic review. J Periodontol 2006; 77(5):753–764.

Desai P, Silver JG. Drug-induced gingival enlargements. J Can Dent Assoc 1998; 64:263–268.

Dental Development and Abnormalities

Michon F. Tooth evolution and dental defects: from genetic regulation network to micro-RNA fine-tuning. Birth Defects Res A Clin Mol Teratol 2011; 91(8):763–769.

Neville BW, Damm DD, Allen CM, et al. Abnormalities of the teeth. In: Oral and maxillofacial pathology. Saunders, Philadelphia, 2002, pp. 45–106.

Shilpa, Mohapatra A, Reddy CP, et al. Congenital absence of multiple primary teeth. J Indian Soc Pedod Prev Dent 2010; 28(4):319–321.

Witkop CJ, Rao S. Inherited defects in tooth structure. In: Bergasma D. Birth defects. Original article series. Williams & Wilkins, Baltimore, 1971, pp. 153–184.

Zhu JF, Marcushamer M, King DL, et al. Supernumerary and congenitally absent teeth: a literature review. J Clin Pediatr Dent 1996; 20:87–95.

10

Genital Disorders

Tina Ho and Kalyani S. Marathe

INTRODUCTION

Children may present to their pediatrician, dermatologist, urologist, or gynecologist with anogenital skin disease. This portion of the chapter highlights some of the most commonly encountered conditions affecting infants, prepubertal children, and adolescents. Recognition of these cutaneous disorders not only enables patients to receive appropriate treatment for their dermatologic disease, but can also alleviate concerns regarding child abuse. However, if child abuse is suspected, a complete physical examination should be performed and documented. Experts in child abuse should be consulted and examination findings reported to the appropriate authorities for further investigation.

ANOGENITAL EXAMINATION

Physical examination of involved skin can provide valuable information regarding the diagnosis and severity of disease; however, not all physicians have experience performing a pediatric anogenital examination.

The purpose of the examination should be explained to children in an age-appropriate manner and permission explicitly obtained from children and parents. Patients should always feel in control of their body and allowed to ask questions, examine swabs or other instruments prior to the examination, and assume the appropriate position on their own. Male children can be examined standing or lying down. Penile length, testicular size, foreskin anatomy, location of the urethral meatus, and the presence and extent of pubic hair should be noted.

Female children can be examined in a supine position with knees bent and feet together in a "butterfly" position. Pressure then can be placed laterally and posteriorly on both buttocks to visualize the architecture of the labia, hymen shape and patency (in prepubertal girls), clitoral size, pubic hair, and presence and color of discharge.

The wishes of the child should always be respected. Children who refuse to be examined can be treated based on history for minor complaints. For more serious conditions, the anogenital examination may be performed with partial sedation or anesthesia.

NON-SPECIFIC VULVOVAGINITIS

Non-specific vulvovaginitis is the most common cause of vulvovaginitis in prepubertal girls. In newborn infants, the vulva is edematous and vaginal mucosa is thickened as a result of the effects of maternal estrogen. However, as maternal hormone levels start to fall, the labia minora and vaginal mucosa become thin and relatively susceptible to irritation. Other factors that contribute to the development of vulvovaginitis in prepubertal girls include lack of pubic hair, minimal adipose tissue in the labia majora, and close proximity of the vagina to the anus.

Non-specific vulvovaginitis is characterized by pruritus, burning, dysuria, and erythema of the vulva and vagina. It can also be associated with atrophy, erythema, excoriations, abnormal vaginal discharge, or vaginal bleeding. Treatment is focused on minimizing irritation from occlusive clothing, detergents, fragrances, urine, and feces. Wiping from front to back, urinating with legs spread apart to prevent urine from becoming trapped in the vagina (vaginal voiding), and sitting in a bathtub of plain water for 10 min daily can improve vulvar hygiene. Avoidance of tight clothing, rapid removal of wet swimsuits, and use of laundry detergents without added dyes or fragrances can also help reduce irritation. Children may also benefit from wearing cotton underwear during the day and a nightgown without underwear prior to bed.

Bacterial vulvovaginitis should be considered and a culture obtained if symptoms persist despite conservative treatment measures. Other conditions to consider include foreign body, pinworms, lichen sclerosus, Mullerian anomalies associated with partial outflow tract obstruction, rectovaginal fistula, and ectopic ureter. Of note, yeast infections are uncommon in prepubertal children.

PERINEAL PYRAMIDAL PROTRUSION

Perineal pyramidal protrusion, also known as infantile perianal pyramidal protrusion, infantile perianal protrusion, or infantile perineal protrusion, is a benign skin finding commonly seen in female infants. These skin-colored to erythematous protrusions are typically located on the midline of the perineum anterior to the anus and may be shaped like a pyramid, peanut, tongue tip, cigar, leaf, or hen's crest (Fig. 10.1). Perineal pyramidal protrusions are thought to occur as a result of congenital weakness of the median raphe and have been associated with constipation and changes in stool consistency associated with the administration of oral antibiotics and viral gastroenteritis. A subset of lesions may occur in a familial pattern.

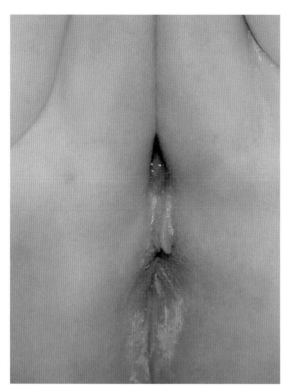

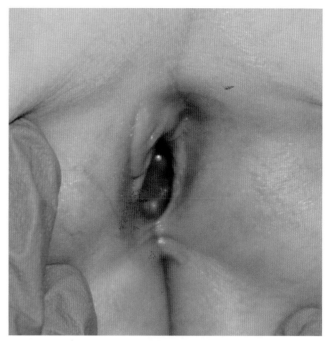

Fig. 10.2 Labial adhesion. Note the more common posterior location of this partial labial adhesion.

Fig. 10.1 Perineal pyramidal protrusion. This healthy 3-year-old girl developed this fleshy pyramidal lesion in the perineal area after antibiotic treatment of otitis media.

Treatment of the underlying constipation with dietary changes or polyethylene glycol (e.g. MiraLAX) may lead to rapid resolution of the perineal pyramidal protrusion. Otherwise, treatment is usually not necessary as the lesions themselves are asymptomatic and often resolve spontaneously. Those removed by surgical excision and examined by histopathology demonstrate normal skin, sometimes with acanthosis, dermal edema, or a mild inflammatory infiltrate.

LABIAL ADHESION

Labial adhesion, also known as labial agglutination, results from postnatal fusion of the labia minora (Fig. 10.2). Toddlers aged 13–23 months have the highest incidence of labial adhesions, possibly as a result of chronic irritation and physical apposition of the labia minora from wearing diapers. Low estrogen levels may also play a role in the pathogenesis of labial adhesions as the condition is rare at birth and in children after puberty.

Labial adhesions may be asymptomatic or present with vaginitis, dysuria, urinary frequency, a painful or altered urinary stream, post-void urinary dribbling, recurrent urinary tract infections, or urinary retention as a result of complete obstruction. Asymptomatic patients may be treated with vaginal hygiene (see section Non-Specific Vulvovaginitis). Children with symptoms can be treated with estrogen cream, betamethasone dipropionate 0.05% cream or ointment, manual separation in the office, or surgical lysis of adhesions in an operating room setting. Unfortunately, there is a high rate of recurrence

regardless of treatment modality. Indications for surgical treatment include acute urinary retention as a result of complete agglutination, recurrent infections, and failure of medical therapy. Side effects of estrogen cream include local irritation, formation of breast buds, vulvar hyperpigmentation, and rarely vaginal bleeding, while side effects of betamethasone dipropionate 0.05% cream or ointment include local irritation and, rarely, growth of fine pubic hair.

DIAPER DERMATITIS

Eruptions that occur on diaper-covered skin include irritant contact dermatitis, allergic contact dermatitis, seborrheic dermatitis, psoriasis, candidiasis, Langerhans cell histiocytosis, and acrodermatitis enteropathica, all of which are discussed in detail in Chapter 2. Severe irritant contact dermatitis, however, may also manifest as pseudoverrucous papules and nodules or Jacquet erosive diaper dermatitis.

Pseudoverrucous papules and nodules typically occur in children and adults with persistent skin irritation from prolonged exposure to urine or liquid stool in a warm, moist environment. They appear as multiple, shiny, smooth or verrucous, brightly erythematous, grey or reddish-brown, moist, flat-topped papules and nodules on perianal, genital, suprapubic, or peristomal skin (Fig. 10.3a) and have been described in patients with a history of Hirschsprung's disease, spina bifida, urethrovaginal fistula, severe constipation with encopresis, and around urostomies and colostomies. Frequent diaper changes, superabsorbent diapers, and use of topical emollients and barrier pastes can help reduce skin irritation; however, pseudoverrucous papules and nodules may not fully resolve until the incontinence improves.

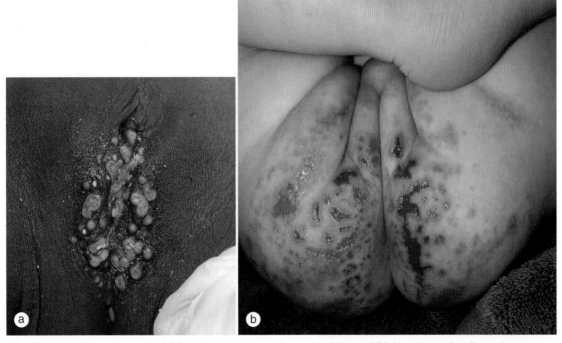

Fig. 10.3 Diaper dermatitis. **(a)** Pseudoverrucous papules and nodules and **(b)** Jacquet erosive diaper dermatitis with perianal erosions and ulcers with elevated borders that developed in a child with loose stools secondary to viral gastroenteritis.

Jacquet erosive diaper dermatitis is characterized by well-demarcated ulcers and erosions with elevated borders (Fig. 10.3b). The condition is believed to be a result of infrequent diaper changes, as well as residual detergent on cloth diapers washed at home, and has become much less common with widespread use of superabsorbent disposable diapers. Treatment involves generous use of zinc oxide cream and avoidance of disposable baby wipes. Instead, the skin should be cleaned using plain water, cloth-like paper towels soaked in water, or laxative-grade mineral oil on cotton squares. Superinfection with *Candida* species is common and can be treated with azole antifungal creams.

INFANTILE HEMANGIOMA

As mentioned in Chapter 2, lower body infantile hemangiomas and other cutaneous defects have been associated with urogenital anomalies, ulceration, myelopathy, bony deformities, anorectal malformations, arterial anomalies, and rectal anomalies in LUMBAR syndrome. Therefore, spinal imaging is recommended for infants with perineal infantile hemangiomas.

Infantile hemangiomas present on anogenital skin (Fig. 10.4) are also more likely to ulcerate because of friction, maceration, and irritation from urine and stool. Therefore, anogenital infantile hemangiomas may be treated more aggressively with topical or systemic beta-blockers than similar-appearing lesions on non-genital skin. Systemic treatment with oral propranolol is also indicated for anogenital infantile hemangiomas that would otherwise delay surgical repair of an underlying congenital anomaly.

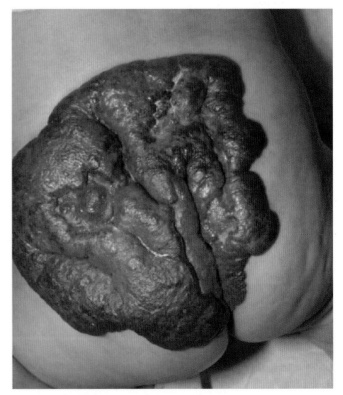

Fig. 10.4 Infantile hemangioma. A 6-month-old boy developed a large hemangioma on his buttocks associated with an ulceration, which healed after starting oral propranolol.

LICHEN SCLEROSUS/BALANITIS XEROTICA OBLITERANS

As previously described in Chapter 7, lichen sclerosus has a bimodal age distribution in female patients, with peak incidence in prepubertal children and postmenopausal adults. In one study, the mean age of diagnosis in female children was 6.7 years.

Children with anogenital lichen sclerosus may be asymptomatic or have soreness, dryness, pruritus, dysuria, dyspareunia, or pain with defecation that can lead to constipation. While adults typically present with pruritus and dyspareunia,

children with lichen sclerosus will very commonly present with a primary complaint of constipation. On physical examination, lichen sclerosus is classically characterized by sclerotic white atrophic plaques with a shiny or wrinkled appearance on the vulva and perianal skin in a figure-of-eight configuration (Fig. 10.5). However, telangiectasias, purpura, erosions, and fissures are also common, and severe disease may demonstrate scarring with burying of the clitoris, loss of the labia minora, and narrowing of the introitus. Superpotent topical steroids are first-line treatment for lichen sclerosus. Topical calcineurin inhibitors can also be used as a steroid-sparing agent, especially to maintain disease remission. Constipation, if present,

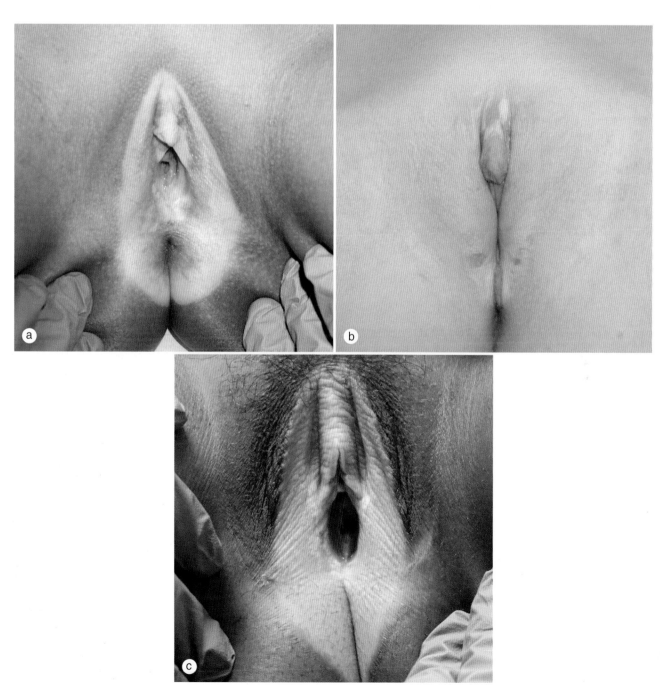

Fig. 10.5 Lichen sclerosus. Note the scarring **(a,c)** and erosions **(b)**.

should be addressed and treated with polyethylene glycol if appropriate.

Balanitis xerotica obliterans is characterized by white atrophic plaques located on the foreskin, frenulum, glans, meatus, and urethra of male patients. Unlike lichen sclerosus in female patients, perianal involvement is rare. Children with balanitis xerotica obliterans can present with pruritus, soreness, phimosis, pain on erection, dysuria, and even urinary obstruction. Topical or intralesional steroids may be of benefit in early disease; however, patients with more severe disease frequently require surgical intervention (e.g. circumcision).

VITILIGO

Vitiligo is an acquired disorder of pigmentation discussed in greater detail in Chapter 6. In children with vitiligo, well-demarcated depigmented patches can be found on any cutaneous surface, including the face, hands and feet, elbows and knees, and anogenital skin (Fig. 10.6). One study showed that 14% of patients with vitiligo had involvement of their genitals. This can affect self-esteem in both male and female children, and unfortunately, treatments such as phototherapy, topical steroids, and topical calcineurin inhibitors are less effective on glabrous skin.

CUTANEOUS CROHN DISEASE

Specific skin manifestations of Crohn disease share the same histopathological findings as the gastrointestinal disease. Namely, biopsies show non-caseating granulomas with foreign body or Langerhans giant cells, epithelioid histiocytes, and plasma cells. Crohn disease–specific skin findings can be categorized into those that result from direct extension of the gastrointestinal disease onto nearby skin and those that are separated from the gastrointestinal tract by normal skin, the latter of which is commonly called non-contiguous or metastatic Crohn disease. Of note, cutaneous manifestations of Crohn disease are more common in patients who have colorectal disease. Moreover, perianal Crohn disease is strongly associated with distal colonic inflammation.

Cutaneous Crohn disease may present with perianal skin tags and fissures, "knife-like" erosions and ulcerations, or erythematous and violaceous nodules and plaques (Fig. 10.7). Abscesses, fistulas, draining sinuses, scarring, or lymphedema can also occur. Particularly in children, cutaneous Crohn disease may manifest as unilateral or bilateral edema or induration without discrete lesions. The skin findings may be asymptomatic, pruritic, tender, or painful and are most commonly located on the penis, scrotum, vulva, buttocks, and perianal skin.

A high index of suspicion for cutaneous Crohn disease is especially important in pediatric dermatology because children are more likely to present with metastatic Crohn disease without a prior diagnosis of inflammatory bowel disease. Asking about weight loss, diarrhea, bloody stools, frequent bowel movements, joint pain, eye pain, blurry vision, photophobia, and family history of inflammatory bowel disease can aid in making the diagnosis. While the clinical course of metastatic Crohn disease is independent of intestinal disease, most children have gastrointestinal symptoms at presentation.

Children without an established diagnosis of gastrointestinal Crohn disease should be referred to gastroenterology for evaluation and management. If possible, biopsy of anogenital Crohn disease should be avoided because of pathergy and poor wound healing. Depending on severity, the cutaneous disease may be

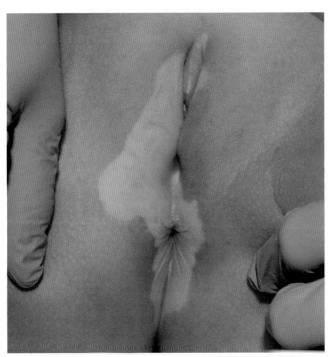

Fig. 10.6 Vitiligo. A well-demarcated depigmented patch on the labia, perineum, and perianal skin.

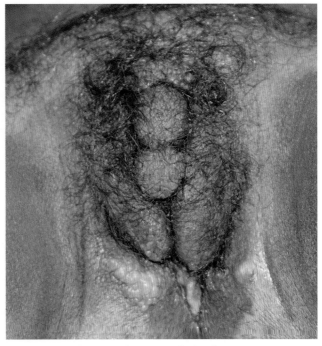

Fig. 10.7 Cutaneous Crohn disease.

treated with topical steroids, topical calcineurin inhibitors, metronidazole, systemic steroids, methotrexate, azathioprine, or tumor necrosis factor-alpha (TNF-α) inhibitors. Abscesses are frequently drained prior to the initiation of immunosuppressive medications, but major surgery such as vulvectomy, ileostomy, or colectomy is typically reserved for cases refractory to medical management.

MOLLUSCUM CONTAGIOSUM

Molluscum contagiosum is a common childhood infection that is discussed in greater detail in Chapter 5. It is caused by the molluscum contagiosum virus, a member of the poxvirus family that is transmitted by direct skin contact or contact with contaminated fomites.

In adults and sexually active adolescents, molluscum contagiosum is generally regarded as a sexually transmitted disease because of the close contact required for viral transmission. In young children, however, the appearance of pearly white, skin-colored, or lightly erythematous dome-shaped papules with central umbilication on anogenital skin usually results from autoinoculation, especially in children with molluscum dermatitis or atopic dermatitis that are frequently scratching (Fig. 10.8; see Fig. 5.12).

Molluscum should be distinguished from pearly penile papules that develop in up to 15% of young men in the second and third decades of life. Pearly penile papules appear as multiple 1–3 mm uniform pale, skin-colored papules in one to two rows on the ridge of the glans penis (Fig. 10.9). They are asymptomatic, and non-infectious, and may also be confused with anogenital warts. They develop more commonly in uncircumcised males, and a similar variant may occur in young women at the perivaginal orifice.

HERPES SIMPLEX VIRUS

As described in Chapters 2 and 4, herpes simplex virus (HSV) is characterized by a cluster of vesicles or erosions on an erythematous base. In contrast to molluscum contagiosum,

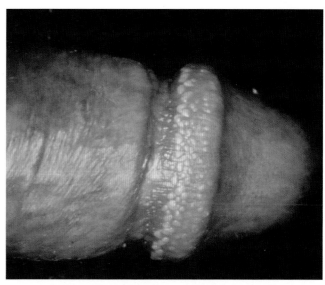

Fig. 10.9 Pearly penile papules. Asymptomatic pearly papules were noted on the base of the glans penis of this 13-year-old boy during a routine physical examination.

anogenital HSV in a child not yet engaging in consensual sexual activity is suspicious for abuse. However, HSV1 has a seroprevalence of 47.8% and HSV-2 has a seroprevalence of 11.9% in people aged 14–49 years in the United States, making it possible for both HSV1 and HSV2 to be transmitted by autoinoculation, close contact with caregivers, and interaction with other children.

HUMAN PAPILLOMAVIRUS

As mentioned in Chapter 5, all warts are caused by infection with human papillomavirus (HPV). Anogenital warts in children not yet old enough to be engaging in consensual sexual activity (Fig. 10.10; see Fig. 5.6a) was once considered to be highly suspicious for sexual abuse; however, more recent studies have shown low rates of sexual abuse in infants and toddlers with anogenital warts, as well as a high rate of vertical transmission in infants born to mothers with HPV. The risk of sexual abuse in children with HPV does increase with age, and most guidelines recommend thorough evaluation for other signs and symptoms of abuse in children with anogenital HPV with no consensus on whether the presence of anogenital HPV alone is sufficient to warrant a report to child protective services.

PINWORMS

Pinworms are common in children across all socioeconomic groups. Symptoms occur weeks to months after infection with *Enterobius vermicularis*, a roundworm that can be transmitted via the fecal–oral route, contact with fomites, or inhalation of airborne organisms.

Once in the gastrointestinal tract, larvae hatch in the duodenum and migrate to the cecum. Gravid female pinworms are white and approximately 5–13 mm in length and emerge from the rectum at night to deposit thousands of ova on perianal

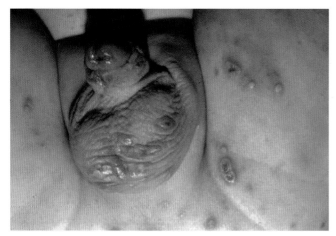

Fig. 10.8 Molluscum contagiosum. Note the umbilicated papules on the penis, scrotum, and thighs of this young boy.

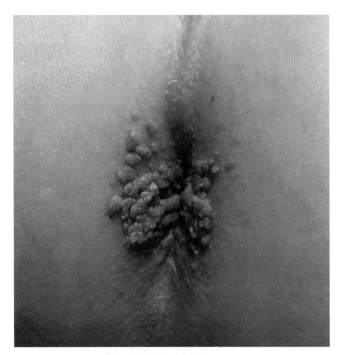

Fig. 10.10 Anogenital warts.

skin. Ova are approximately 55 × 25 µm in size and appear flattened on one side. The ova mature in 4–6 h and can remain viable for as long as 3 weeks at 3–5°C in moist environments.

Children classically present with nocturnal pruritus ani, but may be asymptomatic or simply restless and irritable. Less commonly, patients may also have insomnia, dysuria, enuresis, anorexia, abdominal pain, nausea, vomiting, urinary tract infections, vulvovaginitis, or epididymitis, especially if pinworms have taken up residence in the genitourinary tract, as well as the gastrointestinal tract. Diagnosis is confirmed by identification of the pinworm or ova on adhesive tape applied early in the morning before defecation or bathing, with eosinophilia present only in patients with ectopic infection outside the lumen of the gastrointestinal tract.

Options for treatment include mebendazole, albendazole, and pyrantel pamoate. Albendazole is the treatment of choice in patients with genitourinary infection as mebendazole has poor systemic adsorption. Clothes and bedding should be washed and a second dose of medication given in two weeks to prevent reinfection. Given high rates of transmission among household contacts, it is recommended that everyone be treated simultaneously, even if asymptomatic.

NON-SEXUALLY ACQUIRED GENITAL ULCERATION (NSAGU)

Non-sexually acquired genital ulceration (NSAGU), also known as Lipschütz ulcer or ulcus vulvae acutum, is characterized by exquisitely painful, single or multiple, well-demarcated shallow ulcers with a fibrinous base and surrounding erythematous halo. They are most commonly located on the labia minora but may also occur on the labia majora, lower vagina, and perineum.

The etiology of these ulcerations is unknown; however, the disease is often preceded by a viral prodrome with fever and malaise, and individual cases have been variably associated with Epstein–Barr virus (EBV), cytomegalovirus (CMV), mycoplasma, influenza, and mumps virus. Because the differential diagnosis includes HSV, fixed drug eruption, Behçet disease, and Crohn disease, a complete mucocutaneous examination, medication history, and HSV polymerase chain reaction (PCR) should be obtained in any child suspected to have NSAGU. A biopsy may be needed to rule out other conditions, but NSAGU exhibit only non-specific acute and chronic inflammation with superficial edema, dilated capillaries, epithelial hyperplasia, ulceration, and possible necrosis on histopathology.

Management of NSAGU is largely supportive, with lesions healing in several weeks regardless of treatment. Patients and families should be reassured that the disease is neither contagious nor sexually transmitted. Sitz baths, topical lidocaine, and topical steroids may provide some relief. Urinating in a bath of warm water can also help if dysuria is present. In severe cases, however, urinary catheterization, oral pain medications, and systemic steroids may be required.

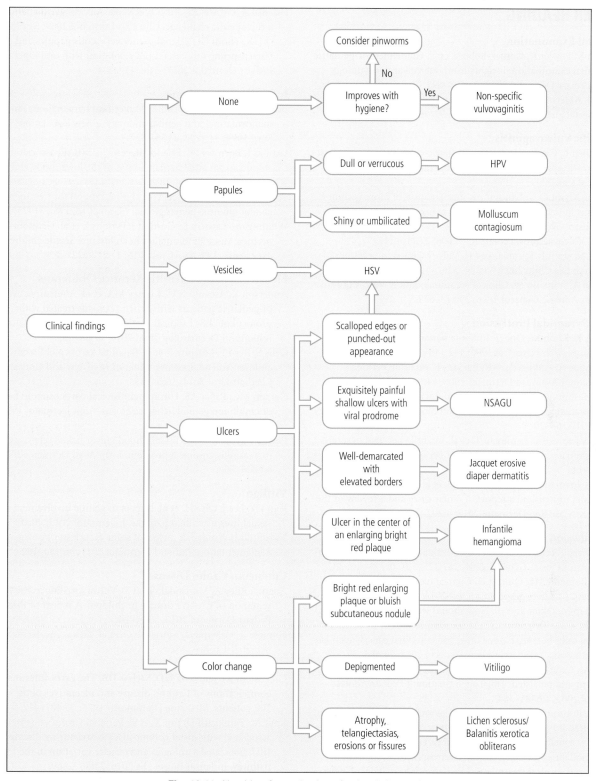

Fig. 10.11 Algorithm for evaluation of vulvar itch or pain.

FURTHER READING

Anogenital Examination

Habeshian K, Fowler K, Gomez-Lobo V, et al. Guidelines for pediatric anogenital examination: insights from our vulvar dermatology clinic. Pediatr Dermatol 2018; 35:693–695.

Jacobs AM, Alderman EM. Gynecologic examination of the prepubertal girl. Pediatr Rev 2014; 35:97–104.

Nonspecific Vulvovaginitis

Eyk NV, Allen L, Giesbrecht E, et al. Pediatric vulvovaginal disorders: a diagnostic approach and review of the literature. J Obstet Gynaecol Can 2009; 31:850–862.

Loveless M, Myint O. Vulvovaginitis- presentation of more common problems in pediatric and adolescent gynecology. Best Pract Res Clin Obstet Gynaecol 2018; 48:14–27.

Kokotos F. Vulvovaginitis. Pediatr Rev 2006; 27:116–117.

Stricker T, Navratil F, Sennhauser FH. Vulvovaginitis in prepubertal girls. Arch Dis Child 2003; 88:324–326.

Zuckerman A, Romano M. Clinical recommendation: vulvovaginitis. J Pediatr Adolesc Gynecol 2016; 29:673–679.

Perineal Pyramidal Protrusion

Kayashima K, Kitoh M, Ono T. Infantile perianal pyramidal protrusion. Arch Dermatol 1996; 132:1481–1484.

Khachemoune A, Guldbakke KK, Ehrsam E. Infantile perineal protrusion. J Am Acad Dermatol 2006; 54:1046–1049.

Konta R, Hashimoto I, Takahashi M, et al. Infantile perineal protrusion: a statistical, clinical, and histopathologic study. Dermatology 2000; 201:316–320.

Merigou D, Labreze C, Lamireau T, et al. Infantile perianal pyramidal protrusion: a marker of constipation? Pediatr Dermatol 1998; 15:143–144.

Zavras N, Christianakis E, Tsamoudaki S, et al. Infantile perianal pyramidal protrusion: a report of 8 new cases and a review of the literature. Case Rep Dermatol 2012; 4:202–206.

Labial Adhesion

Bacon JL. Prepubertal labial adhesions: evaluation of a referral population. Am J Obstet Gynecol 2002; 187:327–331, discussion 332.

Bacon JL, Romano ME, Quint EH. Clinical recommendation: labial adhesions. J Pediatr Adolesc Gynecol 2015; 28:405–409.

Eroglu E, Yip M, Oktar T, et al. How should we treat prepubertal labial adhesions? Retrospective comparison of topical treatments: estrogen only, betamethasone only, and combination estrogen and betamethasone. J Pediatr Adolesc Gynecol 2011; 24:389–391.

Kumetz LM, Quint EH, Fisseha S, et al. Estrogen treatment success in recurrent and persistent labial agglutination. J Pediatr Adolesc Gynecol 2006; 19:381–384.

Leung AK, Robson WL, Tay-Uyboco J. The incidence of labial fusion in children. J Paediatr Child Health 1993; 29:235–236.

Mayoglou L, Dulabon L, Martin-Alguacil N, et al. Success of treatment modalities for labial fusion: a retrospective evaluation of topical and surgical treatments. J Pediatr Adolesc Gynecol 2009; 22:247–250.

Diaper Dermatitis

Askin U, Ada S, Bilezikci B, et al. Erosive papulonodular dermatosis in an adolescent with encopresis. Br J Dermatol 2008; 158:413–415.

Garrido-Ruiz MC, Rosales B, Luis Rodriguez-Peralto J. Vulvar pseudoverrucous papules and nodules secondary to a urethral—vaginal fistula. Am J Dermatopathol 2011; 33:410–412.

Paradisi A, Capizzi R, Ghitti F, et al. Jacquet erosive diaper dermatitis: a therapeutic challenge. Clin Exp Dermatol 2009; 34:e385–386.

Yap FHX, Thom G. Perianal pseudoverrucous papules and nodules in Hirschsprung's disease: rapid resolution with oral loperamide. Pediatr Dermatol 2017; 34:e343–e344.

Infantile Hemangioma

Bouchard S, Yazbeck S, Lallier M. Perineal hemangioma, anorectal malformation, and genital anomaly: a new association? J Pediatr Surg 1999; 34:1133–1135.

Iacobas I, Burrows PE, Frieden IJ, et al. LUMBAR: association between cutaneous infantile hemangiomas of the lower body and regional congenital anomalies. J Pediatr 2010; 157:795–801 e791–797.

Tran C, Tamburro J, Rhee A, et al. Propranolol for treatment of genital infantile hemangioma. J Urol 2016; 195:731–737.

Willihnganz-Lawson K, Gordon J, Perkins J, et al. Genitourinary and perineal vascular anomalies in children: a Seattle children's experience. J Pediatr Urol 2015; 11:227.e221–226.

Lichen Sclerosus/Balanitis Xerotica Obliterans

Anderson K, Ascanio NM, Kinney MA, et al. A retrospective analysis of pediatric patients with lichen sclerosus treated with a standard protocol of class I topical corticosteroid and topical calcineurin inhibitor. J Dermatolog Treat 2016; 27:64–66.

Celis S, Reed F, Murphy F, et al. Balanitis xerotica obliterans in children and adolescents: a literature review and clinical series. J Pediatr Urol 2014; 10:34–39.

Garzon MC, Paller AS. Ultrapotent topical corticosteroid treatment of childhood genital lichen sclerosus. Arch Dermatol 1999; 135:525–528.

Powell J, Wojnarowska F. Childhood vulvar lichen sclerosus: an increasingly common problem. J Am Acad Dermatol 2001; 44:803–806.

Vitiligo

Kim DY, Lee J, Oh SH, et al. Impact of genital involvement on the sexual lives of vitiligo patients. J Dermatol 2013; 40:1065–1067.

Nordlund JJ. Vitiligo: a review of some facts lesser known about depigmentation. Indian J Dermatol 2011; 56:180–189.

Cutaneous Crohn Disease

Ahad T, Riley A, Martindale E, et al. Vulvar swelling as the first presentation of Crohn's disease in children-A report of three cases. Pediatr Dermatol 2018; 35:e1–e4.

Granese R, Calagna G, Morabito G, et al. Vulvar involvement in pediatric Crohn's disease: a systematic review. Arch Gynecol Obstet 2018; 297:3–11.

Greenstein AJ, Janowitz HD, Sachar DB. The extra-intestinal complications of Crohn's disease and ulcerative colitis: a study of 700 patients. Medicine (Baltimore) 1976; 55:401–412.

Kaur M, Panikkath D, Yan X, et al. Perianal Crohn's disease is associated with distal colonic disease, stricturing disease behavior, IBD-associated serologies and genetic variation in the JAK-STAT pathway. Inflamm Bowel Dis 2016; 22:862–869.

Schneider SL, Foster K, Patel D, et al. Cutaneous manifestations of metastatic Crohn's disease. Pediatr Dermatol 2018; 35:566–574.

Seemann NM, Elkadri A, Walters TD, et al. The role of surgery for children with perianal Crohn's disease. J Pediatr Surg 2015; 50:140–143.

Molluscum Contagiosum

Dohil MA, Lin P, Lee J, et al. The epidemiology of molluscum contagiosum in children. J Am Acad Dermatol 2006; 54:47–54.

Neinstein LS, Goldenring J. Pink pearly papules: an epidemiologic study. J Pediatr 1984; 105:594–595.

Sarifakioglu E, Erdal E, Gunduz C. Vestibular papillomatosis: case report and literature review. Acta Derm Venereol 2006; 86:177–178.

Herpes Simplex Virus

McQuillan G, Kruszon-Moran D, Flagg EW, et al. Prevalence of herpes simplex virus type 1 and type 2 in persons aged 14–49: United States, 2015–2016. NCHS Data Brief 2018:1–8.

Reading R, Rannan-Eliya Y. Evidence for sexual transmission of genital herpes in children. Arch Dis Child 2007; 92:608–613.

Human Papillomavirus

Cohen BA, Honig P, Androphy E. Anogenital warts in children. Clinical and virologic evaluation for sexual abuse. Arch Dermatol 1990; 126:1575–1580.

Koskimaa HM, Waterboer T, Pawlita M, et al. Human papillomavirus genotypes present in the oral mucosa of newborns and their concordance with maternal cervical human papillomavirus genotypes. J Pediatr 2012; 160:837–843.

Sinclair KA, Woods CR, Kirse DJ, et al. Anogenital and respiratory tract human papillomavirus infections among children: age, gender, and potential transmission through sexual abuse. Pediatrics 2005; 116:815–825.

Sinclair KA, Woods CR, Sinal SH. Venereal warts in children. Pediatr Rev 2011; 32:115–121, quiz 121.

Pinworms

Jones MF, Jacobs L. The survival of eggs of Enterobius vermicularis under known conditions of temperature and humidity. Am J Hyg 1941; 33:88–102.

Ni Raghallaigh S, Powell FC. Enterobius vermicularis dermatitis. Clin Exp Dermatol 2010; 35:e32–33.

Sinikumpu JJ, Serlo W. Persistent scrotal pain and suspected orchido-epididymitis of a young boy during pinworm (*Enterobius vermicularis*) infection in the bowel. Acta Paediatr 2011; 100:e89–e90.

Non-Sexually Acquired Genital Ulceration

Lehman JS, Bruce AJ, Wetter DA, et al. Reactive nonsexually related acute genital ulcers: review of cases evaluated at Mayo Clinic. J Am Acad Dermatol 2010; 63:44–51.

Rosman IS, Berk DR, Bayliss SJ, et al. Acute genital ulcers in nonsexually active young girls: case series, review of the literature, and evaluation and management recommendations. Pediatr Dermatol 2012; 29:147–153.

11

Psychodermatology

Sherry Guralnick Cohen and Bernard A. Cohen

INTRODUCTION

Psychodermatologic disorders include psychophysiologic skin conditions that compromise quality of life and primary psychiatric disorders associated with somatic expression of stress that results in skin findings. A number of primary psychodermatoses are reviewed, including trichotillomania, delusions of parasitosis, skin picking, and other self-induced skin lesions.

After a discussion of disorders with psychiatric implications, the cutaneous findings of other "outside disorders" including child abuse, graft-vs-host disease, and acquired immunodeficiency syndrome are reviewed. An algorithmic approach to psychodermatoses is summarized at the end of the chapter (see Fig. 11.24).

Psychophysiologic Disorders

Localized skin conditions, which involve cosmetically important areas such as the head and neck, and chronic, widespread rashes such as atopic dermatitis, psoriasis, acne, and vitiligo, may be distressing enough to trigger psychophysiologic disorders. In this group of diseases, disfigurement can result in low self-esteem, social phobia, paranoia, and major depression.

Disfiguring lesions in infants and young children are a source of parental stress. However, if the lesions are treated before a critical period in psychologic development, long-term sequelae may be avoided. Although these critical periods are not well defined, many pediatricians agree that, if possible, treatment should be completed before patients begin school. For instance, large facial congenital pigmented nevi may be excised before kindergarten, and pulsed-dye laser treatment of port-wine stains may begin shortly after birth (see Figs. 2.64–2.66).

Quality of life studies show that patients with eczema and psoriasis have significantly higher rates of anxiety, depression, and sleep disorders, as well as more absenteeism. Treatment is designed to eradicate the lesions that are most visible or symptomatic and minimize school absence. In adolescents, even mild acne may trigger a great deal of anxiety, and cystic acne is treated early and aggressively to avoid permanent scarring.

Periodic reassurance from the practitioner provides adequate support for many patients. Others may find participation in support-oriented groups, such as the National Vitiligo Foundation, National Alopecia Areata Foundation, and the Vascular Birthmarks Foundation, particularly helpful. However, when normal relationships with family and friends are disrupted, psychiatric consultation and counseling may be necessary.

Primary Psychiatric Disorders

In this category of psychodermatoses, the skin becomes the focus of a primary psychosis. In most cases, either no true dermatologic disorder is present or minor findings are misinterpreted by the patient in accordance with his or her underlying psychopathology. Although subtle symptoms may develop in childhood, most cases become manifest in adolescence or young adulthood.

Trichotillomania

Trichotillomania is a compulsive urge to pull out one's own hair. It clinically looks like patchy hair loss that does not follow anatomic or physiologic landmarks. The scalp is most commonly affected, but other areas can be involved. On dermoscopy the most common findings are decreased hair density, broken hairs at different lengths, trichoptilosis (split ends), irregular coiled hairs, upright regrown hairs, and black dots showing perifollicular hemorrhages. Malakar and Mukherjee described a dermoscopy finding of a dark bulbar proximal tip with a linear stem of variable lengths looking like a burnt matchstick. Trauma and traction cause this finding.

Unlike innocent hair pulling, which occurs commonly in toddlers and preschoolers, children with trichotillomania demonstrate obsessive-compulsive symptoms.

The *Diagnostic and Statistical Manual of Mental Disorders, fifth edition (DSM-5)* describes trichotillomania as an impulse control disorder affecting 1.5–2% of the general population. In adults there is a female-to-male ratio of 4:1; however, in children, girls and boys are equally affected and severity is variable. Observational data show that one-third of affected children have comorbid psychiatric conditions including generalized anxiety, social phobia, major depression, substance-use disorders, attention-deficit/hyperactive disorder, and oppositional defiant disorder.

Trichotillomania differs from other obsessive-compulsive disorders (OCDs) as age of onset is usually early adolescence rather than late adolescence, and individuals with trichotillomania do not have intrusive thoughts like in other OCDs. There are often other repetitive motor symptoms such as skin picking and nail biting. Psychotherapy evidence supports cognitive behavioral therapy, focusing on habit-reversal training, where the emphasis is on replacing hair pulling with more desirable behaviors.

A glutamatergic agent, N-acetyl cysteine, has been found to reduce urges. Olanzapine has also been shown to be effective. There is no evidence that selective serotonin reuptake inhibitors (SSRIs) are beneficial. Trichotillomania is not self-limited and requires long-term psychiatric and medical therapy (see Fig. 8.24).

Delusions of Parasitosis

Delusions of parasitosis, the most common monosymptomatic hypochondriacal psychosis treated by dermatologists, occurs when an individual is convinced that the skin is infested with imaginary mites, worms, or insects. Cutaneous findings range from none to excoriations, lichenification, prurigo nodularis, and ulcerations, which are created by the patient attempting to dig out the parasites. Patients may also present with collections of scale, hair, and/or other debris presumably containing parasites (Fig. 11.1). Other delusional disorders include bromosis (foul odor) and dysmorphosis (abnormal or ugly appearance).

These patients have little insight into their disease and usually refuse consultation with psychiatrists. Unfortunately, the prognosis is guarded, and symptoms may persist indefinitely. Small case studies of delusions of parasitosis showed symptom improvement with pimozide at a dose from 1 to 5 mg daily for 6 weeks before starting to taper and olanzapine at 5 mg daily for 10 weeks, sometimes increasing to 10 mg daily.

Concurrent medications may be beneficial, including anxiolytics, antidepressants, and corticosteroid creams. Aripiprazole, a third-generation antipsychotic, is another potentially safe and effective option.

Skin Picking Disorders

Skin picking disorders and other body-focused repetitive behavior disorders (BFRBD) have been introduced in the DSM-5. These disorders can be expressed in multigenerational families and may have comorbid associations.

In acne excoriée and skin picking, variants of OCDs, patients pick and gouge trivial acne or other skin lesions on the face, arms, or hands, but often at multiple sites, resulting in erosions and ulcerations that may heal with scarring (Fig. 11.2). Acne excoriée occurs most commonly in adolescents. This disorder is triggered by emotional states such as anxiety or boredom. There are two subgroups: those with primary acne and those with no primary lesions. Patients may attempt to stop picking, and acne treatment, when appropriate, is the first line of treatment. Cognitive behavioral therapy, habit reversal training, and N-acetyl cysteine have been shown to have good results. SSRIs and/or low-dose antipsychotics have also been used with variable responses.

A subset of patients with self-induced skin lesions, often referred to as factitious disorders, usually adolescents, develop cutaneous findings such as coining, excoriations, and chemical burns in association with situational stress (Figs. 11.3–11.5). Disordered family dynamics, sexual abuse, school phobia, lost love, and other acute or chronic psychosocial problems may result in this form of attention-seeking behavior. When this diagnosis is suspected, lesions may be covered with occlusive dressings for several weeks to see if healing occurs. When confronted, the patients usually admit to the self-injurious behavior. Counseling and improvement in the situation often result in an end to the lesions.

Pseudopsychiatric Disorders

When patients develop bizarre symptoms with few or confusing clinical findings, a psychiatric source is often considered. However, careful attention to the course of symptoms and development of skin lesions may give a clue to the true dermatologic diagnosis.

Dermatitis herpetiformis (DH) is a good example of a pseudopsychodermatosis. In DH, persistent, intense pruritus and subsequent excoriations, which obliterate the primary vesiculobullous lesions, make diagnosis difficult. Unless DH is considered and confirmed by skin biopsy and/or immunofluorescence studies, the patient may be mistakenly referred to psychiatry for evaluation of "neurotic" excoriations. Scabies, folliculitis, urticaria, and other pruritic dermatoses may also be misdiagnosed as psychogenic pruritus.

Occasionally, children with temporal lobe seizures present with pseudo-delusions of parasitosis. Complaints of bizarre sensations

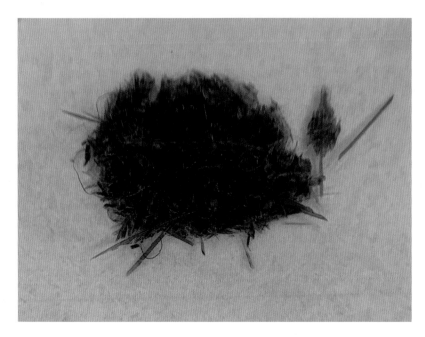

Fig 11.1 An adolescent with delusions of parasitosis presented with a bag of debris collected from the back of his scalp, which on microscopic examination showed shaved hair and scale.

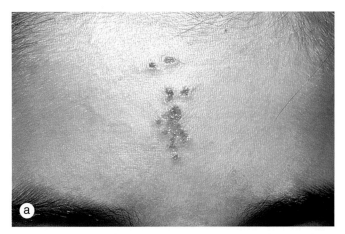

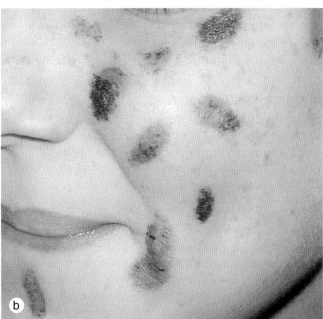

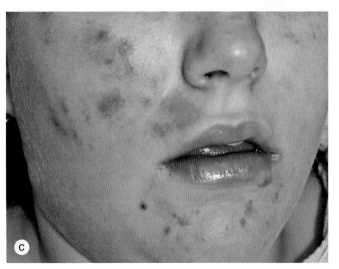

Fig 11.2 Acne excoriée. A 17-year-old girl compulsively picked at subtle comedones, which created punched out ulcerations on **(a)** her forehead. Another adolescent girl **(b)** and boy **(c)** manipulated lesions on their cheeks and chin.

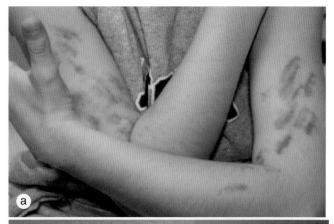

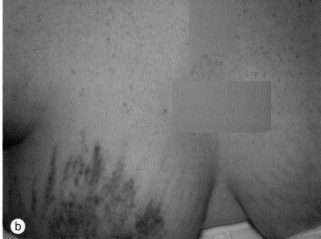

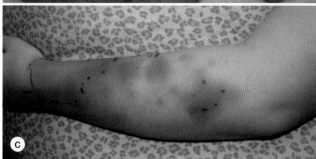

Fig 11.3 Factitial disorders. **(a)** An emotionally disturbed adolescent developed symmetric linear bruises on the arms. During counseling he admitted to producing the lesions with a coin. **(b)** This adolescent girl, who was evaluated for recurrent linear purpura on her breast, admitted to self-injurious behavior in the setting of recurrent sexual abuse by a family member. **(c)** Less well-defined areas of deep purpura developed acutely in a 15-year-old boy. These lesions cleared when the area was covered with a soft cast, only to recur at other unprotected sites.

in the skin also prompt a search for medication overdosage (e.g., diphenhydramine) or illicit drug exposure, or result in excoriations, ulcerations, or other skin findings (Fig. 11.6).

CHILD ABUSE AND NEGLECT

Although the true incidence of child abuse is unknown, over 2 000 000 children are estimated to be abused, or neglected in the United States every year, which results in over 40 000 severely

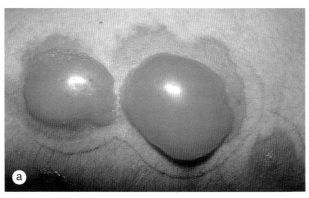

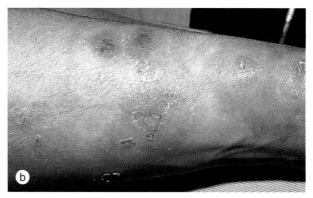

Fig 11.4 Factitial disorders. **(a)** A 15-year-old boy would periodically return from the woods behind his house with large, tense, bullous lesions on his arms. **(b)** Under close observation in the hospital, the lesions healed within several days. Later, in therapy, he admitted to applying a caustic liquid to the skin.

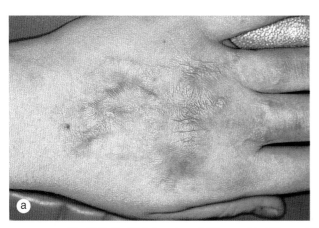

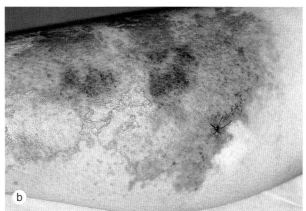

Fig 11.5 Factitial disorders. A 12-year-old girl has evidence of **(a)** old scarring and **(b)** new necrotic crusts on her leg from the application of a solvent to the skin. The fresh lesions healed under an occlusive dressing, which was left in place for 3 days.

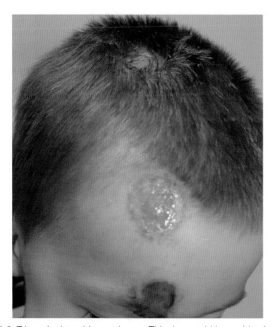

Fig 11.6 Trigeminal trophic syndrome. This 4-year-old boy with trigeminal trophic syndrome experienced intense focal pruritus just to the right of the midline of the scalp and forehead. He was noted to repeatedly scratch these areas.

injured children and 4000 deaths. In many cases, affected children have been evaluated by practitioners who failed to recognize signs and symptoms that suggested the true diagnosis. Frequently, cutaneous findings provide clues to acute or chronic abuse.

Risk Factors

Nearly two-thirds of children who suffer child abuse are under 3 years of age. Premature, disabled, and foster children are also more likely to be abused. About 75% suffer neglect; 15% suffer physical abuse, and 10% of cases involve sexual abuse, of which girls are victims three times more often than boys. However, boys have a higher child fatality rate, at almost 1.5 times that of girls, from abuse and neglect. Parental risk factors include a personal history of child abuse, poor socialization, and limited ability to deal with stress. Healthcare issues including cardiovascular disease, diabetes, and cancer have been linked to adverse childhood experiences. Although families living in poverty have increased exposure to stresses that may result in abuse and neglect, families of all socioeconomic levels may be affected. Alcoholism, addiction, and mental illness are often contributing factors. Families that move frequently and fail to develop support systems in the community are at particularly high risk.

Since 2014, hundreds of thousands of children and families from Guatemala, Honduras, El Salvador, and Mexico have fled to the United States as a result of violence, poverty, and civil wars. The number of immigrants has continued to increase. Detention centers have separated these young children from family members and detained them in deplorable conditions, which has caused significant emotional and physical harm. There is an ongoing battle to try to address these issues because of the abuse it is causing to these young children.

Historical Clues

When the history of how the injury occurred is vague or incompatible with the physical findings, abuse is included in the differential diagnosis. Inconsistencies in the history when parents are interviewed separately and changes in the history when it is taken by different health practitioners should increase the index of suspicion.

Delay between the time of the injury and the visit to the clinician, inappropriate lack of concern for the injury, and abnormal interaction between the parent and child also raise concern.

A review of the primary care or emergency room medical records may reveal a large number of visits for accidental injuries, repeated fractures, and ingestions. Delayed immunizations and health maintenance visits may also serve as a warning. In infants and young children, poor growth or weight gain may be a sign of emotional abuse or neglect.

Clinical Findings

Every child suspected of being abused deserves a thorough physical examination. Care must be taken to peruse the entire skin surface, including the anogenital area, mucous membranes, and scalp. All findings must be documented in the chart. Photographs of suspicious lesions are labeled and dated. The incident must be reported to the appropriate authorities, including Child Protective Services or Social Services and the police if necessary. It is the obligation of healthcare providers to report any suspected child abuse. The Child Abuse Prevention and Treatment Act (CAPTA) of 1974 provides state funding for prevention, assessment, investigation, prosecution, and treatment activities in this context. This has been updated a number of times, most recently in 2018–2019 to provide immunity from civil and criminal liability for people investigating and providing medical evaluations of children reported to have been abused or neglected. Although the practitioner should play the role as an advocate for the family, the primary responsibility is the safety of the child.

Cutaneous Lesions

The distribution and shape of skin lesions may provide a clue to diagnosis. Innocent, play-induced bruises usually appear over bony prominences. Bruises suggestive of abuse occur on the inner and outer thighs, ears, groin, genitals, cheeks, and torso. Thumbprints on the chest and fingerprints on the back of a seizing or floppy infant point to the diagnosis of the so-called shaken-baby syndrome, in which shaking results in subdural hematoma with retinal hemorrhages (Fig. 11.7).

Bruises appear purple and blue for the first 3–5 days and then change through greenish-yellow hues to faded brown at 10 days.

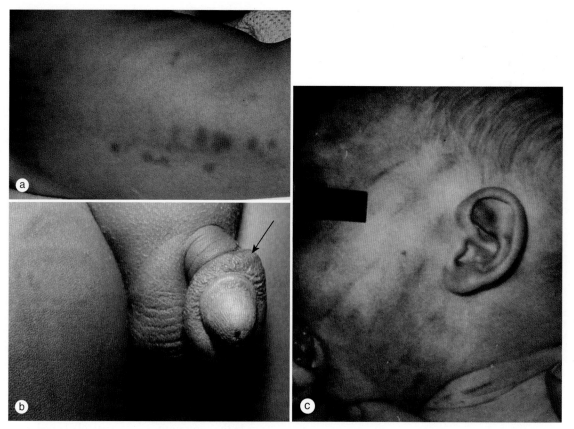

Fig 11.7 Physical abuse. **(a)** Multiple ecchymoses are evident over the back of this child, who presented poorly nourished but with normal coagulation studies. **(b)** This toddler developed edema of the foreskin after a beating with a belt. Note the belt-buckle mark on the right thigh. **(c)** This 8-week-old infant demonstrates linear bruises on the head and neck from physical abuse.

Although it can be difficult to date bruises, multiple bruises of varying intensity and color may suggest an ongoing problem, and the parents' history may not be compatible with the evolution of lesions. Moreover, a complete skin examination with a purple Wood light may reveal old bruises that are no longer clinically visible.

In many cases, the configuration of bruises may conform to the imprint of the object used to induce injury. Linear lesions result from a wooden stick or metal wire. Circumferential bruises or erosions on the arms, legs, or neck may be caused by rope or wire ligatures (Fig. 11.8). Lamp cords (omega-shaped loops), belts ("U"-shaped cuts), belt buckles, and hands often inflict identifiable lesions (Fig. 11.9a,b). However, the clinician should always evaluate these lesions in the proper cultural context. Coining and cupping produce distinctive purpura in a

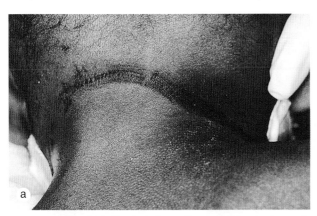
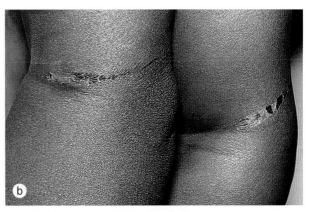

Fig 11.8 Physical abuse. These toddlers had rope tied around **(a)** the neck and **(b)** the legs, which produced circumferential bruising and erosions.

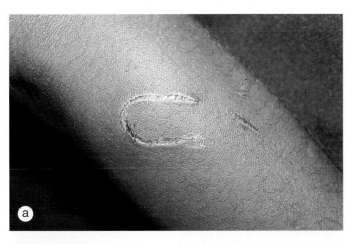
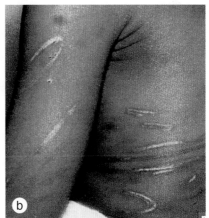
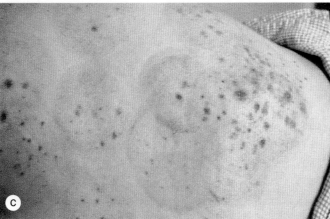

Fig 11.9 Physical abuse. The shape of lesions often gives a clue to the object used to inflict injury. **(a)** The end of a belt produced the "U" shaped cut on the leg of this 5-year-old boy. **(b)** Multiple scars produced by prior whipping with a looped cord are seen in this child. **(c)** Cupping purpura was induced deliberately in this adolescent to treat low back pain. Cupping and coining may be applied in a non-abusive setting and the shape of the lesions is virtually diagnostic.

non-abusive setting and should not be confused with potentially life-threatening non-accidental injury (Fig. 11.9c).

Human bites also have a characteristic appearance. Animal-induced injuries usually produce puncture wounds or tear the skin, while human bites cause crush injuries. Small bite marks may be inflicted by siblings. However, widths of greater than 4 cm occur with bites from adults.

Although burns are fairly common accidental injuries (Fig. 11.10), the shape and distribution of lesions, inconsistent history, and delay in seeking medical care may point to deliberate injuries. Burns from hot-water immersion are a common presentation for abuse. Symmetric lesions on the hands, feet, and diaper area are typical (Fig. 11.11, Fig. 11.12). Frustration with toddlers during toilet training is a common complaint. The tops of the feet and hands may be more severely involved, because the skin on the palms and soles is thicker and may be relatively protected when the extremities are held against the bottom of the sink or tub. Burns from metal objects usually demonstrate the shape of the object (Fig. 11.13). A triangular-shaped injury may occur after branding from a hot iron. A child held against a hot, metal grate may show criss-crossing horizontal and vertical marks. Cigarette burns leave punched-out ulcers with dry, purple crusts (Fig. 11.14). They can be differentiated from impetigo by their uniform size and dry, non-expanding base. Repeated burns may result in lesions at various stages of healing. Some lesions may become impetiginized. Widespread, untreated impetigo and poor hygiene are also signs of child neglect.

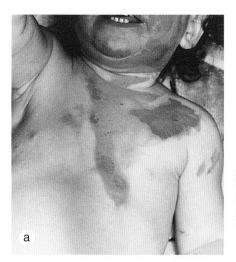
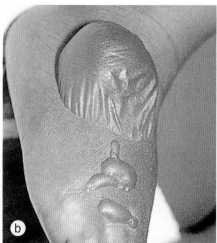
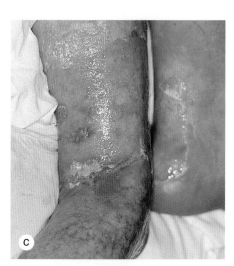

Fig 11.10 Accidental scald. **(a)** A 2-year-old accidentally spilled a teacup filled with hot water onto her face, neck, and chest. Note the irregular, asymmetric, but well-demarcated borders of the burn. **(b)** The accidental splash-and-droplet pattern of blistering is typical of an accidental spill on this toddler, who grabbed a hot cup of tea from the table, while sitting on his grandmother's lap. **(c)** A 12-year-old girl with myelomeningocele and decreased sensation in the lower extremities accidentally dipped her feet into scalding water while preparing to take a bath.

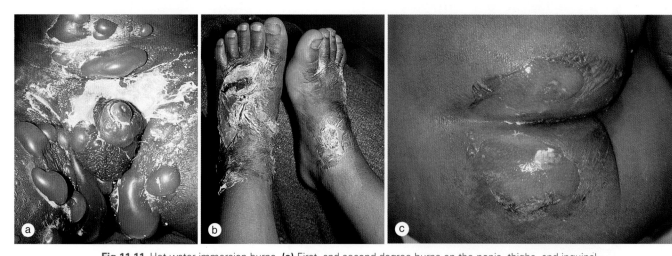

Fig 11.11 Hot water immersion burns. **(a)** First- and second-degree burns on the penis, thighs, and inguinal and suprapubic areas of a toddler who was held under a hot-water spigot. His sacrum and buttocks were spared. **(b)** Symmetric, healing, hot-water burns on the top of the foot of another toddler. Note the sharp line of demarcation at the ankle and sparing of the sole. **(c)** The partial thickness erosion on this toddler's buttocks resulted from a hot-water dip injury.

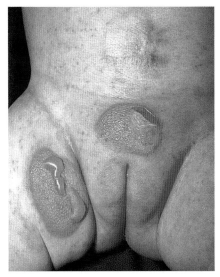

Fig 11.12 Caustic burn. A babysitter was applying a caustic liquid to patches in this child's diaper area. The morphology and course of lesions was not consistent with the history provided by the babysitter. Note the old scar on the abdomen.

Sexual Abuse

Patients evaluated immediately after sexual assault often demonstrate evidence of physical and genital injury. Bruises on the head, neck, torso, and thighs are commonly present. Genital examination may show erythema, bruises, or lacerations (Fig. 11.15). In cases of molestation or incest, which usually occur chronically in a family setting, physical signs are subtle or absent. Patients may present with chronic vaginitis, healed scars in the anogenital area, a patulous introitus, or reflex relaxation of the anal sphincter on perineal stimulation. About 10–15% of these children show evidence of sexually transmitted diseases at the time of diagnosis. Consequently, evaluation includes culturing of the oral pharynx, rectum, and vagina for gonorrhea, chlamydia, and herpes simplex virus and serologic studies for syphilis and human immunodeficiency virus when relevant. Use of the urine nucleic acid amplification tests to confirm the diagnosis of *Chlamydia trachomatis* and *Neisseria gonorrhoeae* is less invasive.

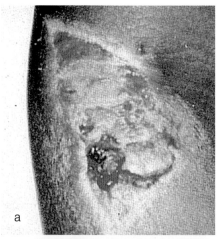

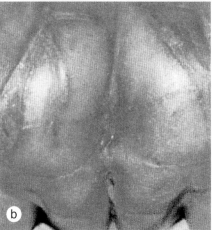

Fig 11.13 Hot-metal burns. **(a)** The pattern of this full-thickness burn to the arm reflects that a hot iron was used on this patient. **(b)** This infant received multiple, linear, full-thickness burns when she was forced to sit on the hot grill of a space heater.

Children who have been sexually assaulted require a thorough examination and collection of forensic data in a medical setting equipped for the special needs of this evaluation.

Occasionally, dermatologic disease can simulate the findings of sexual abuse (see Figs. 4.19 and 7.55). Pyramidal protrusion refers

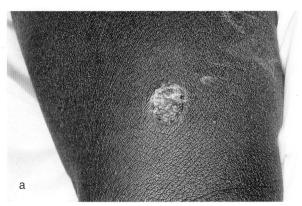

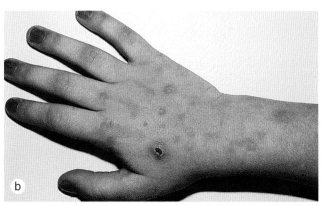

Fig 11.14 Cigarette burns. **(a)** A fresh cigarette burn occurred when this 6-year-old allegedly walked into a lighted cigarette. Note the dry, yellow eschar in the center, with purplish peeled-back scale at the border. **(b)** Cigarette burns in various stages of healing are present on the hand and wrist of this abused 5-year-old child.

to a firm pyramid-shaped congenital or acquired nodule that forms on the perineum after periods of constipation or diarrhea (Fig. 11.16). This smooth skin-colored to pink lesion should not be confused with warts, molluscum, or scars. Bullous pemphigoid and linear immunoglobulin (Ig)A bullous dermatosis have been

misdiagnosed as sexually transmitted herpetic infection. Candidiasis, lichen sclerosus et atrophicus, and inflammatory bowel disease with genital involvement may also mimic sexual abuse.

Other Findings in Abuse

Multiple, unexplained fractures of various ages that involve the long bones and ribs of an infant or young child are a sine qua non of child abuse. Often, the bony injuries are noted as an incidental finding when the child is brought to the practitioner for a single injury or some other, unrelated problem. When child abuse is suspected, a complete skeletal survey is obtained to assess the full extent of the injuries. Blunt objects may cause intra-abdominal injuries, which include duodenal hematomas, small intestinal or mesenteric tears, and lacerations of the liver and spleen. These children may require hospital admission until their safety at home is assured. About 50% of children who are returned to the same environment are eventually killed by the abusive adult.

Innocent Mongolian spots and port-wine stains must not be mistaken for bruises. Past documentation in the child's medical record or observation over several days reveals the proper diagnosis. A bleeding diathesis, which may present with increased bruising, may be quickly excluded by a platelet count and coagulation studies. Insect bites may resemble cigarette burns and, in rare instances, osteogenesis imperfecta may simulate child abuse. Although ligature injuries from hair and cotton fibers around the genitals and digits may be accidental, abuse should always be excluded (Fig. 11.17).

GRAFT-VS-HOST DISEASE

Graft-vs-host disease (GVHD) is an immunologically mediated multisystem disorder caused by injury induced by immunocompetent, histoincompatible donor cells in a compromised recipient. Susceptible immunodeficiency states include the normal developing fetus, congenital immunodeficiency, and acquired

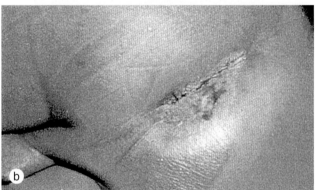
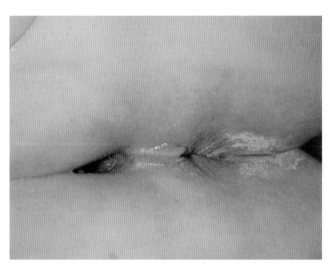

Fig 11.15 Sexual abuse. **(a)** Abrasions, contusions, and punctate tears of the perineum and perianal area can be observed in this prepubescent girl. **(b)** Severe, perianal lacerations, contusions, and abrasions are apparent in this prepubescent boy subjected to sodomy.

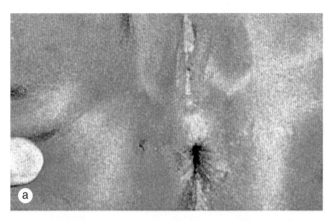

Fig 11.16 Pyramidal protrusion. This pink nodule appeared on the perineum after a 2-week episode of diarrhea in this 6-month-old girl. The lesion resolved without treatment over 4 months.

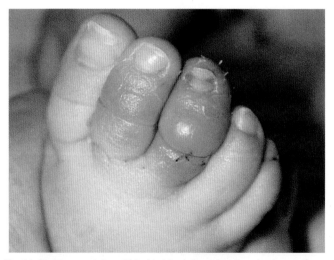

Fig 11.17 Ligature injury. This healthy infant developed edema of several digits after a hair accidentally became entangled around several toes. The hair was removed before the blood supply to the toes was interrupted.

immunodeficiency. Individuals who undergo bone marrow or solid organ transplantation may also be at risk.

When GVHD develops *in utero* in normal fetuses, viable maternal lymphocytes enter the fetal circulation by spontaneous maternal–fetal transfusion. Affected infants usually show signs of chronic disease at delivery. In infants with congenital immunodeficiencies, particularly T-cell deficiencies and severe combined immunodeficiency, the development of GVHD may be the first symptom of the immunodeficiency, which develops about 7–10 days after therapeutic blood transfusion (Fig. 11.18a). In many nurseries, sick infants receive irradiated blood that eliminates the risk of accidental infusion of viable

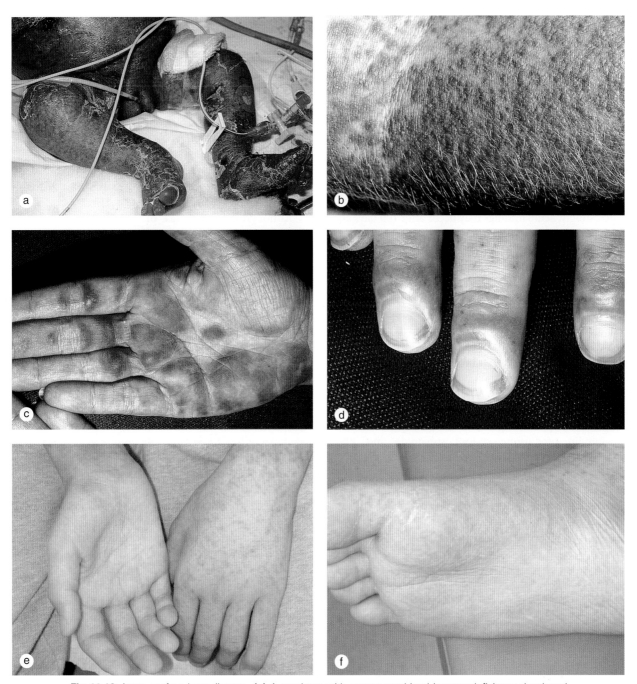

Fig 11.18 Acute graft-vs-host disease. **(a)** A newborn with severe combined immunodeficiency developed graft-vs-host disease after a transfusion with non-irradiated, packed red blood cells. Note the diffuse erythema and scaling. **(b–d)** Severe skin disease developed 3 weeks after allogenic bone marrow transplantation in an adolescent with acute myelogenous leukemia. **(b)** A widespread morbilliform rash became confluent in the skin creases and over the thighs. Necrotic vesicles developed in the center of many red papules, reminiscent of erythema multiforme. Painful, violaceous nodules and plaques appeared on **(c)** the palms and soles, over the knuckles, and **(d)** around the nails. **(e,f)** This adolescent boy developed subtle reticulated erythema on his hands and feet 2 weeks after an autologous bone marrow transplant. The eruption persisted for 4–6 weeks and resolved without changes in his medications.

lymphocytes. The most common group of children at risk for GVHD includes patients with acquired immunodeficiencies that result from chemotherapy, lymphoreticular malignancy, and bone marrow transplantation (Figs. 11.18b–d and 11.19). Virtually every allogenic transplant patient experiences mild GVHD. Although less common, GVHD can also occur in some patients with autologous and syngeneic bone marrow transplantation.

Acute disease usually begins with a widespread, symmetric, pruritic, morbilliform rash within 2–6 weeks and up to 100 days after the introduction of donor cells (Fig. 11.18b–d). The face and neck, and the sides of the palms, soles, and digits are commonly involved. Less commonly, follicular papules erupt, and rarely, necrotic blisters and life-threatening toxic epidermal necrolysis follow (Table 11.1). Hepatic involvement is evident by the presence of elevated liver enzymes, and gastrointestinal symptoms include nausea and vomiting, and often progress to bloody diarrhea.

Chronic disease appears 100–400 days after the introduction of donor cells and may occur without antecedent acute symptoms. Interestingly, acute findings may occur after 100 days and chronic changes may develop earlier than usually anticipated. Chronic GVHD is a multisystem disease with autoimmune-like findings. Early in its course, the skin is involved with diffuse hypo- and hyperpigmentation, a lichenoid rash that resembles lichen planus, and scaly patches. Occasionally, patients develop a diffuse erythroderma. Untreated patients may eventually develop poikiloderma with atrophy, ulcerations, and progressive, widespread sclerodermatous changes (see Fig. 11.19a,b). Other findings include mucositis, cicatricial alopecia, vitiligo, dystrophic nails, Sjögren syndrome, and chronic pulmonary, cardiac, and gastrointestinal disease.

Fortunately, in most transplant patients, aggressive immunosuppressive therapy with cyclosporine, tacrolimus, anti-thymocyte globulin, prednisone, cyclophosphamide, and other agents usually prevents the development of serious GVHD.

The U.S. Food and Drug Administration approved a JAK kinase inhibitor, ruxolitinib, as second-line therapy for patients failing steroids. Routine irradiation of blood products before transfusion also reduces the risk of GVHD in transplant patients and other immunodeficient individuals. In infants with congenital immunodeficiency, mortality is high despite intensive supportive care.

In most patients with GVHD, clinical findings can be used to direct medical therapy. In mild cases, skin biopsies are of little value in distinguishing GVHD from drug reactions and viral exanthems. Although biopsy findings in severe disease may be diagnostic, it is prudent to treat aggressively and promptly, and pathology can be used to confirm the clinical diagnosis. Fortunately, with current prophylaxis for GVHD, most cases are mild, and biopsies are usually unnecessary.

ACQUIRED IMMUNODEFICIENCY SYNDROME

The Centers for Disease Control and Prevention (CDC) reported that in 2017 there were 533 556 adults and adolescents diagnosed with acquired immunodeficiency syndrome (AIDS), and 16 350 died of AIDS or one of the comorbidities. Ages with the highest prevalence were 25–29 years of age, followed by 20–24 years of age.

Although the prevalence of AIDS is relatively low in children, the recent epidemic, which has spread to heterosexual women of child bearing age may in a rise in pediatric cases. In some areas, human immunodeficiency virus (HIV) seroprevalence among pregnant women has dropped to 2%. The rate of transmission from untreated, asymptomatic mothers ranges from 15–35%. Other sources of infection in children include exposure to contaminated blood products, sexual transmission, and intravenous drug use. HIV antivirals have reduced mother-to-child HIV transmission. The recommendation is to get confirmatory studies before treatment is initiated.

Infected infants rarely develop overt disease during the first 3 months of life. However, before 1 year of age, non-specific symptoms commonly include poor growth, generalized lymphadenopathy, hepatosplenomegaly, chronic oral thrush, and recurrent upper respiratory, middle ear, and gastrointestinal infections. At least 50% of infected infants show central nervous system involvement with neurodevelopmental delay or loss of milestones, acquired microcephaly, spastic diplegia, and quadriplegia. Pulmonary disease is the most common manifestation of pediatric AIDS and affects over 75% of infected children during the first several years of life. Atypical tuberculous (TB) symptoms of fever and tachypnea have been seen in children with AIDS. Onset of TB averaged 20 months from diagnosis of AIDS. Interstitial pneumonitis caused by *Pneumocystis carinii* is reported in 60% of patients. Lymphoid interstitial pneumonitis associated with Epstein–Barr virus infection occurs in about half of patients who survive the first year. Other important opportunistic pathogens include cytomegalovirus, *Candida*, *Mycobacterium avium-intracellulare* complex, and *Cryptococcus neoformans*. Patients are also susceptible to bacteremia, severe soft-tissue infection, pneumonitis, and meningitis from encapsulated bacterial organisms, such as *Streptococcus pneumoniae* or *Haemophilus influenzae*.

Skin Lesions

Cutaneous findings may provide an early clue to diagnosis. Cutaneous skin manifestations increase as viral count increases.

Stage	Cutaneous Findings	Grade	Histologic Finding
1	Erythematous macules, papules <25% BSA	1	Basal vacuolar change
2	Erythematous macules, papules 25–50% BSA	2	Dyskeratosis, dermal lymphocyte infiltrate
3	Erythematous macules, papules (>50% BSA) to erythroderma	3	Formation of dermal–epidermal clefts and microvesicles
4	Erythroderma with bulla formation and toxic epidermal necrosis	4	Separation of epidermis from dermis

TABLE 11.1 Clinical Staging and Histologic Grading of Graft-vs-Host Disease

BSA, Body surface area.

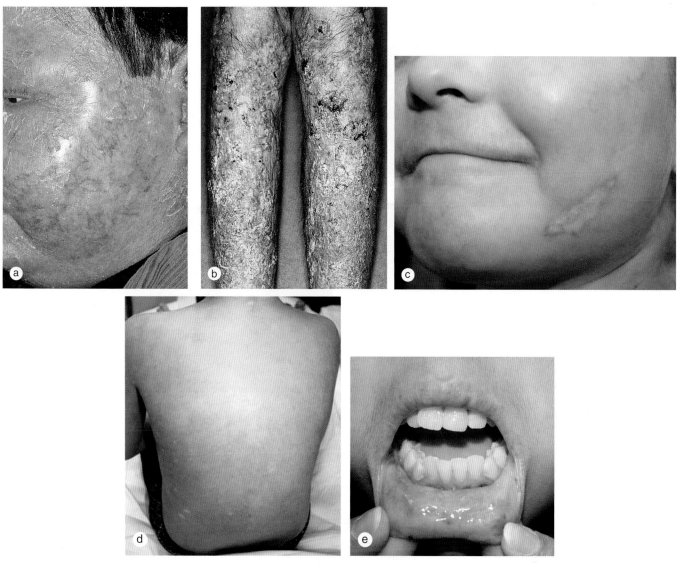

Fig 11.19 Chronic graft-vs-host disease. **(a)** Widespread atrophy, scaling, and fibrosis developed over a year after bone marrow transplantation. This 14-year-old boy had experienced only minimal acute disease after his transplant. **(b)** Recurrent erosions, ulcers, and crusts formed on the arms, trunk, and legs in this 16 year-old boy with chronic disease. **(c,d)** A 6-year-old girl developed diffuse sclerodermatous changes and dyspigmentation typical of chronic graft-vs-host disease a year after bone marrow transplantation for acute lymphocytic leukemia. **(e)** She also developed lichenoid changes with some erosions in her mouth.

Persistent diaper candidiasis and oral thrush recalcitrant to topical therapy occur commonly and prompt a search for HIV infection, especially in a child with growth failure or maternal risk factors. Many children are unable to localize common, usually self-limited, viral infections. Widespread, recurrent herpetic gingivostomatitis and disseminated cutaneous herpes simplex, as well as chronic herpes infections, are a frequent problem. Recurrent, localized herpes zoster and disseminated zoster have also been reported. Widespread, recalcitrant warts or molluscum contagiosum may be the first sign of AIDS in an otherwise asymptomatic child (Fig. 11.20). Persistent and widespread dermatophyte infections that involve the skin, nails, and hair may occur. Disseminated, deep fungal infections with cutaneous involvement, including cryptococcosis (Fig. 11.21) and histoplasmosis, have been described. Skin lesions produced by these fungi may simulate an indolent, bacterial folliculitis or molluscum.

Crusted scabies infestations, with thick, widespread, scaly papules and patches require rapid identification to prevent spread to parents, teachers, and healthcare workers (Fig. 11.22). As in adults, the prevalence of seborrheic dermatitis, particularly widespread, erosive lesions, appears to be high in children with AIDS. Psoriasis, lichen planus, and other dermatoses may also be more common and more resistant to therapy in children and adolescents with HIV infection and AIDS (Fig. 11.23). Cutaneous manifestations of nutritional deficiencies, which include zinc-deficiency dermatitis, pellagra, and scurvy, have been noted, particularly in children with chronic gastrointestinal disease.

An increased frequency of drug eruptions has been reported in adults and children with AIDS. This is a serious problem in

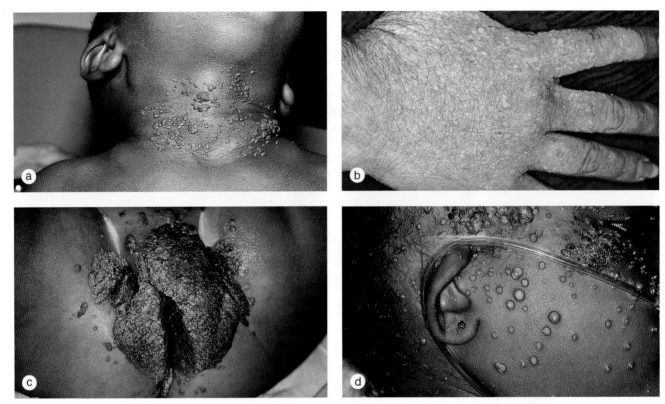

Fig 11.20 Acquired immunodeficiency syndrome (AIDS). **(a)** Multiple, recalcitrant warts developed on the neck of a 2-year-old infant with AIDS. **(b)** This adolescent was plagued with disseminated flat warts, demonstrated here by virtually confluent papules on the top of the hand. **(c)** Large, recalcitrant genital warts were associated with bleeding and recurrent bacterial infections in this toddler. **(d)** Severe molluscum contagiosum became chronically irritated and secondarily infected in this 6-year-old girl with AIDS. When her lymphocyte count rebounded on antiviral therapy, the molluscum regressed.

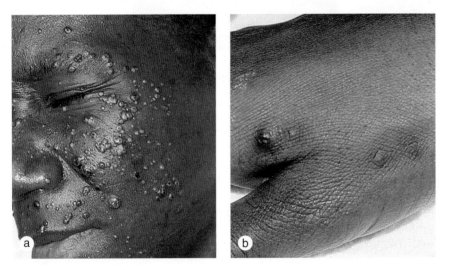

Fig 11.21 *Cryptococcus.* This young woman **(a,b)** with AIDS was initially diagnosed with widespread molluscum. However, a skin biopsy showed *Cryptococcus*, and she died several weeks later of disseminated infection.

patients who require chronic prophylaxis against *Pneumocystis* with trimethoprim-sulfamethoxazole. The incidence of morbilliform drug rashes in adults on this regimen approaches 75%.

Other cutaneous findings in children with AIDS include ecchymoses from idiopathic thrombocytopenic purpura and chronic leukocytoclastic vasculitis. Although cutaneous Kaposi sarcoma is reported frequently in adults, in whom it is an AIDS-defining illness, it occurs only rarely in children.

See Fig. 11.24 for a diagnostic algorithm related to psychodermatologic disorders.

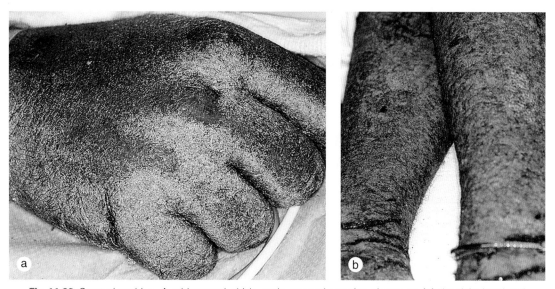

Fig 11.22 Crusted scabies. A widespread, thick, scaly, crusted eruption shown on **(a)** the right hand and **(b)** the legs developed in an adolescent with severe neurologic involvement from AIDS. Scrapings demonstrated multiple scabies mites.

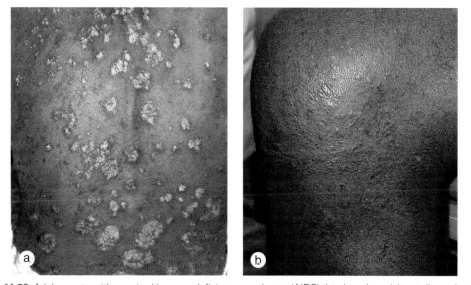

Fig 11.23 Adolescents with acquired immunodeficiency syndrome (AIDS) developed recalcitrant disseminated **(a)** psoriasis and **(b)** lichen planus.

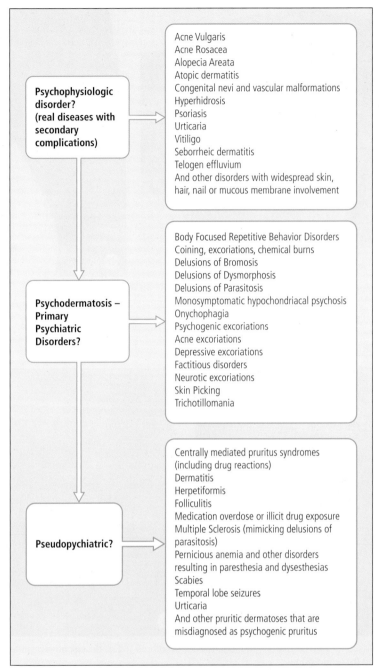

Fig 11.24 Algorithm for the evaluation of psychodermatologic disorders. (From JY, Do JH, Lee CS. Psychodermatology. J Am Acad Dermatol 2000; 43(5 Pt 1):848–853.)

FURTHER READING

Psychodermatology

American Psychiatric Association. Diagnostic and statistical manual of mental disorders, 5th edn. American Psychiatric Publishing, Washington, DC, 2013.

Ankad B, Naidu MV, Beergouder SL, et al. Trichoscopy in trichotillomania: a useful diagnostic tool. Int J Trichology 2014; 6(4):160–163.

Augustin M, Zschocke I, Wiek K, et al. Coping with illness and quality of life of patients with port-wine stains treated with laser therapy. Hautarzt 1998; 49(9):714–718.

Alevizos B, Lykouras L, Zervas IM, et al. Risperidone-induced obsessive-compulsive symptoms: a series of six cases. J Clin Psychopharmacol 2002; 22(5):461–467.

Bloch MH, Landeros-Weisenberger A, Dombrowski P, et al. Systematic review: pharmacological and behavioral treatment for trichotillomania. Biol Psychiatry 2007; 62(8):839–846.

Coric V. Systematic review: pharmacological and behavioral treatment for trichotillomania. Biol Psychiatry 2007; 62:839–846.

Flessner CA. Cognitive behavior therapy for childhood repetitive behavior disorders: tic disorders and trichotillomania. Child Adolesc Psychiatr Clin N Am 2011; 20(2):319–328.

Fried RG. Nonpharmacologic treatment in psychodermatology. Dermatol Clin 2002; 20:177–185.

Eckert L, Gupta S, Amand C, et al Impact of atopic dermatitis on health-related quality of life and productivity in adults in the United States: an analysis using the National Health and Wellness Survey. J Am Acad Dermatol 2017; 77:274–279.e3

Generali J, Cada D. Pimozide: parasitosis (delusional). Hosp Pharm 2014; 49(2):134–135.

Khullar A, Chue P, Tibbo P. Quetiapine and obsessive-compulsive symptoms (OCS): case report and review of atypical antipsychotic-induced OCS. J Psychiatry Neurosci 2001; 26(1):55–59.

Khumalo NP, Shaboodien G, Hemmings SMJ, et al. Pathologic grooming (acne excoriee, trichotillomania, and nail biting) in 4 generations of a single family. JAAD Case Rep 2016; 2(1):51–53.

Kim JH, Ryu S, Nam HJ, et al. Symptom structure of antipsychotic-induced obsessive compulsive symptoms in schizophrenia patients. Prog Neuropsychopharmacol Biol Psychiatry 2012; 39(1):75–79.

Gieler U, Consoli S, Tomas-Aragones L, et al. Self-inflicted lesions in dermatology: terminology and classification—a position paper from the European Society for Dermatology and Psychiatry. Acta Derm Venereol 2013; 93:4–12.

Grant JE, Chamberlain SR. Trichotillomania. Am J Psychiatry 2016; 173(9):868–874.

Ladizinski B, Busse KL, Bhutani T, et al. Aripiprazole as a viable alternative for treating delusions of parasitosis. J Drugs Dermatol 2010; 9(12):1531–1532.

Lee CS. Delusions of Parasitosis. Dermatol Ther. 2008;21:2–7.

Malakar S, Mukherjee SS. Burnt matchstick Sign—a new trichoscopic finding in trichotillomania. Int J Trichology 2017; 9(1): 44–46.

Stamouli S, Lykouras L. Quetiapine-induced obsessive compulsive symptoms: a series of five cases. J Clin Psychopharmacol. 2006;26:396–400.

Meehan WJ, Badreshia S, Mackley CL. Successful treatment of delusions of parasitosis with olanzapine. Arch Dermatol 2006; 142(3):352–355. doi:10.1001/archderm.142.3.352.

Thakkar A, Ooi K, Assaad N, et al. Delusional infestation: are you being bugged? Clin Ophthalmol 2015; 9:967–970.

Ulhaq I, Aji A. Haloperidol induced obsessive compulsive symptom (OCS) in a patient with learning disability and bipolar disorder. BMJ Case Rep 2012; 2012:bcr1120115161.

Child Abuse and Neglect

AlJasser M, Al-Khenaizan S. Cutaneous mimickers of child abuse: a primer for pediatricians. Eur J Pediatr 2008; 167(11):1221–1230.

Andronicus M, Oates RK, Peat J, et al. Non-accidental burns in children. Burns 1998; 24:552–558.

Bechtel K. Sexual abuse and sexually transmitted infections in children and adolescents. Curr Opin Pediatr 2010; 22(1):94–99.

Bell K. Identification and documentation of bite marks. Emerg Nurses Ass 2000; 26:628–630.

Black CM, Driebe EM, Howard LA, et al. Multicenter study of nucleic acid amplification tests for detection of Chlamydia trachomatis and Neisseria gonorrhoeae in children being evaluated for sexual abuse. Pediatr Infect Dis J 2009; 28(7):608–613.

Carpenter RF. The prevalence and distribution of bruising in babies. Arch Dis Child 1999; 80:363–366.

CDC. Adverse childhood experiences reported by adults—five states. MMWR 2009; 59(49):1609–1613.

CDC. Preventing child abuse and neglect. April 7, 2020. www.cdc.gov

Child Welfare Information Gateway. About CAPTA: a legislative history. Factsheet 2/2019. Available at: https://childwelfare.gov/pubPDFs/about.pdf.

Committee on Child Abuse and Neglect. American Academy of Pediatrics. When inflicted skin injuries constitute child abuse. Pediatrics 2002; 110(3):644–645.

Committee on Child Abuse and Neglect. American Academy of Pediatrics. Oral and dental aspects of child abuse and neglect. Pediatrics 2017; 140:e20171487.

Esernio-Jenssen D, Barnes M. Nucleic acid amplification testing in suspected child sexual abuse. J Child Sex Abus 2011; 20(6):612–621.

Hansen KK. Folk remedies and child abuse: a review with emphasis on caida de mollera and its relationship to shaken baby syndrome. Child Abuse Negl 1998; 22:117–127.

Committee on Adolescence. Health care for children and adolescents in detention centers, jails, lock-ups, and other court-sponsored residential facilities. Pediatrics 1989; 84(6):1118–1120.

Linton MJ, Griffin M, Shapiro A. Detention of immigrant children. Pediatrics 2017; 139(5):e201701483. doi:10.1542/peds.2017-0483.

Mok JY. Non-accidental injury in children: an update. Injury 2008; 39(9):978–985.

Montrey JS, Barcia PJ. Nonaccidental burns in child abuse. South Med J 1985; 78:1324–1326.

Myers JE, Berliner L, Briere J, et al. The APSAC handbook on child maltreatment. Sage, Thousand Oaks, 2002.

National Clearinghouse on Child Abuse and Neglect. http://web.archive.org/web/20051215050641/nccanch.acf.hhs.gov/.

Peck M, Priolo-Kapel D. Child abuse by burning: a review of the literature and an algorithm for medical investigations. J Trauma Injury Infect Crit Care 2002; 53:1013–1022.

Preer G, Sorrentino D, Newton AW. Child abuse pediatrics: prevention, evaluation, and treatment. Curr Opin Pediatr 2012; 24(2):266–273.

Scales JW, Fleischer AB, Sinal SH, et al. Skin lesions that mimic abuse. Contemp Pediatr 1999; 16:137–144.

Schwartz AJ, Ricci LR. How accurately can bruises be aged in abused children? Literature review and synthesis. Pediatrics 1996; 97:254–257.

Skellern C, Donald T. Defining standards for medico-legal reports in forensic evaluation of suspicious childhood injury. J Forensic Leg Med 2012; 19(5):267–271.

Stephenson T. Ageing of bruising in children. J Roy Soc Med 1997; 90:312–314.

Sugar NF, Taylor JW, Feldman KW. The Puget Sound Pediatric Research Network. Bruises in infants and toddlers: those who don't cruise rarely bruise. Arch Pediatr Adolesc Med 1999; 153:399–403.

Swerdlin A, Berkowitz C, Craft N. Cutaneous signs of child abuse. J Am Acad Dermatol 2007; 57(3):371–392.

Vogeley JD, Pierce MC, Bertocci G. Experience with Wood lamp illumination and digital photography in the documentation of bruises on human skin. Arch Pediatr Adolesc Med 2002; 156:265.

Woodman J, Lecky F, Hodes D, et al. Screening injured children for physical abuse or neglect in emergency departments: a systemic review. Child Care Health Dev 2010; 36(2):153–164.

Graft-vs-Host Disease

Anderson KC, Weinstein HJ. Transfusion-associated graft-versus-host disease (review article). N Engl J Med 1990; 323:315–321.

Baird K, Cooke K, Schultz KR. Pediatr Clin North Am. 2010; 57:297–322.

Haimes H, Morley KW, Song H, et. al. Impact of skin biopsy on the management of acute graft versus host disease in a pediatric population. Pediatr Dermatol. 2019;36:455–459.

Horn TD. Acute cutaneous eruption after marrow ablation is roses by other names? J Cutan Pathol 1994; 21:385–392.

Nanda A, Husain MAA, et. al. Chronic cutaneous graft verses host disease in children: a report of 14 patients from a tertiary care pediatric dermatology clinic. Pediatr Dermatol. 2018;35:343–353.

Nghiem P. The 'drug vs graft-vs-host disease' conundrum gets tougher, but there is an answer. The challenge to dermatologists. Arch Dermatol 2001; 137:75–76.

Pena PF, Jones-Caballero M, Aragues M, et al. Sclerodermatous graft-vs-host: clinical and pathologic study of 17 patients. Arch Dermatol 2002; 31:189–195.

Wu PA, Cowen EW. Cutaneous graft-versus host disease-clinical considerations and management. Curr Probl Dermatol 2012; 43:101–115.

Acquired Immunodeficiency Syndrome

Carvalho VO, Cruz CR, Marinoni LP, et al. Infectious and inflammatory skin disease in children with HIV infection and their relation with the immune status- evaluation of 127 patients. Pediatr Dermatol 2008; 25(5):571–573.

CDC's Statistic Overview. HIV surveillance report: diagnosis of HIV Infection in the United States and dependent areas, 2018; 30. https://www.cdc.gov/hiv/statistics/overview/index.html.

Chan S, Birnbaum J, Rao M, et al. Clinical manifestation and outcome of tuberculosis in children with acquired immunodeficiency syndrome. Pediatr Infect Dis J 1996; 15(5):443–447.

El Hachem M, Bernarli S, Pianosi G, et al. Mucocutaneous manifestations in children with HIV infections and AIDS. Pediatr 1998; 15:429–434.

Gottschalk GM. Pediatric HIV/AIDS and the skin: an update. Clin Dermatol 2006; 24(4):531–536.

Kaplan MH, Sadick N, McNutt NS, et al. Dermatologic findings and manifestations of acquired immunodeficiency syndrome (AIDS). J Am Acad Dermatol 1987; 16:485–506.

Lambert JS. Pediatric HIV infection. Curr Opin Pediatr 1996; 8:606–614.

Luo R, Boeras D, Broyles L, et al. Use of an indeterminate range in HIV early infant diagnosis: a systematic review of meta-analysis. JAIDS 2019; 82(3):281–286.

Mankahla A, Mosam A. Common skin conditions in children with HIV/AIDS. Am J Clin Dermatol 2012; 13(3):153–166. doi:10.2165/11593900-000000000-00000.

Mendiratta V, Mittal S, Jain A, et al. Mucocutaneous manifestations in children with human immunodeficiency virus infection. Indian J Dermatol Venereol Leprol 2010; 76(5):458–466.

Myskowski PL, Ahkami R. Dermatologic complications of HIV infection. Med Clin North Am 1996; 80:1415–1435.

Prose NS, Mendez H, Menikoff H, et al. Pediatric human immunodeficiency virus infection and its cutaneous manifestations. Pediatr Dermatol 1987; 4:267–274.

Raju PV, Rao GR, Ramani TV, et al. Skin disease: clinical indicator of immune status in human immunodeficiency virus (HIV) infection. Int J Dermatol 2005; 44(8):646–649.

Ramos-Gomez FJ, Hilton JF, Camchola AJ, et al. Risk factors for HIV-related orofacial soft-tissue manifestations in children. Pediatr Dent 1996; 18:121–126.

Shi CR, Huang JT, Nambudiri VE. Pediatric cutaneous graft verses host disease: a review. Curr Pediatr Rev. 2017;13:100–110.

Tschachler E, Bergstresser PR, Stingl G. HIV-related skin diseases. Lancet 1996; 348:659–663.

Umoru D, Oviawe O, Ibadin M, et al. Mucocutaneous manifestation of pediatric human immunodeficiency virus/acquired immunodeficiency syndrome (HIV/AIDS) in relation to degree of immunosuppression: a study of a West African population. Int J Dermatol HYPERLINK "http://www.ncbi.nlm.nih.gov.ezproxy.welch.jhmi.edu/pubmed/22348567" \o "International journal of dermatology." Int J Dermatol 2012; 51(3):305–312. doi:10.1111/j.1365-4632.2011.05077.x.

Vojnov L, Penazzato M, Sherman G, et al. Implementing an indeterminate range for more accurate early infant diagnosis. JAIDS 2019; 82(3):e44–e46.

Wananukul S, Thisyakom U. Mucocutaneous manifestations of HIV infection in 91 children born to HIV-seropositive woman. Pediatr Dermatol 1999; 16:359–363.

Wananukul S, Deekajondech T, Panchareon C, et al. Mucocutaneous findings in pediatric AIDS is related to degree of immunosuppression. Pediatr Dermatol 2003; 20:289–294.

Zuckerman G, Metrou M, Bernstein LJ, et al. Neurologic disorders and dermatologic manifestations in HIV-infected children. Pediatr Emerg Care 1991; 7:99–105.

USEFUL WEBSITES

National Alopecia Areata Foundation: https://www.naaf.org
National Eczema Association: https://nationaleczema.org
National Psoriasis Foundation: https://psoriasis.org
National Vitiligo Foundations: https:// www.vrfoundation.org
The Vascular Birthmark Foundation: https://www.birthmark.org
National Library of Medicine: pubmed.ncbi.nlm.nih.gov
online mendelian inheritance in man: OMIM
DermNet NZ: www.dermnetnz.org
National Center for Biotechnology Information: ncbi.nlm.nih.gov

Notes: vs. indicates a differential diagnosis or comparison. Page numbers followed by 'f' indicate figures and 't' indicate tables.